OXFORD MEDICAL PUBLICATIONS

# Oxford Handbook of
# Midwifery

T0201944

# Published and forthcoming Oxford Handbooks in Nursing

**Oxford Handbook of Adult Nursing**
George Castledine and Ann Close

**Oxford Handbook of Cancer Nursing**
Edited by Mike Tadman and Dave Roberts

**Oxford Handbook of Cardiac Nursing, 2e**
Edited by Kate Olson

**Oxford Handbook of Children's and Young People's Nursing, 2e**
Edited by Edward Alan Glasper, Gillian McEwing, and Jim Richardson

**Oxford Handbook of Clinical Skills for Children's and Young People's Nursing**
Paula Dawson, Louise Cook, Laura-Jane Holliday, and Helen Reddy

**Oxford Handbook of Clinical Skills in Adult Nursing**
Jacqueline Randle, Frank Coffey, and Martyn Bradbury

**Oxford Handbook of Critical Care Nursing, 2e**
Sheila Adam and Sue Osborne

**Oxford Handbook of Dental Nursing**
Elizabeth Boon, Rebecca Parr, Dayananda Samarawickrama, and Kevin Seymour

**Oxford Handbook of Diabetes Nursing**
Lorraine Avery and Sue Beckwith

**Oxford Handbook of Emergency Nursing, 2e**
Edited by Robert Crouch, Alan Charters, Mary Dawood, and Paula Bennett

**Oxford Handbook of Gastrointestinal Nursing**
Edited by Christine Norton, Julia Williams, Claire Taylor, Annmarie Nunwa, and Kathy Whayman

**Oxford Handbook of Learning and Intellectual Disability Nursing**
Edited by Bob Gates and Owen Barr

**Oxford Handbook of Mental Health Nursing, 2e**
Edited by Patrick Callaghan and Catherine Gamble

**Oxford Handbook of Midwifery, 3e**
Janet Medforth, Linda Ball, Angela Walker, Susan Battersby, and Sarah Stables

**Oxford Handbook of Musculoskeletal Nursing**
Edited by Susan Oliver

**Oxford Handbook of Neuroscience Nursing**
Edited by Sue Woodward and Catheryne Waterhouse

**Oxford Handbook of Nursing Older People**
Beverley Tabernacle, Marie Barnes, and Annette Jinks

**Oxford Handbook of Orthopaedic and Trauma Nursing**
Rebecca Jester, Julie Santy, and Jean Rogers

**Oxford Handbook of Perioperative Practice**
Suzanne Hughes and Andy Mardell

**Oxford Handbook of Prescribing for Nurses and Allied Health Professionals**
Sue Beckwith and Penny Franklin

**Oxford Handbook of Primary Care and Community Nursing, 2e**
Edited by Vari Drennan and Claire Goodman

**Oxford Handbook of Renal Nursing**
Edited by Althea Mahon, Karen Jenkins, and Lisa Burnapp

**Oxford Handbook of Respiratory Nursing**
Terry Robinson and Jane Scullion

**Oxford Handbook of Surgical Nursing**
Edited by Alison Smith, Maria Kisiel, and Mark Radford

**Oxford Handbook of Women's Health Nursing**
Edited by Sunanda Gupta, Debra Holloway, and Ali Kubba

# Oxford Handbook of
# Midwifery

**THIRD EDITION**

Edited by

## Janet Medforth
Senior Midwifery Lecturer, Sheffield Hallam University,
UK (retired)

## Linda Ball
Senior Midwifery Lecturer, Sheffield Hallam University
(retired), Research Midwife, Chesterfield Royal Hospital
NHS Foundation Trust, UK

## Angela Walker
Senior Midwifery Lecturer and Supervisor of Midwives,
University of Sheffield (retired), Clinical Nurse Specialist,
Contraception and Sexual Health, and Independent
Prescriber, Derbyshire Community Health Services NHS
Foundation Trust, UK (retired)

## Sue Battersby
Independent Researcher/Lecturer Infant Feeding, formerly
of University of Sheffield, UK

## Sarah Stables
Senior Midwifery Lecturer, Sheffield Hallam University,
Supervisor of Midwives, Consultant Midwife for Normality,
Barnsley NHS Foundation Trust, UK

OXFORD
UNIVERSITY PRESS

# OXFORD
### UNIVERSITY PRESS

Great Clarendon Street, Oxford, OX2 6DP,
United Kingdom

Oxford University Press is a department of the University of Oxford.
It furthers the University's objective of excellence in research, scholarship,
and education by publishing worldwide. Oxford is a registered trade mark of
Oxford University Press in the UK and in certain other countries

© Oxford University Press 2017

The moral rights of the authors have been asserted

First Edition published in 2006
Second Edition published in 2011
Third Edition published in 2017

Impression: 3

Published in the United States of America by Oxford University Press
198 Madison Avenue, New York, NY 10016, United States of America

British Library Cataloguing in Publication Data
Data available

Library of Congress Control Number: 2016945508

ISBN 978–0–19–875478–7

Printed and bound in Great Britain by
Ashford Colour Press Ltd.

# Foreword

It gives me great pleasure to write a foreword for the new third edition of the *Oxford Handbook of Midwifery*. Previous editions have proven to be an excellent resource for midwifery practice and I have no doubt that the new edition will take this to a new height with the rigorous updating of the included chapters.

The authors, whom I have the privilege of knowing and working with, for many years, have conveyed their long years of experience and evidence-based knowledge into a compact midwifery book which has been highly popular so far in its previous editions.

Acknowledging both paradigms of midwifery science and art, the *Oxford Handbook of Midwifery* encompasses key information on basic physiological aspects of pregnancy and birth with practical recommendations on all aspects of midwifery care. This carefully designed book, providing all the essentials for successful midwifery practice, covers a wide range of the maternal and neonatal care continuum, including preconception and the antenatal, post-partum, and neonatal period.

With a great deal of enthusiasm and remarkable efforts, the authors have produced yet another edition of this book which is up-to-date and comprehensive. Similar to its previous editions, this is presented in a very well-structured, user-friendly, and small size, making it a portable knowledge tool for students and professionals alike with their everyday busy lifestyles.

In the face of complex and competing demands on professionals' time, access to reliable and readily available sources of knowledge is paramount. As a Professor of Midwifery having worked within various academic and practice settings, I foresee a continued enthusiasm amongst midwifery students and practitioners to embrace the new edition, as an accessible source for daily practice not just in the UK, but also internationally.

Professor Hora Soltani
Professor of Maternal and Infant Health
Centre for Health and Social Care Research
Faculty of Health and Wellbeing
Sheffield Hallam University

# Preface

Since the previous edition of the *Oxford Handbook of Midwifery* (2011), the maternity services in the UK have undergone a number of challenges mainly in the reconfiguration of the NHS into commissioning bodies for care services and health education. The Kirkup report (2015) has led to the need for updated regulations for midwifery practice and the need for new standards for midwifery education in the UK. These are in progress with implementation planned in 2017. A recent report of a review of the UK maternity services in 2015 suggests that, although numbers of midwife appointments in the UK have risen, there is still a shortage of midwives. According to this report, the UK birth rate fluctuates each year and the service is said to be under strain. Future midwives will contribute significantly to a safe and effective maternity service, hence the decision to update this handbook in support of their understanding of key principles of midwifery care and management of pregnancy, birth, and beyond.

The third edition continues in its previous format as a handy reference guide. The *Oxford Handbook of Midwifery* is therefore a pocket-sized handy reference guide to providing care to women during pregnancy, birth, and the postnatal period with sections on sexual health, contraception, neonatal care, and infant feeding. The chapters contain an introduction to the section, assessment, diagnosis, and management of care with treatment interventions as recommended in national guidelines and protocols. There is new information in the section on initiation of breastfeeding with biological nurturing included. A highlighted section on how to manage obstetric emergencies is central in the book and important psychosocial care issues are addressed. Our aim is to provide concise, practical, and accessible information in a logical sequence; therefore, the layout follows the woman's journey through pregnancy, birth, and early motherhood. The page-to-a-topic format is in place for most of the book so that information is found easily. Key illustrations are provided where these will be helpful in visualizing concepts.

Although the main target of the book is the student midwife, others who work with women and families will find this a useful quick reference guide in practice.

# Acknowledgements

It has been a privilege to edit the third edition of the *Oxford Handbook of Midwifery*. As always it is nearly impossible to produce a book without a lot of support from others. Firstly, we would like to thank previous editors Beverley Marsh and Maggie Evans, for their original contributions which provided some firm foundations for parts of this edition.

We have welcomed two new editors for this edition, Linda Ball and Sarah Stables, who have proved to be a great addition to the team. Thank you both for your hard work.

Our thanks also go to our work colleagues, both at the Universities and in the clinical areas, who supported this endeavour. We would like to give a special mention to the Head of Midwifery at Sheffield Teaching Hospitals NHS Foundation Trust, Paula Schofield and to Sue Gibson, former Head of Midwifery at Barnsley NHS Foundation Trust, for their kind permission to use Trust guidelines for evidence-based care management aspects within the book. Many thanks to the Barnsley Supervisor of Midwives team who gave invaluable help with the midwifery supervision pages.

Our back-up team at Oxford University Press has again been so supportive and helpful in guiding us through the process. Thank you to Michael Hawkes, Fiona Chippendale, and Angela Butterworth for your advice and for keeping everything on track.

Lastly, thanks to all our families, in particular Linda's husband James and son Liam and also Janet's daughter Stella, who have kindly provided us with some lovely illustrations. We are deeply indebted.

# Contents

Symbols and abbreviations *xi*

# Symbols and abbreviations

| | |
|---|---|
| ▶ | important |
| ▶▶ | very important |
| ❶ | warning |
| ↓ | decrease |
| ↑ | increase |
| α | alpha |
| β | beta |
| °C | degree Celsius |
| = | equal to |
| > | greater than |
| < | less than |
| ≥ | equal to or greater than |
| ≤ | equal to or less than |
| % | per cent |
| ® | registered trademark |
| £ | pound |
| ➔ | cross reference |
| ﷼ | online resource/web address |
| AABR | automated auditory brainstem response |
| ABV | alcohol by volume |
| ACE | angiotensin-converting enzyme |
| ACTH | adrenocorticotropic hormone |
| AED | anti-epileptic drug |
| AFE | amniotic fluid embolism |
| AFP | α-fetoprotein |
| AIDS | acquired immune deficiency syndrome |
| ALT | alanine aminotransferase |
| APH | antepartum haemorrhage |
| APT | alkaline phosphatase |
| APTT | activated partial thromboplastin time |
| ARBD | alcohol-related birth defect |
| ARM | artificial rupture of the membranes |

| AST | aspartate aminotransferase |
| β-hCG | β-human chorionic gonadotrophin |
| BFI | Baby Friendly Initiative |
| BFN | *British National Formulary* |
| BFR | Bach flower remedy |
| BHIVA | British HIV Association |
| BMI | body mass index |
| BP | blood pressure |
| BPD | biparietal diameter; biliopancreatic diversion |
| BPI | brachial plexus injury |
| bpm | beat per minute |
| BV | bacterial vaginosis |
| CAF | Common Assessment Framework |
| cal | calorie |
| CCT | controlled cord traction |
| CF | cystic fibrosis |
| CHIVA | Children's HIV Association |
| cm | centimetre |
| $cmH_2O$ | centimetre of water |
| CMP | clinical management plan |
| CMV | cytomegalovirus |
| CNS | central nervous system |
| CO | carbon monoxide |
| $CO_2$ | carbon dioxide |
| CODAC | Cause of Death and Associated Conditions |
| CPAP | continuous positive airway pressure |
| CPR | cardiopulmonary resuscitation |
| CRP | C-reactive protein |
| CSF | cerebrospinal fluid |
| CT | complementary therapy; computed tomography |
| CTG | cardiotocograph |
| CVP | central venous pressure |
| DDH | developmental dysplasia of the hip |
| DIC | disseminated intravascular coagulation |
| dL | decilitre |
| DMP | designated medical practitioner |
| DNA | deoxyribonucleic acid |

| DPPI | Disability, Pregnancy & Parenthood International |
|------|--------------------------------------------------|
| DS | duodenal switch |
| DVT | deep vein thrombosis |
| EAR | estimated average requirement |
| EBM | expressed breast milk |
| ECG | electrocardiogram |
| ECV | external cephalic version |
| EDD | expected (or estimated) date of delivery |
| EDV | end-diastolic flow velocity |
| EFM | electronic fetal monitoring |
| eGFR | estimated glomerular filtration rate |
| EOGBS | early-onset group B haemolytic *Streptococcus* |
| EPAU | early pregnancy assessment unit |
| EPO | Emergency Protection Order |
| FBC | full blood count |
| FBS | fetal blood sampling |
| FDP | fibrin degradation product |
| Fe | iron |
| FFP | fresh frozen plasma |
| FGM | female genital mutilation |
| FHR | fetal heart rate |
| FMH | feto–maternal haemorrhage |
| FSH | follicle-stimulating hormone |
| G6PD | glucose-6-phosphate dehydrogenase |
| G&S | group and save |
| g | gram |
| GAS | group A streptococcal (infection) |
| GBS | group B haemolytic *Streptococcus* |
| GDM | gestational diabetes mellitus |
| GFR | glomerular filtration rate |
| GP | general practitioner |
| GUM | genitourinary medicine |
| h | hour |
| Hb | haemoglobin |
| $HbA_{1c}$ | glycosylated haemoglobin |
| HBIg | hepatitis B-specific immunoglobulin |
| HbS | sickle haemoglobin |

| HBV | hepatitis B virus |
| hCG | human chorionic gonadotrophin |
| HDL | high-density lipoprotein |
| HDN | haemolytic disease of the newborn |
| HDU | high dependency unit |
| HEI | higher education institution |
| HELLP | haemolysis, elevated liver enzymes, and low platelet count |
| HFOV | high-frequency oscillation ventilation |
| HIV | human immunodeficiency virus |
| HPV | human papillomavirus |
| HRT | hormone replacement therapy |
| HSV | herpes simplex virus |
| HTLV | human T-cell lymphotropic virus |
| IAP | intrapartum antibiotic prophylaxis |
| ICM | International Confederation of Midwives |
| ICS | intraoperative cell salvage |
| ICU | intensive care unit |
| Ig | immunoglobulin |
| IgM | immunoglobulin M |
| IM | intramuscular(ly) |
| INR | international normalized ratio |
| IQ | intelligence quotient |
| IRT | immune reactive trypsinogen |
| IU | international unit |
| IUD | intrauterine device |
| IUFD | intrauterine fetal death |
| IUGR | intrauterine growth restriction |
| IUS | intrauterine system |
| IV | intravenous(ly) |
| IVF | *in vitro* fertilization |
| kcal | kilocalorie |
| KCl | potassium chloride |
| kJ | kilojoule |
| kPa | kilopascal |
| L | litre |
| LAM | lactational amenorrhoea method |
| lb | pound |

| LCP | long-chain polyunsaturated fatty acid |
| LFT | liver function test |
| LH | luteinizing hormone |
| LMP | last menstrual period |
| LNU | local neonatal unit |
| LOP | left occipito-posterior |
| LSA | local supervising authority |
| LSAMO | local supervising authority midwifery officer |
| LSCB | Local Safeguarding Children Board |
| LSCS | lower segment Caesarean section |
| m | metre |
| MAP | mean arterial pressure |
| MAS | meconium aspiration syndrome |
| MCADD | medium-chain acyl CoA dehydrogenase deficiency |
| MEOWS | modified early obstetric warning system |
| mg | milligram |
| $MgSO_4$ | magnesium sulfate |
| micromol | micromole |
| min | minute |
| mL | millilitre |
| mm | millimetre |
| mmHg | millimetre of mercury |
| mmol | millimole |
| MMR | measles, mumps, rubella |
| MRI | magnetic resonance imaging |
| MRSA | meticillin-resistant *Staphylococcus aureus* |
| MSH | melanocyte-stimulating hormone |
| MSU | mid-stream urine sample |
| NAAT | nucleic acid amplification test |
| NEC | necrotizing enterocolitis |
| ng | nanogram |
| NHS | National Health Service |
| NICE | National Institute for Health and Care Excellence |
| NICU | neonatal intensive care unit |
| nm | nanometre |
| NMC | Nursing and Midwifery Council |
| NRT | nicotine replacement therapy |

| NSAID | non-steroidal anti-inflammatory drug |
| NST | non-shivering thermogenesis |
| NTD | neural tube defect |
| OAE | oto-acoustic emission |
| ODP | operating department practitioner |
| OGTT | oral glucose tolerance test |
| OR | odds ratio |
| oz | ounce |
| PC | pubo-coccygeous |
| $pco_2$ | partial pressure of $CO_2$ |
| PCR | protein:creatinine ratio |
| PE | pulmonary embolism |
| PET | pre-eclamptic toxaemia |
| PGD | patient group direction/directive |
| PGE | prostaglandin E |
| PGE2 | prostaglandin E2 |
| PID | pelvic inflammatory disease |
| PIH | pregnancy-induced hypertension |
| PKU | phenylketonuria |
| POCT | point-of-care test |
| POP | progesterone-only pill |
| PPH | post-partum haemorrhage |
| PPHN | persistent pulmonary hypertension of the newborn |
| ppm | part per million |
| PPROM | preterm, pre-labour rupture of the membranes |
| PT | prothrombin time |
| PTV | patient-triggered ventilation |
| PV | per vaginum |
| RBC | red blood cell |
| RCM | Royal College of Midwives |
| RCoA | Royal College of Anaesthetists |
| RCOG | Royal College of Obstetricians and Gynaecologists |
| RDS | respiratory distress syndrome |
| Rh | rhesus |
| RNA | ribonucleic acid |
| RNI | reference nutrient intake |
| ROP | right occipito-posterior |

| s | second |
| --- | --- |
| SANDS | Stillbirth and Neonatal Death Society |
| SCBU | special care baby unit |
| SCD | sickle-cell disease |
| SCU | special care unit |
| SD | shoulder dystocia |
| SFH | symphysis–fundal height |
| SGA | small-for-gestational age |
| SHO | senior house officer |
| SIDS | sudden infant death syndrome |
| SIMV | synchronous intermittent ventilation |
| SoM | supervisor of midwives |
| sp. | species |
| SPC | Summary of Product Characteristics |
| SROM | spontaneous rupture of the membranes |
| TBM | transcutaneous bilirubinometer |
| TCU | transitional care unit |
| tds | three times daily |
| TEDS | thromboembolic deterrent stockings |
| TENS | transcutaneous electrical nerve stimulation |
| TPHA | *Treponema pallidum* haemagglutination |
| TSH | thyroid-stimulating hormone |
| TTTS | twin-to-twin transfusion syndrome |
| TXA | tranexamic acid |
| U/E | urea and electrolytes |
| UK | United Kingdom |
| USA | United States |
| VBAC | vaginal birth after a previous Caesarean |
| VDRL | Venereal Disease Research Laboratory |
| VTE | venous thromboembolism |
| VZIG | varicella-zoster immunoglobulin |
| VZV | varicella-zoster virus |
| WHO | World Health Organization |

# Part 1

# Introduction

# Introduction

# Definition of a midwife

The official definition of a midwife comes from the International Confederation of Midwives (ICM):[1]

'A midwife is a person who has successfully completed a midwifery education programme that is duly recognized in the country where it is located and that is based on the ICM Essential Competencies for Basic Midwifery Practice and the framework of the ICM Global Standards for Midwifery Education; who has acquired the requisite qualifications to be registered and/or legally licensed to practice midwifery and use the title 'midwife'; and who demonstrates competency in the practice of midwifery.

*Scope of Practice*

The midwife is recognized as a responsible and accountable professional who works in partnership with women to give the necessary support, care and advice during pregnancy, labour and the postpartum period, to conduct births on the midwife's own responsibility and to provide care for the newborn and the infant.

This care includes preventative measures, the promotion of normal birth, the detection of complications in mother and child, the accessing of medical care or other appropriate assistance and the carrying out of emergency measures.

The midwife has an important task in health counselling and education, not only for the woman, but also within the family and the community. This work should involve antenatal education and preparation for parenthood and may extend to women's health, sexual or reproductive health and child care.

A midwife may practice in any setting including the home, community, hospitals, clinics or health units.'

This definition tells us that midwives have a very diverse role, and it is one that is expanding to meet the needs of modern society.

There are a number of little known facts about what midwives do, and these are just a few examples based on United Kingdom (UK) midwifery practice.

- The midwife is the senior professional attendant at over 50% of births in the UK.
- Midwives can give continuous care to mother and baby from early pregnancy onwards, throughout childbirth, and until the baby is 28 days old.
- Midwives may legally set up in practice and advertise their midwifery services, either alone or in partnerships.
- It is not necessary to be a nurse in order to become a midwife, although many practising midwives also hold nurse qualifications, in addition to their midwifery registration.
- Midwives are the only professionals concerned solely with maternity care. The only other people legally allowed to deliver babies in the UK are doctors (who need not have had specialist training in this field).

### Reference

1 International Confederation of Midwives (2011). *ICM international definition of the midwife*. Available at: ℳ www.internationalmidwives.org/assets/uploads/documents/Definition%20 of%20the%20Midwife%20-%202011.pdf.

# Role of the midwife

The Nursing and Midwifery Council (NMC, 2012)[2] sets out standards of practice for midwives, including being able to deliver the following:

- Safe and effective practice
- Woman-centred care
- Meeting ethical and legal requirements
- Respect for individuals and communities
- Quality and excellence
- Lifelong learning
- Evidence-based practice
- Reflecting the changing nature of new practice.

In 2014, in England and Wales, there were 777 400 live births.[3] This is a decrease of 1.9% from the previous year. In 2012, there were 21 132 full-time equivalent midwives working in the National Health Service (NHS).[4] This represents that for each of these working midwives there were 36 births. However, not all working midwives offer the full range of services to women. This is because midwives fulfil many varied roles such as managerial, research, education, or other specialist roles.

According to the National Audit Office,[4] midwives should be responsible for 29 births per year using Birthrate Plus, a workforce planning tool. This means that over 2000 additional midwives are needed to provide the commitment to continuity of care for all women.

So the midwife's role is adapting to meet significant challenges within the childbearing population. Although the birthrate has fallen, the complexity facing women and midwives is on the increase from underlying medical conditions and women who face increased risks in childbirth due to a raised body mass index (BMI).[5]

Despite this, midwives remain the lead professional for normal birth in the UK and midwife-led care is deemed as safe as other care options.[6]

## References

2 Nursing and Midwifery Council (2012). *Midwives rules and standards 2012*. Available at: ℘ www. nmc.org.uk/globalassets/sitedocuments/standards/nmc-midwives-rules-and-standards.pdf.

3 Office for National Statistics (2015). *Annual mid-year population estimates: 2014*. Available at: ℘ www.ons.gov.uk/peoplepopulationandcommunity/populationandmigration/populationestimates/bulletins/annualmidyearpopulationestimates/2015-06-25.

4 National Audit Office (2013). *Maternity services in England*. Available at: ℘ www.nao.org.uk/wp-content/uploads/2013/11/10259-001-Maternity-Services-Book-1.pdf.

5 Knight M, Kenyon S, Brocklehurst P, Neilson J, Shakespeare J, Kurinczuk JJ (eds.) on behalf of MBRRACE-UK (2014). *Saving Lives, Improving Mothers' Care: Lessons Learned to Inform Future Maternity Care from the UK and Ireland Confidential Enquiries into Maternal Deaths and Morbidity 2009–2012*. Oxford: National Perinatal Epidemiology Unit, University of Oxford.

6 Sandall J, Soltani H, Gates S, Shennan A, Devane D (2013). Midwife-led continuity models versus other models of care for childbearing women *Cochrane Database Syst Rev* 8: CD004667.

# Principles for record-keeping

Record-keeping is an integral part of midwifery practice, designed to assist the care process and enhance good communication between professionals and clients. The NMC (2015)[7] as part of the Code of Practice for Nurses and Midwives includes instructions for record-keeping, the main recommendations of which are given below.

- Keep clear and accurate records relevant to your practice. This includes, but is not limited to, patient records. It includes all records that are relevant to your scope of practice. To achieve this, you must:
  - Complete all records at the time of, or as soon as possible after, an event, recording if the notes are written some time after the event
  - Identify any risks or problems that have arisen and the steps taken to deal with them, so that colleagues who use the records have all the information they need
  - Complete all records accurately and without any falsification, taking immediate and appropriate action if you become aware that someone has not kept to these requirements
  - Attribute any entries you make in any paper or electronic records to yourself, making sure they are clearly written, dated, and timed, and do not include unnecessary abbreviations, jargon, or speculation
  - Take all steps to make sure that all records are kept securely
  - Collect, treat, and store all data and research findings appropriately.

## Reference

7 Nursing and Midwifery Council (2015). *The Code: Professional Standards of Practice and Behaviour for Nurses and Midwives*. Section 10. Available at: ℘ www.nmc.org.uk/globalassets/sitedocuments/nmc-publications/nmc-code.pdf.

# Statutory midwifery supervision

Statutory supervision of midwives has three distinct functions:
1. To provide a system of support and guidance for every practising midwife in the UK
2. To protect women and babies by actively promoting a safe standard of midwifery practice
3. To provide a regulatory aspect; this involves investigating substandard midwifery practice and/or poor outcomes to the mother and/or baby. Following investigations, supervisors make recommendations to resolve the issues found whilst supporting all involved.

The supervision framework has historically been a legal requirement[8] which all maternity services have been obliged to provide to midwives and service users. However, more recently, the effectiveness of the existing model of supervision has been challenged with the publications of the Kings Fund report[9] and the Kirkup report.[10] Within each of the report's recommendations it is suggested that the current arrangement of supervision is not appropriate for public protection and that the NMC should manage the regulatory aspect of midwives.

The Secretary of State for Health in England announced on 16 July 2015 that the government will change the legislation governing their regulation of midwives. The main effect of the changes will be to take supervision out of the NMC regulatory legislation. Ultimately this change will ensure that, as the regulator, the NMC is responsible for all regulatory decisions regarding midwives. It is likely that the proposed legislative change will take 12–18 months to complete. In the meantime, the current *Midwives Rules and Standards*[11] remain in force. It is important that, during this time of transition, the NMC, along with employers of midwives and the midwifery community, continue to uphold them in the interest of women and babies.

Supervision currently covers a wide range of activity beyond regulatory investigations, including support, development and leadership. The above decision need not affect those activities.

The current purpose of supervision of midwives is to protect women and babies by:
• Promoting best practice and excellence in care
• Preventing poor practice
• Intervening in unacceptable practice.

The practising midwife's responsibilities are to:
• Ensure safe and effective care of mothers and babies
• Maintain fitness to practice
• Maintain registration with the NMC.

Your responsibility in maintaining current registration with the NMC is to:
• Identify and meet the NMC requirements for revalidation
• Meet at least annually with your named supervisor of midwives (SoM)
• Notify your intention to practice annually to the local supervising authority (LSA) via your named SoM
• Have a working knowledge of how NMC publications affect your practice.[12]

## References

8  Statutory Instruments 2002 No. 253 (2002). *The Nursing and Midwifery Order 2001*. Available at: 🔗 www.legislation.gov.uk/uksi/2002/253/contents/made.

9  Baird B, Murray R, Seale B, Foot C (2015). *Midwifery Regulation in the United Kingdom*. London: The Kings Fund.

10  Kirkup B (2015). *The Report of the Morecambe Bay Investigation*. Available at: 🔗 www.gov.uk/government/uploads/system/uploads/attachment_data/file/408480/47487_MBI_Accessible_v0.1.pdf.

11  Nursing and Midwifery Council (2012). *Midwives Rules and Standards 2012*. Available at: 🔗 www.nmc.org.uk/globalassets/sitedocuments/standards/nmc-midwives-rules-and-standards.pdf.

12  Nursing and Midwifery Council (2015). *The Code: Professional Standards of Practice and Behaviour for Nurses and Midwives*. Available at: 🔗 www.nmc.org.uk/globalassets/sitedocuments/nmc-publications/nmc-code.pdf.

## Further reading

Nursing and Midwifery Council. *Revalidation*. Available at: 🔗 www.nmc.org.uk/standards/revalidation/.

# Role of the supervisor of midwives

As previously mentioned, the role of the SoM is under review. Future models for supervision, along with future names for supervisors, are being reviewed and discussed. Until there is a conclusive agreement from all stakeholders involved the NMC has requested that the existing model set out within the *Midwives Rules and Standards*[13] be upheld until further notice. Below is an overview of what the role of the SoM is currently and what qualities a midwife considering the role of the SoM is required to demonstrate.

The potential SoM is nominated by peers and supervisors in their place of work and must undergo a selection process led by the LSA midwifery officer (LSAMO) and university programme leader and which must include a user representative.

The midwife must:
- Have credibility with the midwives she/he will potentially supervise and with senior midwifery management
- Be practising, having at least 3 years' experience, at least one of which shall have been in the 2-year period immediately preceding the appointment
- Be academically able—the supervision programme is currently delivered at Masters level
- Have demonstrated ongoing professional development[13, 14]
- Having successfully completed the preparation programme; the midwife must then be appointed by the LSAMO as a supervisor to the LSA and to whom the SoM is responsible in that role[14]
- Have good communication skills and an approachable manner as being essential to the role.

The SoMs:
- Receive and process notification of intention-to-practise forms
- Provide guidance on the maintenance of registration
- Work in partnership with mothers, midwives, and student midwives
- Create an environment that supports the midwife's role and empowers practice through evidence-based decision-making
- Monitor standards of midwifery practice through audit of records and assessment of clinical outcomes
- Are available for midwives to discuss issues relating to their practice and provide appropriate support
- Are available to mothers to discuss any aspects of their care
- Arrange regular meetings with individual midwives at least once a year, to help them evaluate their practice and identify areas of development
- Investigate critical incidents and identify any action required
- Report to the LSAMO serious cases involving professional conduct and when it is considered that local action has failed to achieve safe practice
- Contribute to confidential enquiries, risk management strategies, clinical audit, and clinical governance

The ratio of SoMs to midwives should reflect local needs and circumstances and should not compromise the safety of women. This ratio will not normally exceed 1:15.

It is recommended that a named SoM be available to all student midwives and that the student is aware of how and when they can contact an SoM for support.

## References

13  Nursing and Midwifery Council (2006). *Standards for the Preparation and Practice of Supervisors of Midwives*. London: Nursing and Midwifery Council.
14  Nursing and Midwifery Council (2012). *Midwives Rules and Standards 2012*. Rules 9–16. Available at: www.nmc.org.uk/globalassets/sitedocuments/standards/nmc-midwives-rules-and-standards.pdf.

# Role of the LSA and LSA midwifery officer

The LSA is a body responsible in law for ensuring that statutory supervision of midwives and midwifery practice is employed, within its boundaries, to a satisfactory standard, in order to secure appropriate care for every mother.[15] However, as previously discussed on ➔ p. 8 and p. 10, the statutory function of the SoM is currently under review with the aim of its removal from the SoM's remit. When the law is changed, the role of the LSA and LSAMO will also change dramatically. It is thought that their future role will remain one of leadership to other midwives and one which is key to delivering a national midwifery strategy, but the full extent and remit of the new LSA and LSAMO are yet unknown. Due to this the following information is an overview of the current roles and responsibilities.

Each LSA appoints an LSAMO to undertake the statutory function on its behalf. This must be a suitably experienced SoM,[15] who has the skills, experience, and knowledge to provide expert advice on issues such as structures for local maternity services, human resources planning, student midwife numbers, and post-registration education opportunities. The role of the LSAMO is unique as it does not represent the interests of either the commissioners or providers of NHS maternity services.[16]

The functions of the LSA and the LSAMO are to:
- Be available to women if they wish to discuss any aspect of their midwifery care that they do not feel had been addressed through other channels
- Compile an annual report for the NMC, which outlines supervisory activities over the past year, key issues, audit outcomes, and emerging trends affecting maternity services
- Appoint SoMs and publish a list of current supervisors
- Ensure that every practising midwife has a named SoM
- Determine the appropriate number of supervisors to reflect local circumstances
- Receive annual notification of intention to practice from all midwives within the LSA boundary and forward the completed forms to the NMC
- Operate a system to ensure that each midwife meets the statutory requirements for practice
- Provide continuing professional development and updating for all SoMs for a minimum of 15h in each registration period
- Ensure that systems are in place to investigate alleged suboptimal care or possible misconduct, in an impartial and sensitive manner
- Determine whether to suspend a midwife from practice
- Where appropriate, proceed to suspend a midwife from practice whom it has reported to the NMC
- Investigate and initiate legal action in cases of midwifery practice by unqualified persons.

## References

15 Nursing and Midwifery Council (2012). *Midwives Rules and Standards 2012*. Rules 9–16. Available at: ℘ www.nmc.org.uk/globalassets/sitedocuments/standards/nmc-midwives-rules-and-standards.pdf.

16 Nursing and Midwifery Council (2009). *Modern Supervision in Action: A Practical Guide for Midwives*. London: Nursing and Midwifery Council.

# Drug administration in midwifery

Under the Human Medicines Regulations (2012),[17] medicines can only be supplied and administered under the directions of a doctor.

Student midwives can administer any medicine prescribed by a doctor under the direct supervision of a registered midwife.

These regulations permit exemptions which allow other professionals to supply and administer medicines in specific circumstances. Midwives are exempt under Section seventeen, Part three from this requirement in relation to certain specified medicines, provided they have notified their intention to practice and the drugs are for use only within their sphere of practice. This allows midwives to supply and administer these drugs without the direction of a doctor.

This is known as the midwives exemptions list (see below) updated in these regulations. This ensures appropriate and responsive care can be given to women safely as part of a midwife's normal sphere of practice and especially during emergencies. The regulation exemption allows student midwives to administer medicines from this list under the direct supervision of a registered midwife, with the exception of diamorphine, morphine, or pethidine.

The medicines to which this exemption applies are as follows:
• Adrenaline
• Anti-D immunoglobulin
• Carboprost
• Cyclizine lactate
• Diamorphine
• Ergometrine maleate
• Hepatitis B vaccine
• Hepatitis B immunoglobulin
• Lidocaine hydrochloride
• Morphine
• Naloxone hydrochloride
• Oxytocins, natural and synthetic
• Pethidine hydrochloride
• Phytomenadione
• Prochlorperazine
• Sodium chloride 0.9%
• Gelofusine®
• Haemaccel®
• Hartmann's solution.

Midwives can also supply and administer all non-prescription medicines, including all pharmacy and general sales list medicines, without a prescription. These medicines do not have to be in a patient group direction (PGD) for a midwife to be able to supply them.

## Patient group directions

PGDs are detailed documents compiled by a multidisciplinary group of a local trust or hospital. They allow certain drugs to be given to particular groups of clients without a prescription to a named individual.

This arrangement is very useful, as it allows the midwife to give a drug listed in the PGD to a woman, without having to wait for a doctor to come and prescribe it individually. The midwife is responsible for following the instructions related to dosage and contraindications provided in the PGD.

Examples of drugs included in a PGD are:
- Dinoprostone (Prostin E2® gel) for induction of labour; 1mg or 2mg gel can be repeated after 6h. Give a lower dose if the cervix is favourable
- Ranitidine 150mg tablets.

It is recommended that, if a drug is on the midwives exemption list, it does not need to appear in a PGD. Under medicines legislation, there is no provision for 'standing orders'; therefore, these have no legal basis.

The NMC (2015)[18] has published *Standards for Medicines Management* which includes dispensing, storage and transportation, administration, delegation, disposal, and management of adverse events and controlled drugs. Registered midwives must only supply and administer medicines for which they have received appropriate training.

There is clear instruction on the role of the midwife in *directly supervising student midwives during drug administration* and that only a registered midwife may administer a drug which is part of PGD arrangements.

## References

17 Statutory Instruments 2012 No. 1916 (2012). *The Human Medicines Regulations 2012.* Available at: ℛ www.legislation.gov.uk/uksi/2012/1916/made.
18 Nursing and Midwifery Council (2015). *Standards for Medicines Management.* London: Nursing and Midwifery Council.

# Independent midwife prescribing

Current legislation gives independent prescribing rights, including for some controlled drugs, to midwives, nurses, and other health-care professionals *within the individual practitioner's sphere of competence*. Whilst the midwife has a wide range of drugs which can be administered within the Midwives Exemptions (UK), there are situations where to be able to independently prescribe has a real advantage for prompt and appropriate action and continuity of care for mothers by experienced, suitably qualified midwives. For example, prescription of antibiotics for mastitis, infected perineum, or urinary tract infection. The drugs to be prescribed will be agreed within the NHS trust, as the employer, for the individual midwife's sphere of practice, e.g. the labour ward or the community. In this way, the midwife's personal practice can be enhanced by making effective use of prescribing.

If the midwife is going to prescribe for the newborn baby, the same principles apply, but the midwife must also demonstrate prescribing competency for this special group as overseen and assessed by an experienced paediatrician.

In the UK, the midwife must undertake an NMC-approved programme at a university approved to run the course at degree or normally Masters degree level. For midwives, the lead midwife for education will oversee the mentoring and assessment process to ensure the principles and practice of prescribing are applied to midwifery practice. Once achieved, the qualification is recordable on the NMC professional register. As with other aspects of professional practice, evidence of continuing professional development in prescribing must be kept in the midwife's professional portfolio.

A designated medical practitioner (DMP) will mentor and assess the required competencies, supported by an experienced midwife prescriber/ SoM to support the midwifery perspective.

The programme and assessment are based on:
- An in-depth knowledge of pharmacology, modes of action, side effects, contraindications, and drug interactions of individual drugs
- An in-depth knowledge and ability to accurately diagnose the conditions being prescribed for
- Safe, effective, and cost-effective prescribing
- Legal and ethical aspects of prescribing
- Evidence-based practice
- Record-keeping
- The seven steps to safe prescribing
- The single competency framework for all prescribers.

## Supplementary prescribing

In some circumstances the midwife may be a supplementary midwife prescriber to an independent medical prescriber, working within the terms of an agreed clinical management plan (CMP). This allows the midwife to make changes to the prescribed dose or drug without the need to see the doctor, providing the criteria of the CMP are met.

**Further reading**

Beckwith S, Franklin P (2011). What is a non-medical prescriber? In: Beckwith S, Franklin P. *Oxford Handbook of Prescribing for Nurses and Allied Health Professionals*, 2nd edn. Oxford: Oxford University Press, pp. 3–17.

National Prescribing Centre (1999). Signposts for prescribing nurses—general principles of good prescribing. *Nurse Prescribing Bulletin* **1**: 1–4.

National Prescribing Centre (2012). *A Single Competency Framework for All Prescribers*. London: National Institute for Health and Care Excellence. Available at: ℅ med.mahidol.ac.th/nursing/sites/default/files/public/knowledge/doc/3.pdf.

Nursing and Midwifery Council (2006). *Standards of Proficiency for Nurse and Midwife Prescribers*. London: Nursing and Midwifery Council. Available at: ℅ www.nmc.org.uk/standards/additional-standards/standards-of-proficiency-for-nurse-and-midwife-prescribers/.

Nursing and Midwifery Council (2010). *Nurse and Midwife Independent Prescribing of Unlicensed Medicines*. London: Nursing and Midwifery Council. Available at: ℅ www.nmc.org.uk/globalassets/sitedocuments/circulars/2010circulars/nmccircular04_2010.pdf.

# Preconception care

# Taking a menstrual history

### Important points to remember

- A menstrual history is usually undertaken as part of the initial booking interview, ensuring privacy for the discussion.
- Allow sufficient time for discussion.
- Find out whether the woman has been keeping a recent diary record of her menstrual pattern or knows her normal menstrual cycle—the number of days between the first day of one menstrual period and the next.
- Find out what form of contraception, if any, she has been using—most hormonal methods will influence the menstrual pattern, which may take several months to return to normal after discontinuation.
- An accurate menstrual history is essential to calculate the expected birth date, or the expected date of delivery (EDD), as accurately as possible. This is a particularly important consideration where ultrasound examination to determine dates is not available or the woman makes an informed choice to decline this procedure.
- An accurate calculation of the expected birth date, as near to the beginning of pregnancy as possible, will subsequently allow you to calculate the gestational age accurately at any point in the pregnancy and assess fetal growth.
- Abdominal assessment of uterine growth at each antenatal visit takes into account the estimated gestational age calculated from the expected birth date.
- It is important that the woman understands that her baby may be born anywhere between the beginning of the 38th week and the end of the 42nd week and be at term. The calculated expected birth date is only 1 day within that time frame.

### Calculation of expected birth date

- Conventionally undertaken using Naegele's rule, which calculates the duration of pregnancy as 280 days.
- Nine calendar months and 7 days are added to the first day of the last menstrual period (LMP).
- Research by Nguyen et al.[1] into the accuracy of this method of calculation, compared with that of ultrasound measurement of fetal biparietal diameter (BPD), recommended that dating is more accurate by adding 282 days to the LMP.

### Naegele's rule

- To the first day of the LMP add 9 months and 7 days.
- Or subtract 3 months and add 7 days (not forgetting to add a year!).
- To be more accurate, as discussed above, add 9 days instead of 7.
- If available, use an obstetric calendar, but add an additional 2 days.
- Naegele's rule assumes a 28-day menstrual cycle.

- Ovulation occurs 14 days before menstruation; in a 28-day cycle that is day 14.
- If the woman's normal menstrual cycle is shorter or longer than this, you will need to add or subtract days accordingly. Calculate according to Naegele's rule above, then add or subtract the required days.

*Examples*
- For a regular 25-day cycle, subtract 3 days from the calculated expected birth date.
- For a regular 35-day cycle add 7 days to the calculated expected birth date.
- For an irregular cycle that has no definite pattern, it is advisable to send a woman for an early dating scan, before 12 weeks of pregnancy, if this service is available; or do your best to calculate and use other clinical signs and symptoms of early pregnancy to help you.
- Remember that a woman may be quite clear that she knows exactly when she conceived. Use this information as part of your judgement.

*When calculation is difficult*
- The woman does not know the date of her LMP.
- Cycles are irregular.
- A normal cycle has not resumed since she stopped using hormonal contraception:
  - Combined oral contraception—'the pill'—may confuse withdrawal bleeding with a normal period; anovular cycles may lead to inaccuracy in calculation of the expected birth date
  - Desogestrel progesterone-only pill (POP) may have the same effect—it is designed to inhibit ovulation, unlike other POPs.
  - After Depo-Provera® injections, it may take several months before menstrual bleeding and ovulation return; anovular cycles may lead to inaccuracy in calculating the expected birth date.
  - After the removal of the Mirena® intrauterine system (IUS) or a Nexplanon® implant, the woman's hormonal levels return to normal with 72h of removal and will not inhibit early conception.
  - A copper intrauterine device (IUD) does not affect the woman's hormonal levels.

## Reference
1 Nguyen T, Larsen T, Engholm G, et al. (1999). Evaluation of ultrasound-estimated date of delivery in 17,450 spontaneous singleton births: do we need to modify Naegele's rule? *Ultrasound Obstet Gynaecol* 14: 223–8.

## Nutrition

For women of childbearing age, the estimated average requirement (EAR) for energy is approximately 2000kcal/day. A healthy diet contains a variety of foods including protein and starchy carbohydrates such as bread, breakfast cereals, potatoes, pasta, rice, and a daily helping of at least five fruits or vegetables. Foods containing excess fat should be used sparingly and foods containing sugar should be eaten infrequently in small amounts. (➔ See also Chapter 4.)

Good nutrition is an essential requirement to a successful outcome of pregnancy. In an ideal situation, the woman will have good body stores of the vitamins and minerals the embryo requires in order to develop into a healthy fetus. Poor nutritional status can cause problems with fertility and conception, and the extremes of body weight, e.g. being underweight or very overweight, are associated with adverse pregnancy outcomes, such as low birthweight, or developing complications of pregnancy such as high blood pressure (BP), gestational diabetes, and preterm labour. Women in these categories are advised to take steps to modify their body weight towards the normal range in preparation for pregnancy.

Other categories of women who may be in need of nutritional counselling include:

- Those with *closely spaced pregnancies*. If the gap between births is only about 1 year, there is an increased risk of the next baby being born prematurely and/or of low birthweight. Two or 3 years between births allows the repletion of body stores. Until then, vitamin and/or mineral supplements may be appropriate
- *Vegans/vegetarians*. These diets can be extremely healthy; however, if meat or fish or dairy foods are avoided, essential nutrients must be replaced from other food sources such as cereals and pulses, nuts, and seeds. Yeast extracts, such as Marmite®, are fortified with vitamin $B_{12}$
- *Adolescents*. A main influence on pregnancy outcome is the number of years between the menarche and pregnancy—the shorter this interval, the greater the potential for nutritional deficiencies. Nutritional deficiencies are also more likely during pregnancy, as adolescents need enough nutrients to complete their own growth as well as to fulfil the demands of a growing baby
- Those with *a low income*. Several surveys have shown that women tend to 'go without' food themselves in order to ensure that other members of their family get enough to eat
- Those with *a pre-existing disease*, e.g. diabetes and epilepsy. Food allergies should always be diagnosed medically, and malabsorption syndromes, such as Crohn's disease, ulcerative colitis, or cystic fibrosis, require dietetic consultation
- Those with *eating disorders*—anorexia nervosa, bulimia nervosa, or binge eating

- *Immigrants/ethnic minorities*. Vegetarianism and fasting are common practices in those of Asian origin. Their diets are often low in calcium, with a low intake of dairy foods and a higher intake of wholewheat cereals, which are high in phytate, an inhibitor of calcium absorption. Because many Asian women cover their head and body, they do not manufacture much vitamin D in their skin, so they may require a supplement of 10 micrograms/day.

## Women planning a pregnancy

- *Take a folic acid supplement.* Take a 400-microgram (or more if advised by your doctor) folic acid supplement each day and continue to take this until 12 weeks pregnant. Eat more foods that contain natural folates, e.g. green leafy vegetables, fruit, bread, and fortified breakfast cereals. Folate/folic acid is important during preconception and early pregnancy as it can reduce the risk of neural tube defects (NTDs) such as spina bifida.

- *Vitamin D.* Vitamin D is important during pregnancy to help build the fetus's growing bones and all pregnant and breastfeeding women are advised to take a vitamin D supplement (10 micrograms per day).

  Low vitamin D status is relatively common in the UK population. Women with darker skin, e.g. those of South Asian, African, or Caribbean origin, and women who rarely expose themselves to sunlight, because they cover their skin or spend long periods indoors, are recommended to take a vitamin D supplement. For those planning to conceive, consider taking a vitamin D supplement to ensure stores are sufficient for pregnancy.

- *Fish.* Oily fish is a good source of omega-3 fats and other nutrients and should be eaten as part of a healthy varied diet. Omega-3 fats have an important role in the development of the central nervous system (CNS), the brain, and the retina of the fetus as well as supporting a healthy heart in the mother.

  It is recommended that women eat two portions of fish (one portion is 140g, cooked weight) a week, one of which should be oily fish. However, avoid shark, swordfish, and marlin, and limit the amount of tuna to no more than two tuna steaks a week or four cans of tuna a week. This is because the mercury in these fish could build up and subsequently damage the baby's developing nervous system. Also, limit the intake of oily fish (e.g. salmon, fresh tuna, sardines, trout, and mackerel) to no more than two portions a week.

- *Avoid drinking alcohol.* High intakes of alcohol may affect fetal development, particularly in the early stages of pregnancy. As there may be a gap between conception and confirmation of pregnancy, it is best to simply avoid drinking alcohol during this time.

  It is recommended not to drink more than one to two units of alcohol once or twice a week and to avoid getting drunk. One unit is 100mL of 10% alcohol by volume (ABV) wine, half a pint of ordinary-strength beer, lager, or cider, or a single pub measure (25mL) of spirits.

## Further reading

British Nutrition Foundation (2016). *Pregnancy and pre-conception*. Available at: ℘ www.nutrition.org.uk/nutritionscience/life/pregnancy-and-pre-conception.html.

# Lifestyle

### Changes in lifestyle

A person's lifestyle can impact on their health and well-being, and a healthy lifestyle is the ideal for everyone. It is even more appropriate during pregnancy to consider the impact of lifestyle choices. Couples who are planning a pregnancy may seek advice prior to conception.

The aim of preconception care is to prepare the body for a successful pregnancy. This preparation should take place at least 3–4 months prior to conception. The following lifestyle changes may be suggested.

- Advise the woman and her partner to give up smoking, as women who smoke reduce their chance of a successful pregnancy by 40%, compared with non-smokers. Smoking reduces sperm motility and can lead to higher numbers of abnormal sperm. Offer referral to a smoking cessation programme (the NHS smoking helpline is 0800 169 0169).
- Advise a reduction or elimination of alcohol from the diet. Women who drink more than 10 units per week have a reduced chance of successful pregnancy and an increased risk of miscarriage, compared with women who drink fewer than 5 units per week. Excess alcohol consumption by the mother is associated with fetal alcohol syndrome.
- Advise the woman to avoid using illegal drugs and if she is taking prescribed medications to ask for her general practitioner's (GP's) advice.
- Some occupations may reduce male and female fertility. Exposure to heat, X-rays, chemical pesticides, or solvents may contribute to reduced fertility. Advise avoiding such exposure as far as possible.
- If the man or woman is obese, advise weight reduction prior to pregnancy as excessive weight reduces fertility in both men and women, and the woman is at a greater risk of pregnancy and delivery complications.

### Medical considerations

- Check the status of the woman's measles, mumps, rubella (MMR) history and offer two doses if not previously vaccinated. Can also be offered postnatally.
- Perform a full blood count (FBC) to screen for anaemia, which can be corrected prior to pregnancy.
- Measure the BP to screen for hypertension.
- Perform a cervical smear test if more than 5 years have elapsed since her last test.
- Test a urine sample for the presence of protein (indicator of renal disease or infection) and glucose (indicator of diabetes).
- Offer the couple screening for genital infection as many of these are asymptomatic.

# Medical conditions

Certain medical conditions may complicate pregnancy, and women who have these should be referred to their GP before embarking on a pregnancy so that any concerns can be addressed, medications reviewed, and treatment adjusted to enable a successful pregnancy to be achieved.

## Type 1 diabetes

- Diabetes can have serious consequences for the mother and fetus, and the severity of the problems is linked directly to the degree of the disease and the mother's blood glucose control.
- High blood glucose levels prior to, and around the time of, conception increase the risk of fetal abnormality and intrauterine death in macrosomic babies.
- Women planning a pregnancy should have a medical, dietetic, educational, drug, obstetric, and gynaecological history taken. Metformin may be used together with, or in place of, insulin during preconception and throughout pregnancy. All other blood glucose-lowering medications should be stopped before pregnancy and replaced with insulin. If the woman is taking any other medication that is not recommended in pregnancy, e.g. angiotensin-converting enzyme (ACE) inhibitors, statins, diuretics, or β-blockers, steps should be taken to remedy this before conception or as soon as pregnancy is confirmed.[2]
- Advise the mother to aim to keep her blood glucose within the range of 4–7mmol/L before she conceives and during the pregnancy.
- Fetal macrosomia results from high blood glucose in the mother and increased insulin levels in the fetus. This promotes excessive growth of the fetus and can lead to delivery problems (shoulder dystocia) and early problems for the newborn such as respiratory difficulties and hyperglycaemia.

## Hypertension

- Pre-existing hypertension can cause problems in the mother and fetus during pregnancy.
- Hypertension can lead to placental complications, slow growth of the fetus, and renal complications in the mother.
- Pregnancy-induced hypertension (PIH) can occur alongside existing hypertension, requiring earlier intervention or antenatal admission.
- Women with hypertension need to continue taking antihypertensive medication and may need to switch to a safer drug during pregnancy.

## Epilepsy

- Advise women with epilepsy to seek advice prior to becoming pregnant, so that their anti-epileptic drugs (AEDs) can be adjusted, if necessary. This is because there is a threefold increase of congenital malformations in babies of women with epilepsy.
- Advise the woman not to stop taking her medication unless otherwise directed by the specialist.[3]

- AEDs are known to cause folic acid deficiency. Therefore, women with epilepsy should take folic acid supplements preconceptually and during the first 12 weeks of pregnancy. They will require a higher dose than normal of 5mg/day.

## Infections

- Screening for rubella is no longer offered. Check the status and administration of MMR vaccine and offer 2 doses if the woman has not been vaccinated.
- Hepatitis B vaccine and a tetanus booster should also be available.
- Sexually transmitted diseases, such as herpes, genital warts, and chlamydiosis, can be screened for and treated prior to pregnancy.

## References

2 Diabetes UK (2015). *Preconception care for women with diabetes.* Available at: ℘ www.diabetes. org.uk/About_us/What-we-say/Specialist-care-for-children-and-adults-and-complications/ Preconception-care-for-women-with-diabetes/.

3 National Institute for Health and Care Excellence (2012). *Pre-conception—advice and management.* Clinical Knowledge Summaries. Available at: ℘ cks.nice.org.uk/pre-conception-advice-and-management.

# Sexual health

# Vaginal infections

During pregnancy an increased vaginal discharge is commonly experienced and is the result of normal physiological changes related to increased blood flow in the reproductive organs and a decrease in the acidity of the vaginal discharge. Investigation should be considered if the woman reports itching, soreness, offensive smell, or pain on passing urine.

It is important to remember that *Chlamydia trachomatis* is the most common cause of infection and 70–80% of infected women are asymptomatic. All women should be offered a routine urine-based screening test in early pregnancy and at any other time, as required.

For specific infections see the relevant sections in this chapter.

## Obtaining a vaginal swab

* There are two methods to obtain a vaginal swab: high and low vaginal.
* A *self-taken low vaginal swab* for chlamydia and gonorrhoea is as effective as an endocervical swab and preferable in pregnancy. Tell the woman to rotate the swab at least ten times in the lower vagina, using a circular movement to ensure she gets adequate sampling from the lower vaginal walls.
* A swab for group B haemolytic *Streptococcus* (GBS) is obtained from just inside the vaginal opening. At the same time, a rectal swab is usually taken. There is less emphasis on avoiding contamination, as the organism inhabits both the rectum and lower genital tract.
* A *high vaginal swab* is obtained by viewing the upper vagina with a speculum and a good light.
  * For a high vaginal swab, having consented to the procedure and removed the necessary undergarments, the client should lie on an examination couch, bend her knees, and with her heels together let her knees fall apart. Lighting and couch height should be adjusted to give a good view of the vulva and vagina.
  * The speculum should ideally be disposable, lubricated with a water-based lubricant, and inserted gently into the vagina with closed blades orientated in the same direction as the vaginal opening. Once inserted, the blades should be slowly rotated until they are horizontal and opened slowly, bringing the cervix into view. If not immediately visible, be patient and allow it to slowly come into view with minimal movement of the speculum.
  * The swab can now be taken from the fornices of the upper vagina, avoiding contamination from the vaginal entrance.
  * Note the condition of the vagina and cervix. What does the vaginal discharge look like and is there any evidence of cervical inflammation or excoriation?

# Bacterial vaginosis

- Bacterial vaginosis (BV) is the most common cause of vaginal discharge in women of childbearing age.[1]
- It is caused when the normal lactobacilli of the vaginal flora are replaced with anaerobic flora such as *Gardnerella vaginalis*.
- It often coexists with other sexually transmitted infections (STIs) but may occur spontaneously, often repeatedly, in both sexually active and non-sexually active women.
- It is often diagnosed in an asymptomatic form by the detection of 'clue cells' when analysing a high vaginal swab taken for an STI screen.
- Commonly, women report it to be more of a problem in the perimenstrual period.
- It is more common in black women than white, those with an IUD, and women with pelvic inflammatory disease (PID).
- In those who have undergone termination of pregnancy it may cause post-termination endometritis.
- On examination the vaginal mucosa is not inflamed.
- The main symptom is a malodorous, greyish, watery discharge, although 50% of women are asymptomatic. In practice, it is not usually treated unless there are symptoms.
- The 'fishy' odour is characteristic and more pronounced following sexual intercourse, due to the alkaline semen.
- About one-third of women with active BV may also have vulval irritation.
- Treatment is usually metronidazole 2g stat or alternatively a course of clindamycin may be given.
- All these treatments have been shown to be 70–80% effective in controlled trials; however, recurrence of infection is common.
- Whilst undergoing treatment, the woman should avoid drinking alcohol for the duration of the treatment and for the next 48h, as it may cause nausea and vomiting.
- She should also abstain from sexual intercourse for the duration of the treatment and the next 7 days.
- In order to preserve vaginal acidity, the woman should be advised to avoid the use of shower gel in the vulval area or of bath foam, antiseptic agents, or shampoo in the bath. Similarly, she should avoid vaginal douching. Laundry products also need to be considered, and use those recommended for babies.
- Long-term use of a gel, such as Balance Activ™, will help to maintain normal vaginal pH and reduce recurrence rates—widely available over the counter.

## Bacterial vaginosis in pregnancy

- About 20% of pregnant women have BV, with the majority being asymptomatic.
- There is substantial evidence that BV is associated with preterm rupture of the membranes, preterm labour, and birth.
- Other evidence suggests an association with late spontaneous abortion, intra-amniotic infection, and postnatal endometritis.

- It is recommended that women with a history of repeat second-trimester miscarriage or preterm birth be screened for BV.
- The manufacturers of the treatment recommend caution in pregnancy, but only against high doses and there is no evidence of teratogenic effects.

## Fetal and neonatal infection

- There is no evidence of direct fetal or neonatal infection.
- Care should be taken when prescribing treatment whilst breastfeeding.

## Reference

1 Brocklehurst P, Gordon A, Heatley E, Milan SJ (2013). Antibiotics for the treatment of BV in pregnancy. *Cochrane Database Syst Rev* 1: CD000262. Also available at: ℘ onlinelibrary.wiley.com/enhanced/doi/10.1002/14651858.CD000262.

# Candidiasis

- The causative organism is usually *Candida albicans*, normally a commensal organism found in the flora of the mouth, gastrointestinal tract, and vagina, which under certain circumstances becomes pathogenic and can cause symptoms.
- It may be sexually transmitted, but most cases occur spontaneously. Colonization from the lower intestinal tract is common.
- Culture from a high vaginal swab is currently the best method of diagnosis for vulval vaginal infection. Similarly, a mouth/throat swab should be taken for oral infection.
- The condition is not usually treated unless the woman is symptomatic, which is indicated by a thick, white discharge and vaginal and vulval irritation.
- There is no need to treat the partner, unless he is symptomatic.
- Common in diabetes mellitus, due to increased glycogen levels in uncontrolled diabetes.
- Found more commonly in the luteal phase of the menstrual cycle.
- There is no evidence that women using the combined oral contraceptive have an increased incidence of colonization. Other contraceptives, such as diaphragms and caps, may carry the infection and cause reinfection, if not cleaned and stored properly.
- Impaired immunity, such as that found with human immunodeficiency virus (HIV) infection, will increase the incidence.
- Broad-spectrum antibiotics increase yeast carriage by 10–30%.
- Vaginal deodorants, disinfectants, perfumed shower, and bath gels may exacerbate the problem by increasing irritation and vulval excoriation and dermatitis.
- Washing and wiping the vulval area should always be from front to back.
- The wearing of tight, synthetic clothing should be avoided.
- Application of plain yoghurt may soothe the irritation in the short term but has not been shown to be effective as treatment. Daily oral ingestion of 8oz of active yoghurt has been shown to decrease the incidence of candidal colonization and infection, but this has not been replicated in other studies.

## Candidiasis in pregnancy

- Vaginal candidiasis is the most common cause of troublesome vaginal discharge and vulval irritation in pregnancy.
- It occurs 2–10 times more frequently in pregnant than in non-pregnant women and is more difficult to eradicate.
- The problems are worst in the third trimester, with over 50% having significant colonization due to increasing vaginal glycogen and the changing pH of the vagina in pregnancy.
- A Cochrane review of topical treatments for vaginal candidiasis[2] concluded that topical imidazole drugs are more effective than clotrimazole and that treatment over 7 days is more effective than a single dose or 3- to 4-day treatment.
- Refer the woman to the sexual health clinic for management of persistent or recurring *Candida* infection.

## Fetal and neonatal infection
- The baby may become colonized from an infected birth canal but is more likely to become infected from poor handwashing hygiene by those caring for, or handling, the baby, including visitors, or inadequately sterilized or contaminated feeding bottles.
- A breastfeeding baby may become infected from a sore nipple that becomes infected.

## Reference
2 Young GL, Jewell D (2001). Topical treatment for vaginal candidiasis in pregnancy. *Cochrane Database Syst Rev* 4: CD000225. Also available at: ℘ onlinelibrary.wiley.com/enhanced/doi/10.1002/14651858.CD000225/.

# Chlamydia

- *C. trachomatis* is the most common cause of bacterial STI in the UK, affecting both men and women, and a leading cause of PID.
- Prevalence is highest among, but not exclusive to, young sexually active adults, especially those under 25, hence the current National Chlamydia Screening Programme in England for the 16- to 25-year age group.
- Eighty per cent of women and 50% of men have no symptoms, and, left untreated, chlamydia can, in women, lead to infertility, ectopic pregnancy, and chronic pelvic pain. In men, it may cause urethritis and epididymitis. In both sexes, it can cause arthritis—Reiter's syndrome.
- In the symptomatic woman it may cause mucopurulent cervicitis, and post-coital and/or intermenstrual bleeding.
- Because of the prevalence of chlamydia in the sexually active population and the lack of symptoms, *it is good midwifery practice to routinely offer a chlamydia screening test*, using a 'first catch' urine sample or a self-taken low vaginal swab, both at the beginning of pregnancy and again by 36 weeks, to detect and treat affected women. The nucleic acid amplification test (NAAT) is 95% sensitive. The low vaginal swab has now largely replaced the endocervical swab and is easily taken by the woman or the midwife.
- An endocervical swab should only be taken if examining the cervix for another reason.
- It is also good practice to screen the male partner(s) and to refer both partners to the local sexual health service for further STI screening, contact tracing, and follow-up, should there be a positive result.
- Antibiotic treatment in pregnancy is usually with a course of erythromycin 500mg twice daily for 14 days, but exact treatment will be decided by the doctor or specialist nurse with prescribing rights. Azithromycin should be used with caution in pregnancy and breastfeeding,[3] but there is no evidence to date that its unlicensed use is detrimental.

## Chlamydia in pregnancy

- In the pregnant woman, the increased vascularity of the cervix may lead to post-coital or irregular spotting or vaginal bleeding and any woman with such bleeding should be screened for chlamydia.
- Chlamydia in pregnancy can cause amnionitis and postnatal endometritis.
- The evidence on its role in spontaneous abortion, preterm rupture of the membranes, preterm birth, and neonatal death is unclear from studies to date.

## Fetal and neonatal infection

- Although there is some evidence that intrauterine infection can occur, the major risk to the baby is during vaginal birth through an infected cervix.
- Up to 70% of babies born to mothers with untreated chlamydia will become infected; 30–40% will develop chlamydial conjunctivitis and 10–20% a characteristic pneumonia.

- Chlamydial ophthalmia neonatorum is a notifiable infection.
- Chlamydial ophthalmia neonatorum is now much more common than gonococcal ophthalmia, although, in practice, the two may occur together; 50% of those with gonococcal ophthalmia also have chlamydia.
- Chlamydial ophthalmia has an incubation period of 10–14 days, much longer than gonococcal ophthalmia, which is evident in about 48h.
- *It can permanently affect vision and can even cause blindness.*
- The orbit of the eye is swollen and there is a mucoid discharge, often known as a 'sticky eye'.
- The midwife must take swabs from both eyes, for chlamydia, gonococcal infection, and general culture and sensitivity, and ensure they are immediately transported to the laboratory.
- After taking the swab, the eyes are regularly cleansed with normal saline.
- Inform the paediatrician, or the GP in the community, and ensure the baby is examined and treated as a matter of urgency.
- The nasopharynx is also likely to be infected, which may lead to pneumonia unless promptly treated with systemic antibiotics.
- It is important to diagnose and treat any baby with chlamydial infection
- It is thought that the baby who is affected by chlamydia pneumonia is more likely to develop obstructive lung disease and asthma than those with pneumonia from other causes.
- It may be up to 7 months before a chlamydial infection becomes apparent and cultures from the pharynx, middle ear, vagina, and rectum of the baby are positive.
- Knowledge about prevalence in the community and the effects on both mother and baby should encourage the midwife to take a thorough sexual health history, to be proactive in chlamydia testing, and to offer routine testing to all pregnant women in her care.

## Reference

3 *British National Formulary* (2015). Available at: ℬ www.bnf.org.

## Further reading

Brocklehurst P, Rooney G (2009). Interventions for treating genital chlamydia trachomatis infection In pregnancy. *Cochrane Database Syst Rev* **4**: CD000054. Also available at: ℬ onlinelibrary.wiley.com/enhanced/doi/10.1002/14651858.CD000054.

# Genital warts

- Genital warts are caused by the human papillomavirus (HPV) types 6 and 11.
- Sexual transmission is the most usual mode of infection.
- The incidence of genital warts diagnosed has steadily been rising over the past 10 years and the highest rates are seen in the female in the 16- to 24-year age group.
- They are not only uncomfortable, but also psychologically distressing.
- They are difficult and time-consuming to treat and may reoccur months or years later.
- Refer a woman who has genital warts to a specialist sexual health clinic for treatment and further investigation for other STIs.
- Although most genital warts are benign, it is important that an annual liquid-based cytology screen is recommended, as HPV types 16, 18, 31, 33, and 35 are strongly associated with the development of cervical cancer.
- The midwife has an important role in sexual health promotion, encouraging safer sex and promoting participation in the cervical screening programme, particularly if the woman is over 25 and not yet had her first screening test.

## Genital warts in pregnancy

- Genital warts are caused by HPV.
- In pregnancy the warts may increase considerably in size and have a cauliflower-like appearance.
- Occasionally they are so large and widespread that they may obstruct the vulva and lower vagina and prevent a vaginal birth, therefore requiring a Caesarean section.
- The normal treatment is a *drug contraindicated in pregnancy*, because of possible teratogenic effects; therefore, pharmacological treatment is not given until after birth.
- Cryocautery is the only treatment possible during pregnancy, done at a specialist sexual health clinic.

## Fetal and neonatal infection

- Babies and young children may develop laryngeal papilloma after being infected by maternal genital warts during vaginal birth.

# Gonorrhoea

- Gonorrhoea is the second most common STI in the UK.
- Prevalence is highest among sexually active adults under 25 years.
- It is a bacterial infection, caused by *Neisseria gonorrhoeae*.
- The organism adheres to mucous membranes and is more prevalent on columnar, rather than squamous, epithelium.
- The primary sites of infection are the mucous membranes of the urethra, endocervix, rectum, pharynx, and conjunctiva.
- Importantly, gonorrhoea frequently coexists with other genital mucosal infections such as those caused by *C. trachomatis, Trichomonas vaginalis*, and *C. albicans*.
- Most areas are now also testing for gonorrhoea and chlamydia on self-taken low vaginal swabs and urine samples, because of the prevalence of co-infection. Be aware of the testing procedures in your own area.
- Up to 80% of PID in women under 26 is caused by gonorrhoea or chlamydia or both.
- The consequences of untreated gonorrhoea leading to PID include infertility, ectopic pregnancy, and chronic pelvic pain. Although uncommon, it may also cause disseminated general disease and arthritis—Reiter's syndrome.
- Fifty per cent of women may be asymptomatic.
- The most common symptom is increased or altered vaginal discharge (penile discharge in men).
- Other symptoms include lower abdominal pain, dysuria, dyspareunia, intermenstrual uterine bleeding, and menorrhagia.
- It is also good practice to screen the male partner(s) and to refer both partners to the local sexual health service for further STI screening, contact tracing, and follow-up.

## Gonorrhoea in pregnancy

- The incidence of 1–5% is small, *but the incidence of gonorrhoea nationally is rising*. Midwives must therefore be vigilant, as there is evidence that it is detrimental in pregnancy. Refer the woman immediately to the sexual health/genitourinary medicine (GUM) service for investigation and treatment.
- Gonorrhoea is associated with spontaneous abortion, chorioamnionitis, preterm rupture of the membranes, preterm labour, and very low birthweight. Postnatally, it can cause endometritis and pelvic sepsis, which may be severe.
- A Cochrane systematic review of interventions for treating gonorrhoea in pregnancy concluded that the well-established treatment with penicillin and probenecid is effective.[4] However, antibiotic-resistant strains are now becoming apparent and making treatment more difficult.

## Fetal and neonatal infection

- The most common mode of transmission to the baby is through the infected cervix during vaginal birth.
- It may also be transmitted in the uterus, following prolonged rupture of the membranes.

- The risk of vertical transmission from an infected mother is 30–50%.
- The most usual manifestation of neonatal infection is gonococcal ophthalmia neonatorum.
- A profuse, purulent discharge from red and swollen eyes appears usually within 48h of birth.
- *It can permanently affect vision and can even cause blindness* through corneal ulceration and perforation.
- The midwife must take swabs from both eyes, for gonococcal infection and general culture and sensitivity, and ensure they are immediately transported to the laboratory. The swabs are normally specially designated, containing a transport medium to keep the gonococcus alive until it reaches the laboratory.
- After taking the swab, the eyes are regularly cleansed with normal saline.
- Inform the paediatrician, or the GP in the community, and ensure the baby is examined and treated with systemic antibiotics as a matter of urgency.
- The mother and her sexual partner(s) must be screened for infection and treated.

## Reference

4 Brocklehurst P (2002). Interventions for treating gonorrhoea in pregnancy. *Cochrane Database Syst Rev* 2: CD000098. Also available at: ℘ onlinelibrary.wiley.com/enhanced/doi/10.1002/14651858.CD000098.

# Hepatitis B

- The hepatitis B virus (HBV) is the most commonly transmitted blood-borne virus worldwide and a major public health problem.
- It is an important cause of both mortality and morbidity from acute infection and chronic long-term sequelae, including cirrhosis of the liver and primary liver cancer.
- The virus can be transmitted both sexually and parenterally through infected blood and blood products.
- Other body fluids, such as saliva, menstruation, vaginal discharge, seminal fluid, and breast milk, and serous exudates have been implicated, but infection via these routes is far less common.
- Unsterilized equipment, such as that associated with injecting drug users sharing equipment, tattooing, and acupuncture, is a source of infection.
- Importantly, health-care workers may be infected through needlestick injury and must follow local policy for reporting such injuries and subsequent testing. In the UK, all health-care workers at any risk are required to be immunized against HBV.
- Although the initial acute phase is characterized by a flu-like illness, followed by a phase characterized by jaundice, loss of appetite, nausea, and fatigue, it may be asymptomatic in 10–50%.
- In chronic infection, there are often no physical signs or symptoms, but there may be signs of chronic liver disease.
- The midwife has an important health promotion role in careful history taking, detecting risk factors, giving evidence-based information, and encouraging women to participate in antenatal HBV testing.

## Hepatitis B in pregnancy

- If a woman is a carrier of HBV, she has an 85% risk of transmission of the virus to her infant.
- Acute HBV infection occurring during pregnancy is associated with an increased risk of spontaneous abortion and preterm labour and birth.
- The objective of offering HBV screening to pregnant women and immunization of babies born to infected mothers is to reduce the perinatal transmission of this infection.
- All women are offered screening for HBV during early pregnancy.

## Fetal and neonatal infection

- If the mother tests positive for HBV, her baby will be vaccinated shortly after birth.
- Obtain consent for the baby's immunization prior to birth, and give the first dose as early as possible, but always within 24h.
- If the mother became infected during pregnancy or does not have the HBe antibodies, the baby should receive hepatitis B-specific immunoglobulin (HBIg) at birth, injected at a different site to the vaccine. This will give immediate immunity and reduces vertical transmission by 90%.
- Encourage and support breastfeeding, as there is no additional risk of virus transmission to the baby.

- Further doses of the vaccine should be given at 1 month and 6 months of age, and a booster dose at 12 months.
- Give the mother and the GP written information about the number of injections the baby requires, when the injections should be given, and who will be responsible for the administration of each dose.
- Stress the importance of completing the full course of immunization.
- In almost all cases of babies and children being infected, it is almost always asymptomatic.

# Hepatitis C

- The hepatitis C virus occurs throughout the world and is mainly transmitted by infected blood, blood products, and inoculation through the skin.
- With screening of all blood donors in the UK for the past 20 years, the incidence of transmission via infected blood and blood products is virtually nil; however, this may not be true elsewhere.
- In intravenous (IV) drug users, the infection rate is over 60% by contamination from sharing needles and syringes.
- Sexual transmission rates are very low.
- The midwife has an important health promotion role in encouraging positive sexual health.

## Hepatitis C in pregnancy

- Careful sexual health and intravenous drug history taking will indicate possible risk factors for infection.
- As with all other blood-borne viruses, it is important to follow universal safe precautions when handling blood and body fluids, to avoid possible health-care worker infection.
- Find out what special precautions in handling of blood and body fluids are to be taken locally for a person known to be hepatitis C-positive.
- The vertical transmission rate is 5% or less but may be increased in a mother who is also HIV-positive.
- Currently, there is no way of preventing vertical transmission, but avoiding unnecessary procedures, such as rupturing the membranes or applying a fetal scalp electrode, will help.
- Refer to a consultant hepatologist for ongoing management and care.

## Fetal and neonatal infection

- Encourage and support breastfeeding, as there is no evidence that breastfeeding increases the risk of transmission, unless the mother is symptomatic and has a high viral load.
- Encourage high standards of personal hygiene in the mother and the importance of handwashing when handling her baby.

# Herpes simplex virus

- There are two types of herpes simplex virus (HSV):
  - HSV1 is usually acquired in childhood or as a young adult coming into contact with infected oral secretions and it causes 'cold sores'
  - HSV2 is sexually transmitted and is the most common cause of genital herpes.
- Once acquired, HSV remains in the body for life and will cause frequent infection.
- The chance of becoming infected is increased with factors such as early age of initiation of sexual activity, the number of sexual partners, and previous genital infections.
- If the individual already has HSV1, the symptoms of a first HSV2 infection may be less severe.
- Commonly, the infection causes painful, vesicular, or ulcerative lesions of the skin and mucous membranes. Dysuria and increased vaginal discharge may also occur. These are more pronounced in a first infection.
- Systemic infection is characterized by high temperature and myalgia may occur.
- Occasionally, the infection may be asymptomatic in adults.

## Definitions

- *First episode of primary infection*: the first infection with either HSV1 or HSV2. The symptoms tend to be pronounced and the lesions may last 2–3 weeks.
- *First episode of non-primary infection*: the first infection with either HSV1 or HSV2, but the person already has pre-existing antibodies to the other type.
- *Recurrent infection*: recurrence of clinical symptoms.

## Diagnosis

- Viral cultures from open lesions, with a special viral swab, are the easiest and one of the best methods of diagnosing infection. The swab should be sent to the laboratory immediately.
- Other specialist tests may be carried out in a sexual health clinic where the woman should be referred for treatment.

## Herpes simplex virus in pregnancy

- The effects of a first or recurrent infection, as discussed above, on the mother will be treated as in the non-pregnant state, and treatments include antiviral therapy, analgesia, saline baths, and a topical anaesthetic gel to soothe the pain and discomfort.
- If the mother acquires a primary infection in the first or second trimester, oral antiviral therapy with aciclovir will be commenced. Occasionally, the clinical manifestation may warrant IV therapy to reduce virus shedding and promote healing. Although not licensed for use in pregnancy, the clinical evidence is that its use is safe.
- If the mother is immunocompromised, as in HIV, the dose will need to be increased.

- From 36 weeks onwards, continuous aciclovir therapy will reduce the risk of clinical risk of recurrence at the time of birth and allow a normal vaginal birth.
- A woman with active lesions after 34 weeks is delivered by a Caesarean section.
- A Caesarean section is not indicated, unless active genital lesions or symptoms of an impending infection are present.

## Fetal and neonatal infection

- The main danger of primary HSV infection in early pregnancy is congenital herpes that causes severe abnormalities, similar to those caused by rubella, toxoplasmosis, and cytomegalovirus (CMV).
- Active primary infection at the time of birth has a 40% risk of transmission to the newborn.
- Recurrent infection at the time of birth has a transmission risk of <5%, whilst virtually nil with asymptomatic virus shedding.

# Syphilis

- Syphilis remains a high cause of fetal and neonatal loss in developing countries, particularly Africa.
- The overall number of cases of infectious syphilis has increased substantially in 16- to 34-year-old females in the UK in recent years. Congenital syphilis has therefore re-emerged.
- It caused by the bacterium *Treponema pallidum* and is usually acquired by sexual contact.
- Infection causes a complex systemic disease that can involve almost every organ in the body.
- It can be congenitally transmitted across the placenta.
- Because of the increased incidence and its devastating effects, it is still routinely screened for in early pregnancy in the UK (see Screening for syphilis, p. 170)
- The midwife has a responsibility for effective sexual health promotion and encouraging effective long-term contraception for at least 2 years after this pregnancy. Both the woman's contraception and sexual health needs are best dealt with by the local specialist contraception and sexual health clinic.

## Stages of infection

Early infectious stage:
- *Primary*: occurs 9–90 days after exposure (average 21 days)
- *Secondary*: 6 weeks to 6 months after exposure (4–8 weeks after primary lesion)
- *Early latent*: 2 years after exposure.

Late non-infectious stage:
- *Late latent*: >2 years after exposure, with no signs or symptoms
- *Neurosyphilis, cardiovascular syphilis, gummatous syphilis*: 3–20 years after exposure.

## Syphilis in pregnancy

- Untreated syphilis may result in spontaneous abortion, preterm birth, stillbirth, or neonatal death.
- If the infant survives and depending on the stage of infection in the mother, there is a high risk of infant or childhood morbidity.
- Congenital transmission will occur from 4 months onwards, and the highest risk is from 6 months onwards, once the Langhan's layer of the early placenta has completely atrophied, which was the protective mechanism.
- A woman diagnosed in pregnancy is likely to have early infectious syphilis, and early treatment will prevent congenital infection.
- Treatment is usually with a course of intramuscular (IM) penicillin. For a woman with penicillin allergy, erythromycin is the drug of choice. Tetracycline is contraindicated in pregnancy.

- Treatment, follow-up, and contact tracing will usually be led by a consultant in GUM, to whom the woman should be immediately referred.
- If untreated, up to one-third of pregnancies will result in stillbirth, and 70–100% of babies will be infected.

## Congenital syphilis

- Although the incidence of congenital syphilis is estimated at 70 per million births, this is likely to increase, whilst the overall increase in incidence in the childbearing age group continues.
- Classification will depend on the stage of disease reached, with approximately two-thirds of live-born infected babies showing no signs or symptoms at birth.
- Lesions will develop from 4 months onwards.
- Serology at birth is unreliable, because of the presence of passive transfer from the mother; the treponemal-specific immunoglobulin M (IgM) light test is unreliable and can give false-positive or negative results.
- The baby should be further serologically tested at 6 weeks and 3 months of age, allowing time for passive maternal antibodies to disappear.
- In subsequent pregnancies, even if the mother has been followed up for 2 years and discharged, the baby should be tested at 3 months of age, in case any trepenomes have persisted in the maternal circulation.
- If the mother is still being followed up when she becomes pregnant again, she should be immediately referred to the GUM clinic for investigation and management.

# Trichomonas vaginalis

- Common worldwide sexually transmitted flagellated protozoal infection, parasitic in the genital tract of both males and females.
- In the female can be found in the cervix, urethra, bladder, Bartholin's glands in the lower vagina, and Skene's periurethral glands.
- Most common in females during the sexually active years.
- Can be associated with other STIs, therefore full screening required if found.
- High rate of reinfection, unless the partner(s) is treated.

## Signs and symptoms

- Twenty to 50% asymptomatic.
- Altered vaginal discharge in up to 70%, vaginal 'fishy' malodour (similar to bacterial vaginosis).
- Vulvovaginitis.
- Vulval discomfort.
- Dysuria.
- On speculum examination, the typical 'strawberry' cervix may be seen.

## Trichomonas in pregnancy

- Refer her to the local specialist sexual health service for investigation and treatment if symptomatic.
- Co-infection with chlamydia and gonorrhoea is common.
- Treatment is with metronidazole if symptomatic.
- Avoid sexual intercourse during treatment and for 7 days after both partners treated.
- Independent association with premature rupture of membranes, preterm labour and birth, and low birthweight.
- No evidence that antenatal screening and treatment for asymptomatic *T. vaginalis* infection will reduce the risk of preterm birth.

## Fetal and neonatal infection

- Risk of preterm rupture of membranes and preterm birth.
- Neonatal vulvovaginitis acquired during birth may occur in about 5% of babies born to mothers with *T. vaginalis* infection.
- Most commonly asymptomatic and will resolve spontaneously in 3–6 weeks, as the influence of maternal oestrogen levels fall in the newborn baby.

## Further reading

*Books*

Pattman R, Sankar KN, Elawad B, Handy P, Ashley Price D (2010). *Oxford Handbook of Genitourinary Medicine, HIV, and Sexual Health*, 2nd edn. Oxford: Oxford University Press.
Rogstad K (ed.) (2011). *ABC of Sexually Transmitted Infections*, 6th edn. Chichester: Wiley Blackwell.
Wylie K (ed.) (2015). *ABC of Sexual Health*, 3rd edn. Chichester: Wiley Blackwell.

## Websites

British Association for Sexual Health and HIV (BASHH). Available at: ℘ www.bashh.org.

*British National Formulary (BNF)*. Available at: ℘ www.bnf.org.

Chlamydia Professional. Available at: ℘ chlamydiae.com.

Department of Health. Available at: ℘ www.gov.uk/government/organisations/department-of-health.

Faculty of Reproductive Sexual Health. Available at: ℘ www.fsrh.org/home/.

Medical Foundation for HIV & Sexual Health. Available at: ℘ www.medfash.org.uk.

National Institute for Health and Care Excellence. Available at: ℘ www.nice.org.uk.

Pellowe C, Pratt RJ (2006). Neonatal conjunctivitis and pneumonia due to chlamydia infection. *Infant* 2: 16–17. Available at: ℘ www.infantgrapevine.co.uk/pdf/inf_007_cif.pdf.

Public Health England (2003). *National Chlamydia Screening Programme (NCSP)*. Available at: ℘ www.chlamydiascreening.nhs.uk/ps/index.html.

UK STI management guidelines. Available at: ℘ www.bashh.org.uk/guidelines/ceguidelines/htm.

# Antenatal care

# Confirmation of pregnancy

There are a number of options for women wishing to confirm their pregnancy. A range of home pregnancy testing kits are available from pharmacies, and most pharmacies will carry out a test for a small charge.

GP surgeries also provide this service.

The tests are based on detecting the presence of β-human chorionic gonadotrophin (β-hCG) in the woman's urine or blood. This hormone is secreted by trophoblast or placental tissue from around 7–10 days after conception.

Other signs of pregnancy are:
- *Amenorrhoea*: absence of menstrual periods in a woman who normally experiences menstruation
- *Nausea and vomiting*: common in the first trimester from 6 weeks' gestation, peaking at around 10 weeks' gestation and diminishing as the pregnancy reaches 12 weeks and beyond. It persists throughout pregnancy in some women
- *Frequency of micturition*: increased urine production and pressure on the bladder due to the growing uterus
- *Tiredness*: increased metabolic activity and rapid growth of uterine and placental tissue
- *Breast tenderness/changes*: hormonal effects of oestrogen and progesterone. The breasts enlarge and become tender and heavier
- *Fetal movements*: these are a late sign, appearing in the second trimester as the fetus grows and the uterus becomes a larger abdominal organ. Early movements feel like fluttering or bursting bubbles. First-time mothers notice these later (18–20 weeks) than those undergoing a second or subsequent pregnancy (16–18 weeks)
- *Pica*: or craving for unusual foods, or combinations of foods—hormonal influences on the gastrointestinal tract alter the mother's perception of taste.

## Dating the pregnancy

Ascertain the following:
- The first day of the LMP. This may be difficult to ascertain accurately, unless the woman is in the habit of recording this
- The length of the menstrual cycle in days and its regularity
- The number of days of bleeding and if the LMP was a normal bleed
- The woman's usual method of contraception and when this was stopped. If the LMP was a withdrawal bleed after oral contraceptive, this date is unreliable.

Calculate the EDD for a 28-day cycle by adding 7 days and 9 months to the date of the LMP. Make adjustments for shorter or longer cycles. (➔ See also Taking a menstrual history, p. 20.)

Confirm the dates by ultrasound scan. Most women will be offered a scan at around 14 weeks' gestation to coincide with serum fetal screening tests.

The earlier the scan, the more accurate the estimation of the fetal age. If the results differ from the menstrual date by >2 weeks, the scan date should be accepted as the correct date and the EDD adjusted accordingly.

Having accurate dates allows for correct interpretation of fetal screening tests and prevents unnecessary induction of labour for post-maturity.

## Further reading

Debbie Chalk; North Somerset Community Partnership. *Pregnancy testing standards*. Available at: ℘ www.nscphealth.co.uk/pregnancy-testing-standards-public-pdf.

NHS Choices. *Doing a pregnancy test*. Available at: ℘ www.nhs.uk/conditions/pregnancy-and-baby/pages/pregnancy-test.aspx#close.

## Adaptation to pregnancy

Increasing amounts of circulating hormones bring about pregnancy changes throughout the body, and all body systems are affected to a greater or lesser degree. The changes allow the fetus to develop and grow, prepare the woman for labour and delivery, and prepare her body for lactation.

### The reproductive system

- Most of the changes take place in the uterus, which undergoes hypertrophy and hyperplasia of the myometrium. The decidua also becomes thicker and more vascular.
- Progesterone causes the endocervical cells to secrete thick mucus, which forms a plug, called the operculum, in the cervical canal, protecting the pregnancy from ascending infection.
- Muscles in the vagina hypertrophy and become more elastic to allow distension during the second stage of labour.

### The cardiovascular system

- Due to the increasing workload, the heart enlarges.
- Cardiac output increases to accommodate the increasing circulating blood volume.
- Peripheral resistance is lowered, due to the relaxing effect of progesterone on the smooth muscle of the blood vessels, leading to a fall in BP.
- To avoid aorto-caval compression, as the arterial walls are more relaxed, it is important to avoid placing the woman in an unattended supine position during the third trimester.
- Blood flow increases in the uterus, skin, breasts, and kidneys, and blood volume increases by 20–50%, varying according to size, parity, and whether the pregnancy is singleton or multiple.

### The respiratory system

- Oxygen consumption increases by 15–20% at term.
- Tidal volume increases by 40%.
- Residual volume decreases by 20%.
- Alveolar ventilation increases by 5–8L/min, four times greater than oxygen consumption, resulting in enhanced gaseous exchange.
- The amount of air inspired over 1min increases by 26%, resulting in hyperventilation of pregnancy, causing carbon dioxide ($CO_2$) to be removed from the lungs with greater efficiency.
- Oxygen transfer to, and $CO_2$ transfer from, the fetus are facilitated by changes in the maternal blood pH and partial pressure of $CO_2$ ($pCO_2$).

### The urinary system

- Renal blood flow increases by 70–80% by the second trimester.
- The glomerular filtration rate (GFR) increases by 45% by 8 weeks' gestation.
- Creatinine, urea, and uric acid clearance is increased.
- Glycosuria occurs as a result of the increased GFR and is not usually related to increased blood glucose.

- The ureters relax under the influence of progesterone and become dilated. Compression of the ureters against the pelvic brim can lead to urinary stasis, bacteriuria, and infection of the urinary tract.
- As the fetal head engages at the end of pregnancy, the bladder may become displaced upwards.

## The gastrointestinal system

- Nausea is experienced by 70% of pregnant women, beginning at around 4–6 weeks and continuing until 12–14 weeks.
- Most women notice an increased appetite and an increased thirst in pregnancy.
- Reflux of acid into the oesophagus, resulting in heartburn, is common.
- Transit of food through the intestines is much slower and there is increased absorption of water from the colon, leading to an increased tendency to constipation.

## Skeletal changes

- Pelvic ligaments relax under the influence of relaxin and oestrogen, with the maximum effect in the last weeks of pregnancy.
- This allows the pelvis to increase its capacity to accommodate the presenting part during the latter stage of pregnancy and during labour.
- The symphysis pubis widens and the sacro-coccygeal joint loosens, allowing the coccyx to be displaced.
- Whilst these changes facilitate vaginal delivery, they are likely to be the cause of backache and ligament pain.

## Skin changes

- Increased pigmentation of the areola, abdominal midline, perineum, and axillae due to a rise in pituitary melanocyte-stimulating hormone (MSH).
- The 'mask of pregnancy', or chloasma, a deeper colouring of the face, develops in 50–70% of women, is more common in dark-haired women, and is exacerbated by sun exposure.
- Striae gravidarum, commonly called stretch marks, occur as the collagen layer of the skin stretches over areas of fat deposition, e.g. breasts, abdomen, and thighs.
- The stretch marks appear as red stripes and change to silvery white lines within 6 months of delivery.
- Scalp, facial, and body hair become thicker. The excess is shed in the postnatal period.

## The breasts

- Breast changes are one of the first signs of pregnancy noticed by the mother. From around 3–4 weeks' gestation, there is increased blood flow and tenderness; veins become more prominent, and the breasts feel warm.
- Under the influence of oestrogen, fat is deposited in the breasts, increasing their size. The lactiferous tubules and ducts enlarge.
- The pigmented area around the nipple darkens.
- Progesterone causes growth of the lobules and alveoli and develops the secretory ability of these structures, ready for lactation.

- Prolactin stimulates the production of colostrum from the second trimester onwards and, after delivery, is responsible for the initiation of milk production.

## The endocrine system

All the endocrine organs are influenced by secretion of placental hormones during pregnancy.

- *Pituitary hormones*: prolactin, adrenocorticotropic hormone (ACTH), thyroid hormone, and MSH increase. Follicle-stimulating hormone (FSH) and luteinizing hormone (LH) are inhibited. Oxytocin is released throughout pregnancy and increases at term, stimulating uterine contractions.
- *Thyroid hormones*: total thyroxine levels rise sharply from the second month of pregnancy. The basal metabolic rate is increased.
- *Adrenal hormones*: cortisol levels increase, leading to insulin resistance and a corresponding rise in blood glucose, particularly after meals. This makes more glucose available for the fetus.
- *Pancreas*: due to increasing insulin resistance, the β cells are stimulated to increase insulin production by up to four times during pregnancy. In women with borderline pancreatic function, this may result in the development of gestational diabetes, affecting 3–12% of pregnant women.

## Further reading

McNabb M (2011). Maternal and fetal responses to pregnancy. In: Macdonald S, Magill-Cuerden J, eds. *Mayes' Midwifery: A Textbook for Midwives*, 14th edn. Edinburgh: Baillière Tindall, pp. 397–410.

## Blood values in pregnancy

# Blood values in pregnancy

Table 4.1 summarizes the main components of blood and shows the values prior to pregnancy and the changes as a result of the maternal adaptation to pregnancy.

- The main feature is physiological anaemia due to increased plasma volume despite a rise in the red cell mass.
- Decreasing plasma protein concentrations lead to lower osmotic pressure, contributing to oedema seen in the lower limbs during pregnancy. Moderate oedema, when not associated with disease, is an indicator of a favourable pregnancy outcome.

**Table 4.1** The main components of blood

| Component | Non-pregnant | Change in pregnancy |
|---|---|---|
| Plasma volume | 2600mL | 3850mL at 40 weeks |
| Red cell mass | 1400mL | 1650mL at 40 weeks |
| Total blood volume | 4000mL | 5500mL at 40 weeks |
| Haematocrit (PCV) | 35% | 30% at 40 weeks |
| Haemoglobin (Hb) | 125–139g/L | 105–140g/dL at 40 weeks |
| Protein | 65–85g/L | 55–75g/L at 20 weeks |
| Albumin | 35–48g/L | 25–38g/L at 20 weeks |
| Fibrinogen | 15–36g/L | 25–46g/L at 20 weeks |
| Platelets | $150–400 \times 10^3+/mm^3$ | Slight decrease |
| Clotting time | 12min | 8min |
| White cell count | $9 \times 10^9/L$ | $10–15 \times 10^9/L$ |
| Red cell count | $4.7 \times 10^{12}/L$ | $3.8 \times 10^{12}/L$ at 30 weeks |

# The booking interview

The booking interview is a holistic assessment of the woman's social, health, educational, and psychological needs and identifies those needing additional care. The purpose of the interview is to obtain a history and exchange information so that future care during pregnancy and birth can be planned. Both verbal and written information is given to enable parents to make informed decisions about screening tests.

The following is a guide to the information given and obtained and the investigations that can be performed during this appointment. All the information gained and given should be carefully recorded. As the interview proceeds, it will be possible to establish a rapport and judge when it is appropriate to ask some of the more sensitive questions.

Refer to the National Institute for Health and Care Excellence (NICE) antenatal care guidelines for conducting the booking interview.

## Social considerations

- Confirm the woman's name, age, and other relevant biographical details.
- Is she in a stable supportive relationship?
- What is her (and/or her partner's) occupation?
- Sensitive enquiry about whether she has experienced domestic abuse and if she is still in that relationship.

## Emotional and psychological considerations

- Is the pregnancy planned?
- Is she happy to be pregnant?
- Has she any history of mental health problems?
- Has she any concerns about her health or her pregnancy?

## Health considerations

- Ask about present health and the current pregnancy. Are there any problems?
- Ask about previous obstetric history, the number of pregnancies and births (gravida and parity), and whether these were normal.
- Are her previous children healthy?
- Ask about menstrual history, and calculate the EDD.
- Ask about previous medical and family history such as twins, diabetes, epilepsy, hypertension, mental health issues, previous operations, and blood transfusions.
- Verify the blood group and rhesus (Rh) status.
- Measure the BMI and BP, and test the urine for proteinuria.

## Educational considerations

Information and discussion to obtain consent for the following:
- Offer screening for anaemia, red cell antibodies, hepatitis B, HIV, rubella antibodies, and syphilis
- Offer screening for asymptomatic bacteriuria
- Offer screening for Down's syndrome
- Offer an early ultrasound scan for gestational age assessment.

## Further reading

National Institute for Health and Care Excellence (2008). *Antenatal care for uncomplicated pregnancies. Appendix D: antenatal appointments (schedule and content).* NICE guidelines CG62. Available at: ℛ www.nice.org.uk/guidance/cg62/chapter/appendix-d-antenatal-appointments-schedule-and-content.

# Taking a sexual history

- Unprotected sexual intercourse resulting in pregnancy may also put a woman at risk of contracting an STI.
- Sensitive discussion about her past and current sexual health will determine the need for STI testing.
- It is important to raise the issue of sexual health and STIs early in pregnancy to initiate diagnostic testing, appropriate referral to the sexual health service, and sexual health promotion, if applicable.
- The rates of STIs in the UK have risen sharply in the past decade. The highest rates are found in women, gay men, teenagers, young adults, and black and ethnic minority groups.[1]
- Whilst a programme of chlamydia screening in the 16- to 24-year age group has been instituted in the UK, this common STI is by no means limited to this age group and it is good practice to offer every pregnant woman urine-based screening, as a prevention for her ongoing, long-term sexual health and to prevent vertical transmission to her baby during vaginal birth.
- Unrecognized/untreated STIs may be vertically transmitted to the baby, following rupture of the membranes and vaginal birth. (➔ See Chapter 3 for more specific discussion on individual infections.)

## The discussion should include

- Length of current relationship.
- Number of sexual partners in the past 12 months.

## Symptoms

- Change in vaginal discharge.
- Vulval/vaginal soreness or irritation.
- Intermenstrual bleeding.
- Post-coital bleeding.
- Pain during sex (dyspareunia).
- Abdominal pain.
- Contact of STI.
- Past history of STI.
- Contraception method(s).
- Condom use.
- Is she an IV drug user past or present?
- Has she had sex with an IV drug user?
- Has she been paid for sex?
- Is her partner bisexual?
- Has any partner been of non-UK origin, in this country or abroad?

## Investigations

Investigations may include the following.

*Chlamydia*

- Endocervical swab.
- Self-taken swab.
- Urine test (first catch).

*Gonorrhoea*
- Endocervical swab, high vaginal swab: candidiasis ('thrush'), *Trichomonas vaginalis*, bacterial vaginosis.
- Viral culture swab: herpes, HPV.

*Blood testing*
- Syphilis.
- HIV.
- Hepatitis A.
- Hepatitis B.
- Hepatitis C.

*Other*
- Cervical screening:
  - Has the woman been called for screening at all? This will depend on the country in which she resides and the age at which the screening programme commences
  - If appropriate, has she been screened at all and when was her last test?
  - Has she ever been asked to attend for repeat testing within the normal recall time and has she ever had an abnormal result?
- Has she had a colposcopy examination, and, if so, what was the outcome?

## Reference

1 Public Health England (2014). HIV and STIs. In: Public Health England. *Health Protection Report: latest infection reports*. Available at: ℘ www.gov.uk/government/collections/health-protection-report-latest-infection-reports#hiv-and-sti.

# Principles of antenatal screening

As science and technology advance, we are able to elicit more information about pregnancy, the mother, and the fetus than ever before. The scrutiny with which we examine every aspect of pregnancy has never been more detailed. It is very likely that further advances in these techniques will expose women to increasingly difficult choices and dilemmas. The midwife will need to be well prepared and informed to guide her clients through this process.

A range of activities come under the banner of 'antenatal screening'. Certain activities are a fundamental part of midwifery practice, e.g. measuring the fundal height, listening to the fetal heart, and the routine blood tests, including FBC, group and Rh factor, and maternal serum for rubella antibodies. We may classify these as low intervention, unlikely to cause any ethical concern. Other types of screening, such as those undertaken to detect a fetal abnormality, can lead to much moral difficulty.

## Aims of screening

The whole pregnant population is screened because, although collectively this population has a low risk of abnormality, screening aims to identify those at higher risk, so that more specific diagnostic tests can be applied.

## Benefits of screening and diagnosis

- Reduce fetal abnormality.
- Reduce genetic reoccurrence.
- Reduce the incidence of mental handicap.
- Reduce the burden on family and society.
- Increase resources for those disabled individuals who are not detected before birth.

## Adverse effects of screening and diagnosis

- Anxiety provoked by screening procedures.
- Psychological sequelae for parents.
- Risks of diagnostic tests to the woman and fetus.
- Risks to the woman of a late termination of pregnancy.
- Risk of aborting a normal fetus.
- Long-term effects on society's attitude to the disabled.

## Implications

- Inadequate counselling at the time of the test could mean that clients are not prepared for adverse outcomes, such as being recalled with a high-risk result or giving birth to an affected child after having a low-risk result from the screening test.[2]
- No matter how good a test is technically, screening uninformed, unsupported clients by unprepared staff is a recipe for, at best, confusion and, at worst, great distress. This is avoidable.[3]

## Consent and counselling

- Screening tests other than those performed in normal midwifery care are likely to reveal information for which parents need to be prepared and to result in decisions being made about the future of the pregnancy.
- If, on consideration, parents decide not to take up the offer of tests, then this should be respected.
- In practice, it is difficult to ensure that clients are aware of all the ramifications of tests, especially when so many are on offer.
- Where informed consent has not been obtained and a positive result to a screening test is returned, the practitioner is vulnerable to litigation.
- If a client's language barrier or intellect makes understanding difficult, it may not be professionally acceptable to go ahead with tests.
- The use of interpreters is problematic, but there is usually a protocol, and advice can be sought from a specialist midwife.
- If the client is not mentally competent, then she cannot effectively give consent as an autonomous person. The principle of beneficence could be invoked to provide care that is in the best interests of the client. Paternalism may be justified in any number of circumstances, notwithstanding the limited mental capacity of the client.

## References

2  Public Health England (2015). *NHS Screening Programmes: fetal anomaly*. Available at: ℘ www.gov.uk/government/uploads/system/uploads/attachment_data/file/456654/FASP_programme_handbook_August_2015.pdf.
3  Public Health England (2013, updated 2015). *Fetal anomaly screening: providing services*. Available at: ℘ www.gov.uk/government/collections/fetal-anomaly-screening-providing-services.

# Screening for risk in pregnancy

Risk screening during pregnancy aims to identify those women at risk, so that a suitable pattern of care can be planned for the pregnancy with the appropriate professional.

For women deemed to be healthy and at low risk, midwife or midwife/GP care, based in the community, is a suitable alternative to consultant- or hospital-based care programmes.

Assessment of risk should be ongoing, so that deviations from the normal or the development of complications can be identified at any stage of pregnancy and referral to appropriate care arranged. This assessment starts at the booking interview or initial appointment. For many women this takes place in their own home and is conducted by the community midwife.

Women with any of the following need care over and above that recommended for low-risk, healthy women by the NICE guidelines:[4]
- Cardiac disease, including hypertension
- Renal disease
- Endocrine disorder or diabetes requiring insulin
- Psychiatric disorder (on medication)
- Haematological disorder (including thromboembolic disease)
- Epilepsy requiring anticonvulsant medication
- Malignant disease
- Severe asthma
- Drug misuse (heroin, cocaine, ecstasy)
- HIV or hepatitis B
- Autoimmune disorders
- Obesity—BMI 30kg/m$^2$ or above (or underweight—BMI <18kg/m$^2$)
- Women at higher risk, e.g. age >40 or <14 years
- Women who are particularly vulnerable or who lack social support.

Women who have experienced any of the following in previous pregnancies are at higher risk:
- Recurrent miscarriage (three or more)
- Preterm birth
- Severe pre-eclampsia, eclampsia, or HELLP (haemolysis, elevated liver enzymes, and low platelet count) syndrome
- Rh isoimmunization or other significant blood group antibodies
- Uterine surgery—Caesarean section, myomectomy, or cone biopsy
- Ante- or post-partum haemorrhage on two occasions
- Puerperal psychosis
- Grand multiparity (>6)
- A stillbirth or neonatal death
- A small-for-gestational-age (SGA) infant (<5th centile)
- A large-for-gestational age infant (>95th centile)
- A baby weighing <2.5kg or >4.5kg
- A baby with a congenital anomaly (structural or chromosomal).

## Reference

4 National Institute for Health and Care Excellence (2008). *Antenatal care for uncomplicated pregnancies*. NICE guidelines CG62. Available at: ℘ www.nice.org.uk/guidance/cg62.

# The full blood count

- An FBC obtained in the first trimester acts as a baseline against which all other measurements can be compared.
- An FBC should be repeated at 28 weeks' gestation to allow for correction of anaemia prior to term.
- As pregnancy progresses, plasma volume expansion is greater than the corresponding rise in the red cell count; this leads to a haemodilution effect and the haematocrit falls, along with the Hb level. This is called physiological anaemia.
- Apparent anaemia can be a sign of an excellent adaptation to pregnancy. The effect is greatest at around 30–32 weeks' gestation.
- Lower mean Hb concentrations are associated with higher mean birthweights, and higher mean Hb concentrations are associated with an increase in preterm delivery and low-birthweight babies.
- Hb levels outside the normal UK range for pregnancy should be investigated, and iron supplementation considered if indicated.
- The levels are 110g/L at first contact and 105g/L at 28 weeks' gestation.
- In order to correctly assess for anaemia, the impact of gestational age on plasma volume should be considered. Use of Hb level as a sole indicator of anaemia is not recommended.
- Serum ferritin is the most sensitive single screening test to detect adequate iron stores. Using a cut-off point of 30 micrograms/L a sensitivity of 90% has been reported.[5]

## Reference

5 National Institute for Health and Care Excellence (2008). *Antenatal care for uncomplicated pregnancies*. NICE guidelines CG62. Available at: ℵ www.nice.org.uk/guidance/cg62.

# ABO blood group and rhesus factor: anti-D prophylaxis for the Rh-negative mother

At the initial appointment, as well as obtaining a full medical and obstetric history from the woman, venous blood is obtained so that the blood group, the Rh factor, and the presence of red cell antibodies can be determined. This test will identify women who are Rh-negative and who therefore require further antibody testing during pregnancy.

Recording the blood group is necessary for future reference if the mother needs a blood transfusion around the time of birth. Group O is the most common blood type in the UK; 85% of individuals will also have the Rh factor and will therefore be Rh-positive.

## What is the Rh factor?

- The Rh factor is a complex protein antigen carried on the surface of the red blood cell (RBC). It is inherited from three pairs of genes called *cde/CDE*. It is the pair named D that makes an individual Rh-positive and is likely to cause Rh isoimmunization.
- Rh-negative women who carry an RhD-positive fetus may produce antibodies to the fetal RhD antigens after a fetomaternal haemorrhage. These antibodies may cross the placenta in future pregnancies, causing haemolytic disease of the newborn (HDN) if the fetus is RhD-positive.
- HDN can range in severity from stillbirth, severe disabilities, or death to anaemia and jaundice in the neonate. To prevent this from occurring, Rh-negative women who have experienced a suspected or known sensitizing event during pregnancy are given an IM injection of anti-D immunoglobulin (Ig) to prevent antibody production.
- The anti-D Ig works by coating the fetal red cells that have escaped into the mother's circulation so that they cannot be recognized by her immune system. This prevents maternal antibody formation and thus protects the RhD-positive fetus of any subsequent pregnancy.

## What is a sensitizing event?

Very occasionally Rh-negative women may produce antibodies as a result of a mismatched blood transfusion, but fetal red cells from the RhD-positive fetus can cross the placenta and enter the woman's circulation at any time during the pregnancy, particularly if events cause bleeding from the placental site.

▶▶ The most important cause of RhD immunization is during pregnancy where there has been no overt sensitizing event. Sensitizing events include:
- Threatened abortion and abortion after 12 weeks' gestation
- Chorion villus sampling
- Threatened abortion, spontaneous abortion, termination of pregnancy where bleeding is repeated, heavy, or associated with abdominal pain
- Amniocentesis
- Antepartum haemorrhage (APH)
- Abdominal trauma

- Hypertension
- Eclampsia
- Traumatic delivery, including Caesarean section
- Placental separation during the third stage of labour
- Manual removal of the placenta.

In the Rh-negative woman, these events should be followed by prophy-lactic administration of anti-D Ig. The British Committee for Standards in Haematology (2014) has reviewed the advice that recommends that all Rh-negative women receive prophylactic anti-D.[6]

- The treatment regimen may vary, according to local costs, for instance being able to offer a one-visit option, staff costs of administration, and the cost of the Ig.
- The options are:
  - 250IU below 12 weeks, and 500IU at 28 and 34 weeks' gestation;
  - 1000–1650IU at 28 and 34 weeks' gestation
  - a single dose of 1500IU at 28–30 weeks, as well as cover for sensitizing events.
- If a sensitizing event is suspected, Kleihauer's test (on maternal venous blood) estimates the amount of fetal red cells in the maternal circulation, and a measured dose of anti-D can be administered. A 500IU dose is enough to deal with an 8mL transplacental transfusion of fetal blood. Prior to 20 weeks' gestation, it is usual to give 250IU as a prophylactic dose.
- Blood samples are taken within 1h of delivery from the Rh-negative mother to test for maternal antibodies and fetal cells (Kleihauer's).
- Also from the neonate, to discover its blood group and Rh factor. If the neonate is Rh-negative, then the mother requires no further anti-D Ig.
- In the event of an intrauterine death where no sample can be obtained from the baby, an appropriate dose of prophylactic anti-D Ig should be administered to D-negative, previously non-sensitized women within 72h of the *diagnosis of the intrauterine death*, irrespective of the time of subsequent delivery (Grade 1C).
- Where intraoperative cell salvage (ICS) is used during a Caesarean section in D-negative, previously non-sensitized women and where the cord blood group is confirmed as D-positive (or unknown), a minimum dose of 1500IU anti-D Ig should be administered following the reinfusion of salvaged red cells, and a maternal sample should be taken for estimation of feto–maternal haemorrhage (FMH) 30–45min after reinfusion in case more anti-D Ig is indicated. It is important that clinicians inform the transfusion laboratory if ICS has been used to ensure that the correct dose of anti-D Ig is issued (Grade 2C).
- It is the midwife's responsibility to carry out tests during pregnancy to identify women who require anti-D prophylaxis. A full explanation should be given to the woman and her consent obtained for any tests or administration of anti-D Ig.

## Reference

6 Qureshi H, Massey E, Kirwan D, et al.; British Society for Haematology (2014). BSCH guideline for the use of anti-D immunoglobulin for the prevention of haemolytic disease of the fetus and newborn. *Transfus Med* 24: 8–20.

# Screening for Down's syndrome risk

The incidence of Down's syndrome is approximately 1:600 to 1:700 across the age range of the childbearing population. There are variations in incidence according to maternal age:

- At 18 years of age, the incidence is 1:2300
- At 35 years, it is 1:200 to 350
- At 40 years, it is 1:100
- At 45 years, it is 1:45.

Taking age as the only risk factor would mean that <30% of affected fetuses would be detected by diagnostic testing, as it would not be appropriate to offer amniocentesis to all women.

Down's risk screening was developed in the 1980s to enable all pregnant women to be given an estimate of the individual risk if they choose to be screened. The risk is calculated by examining a combination of the following factors:

- Maternal age
- Gestational age in completed weeks
- Maternal body weight
- Serum screening.

## Maternal serum screening

- This enables examination of a combination of hormones and proteins present in the maternal bloodstream during early pregnancy.
- Levels vary according to the fetal gestational age.
- Abnormally low or high levels are linked to genetic, chromosomal, and structural abnormalities of the fetus.
- High levels of $\alpha$-fetoprotein (AFP) are associated with NTDs, and low levels with Down's syndrome.
- NTDs can be confirmed by ultrasound scan and also amniocentesis.

*Recommended screening: aims*

- Screening for Down's syndrome should be performed by the end of the first trimester (13 weeks 6 days), but provision should be made to allow later screening (which could be as late as 20 weeks 0 days) for women booking later in pregnancy.
- The 'combined test' (nuchal translucency, $\beta$-hCG, pregnancy-associated plasma protein-A) should be offered to screen for Down's syndrome between 11 weeks 0 days and 13 weeks 6 days.
- For women who book later in pregnancy the most clinically and cost-effective serum screening test (triple or quadruple test) should be offered between 15 weeks 0 days and 20 weeks 0 days.
- When it is not possible to measure nuchal translucency, owing to fetal position or high BMI, women should be offered serum screening (triple or quadruple test) between 15 weeks 0 days and 20 weeks 0 days.

*Sensitivity*

- The sensitivity of the test is a measurement of how many affected fetuses are detected. This means that around 5% of women having the test will be recalled for further investigation.
- The false-positive rate is between 2.6% and 5%. This percentage of women will be carrying a normal baby despite a high-risk screening result. About 60 women will be recalled for every affected baby diagnosed.
- The false-negative rate is 20%. This percentage of women will be carrying an affected baby despite a low-risk screening result.

*Results and consequences of screening*

- Offer diagnostic testing if a woman's screening result is 1:10 to 1:210.
- If the result is 1:210+, then advise the woman that her screening result is low risk.
- Provide information about what the test involves, how the risk is calculated, and what is meant by a risk factor.
- There needs to be an understanding that low risk is not 'no risk' and that any woman could be the 'one' of the 1:800.
- Explain the nature of the diagnostic test and the risk of miscarriage from this test (1%).
- Discuss options following a diagnosis of Down's syndrome and provide non-directive support to the decision to choose termination or continuation of the pregnancy.

## Further reading

National Institute for Health and Care Excellence (2008). *Antenatal care for uncomplicated pregnancies.* NICE guidelines CG62. Available at: ℘ www.nice.org.uk/guidance/cg62.

# Sickle-cell anaemia

Haemoglobin is a complex molecule, with the ability to absorb oxygen easily and reversibly. The molecule is composed of iron and protein. The protein structure is inherited and is the part affected in haemoglobinopathies, being either abnormal or partly missing.

A normal RBC in an adult is filled with adult Hb. Everyone inherits their Hb type from their parents, half of the responsible gene copies from each, and the usual type is HbAA.

## Sickle-cell trait

- Sickle Hb (abbreviated HbS) has an abnormality of the protein part of the molecule.
- An individual inheriting HbS from one parent and HbA from the other will have Hb type HbSA.
- This is known as the sickle-cell trait.
- The RBCs of such individuals will function normally, and they will have few, if any, symptoms.
- However, these individuals have a 50% chance of passing this type of Hb on to their children.
- This condition confers immunity from the malaria parasite, which explains the prevalence of the condition in areas where malaria infection is endemic.
- Due to population movement, individuals can inherit this type of Hb, even if their ancestry is from malaria-free areas.

## Sickle-cell anaemia

- In this case, the individual inherits HbS from both parents, so the Hb type is HbSS.
- RBCs containing only HbSS react to hypoxia, acidosis, or dehydration by changing shape, from the usual biconcave disc to a crescent or sickle shape.
- These RBCs are more fragile and easily damaged and will clump together, blocking capillaries.
- Painful crises are provoked by the blockage of small blood vessels.
- The overall effect is that the RBCs are haemolysed, rapidly causing chronic haemolytic anaemia.

### Effects on childbearing

Increased incidence of:
- Subfertility
- Spontaneous miscarriage
- APH
- Antenatal hospitalization
- Impaired placental function
- PIH
- Pulmonary and renal problems
- Phlebitis and thromboembolic events
- Fetal growth restriction
- Premature labour

- Caesarean birth
- Infection
- Perinatal mortality.

Women with this type of anaemia need to be well hydrated during labour and need careful monitoring to avoid hypoxia should an anaesthetic be required.

*Screening*

It is estimated that there are 12 000–15 000 affected individuals and over 300 infants born with sickle-cell disease (SCD) in the UK each year who are diagnosed as part of the neonatal screening programme. There are approximately 100–200 pregnancies in women with SCD per year in the UK.

- Information about screening for SCDs and thalassaemias, including carrier status and the implications of these, should be given to pregnant women at the first contact with a health-care professional.
- Screening for SCDs and thalassaemias should be offered to all women as early as possible in pregnancy (ideally by 10 weeks). The type of screening depends upon the prevalence and can be carried out in either primary or secondary care.
- If the woman has not been seen preconceptually, she should be offered partner testing. If the partner is a carrier, appropriate counselling should be offered as early as possible in pregnancy—ideally by 10 weeks of gestation—to allow the option of first-trimester diagnosis and termination if that is the woman's choice.

**Further reading**

Royal College of Obstetricians and Gynaecologists (2011). *Sickle cell disease in pregnancy, management of (Green-top guideline No. 61).* Available at: ℝ www.rcog.org.uk/en/guidelines-research-services/guidelines/gtg61/.

# Thalassaemia

In this recessively inherited condition part of the Hb protein is missing. The protein is made from structures called α and β chains. As several genes are responsible for the structure of these chains, it is possible to have varying degrees of the condition.

## β-thalassaemia minor

The individual inherits one normal gene from one parent and one affected gene from the other parent. This is a carrier state and has little effect on health, other than mild anaemia. Affected individuals can pass on the defective gene to their children.

## β-thalassaemia major

The individual inherits defective genes from both parents and can make no, or very few, β chains, so does not produce sufficient Hb. This results in severe anaemia, requiring regular blood transfusions and therapy to remove excess iron from the blood.

## α-thalassaemia

People with normal Hb carry four α globin genes, two from each parent. α-thalassaemia results from the deletion of one or more of these genes. Table 4.2 shows the result of deletions of one or more of the genes and the effect on the type of Hb produced.

## Screening for thalassaemia

- As with sickle-cell anaemia, antenatal screening should be offered to all pregnant women, as recommended.[7]
- A routine FBC will identify women with hypochromic, microcytic anaemia. Hb electrophoresis will then identify the underlying haemoglobinopathy.
- Knowing the carrier state of each parent allows counselling about the risks to the fetus of being a carrier or having the disease.
- Haemoglobinopathy screening is carried out on newborns as part of the neonatal blood spot test.

Table 4.2 Effect of gene deletions

| Gene deletions | Diagnosis | Adult blood |
|---|---|---|
| (aa/−a) | α² thalassaemia | Normal |
| (aa/− −) or (a−/a−) | α¹ thalassaemia | Small RBCs |
| (−a/− −) | Hb H disease | Moderate anaemia |
| (− −/− −) | Hydrops fetalis | Not compatible with life |

## Impact of maternal thalassaemia major on pregnancy

- Depends on the degree of chronic anaemia and the oxygen deprivation that results from this.
- If the woman cannot adequately meet her own oxygen needs, the fetus becomes progressively hypoxic.
- Fetal survival may be threatened with spontaneous abortion, intrauterine growth restriction (IUGR), preterm birth, or intrauterine death.
- Women who are carriers ($\alpha$- and $\beta$-thalassaemia trait) may be only mildly anaemic and require only supportive care.

## Management of thalassaemia major during pregnancy

- Specialist medical and obstetric supervision is required.
- Blood transfusion therapy continues.
- Use of iron chelation therapy is not without risk and needs to be individualized. Desferrioxamine should be avoided in the first trimester, owing to a lack of safety data. It has been used safely after 20 weeks of gestation at low doses.[7]
- Iron deposition in the pancreas and thyroid increases the risk of the woman developing diabetes, so a glucose tolerance test would be indicated.
- Blood transfusion, whilst vital, increases the risk of cardiac failure, which, in turn, increases the risk of maternal mortality by as much as 50%.

Women who are asymptomatic before pregnancy may find the added stresses of pregnancy can cause deterioration of their health status. The more severe the syndrome, the more significant the consequences for the woman and fetus.

## Reference

7 Royal College of Obstetricians and Gynaecologists (2014). *Management of beta thalassaemia in pregnancy (Green-top guideline No. 66)*. Available at: ℐ www.rcog.org.uk/globalassets/documents/guidelines/gtg_66_thalassaemia.pdf.

## Antenatal examination

The purpose of the antenatal examination depends on the length of gestation at which it takes place.

NICE (2008) has published guidelines for the routine care of women who are experiencing a healthy, low-risk pregnancy.[8] The recommended number of scheduled appointments is determined by parity and the function of the appointment. For the primigravida with an uncomplicated pregnancy, ten visits are adequate, and, for the parous woman with an uncomplicated pregnancy, seven visits should be adequate.

Throughout the antenatal period, be alert to the signs and symptoms of conditions that affect the health of the mother and fetus such as preeclampsia, diabetes, and domestic abuse.

- After the first appointment or booking visit, use the next visit to review, discuss, and document the results of all the screening tests undertaken earlier and to identify women who need additional care.
- Arrange further investigations for a woman with a Hb level of <110g/L, and offer iron supplementation.
- At each visit, measure the BP and test the urine for protein.
- At each visit, be prepared to ask questions; give information and discuss issues about the woman's physical and emotional/psychological well-being; and use the available time to provide education, supported by antenatal classes and written information.
- After 20 weeks, measure and plot the symphysis–fundal height (SFH) to detect small- or large-for-dates pregnancies.
- If requested by the mother, auscultate the fetal heart sounds by handheld ultrasound.
- Offer anti-D prophylaxis to Rh-negative women at 28 and 34 weeks' gestation.
- Offer a second screening for anaemia and atypical red cell antibodies at 28 weeks' gestation. Investigate a Hb level of <105g/L and provide iron supplementation if necessary.
- At 36–37 weeks' gestation, confirm the lie and presentation of the fetus, and offer external cephalic version for women whose babies are in the breech position.
- If an earlier report showed the placenta extending over the internal cervical os, a further scan should be arranged and reviewed at 36 weeks.
- A further appointment should be arranged for women who have not given birth by 41 weeks, to offer a membrane sweep and induction of labour if this is unsuccessful.

### Reference

8 National Institute for Health and Care Excellence (2008). *Antenatal care for uncomplicated pregnancies.* NICE guidelines CG62. Available at: 🔗 www.nice.org.uk/guidance/cg62.

## Abdominal examination

### Inspection

### Palpation

# Abdominal examination

An abdominal examination can be carried out at any stage of pregnancy and is used to determine the progress of pregnancy or labour and fetal well-being.

The examination is in three parts: inspection, palpation, and auscultation.

Ask for the woman's consent before the examination. Make her comfortable on the examination couch, lying supine with her head supported by one pillow. Her arms should be relaxed by her sides. Expose her abdomen, but use a sheet or towel to cover her pelvic area and legs, preserving her privacy and dignity.

## Inspection

- Inspect the abdomen for size and shape. In the primigravida, the shape is oval, due to abdominal muscle tone. In the parous client, the shape may be more rounded.
- There may be a saucer-shaped depression below the umbilicus if the fetus is presenting in an occipito-posterior position.
- A heart-shaped uterus may indicate a transverse lie.
- The umbilicus may protrude, and the linea nigra, which is the pigmented midline of the rectus sheath, may be apparent.
- Other abdominal scars may be apparent, as will striae gravidarum or stretch marks, which are pink at first, turning to silvery white as they age.
- Size should indicate the stage of pregnancy, which will be confirmed by measuring the SFH.
- Observe for fetal movements—this confirms a live fetus.

## Palpation

- Serial SFH measurements should be recorded at each antenatal appointment from 24 weeks' gestation.[9]
- Measure using a non-elastic tape measure.[10]
- To enable an accurate identification of the uterine fundus, use both hands to locate the fundus.[10]
- Use the tape measure with the centimetres on the underside to reduce bias, and measure from the top of the fundus to the top of the symphysis pubis, keeping the tape in contact with the skin.[10]

The measurement should be plotted on a customized chart to improve prediction of an SGA infant.[9]

- The lie of the fetus is normally longitudinal, with the long axis of the fetus lying along the long axis of the mother.
- The presenting part is normally the fetal head. Breech presentation occurs in approximately 3% of pregnancies at term.
- Determine the position of the fetus:
  - The position of the occiput can be found by locating the fetal back, which feels smooth and firm and will lie anteriorly on the left or right side of the uterus if the occiput is anterior
  - In posterior position, the back may be felt in the left or right flank, or it may not be palpable. If fetal limbs are felt on both sides of the midline, it is likely that the fetus is lying in an occipito-posterior position.

- Establish the relationship of the presenting part to the pelvic brim. The fetal head is engaged in the pelvis when the widest diameter of the fetal head has entered the pelvic brim.

## Auscultation

- Hearing the fetal heart will confirm that the fetus is alive, but it does not have any proven predictive value. Routine listening is not recommended, but if the mother requests it, auscultation may provide reassurance.
- Explain the findings of the examination to the mother and record them in her notes.

## References

9  Royal College of Obstetricians and Gynaecologists (2014). *The investigation and management of the small-for-gestational-age fetus (Green–top guideline No. 31)*. Available at: ℳ www.rcog.org.uk/globalassets/documents/guidelines/gtg_31.pdf.
10 Perinatal Institute. *Fetal growth: fundal height measurements*. Available at: ℳ www.perinatal.org.uk/fetalgrowth/FundalHeight.aspx.

## Further reading

National Institute for Health and Care Excellence (2008). *Antenatal care for uncomplicated pregnancies*. NICE guidelines CG62. Available at: ℳ www.nice.org.uk/guidance/cg62.

# Monitoring fetal growth and well-being

As part of the overall antenatal assessment, the midwife is responsible for monitoring the growth and well-being of the fetus. Maternal well-being is the best indicator of fetal well-being, so evaluate the mother closely, looking for any problems that are likely to affect the fetus, e.g. hypertension, infection, diabetes, and environmental factors such as smoking, substance misuse, and dietary inadequacies.[11]

- Ask about fetal patterns of movement and activity. All fetuses are active at some stage during a 24h period. The standard is to ask whether there are ten movements in a 12h period. Ask about strength of movements. This may change towards the end of pregnancy, as the fetus has less room to move about. Determine whether the mother is aware of all of the fetal activity.
- Most mothers tend to know their baby's activity pattern well. Ask them to report any concerns, such as reduced activity, especially after 40 weeks' gestation.
- If, during an antenatal visit, a mother reports diminished or absent movements, listen to the fetal heart with a Pinard stethoscope or an ultrasound transducer, and reassure the mother. (*Intrauterine death is an uncommon, but possible, occurrence. If you do not hear the fetal heart, explain this in an honest and sensitive way and make arrangements to confirm the absence of the heartbeat by ultrasound scan.*)
- If a mother seeks advice over the telephone, you may want to arrange a cardiotocograph (CTG) of the fetal heart. This would be carried out in hospital and a non-reassuring trace referred to the obstetrician.
- Carry out an abdominal examination at prescribed times, according to whether the mother has been assessed as low or high risk. A more accurate assessment of fetal growth can be obtained if the same person examines the mother on each occasion.
- Overall growth of the uterus is estimated and the fundal height measured in centimetres. This should correspond roughly to the number of weeks' gestation, plus or minus 2cm, taking into account maternal height and build.
- Assess the volume of amniotic fluid surrounding the fetus and note increased or diminished amounts. Each pregnancy is assessed on its individual merits and over- or underproduction of amniotic fluid may be pathological or entirely innocent. If you are concerned, refer the woman to an obstetrician.
- When IUGR or large-for-gestational-age fetuses are suspected, decide whether to refer for further investigation.
- A large-for-date uterus may be due to a multiple pregnancy. The advent of routine dating scans has meant that multiple pregnancy is now diagnosed early, unless there has been an operator error or the woman has declined a scan.
- An ultrasound scan may be arranged, but take care not to make the mother overanxious. These conditions are often overdiagnosed, leading to much unnecessary worry for mothers.

- A scan to measure the head-to-abdomen ratio, performed on >1 occasion, will distinguish between symmetrical and asymmetrical growth restriction.
- Scans estimating fetal weight are not reliable enough to predict an accurate birthweight, but they do provide a reasonable estimate to within 500g on either side of a given figure.

## Reference

11 National Institute for Health and Care Excellence (2008). *Antenatal care for uncomplicated pregnancies*. NICE guidelines CG62. Available at: ℬ www.nice.org.uk/guidance/cg62.

# Health advice in pregnancy

# Preconception care

The period before conception is increasingly regarded as important for the health of pregnant women and future generations. Successive reports from the Centre for Maternal and Child Enquiries[1,2] conclude that lack of preconception care is a contributory factor in maternal deaths, whilst evidence from life course epidemiology[3,4] and epigenetics[5] highlights the importance of the intrauterine environment in determining chronic disease risk in childhood and adulthood. Factors, such as maternal diet and nutritional status, which can be modified before conception, have an important influence on the intrauterine environment and fetal development. Consequently, the preconception period is seen as a critical period where intervention can lead to both short-term benefit, by reducing pregnancy complications and adverse birth outcomes, and long-term health gain, as emphasized in the WHO Global Action Plan for the Prevention and Control of Noncommunicable Diseases 2013–2020.[6]

## Fetal programming

Pregnancy is a critical time for healthy fetal development as the fetus relies heavily on maternal stores and nutrient intake for optimal growth. Nutrition and weight management before and during pregnancy are already known to have a profound effect both on the development of the fetus and health outcomes later in life. However, fetal programming (based on Barker's hypothesis)[7] is an emerging concept discovering links between environmental conditions during embryonic and fetal development and the risk of diseases later in life.

The fetal environment is influenced by several factors, including the intake of macro- and micronutrients and toxic compounds by the mother. The genome as such is not changed in the programmed individual, but the causative factors may affect the expression of genes in a way that has lasting effects on the metabolic functions. The critical issue is that fetal programming is even transmitted to the next generations. However, the molecular mechanisms that are involved in this fetal programming are far from understood, and the Centre for Fetal Programming[8] is aiming to unravel the impact of maternal dietary factors on childhood health.

The concept of fetal programming has gained increased credence supported by strong findings from human epidemiologic studies and animal models.[9] Specifically, *in utero* exposures to altered maternal nutrition (excess and deficient), stress (e.g. glucocorticoids), or environmental toxins, among others, may alter organ structure or function. As approximately 50% of all cell divisions for growth occur from conception to birth, it is not surprising that environmental stresses may impact cell number. Although the genotype of programmed offspring does not change, modified gene expression may be a consequence of exposure-mediated epigenetic changes, thus altering the expression of regulatory peptides and organ function.

The word '*programming*' illustrates the idea that during critical periods in early fetal development, there are persisting changes in fetal body structure and function that are caused by environmental stimuli.

This theory links to the concept of '*developmental plasticity*' where our genes are believed to express different ranges of physiological or morphological states, in response to the environmental conditions which were encountered during our fetal development.[9] For example, if the mother has an inadequate diet whilst pregnant, then this signals that living conditions in the long term will be impoverished; consequently the fetus adapts by changing its body size and metabolism to prepare for food shortages after birth. Physiological and metabolic processes in the body subsequently undergo long-term changes as a result of this restricted fetal growth.[10]

Epidemiological observations as well as clinical and experimental studies support the concept of fetal programming as the origin of a number of diseases, including obesity, type 2 diabetes, and allergic diseases. It is also believed that maternal conditions, such as cardiovascular disease and hypertension, during pregnancy can have long-term effects upon the adult health of the fetus. Several exposures during pregnancy have already been indicated to have an impact.[8]

## Asthma and allergic disease
- Environmental: exposure to polychlorinated biphenyl compounds in pregnancy is associated with an increased risk of asthma in the children at age 20 years.
- Diet: peanut, nut, and fish consumption in pregnancy are found to be associated with a lower risk of child asthma and allergic rhinitis; conversely, intake of low-fat yoghurt and artificially sweetened beverages were identified as risk factors.
- Vitamin D: a high maternal vitamin D concentration might be associated with an increased risk of allergic diseases in offspring.[11]

## Metabolic disease
- Maternal exposure to perfluorinated compounds (environmental pollutants) may be associated with an increased propensity for obesity in young adult women.
- Protein intake: high maternal protein intake in pregnancy may increase the risk of overweight children.

## Reproductive outcomes
- Maternal smoking in pregnancy was associated with an earlier age of menarche in their daughters.
- Fetal exposure to perfluorinated compounds resulted in altered reproductive function later in life. This was specifically related to poorer semen quality and reproductive hormone profile measures in young men.

## Epigenetics
As more is understood about the human genetic make-up, a number of genes (alleles) that determine how individuals respond to various exposures have been identified. It is already known that there are differences in the type of gene that individuals have—one person may have type 1 of a particular gene, whilst another person has type 2 or type 3 of that same gene. Scientists have now discovered that these different gene types react in different ways to prenatal exposures and events. For example, it has been

shown that a person with a type 1 gene may deal very well with stress and the child will be of normal birthweight, while the type 2 person will have an excessive amount of cortisol and this infant will be programmed for later anxiety problems.

The fetal environment is influenced by several factors, including the intake of macro- and micronutrients and toxic compounds by the mother. The genome as such is not changed in the programmed individual, but the causative factors may affect the expression of genes in a way that has lasting effects on the metabolic functions. The critical issue is that fetal programming is even transmitted to the next generations. There is thus much current research to explore, examine, and understand the impact of environmental factors working during the fetal period and how these factors may interact with genetic factors and with environmental factors working prior to or after this period in determining the development, the health, and specific diseases appearing during the life course of the individual.

The genotype of the mother has also been shown to be related to the number of alcohol-related physical features that the baby will show. In particular, if the mother has the ADH2-2 allele, which leads to a more rapid clearing out of alcohol from her body, then her infant is not likely to have alcohol-related birth defects.

Studies of this kind will help to determine which women are at high risk for having a baby with later problems.

## Relevance to midwifery care

Many women are motivated to adopt healthier behaviours in the preconception period and yet, despite a high level of pregnancy planning, awareness of preconception health among women and health professionals is low, whilst the individual responsibility for providing preconception care is sometimes unclear.[12] However, as both epidemiologic and epigenetic research findings suggest that focusing on pre-pregnancy intervention by health professionals would not merely benefit the 'worried well' or women with specific medical disorders but could be an effective approach to addressing important health inequalities relating to smoking, alcohol, obesity, and other risky behaviours, it must be a priority in contemporary midwifery care.

## References

1  Lewis G (ed.) (2007). *The Confidential Enquiry into Maternal and Child Health (CEMACH). Saving Mothers' Lives: reviewing maternal deaths to make motherhood safer: 2003–2005. The Seventh Report on Confidential Enquiries into Maternal Deaths in the United Kingdom.* London: CEMACH.

2  Centre for Maternal and Child Enquiries (CMACE) (2011). *Saving Mothers' Lives. Reviewing maternal deaths to make motherhood safer: 2006–2008. The Eighth Report of the Confidential Enquiries into Maternal Deaths in the United Kingdom.* BJOG **118**(Suppl 1): 1–203.

3  Hanson M, Fall C, Robinson S, Baird J, BMA Board of Science (2009). *Early Life Nutrition and Lifelong Health.* London: British Medical Association.

4  Ben-Shlomo Y, Kuh D (2002). A life course approach to chronic disease epidemiology: conceptual models, empirical challenges and interdisciplinary perspectives. *Int J Epidemiol* **31**: 285–93.

5  Gluckman P, Hanson M, Buklijas T, Low F, Beedle A (2009). Epigenetic mechanisms that underpin metabolic and cardiovascular diseases. *Nat Rev Endocrinol* **5**: 401–8.

6  World Health Organization (2013). *Global Action Plan for the Prevention and Control of Noncommunicable Diseases 2013–2020.* Geneva: World Health Organization.

7  Barker DJP (2004). The developmental origins of adult disease. *J Am Coll Nutr* **23**: 588S–95S.

8  Centre for Fetal Programming (2014). *About fetal programming.* Available at: ℜ www.cfp-research.com/About%20CFP/About%20fetal%20programming.aspx.

9  Bateson P (2001). Fetal experience and good adult design. *Int J Epidemiol* 30: 928–34.
10 Jørgensen SW, Brøns C, Bluck L, et al. (2015). Metabolic response to 36 hours of fasting in young men born small vs appropriate for gestational age. *Diabetologia* 58: 178–87.
11 Hansen S, Maslova E, Strom M, et al. (2015). The long-term programming effect of maternal 25-hydroxyvitamin D in pregnancy on allergic airway disease and lung function in offspring after 20 to 25 years of follow-up. *J Allergy Clin Immunol* 136: 169–76.e2.
12 Royal College of Midwives (2012). *Maternal Emotional Wellbeing and Infant Development: A Good Practice Guide for Midwives*. London: Royal College of Midwives.

# Smoking

As smoking is a potentially preventable activity, it is a significant public health issue in pregnancy. There are a number of risks associated with smoking during pregnancy. Although the risks are well known, many women still require specific information about the effects and support to give up or reduce the number of cigarettes smoked. It is estimated that 25% of pregnant women who smoke stop before their first antenatal appointment, and 27% of women report that they are current smokers at the time of the birth of their baby.[13]

- Cigarette smoke contains carbon monoxide (CO) and nicotine. The Hb in RBCs combines with oxygen, but if CO is present, this replaces the oxygen in the cell.
- During gaseous exchange in the placenta, the oxygen levels are reduced whilst the cigarette is being smoked and less oxygen is transferred to the fetus.
- Each time a cigarette is smoked, the fetus can become hypoxic.
- Nicotine acts on the blood vessels, making them narrow. This decreases the blood flow, reducing oxygen and nutrient supply in the body.
- Blood vessels in the placenta will be affected at the same time, reducing oxygen and nutrient supply to the fetus.

## These effects cause damage in several ways

- Low birthweight due to reduced nutrition.
- Preterm birth.
- Stillbirth.

Babies born to smokers may have the following problems:

- Decreased physical growth
- Decreased intellectual development
- Increased risk of sudden infant death syndrome (SIDS)
- Behavioural problems
- Asthma and respiratory problems
- Poor lung development.

## The mother may also experience problems during pregnancy as a result of smoking

- Increased risk of early miscarriage.
- Placental complications such as placenta praevia and placental abruption.
- Preterm labour.
- Intrauterine infection.

The midwife is in a unique position to offer information and support to the mother who smokes. If the mother is able to give up early in pregnancy, she will greatly increase her chances of delivering a healthy baby. Many localities now have a midwife dedicated to smoking cessation support and mothers can be referred to this service to receive the help they need. Women who are unable to quit should be encouraged to reduce smoking.

## All women should be offered

- *A carbon monoxide test.* A CO test is an immediate and non-invasive biochemical method for helping to assess whether or not someone smokes. However, it is unclear as to what constitutes the best cut-off point for determining the smoking status. Some suggest a CO level as low as 3 parts per million (ppm); others use a cut-off point of 6–10 ppm.[14]

- Advice about the specific risks of smoking during pregnancy.
- Encouragement to use the NHS Stop Smoking Services and the NHS pregnancy smoking helpline (0800 169 9 169).
- Group support for the family.

## Recommended approach for women who smoke

- Assess the woman's exposure to tobacco smoke through discussion and use of a CO test.
- Explain that the CO test will allow her to see a physical measure of her smoking and her exposure to other people's smoking. Ask the woman if she or anyone else in her household smokes. Advise that if her partner or others in the household smoke, they should also contact NHS Stop Smoking Services (if no one smokes, give positive feedback).
- To help interpret the CO reading, establish whether she is a light or an infrequent smoker. Other factors to consider include the time since she last smoked and the number of cigarettes smoked (and when) on the test day. (Note: CO levels fall overnight so morning readings may give low results.)
- Provide information (e.g. a leaflet) about the risks to the unborn child of smoking when pregnant and the hazards of exposure to second-hand smoke for both the mother and baby. Information should be available in a variety of formats.
- Explain about the health benefits of stopping for the woman and her baby. Advise her to stop—not just cut down.
- Explain that it is normal practice to refer all women who smoke for help to quit and that a specialist midwife or adviser will phone and offer her support. (Note: a specialist adviser needs to offer this support to minimize the risk of her opting out.)
- Refer all women who smoke, or have stopped smoking within the last 2 weeks, to NHS Stop Smoking Services. Also refer those with a CO reading of 7 ppm or above. (Note: light or infrequent smokers should also be referred, even if they register a lower reading, e.g. 3 ppm.) If they have a high CO reading (>10 ppm) but say they do not smoke, advise them about possible CO poisoning, and ask them to call the free Health and Safety Executive gas safety advice line on 0800 300 363.[14]

## Nicotine replacement therapy

The midwife should discuss the risks and benefits of nicotine replacement therapy (NRT). For those women who use NRT patches, advice should be given on the importance of removing them before going to bed.

## E-cigarettes

Women should be advised to avoid electronic cigarettes (e-cigarettes) during pregnancy; e-cigarettes are electrical devices that mimic real cigarettes by producing a vapour that is potentially less harmful than tobacco smoke. However, many e-cigarettes contain nicotine but are not currently regulated, hence the level of nicotine they contain is unclear.

## References

13 National Institute for Health and Care Excellence (2008). *Antenatal care for uncomplicated pregnancies*. NICE guidelines CG62. Available at: ℘ www.nice.org.uk/guidance/cg62.
14 National Institute for Health and Care Excellence (2010). *Smoking: stopping in pregnancy and after childbirth*. NICE guidelines PH26. Available at: ℘ www.nice.org.uk/guidance/ph26.

# Alcohol

When alcohol consumption is either occasional or moderate, it is recognized as a socially acceptable behaviour. Over 90% of the population consumes alcohol, but the quantity and frequency of alcohol consumption in women of reproductive age is increasing.

The consequences of alcohol consumption on pregnancy are difficult to study, due to confounding variables such as smoking, diet, socio-economic status, and other substance misuse. The effect of alcohol consumption on the developing fetus depends on:

- The timing in relation to the period of gestation
- The amount of alcohol consumed.

Effects can range from organ damage in the first trimester of pregnancy to growth restriction and inhibited neurobehavioural development in the second and third trimesters.

Fetal alcohol syndrome describes the complete form of the condition and has become recognized as the foremost preventable, non-genetic cause of intellectual impairment. Another term used to describe various types of this condition is 'alcohol-related birth defects' (ARBDs).

NICE[15] states that there is no conclusive evidence of adverse effects on either fetal growth or childhood intelligence quotient (IQ) at levels of consumption below 1–2 units of alcohol once or twice per week, but it recommends that women should avoid alcohol if planning a pregnancy and in the first trimester in particular, because of the increased risk of miscarriage.

There is uncertainty about what constitutes a safe level of alcohol consumption during pregnancy, but women should be informed that getting drunk or binge drinking (five drinks/7.5 units on a single occasion) may be harmful to the unborn baby.

One unit of alcohol equates to approximately 8g of absolute alcohol. The following measures are used as guides when discussing alcohol consumption (although it is recognized that 'home measures' are often larger than pub measures):

- 1 unit alcohol = 10g alcohol
- 1 unit alcohol = 1 pub measure of spirits
- 1 unit alcohol = 1/2 pint of ordinary-strength beer/lager
- 1 unit alcohol = 1 small glass of red or white wine.

There is no proven safe amount of alcohol that a woman can drink during pregnancy. The only way to be certain of reducing harm from alcohol is not to drink at all during pregnancy or while breastfeeding.

It is recommended not to drink alcohol when planning a pregnancy or during the first 3 months of pregnancy. Drinking small amounts of alcohol after this time does not appear to be harmful for the unborn baby, but not more than 1 or 2 units, and then not more than once or twice per week.

Advise women to check how strong the drink is, how large the glass is, and how full the glass is.[15]

## Binge drinking

Binge drinking (which, for a woman, is when she has 6 units or more of alcohol on any one occasion) is not recommended in pregnancy.

## Reference

15 National Institute for Health and Care Excellence (2008). *Antenatal care for uncomplicated pregnancies*. NICE guidelines CG62. Available at: ⅃℧ www.nice.org.uk/guidance/cg62.

# Nutrition during pregnancy

Good nutrition is essential for a successful and healthy pregnancy, as poor nutrition is associated with adverse pregnancy outcomes. Increases in specific nutrients are recommended during pregnancy, but these are not difficult to attain in a well-balanced diet. The EAR for energy during pregnancy is 2000kcal/day in the last trimester only;[16] therefore, it is not necessary for a woman to 'eat for two'. Nutritional requirements also vary due to changes in basal metabolic rate, which varies widely, increasing in some women and decreasing in others. Eating a healthy, varied diet in pregnancy will help ensure an adequate supply of vitamins and minerals. There are some vitamins and minerals that are especially important when pregnant, however, whilst certain women may need to take supplements as well.[17]

### What action should be taken?

Early in pregnancy, discuss the woman's diet and eating habits, and find out and address any concerns she may have about her diet. Provide information on the benefits of a healthy diet and practical advice on how to eat healthily throughout pregnancy. This should be tailored to the woman's circumstances but should include: eat five portions of fruit and vegetables a day and one portion of oily fish (e.g. mackerel, sardines, pilchards, herring, trout, or salmon) a week.

### Folic acid

Folic acid is important for pregnancy, as it can help to prevent NTDs. Women who are planning a pregnancy or are in the early stages of pregnancy should be advised to take 400 micrograms of folic acid daily until they are 12 weeks pregnant. Women should also be advised to eat foods that contain folate (the natural form of folic acid) such as green leafy vegetables and brown rice. Some breakfast cereals and some fat spreads, such as margarine, have folic acid added to them.

Women should be prescribed 5mg of folic acid a day if they (or their partner) have an NTD, they have had a previous baby with an NTD, they (or their partner) have a family history of NTDs or they have diabetes. Women with a raised BMI should also receive a higher dose.

### Calcium

Calcium needs are highest during the last trimester. Calcium absorption is more efficient during pregnancy, but it is still important to eat plenty of calcium-rich foods. The best sources are dairy products such as milk, cheese, yoghurt, dark green vegetables, sardines, pulses, tofu, nuts, and seeds.

### Iron

Iron is needed by the fetus during pregnancy and by the mother as a reserve for blood loss during birth. Needs are normally met by an increase in absorption and the absence of menstruation. Good maternal iron stores and a good dietary intake are needed throughout pregnancy. Lean red meat, chicken to a lesser extent, and fish are the best sources. Iron from animal sources is better absorbed than that from green vegetables, fortified breakfast cereals, bread, pulses, and dried fruit. Vitamin C helps the absorption of iron if taken at the same time. Tannin in tea prevents the absorption of iron.

## Zinc

Zinc is involved in over 200 enzyme reactions in the body, including a key role in stabilizing the structure of DNA and RNA; therefore, in conjunction with folic acid, it helps to prevent NTDs. It is also an important mineral for fertility in both men and women. Although zinc is widespread in many foods, it may be deficient in some diets due to a high consumption of highly processed foods.

## Essential fatty acids

Essential fatty acids are particularly important during periods of rapid fetal brain growth and in early neonatal life. During pregnancy they are responsible for the production of prostaglandins and steroid hormones. Dietary sources include vegetable oils, oily fish (mackerel, tuna, and sardines) and lean red meat.

## Vitamin D

Vitamin D is produced within the skin in response to sunlight. The majority of women have no difficulty in maintaining their own vitamin D levels, but, for vulnerable groups which include women whose cultural practices include covering the head and body, vitamin D synthesis may be reduced. For these women, a 10 micrograms/day supplement is recommended.[17]

## Vitamin $B_{12}$

Vitamin $B_{12}$ stores are not usually depleted as a result of pregnancy and lactation, but they can be impaired in vegetarians, as vitamin $B_{12}$ is exclusively of animal origin. Vitamin $B_{12}$ levels can be maintained by consuming fortified products such as Marmite®, breakfast cereals, and soya products.

## Vitamin C

Vitamin C protects cells and helps to keep them healthy. A balanced diet containing fruit and vegetables, including broccoli, citrus fruits, tomatoes, bell peppers, and blackcurrants, will provide all the vitamin C needed.

## Healthy Start vitamin tablets

These are specially designed for pregnant and breastfeeding women and contain vitamins C and D and folic acid (see ℳ www.healthystart.nhs.uk).

## References

16  Department of Health (1991). *Report on Health and Social Subjects 41. Dietary Reference Values for Food Energy and Nutrients for the United Kingdom. Dietary Reference Values for the United Kingdom.* London: HMSO.

17  National Institute for Health and Care Excellence (2008). *Maternal and child nutrition.* NICE guidelines PH11. Available at: ℳ www.nice.org.uk/guidance/ph11.

## Further reading

NHS Choices. *Food to avoid in pregnancy.* Available at: ℳ www.nhs.uk/Conditions/pregnancy-and-baby/pages/foods-to-avoid-pregnant.aspx#Liquorice.

# Weight gain in pregnancy and body mass index

Weight gain during pregnancy is extremely variable and can be influenced by factors such as maternal age, parity, BMI, diet, smoking, pre-pregnancy weight, size of the fetus, and maternal illness such as diabetes. The weight gain is distributed between the fetus, placenta, membranes, amniotic fluid, and the physiological development of maternal organs, e.g. uterus and breasts (blood and fat deposition in preparation for lactation). Most healthy women in the UK gain between 11 and 16kg, although young mothers and primigravidae usually gain more than older mothers and multigravidae.[18]

An optimal weight gain of 12.5kg is the figure used for an average pregnancy. This is associated with the lowest risk of complications during pregnancy and labour and of low birthweight babies.[19] Maternal weight gain tends to be more rapid from 20 weeks onwards, although excessive weight gain during pregnancy is associated with post-partum weight retention, as is increased weight gain in early pregnancy compared with late pregnancy. Weight gains above 12.5kg in women of normal pre-pregnancy BMI are unlikely to reflect an increase in fetal weight, maternal lean tissue, or water.

Perinatal outcome has a complex relationship with maternal pre-pregnancy BMI, as well as with antenatal weight gain. Calculating the BMI is a method of estimating the amount of body fat, based on the weight and height. The index is calculated by dividing the individual's weight in kilograms by the square of his or her height in metres. Many charts are available for instant grading.

The WHO[20] has defined BMI classifications to represent the risk of associated co-morbidities (Table 5.1).

## Weight gain for individual women

Recommended weight gain should be based on the pre-pregnancy BMI (Table 5.2), as lower perinatal mortality rates are associated with underweight women who achieve high weight gains and overweight women who achieve low gains. The number of women in the obese category of BMI

Table 5.1  BMI classification

| Classification | BMI (kg/m²) | Risk of co-morbidities |
|---|---|---|
| Underweight | <18.5 | Low, but the risk of other clinical problems is increased |
| Ideal range | 18.5–24.9 | Average |
| Overweight | 25.0–29.9 | Mildly increased |
| Obese | >30.0 | Increased |
| Class I (moderately obese) | 30.0–34.9 | Moderate |
| Class II (severely obese) | 35.0–39.9 | Severe |
| Class III (morbidly obese) | >40.0 | Very severe |

Table 5.2 Weight gain in pregnancy and BMI

| Pre-pregnancy BMI [weight (kg)/height (m²)] | Recommended weight gain | |
|---|---|---|
| | (kg) | (lb) |
| Low (<19.8) | 12.5–18.0 | 28–40 |
| Normal (19.8–26) | 11.5–16.0 | 25–35 |
| High (26.0–29.0) | 7–11.5 | 15–25 |
| Obese (>29) | 6 (min) | 14 (max) |

is escalating and rapidly becoming a major public health problem within maternity care.[21] Maternal and perinatal complications are much more prevalent such as an increased risk of gestational diabetes, pre-eclampsia, macrosomia, and perinatal mortality.[21,22]

## Weight management in pregnancy

During and after pregnancy are vulnerable life stages for weight gain, which makes them a good time for health-care professionals to discuss diet and physical activity. Dieting during pregnancy is not recommended, as weight loss may harm the health of the unborn child. But there are no guidelines on recommended weight gain in the UK which are broken down by pre-pregnancy BMI category.

• The British Dietetic Association[23] recommends that pregnant women should gain at least 6kg if overweight.
• The USA Institute of Medicine[24] recommends that obese women should gain between 5 and 9kg over the course of their pregnancy.

## Pregnancy after weight loss surgery

The prevalence of obesity among women of reproductive age is 19%.[25] As four times as many women have weight loss surgery than men, there are a growing number of women presenting for antenatal care having had weight loss surgery. Women are advised not to become pregnant within 12 months of having had weight loss surgery. Despite this advice, many women do become pregnant and go on to have a successful pregnancy.

There are various surgical procedures available. A full description is available from the NHS website (available at: ℅ www.nhs.uk/conditions/weight-loss-surgery/Pages/Introduction.aspx). Procedures are either restrictive (gastric band, sleeve gastrectomy) or malabsorptive (biliopancreatic diversion (BPD), duodenal switch (DS)) or have an element of both (Roux-en-Y gastric bypass).

## Antenatal care after weight loss surgery should consider

• Nutritional deficiencies can occur after bariatric surgery and it is usual for all patients to be prescribed multivitamin and mineral supplements, and sometimes at higher doses than usually observed in the general population.

- A higher level of folic acid (5mg) and a vitamin D supplement are also advised during pregnancy.
- Women who had bypass surgery are at the greatest risk of nutritional deficiencies, particularly vitamin D, calcium, vitamin $B_{12}$, and iron, and they should be monitored closely during their pregnancy for nutritional deficiencies.

## References

18 Webster-Gandy J, Madden A, Holdsworth M (2006). *Oxford Handbook of Nutrition and Dietetics*. Oxford: Oxford University Press.

19 Hytten FE (1991). Weight gain in pregnancy. In: Hytten FE, Chamberlain G, eds. *Clinical Pathology in Obstetrics*. London: Blackwell Scientific, pp. 173–203.

20 World Health Organization (2000). *Obesity: Preventing and Managing the Global Epidemic: Report of a WHO Consultation (WHO Technical Report Series 894)*. Geneva: World Health Organization.

21 Veerareddy S, Khalil A, O'Brien P (2009). Obesity implications for labour and the puerperium. *Br J Midwifery* 17: 360–2.

22 Stewart FM, Ramsay JE, Greer IA (2009). Obesity: impact on obstetric practice and outcome. *Obstet Gynaecol* 11: 25–31.

23 British Dietetic Association (2016). *Food fact sheet: pregnancy*. London: British Dietetic Association. Available at: ℔ www.bda.uk.com/foodfacts/pregnancy.pdf.

24 Institute of Medicine (2009). *Weight Gain during Pregnancy: Re-examining the Guidelines*. Washington DC: US Department of Health and Human Services.

25 Centre for Maternal and Child Enquiries (CMACE) (2010). *Maternal obesity in the UK; findings from a national project*. London: CMACE. Also available at: ℔ www.publichealth.hscni.net/sites/default/files/Maternal%20Obesity%20in%20the%20UK.pdf.

## Further reading

Goldberg GR (2000). Nutrition in pregnancy. *Advisa Medica (London)* 1: 1–3.

National Institute for Health and Care Excellence (2006). *Obesity prevention*. NICE guidelines CG43. Available at: ℔ www.nice.org.uk/guidance/cg43.

National Obesity Observatory (2010). *Bariatric surgery for obesity*. Available at: ℔ www.noo.org.uk/uploads/doc/vid_8774_NOO%20Bariatric%20Surgery%20for%20Obesity%20FINAL%20MG%20011210.pdf.

UK Obstetric Surveillance System (2015). *Pregnancy following gastric bypass surgery: study protocol*. Available at: ℔ www.npeu.ox.ac.uk/ukoss/current-surveillance/gby.

# Food safety

## Foods to avoid during pregnancy

Advice from the Department of Health[26] for pregnancy includes avoiding the following foods:

- Raw or partly cooked eggs
- Mould-ripened soft cheeses (when uncooked), such as Brie and Camembert, and blue-veined cheeses, such as Danish Blue or Stilton
- Caffeine (maximum of 200mg daily)
- Pâté: meat, fish, or vegetable, unless it is tinned or marked pasteurized
- Liver sausage/haggis
- Raw or rare meats
- Liver
- Fish oil supplements and other vitamin supplements containing vitamin A
- Shark, swordfish, or marlin
- Cold cured meats such as Parma ham
- Foods with soil on them
- Raw fish/raw shellfish/wild fish sushi
- Some unpasteurized ice cream/yoghurts
- Liquorice.

## The risks of these foods are summarized as follows

*Listeriosis*

*Listeria monocytogenes* is a Gram-positive bacterium that is normally found in soil and water, on plants, and in sewage. The incidence of listeriosis in adults is 0.5:100 000 and the mortality rate is about 26% in vulnerable groups, such as babies, the elderly, and immunocompromised individuals (such as those with acquired immune deficiency syndrome (AIDS)), and during pregnancy. Infection is usually asymptomatic in healthy adults.

Currently, it is thought to affect approximately 1 in 20 000 pregnancies and, due to the suppressed immune response in pregnancy, the bacteria can cross the placenta. Infection during pregnancy is serious and can lead to spontaneous abortion, stillbirth, preterm labour, congenital infection, or infection after birth. Affected babies often develop pneumonia, septicaemia, or meningitis, depending on when the infection occurred. Case studies of pregnancies complicated by listeriosis report a history of having had a flu-like illness up to 2 weeks before the onset of labour and of eating soft French cheeses, pre-packaged salads, or pre-cooked chicken.

Advice from the Department of Health[26] is to thoroughly re-heat cooked/chilled foods and ready-cooked poultry.

*Toxoplasmosis*

Toxoplasmosis is an infection caused by the parasite *Toxoplasma gondii*, a microscopic, single-celled organism that can be found in raw and inadequately cooked/cured meat, cat faeces, the soil where cats defecate, and unpasteurized goats' milk. Infection is often asymptomatic, although, if symptoms do present, they are of a mild flu-like illness. Infection produces lifelong immunity. It is predicted that 30% of people will have had toxoplasmosis by the age of 30 years.

Vulnerable groups are babies, the elderly, immunocompromised individuals, and pregnant women. The risk of vertical transmission ranges from 15% in the first trimester to 65% in the third trimester.[27] If the infection is contracted during the first trimester of pregnancy, then severe fetal damage is likely and may result in miscarriage or stillbirth. If it is contracted during the third trimester, then the risk of the fetus being infected is higher. Babies with congenital toxoplasmosis may develop encephalitis, cerebral calcification, convulsions, and chorioretinitis.

Immune status can be determined by serological screening, although routine testing in the UK is not offered, as it is predicted that 80% of women would be negative.[28] If infection during pregnancy is suspected, blood tests for antibodies will be able to detect whether the infection is recent, and amniocentesis or cordocentesis will determine whether the fetus is affected. Management may include antibiotic therapy. Termination of pregnancy may be offered when there is evidence of fetal damage or infection.

Avoiding the infection is the simplest and best way to prevent congenital toxoplasmosis; therefore, the following advice should be given to pregnant women.

- Only eat well-cooked meat which has been cooked thoroughly right through (i.e. no traces of blood or pinkness).
- Avoid cured meats such as Parma ham.
- Wash hands and all cooking utensils thoroughly after preparing raw meat.
- Wash fruit and vegetables thoroughly to remove all traces of soil.
- Take care with hygiene when handling dirty cat litter. Wear rubber gloves when clearing out cat litter and wash hands and gloves afterwards. If possible, get someone else to do the job.
- Cover children's outdoor sandboxes to prevent cats from using them as litter boxes.
- Wear gloves when gardening, and avoid hand-to-mouth contact. Wash hands afterwards.
- Avoid unpasteurized goats' milk or goats' milk products (although this route of transmission is rare).
- Avoid sheep that are lambing or have recently given birth.

There is no contraindication to breastfeeding by a woman who has, or is undergoing treatment for, toxoplasmosis.

### Vitamin A

Vitamin A is a fat-soluble vitamin that is essential for embryogenesis, growth, and epithelial differentiation. The retinol form of vitamin A is found chiefly in dairy products, such as milk, butter, cheese, and egg yolk, in some fatty fish, and in the liver of farm animals and fish. Experiments in animals have shown that retinoids, but not carotenoids, can be teratogenic.[29]

A high dietary intake of vitamin A before the seventh week of pregnancy has produced an increased frequency of birth defects, including cleft lip, ventricular septal defect, multiple heart defects, transposition of the great vessels, hydrocephaly, and NTDs.

Retinol is given to animals as a growth promoter, and any excess is stored in the liver. Since 1990, women who are pregnant or planning a pregnancy have been advised to avoid eating liver and liver products, such as pâté or liver sausage, as they contain large amounts of retinol.

Vitamin A deficiency is largely a problem of developing countries and is relatively uncommon in the developed world in the absence of disease. In the UK, the reference nutrient intake (RNI) is 600 micrograms/day, with a 100 micrograms/day increase during pregnancy.[30] Most women in the UK have a vitamin A intake in excess of the RNI.

Cod liver oil supplements may contain large amounts of vitamin A and should not be taken during pregnancy, except on medical advice.

### Caffeine

Caffeine is a methyl xanthine, a naturally occurring compound found in plants. It is present in tea, coffee, and chocolate and acts as a stimulant. It is also added to some soft drinks and so-called 'energy' drinks, as well as over-the-counter antiemetics and analgesics.[31] In pregnant women, it is metabolized more slowly, and studies have suggested an association between the ingestion of caffeine and an increased risk of spontaneous abortion.[32] During breastfeeding an excessive intake can cause irritability and sleeplessness in both the mother and the baby.

The Committee on Toxicity of Chemicals in Food, Consumer Products and the Environment looked at the effects of caffeine on reproduction and concluded that caffeine intakes above 200mg/day may be associated with low birthweight and, in some cases, miscarriage. Therefore, the Food Standards Agency[33] has issued advice to pregnant women to limit their intake of caffeine to less than the equivalent of two mugs of coffee a day.

It is not necessary for women to cut out caffeine in the diet completely, but it is important that they are aware of the risks, so they can ensure that they do not have more than the recommended amount. A total of 200mg of caffeine is roughly equivalent to:

• Two mugs of instant coffee (100mg each)
• 2 1/2 cups of instant coffee (75mg each)
• Two cups of brewed coffee (100mg each)
• Four cups of tea (50mg each)
• Three cans of cola (up to 80mg each)
• Four (50g) bars of chocolate (up to 50mg each).

### References

26 Food Standards Agency (2016). *Listeria Guidance*. Available at: ℘ https://www.food.gov.uk/news-updates/news/2016/15253/listeriosis-guidance-published in Scotland available at: ℘ www.foodstandards.gov.scot.

27 Tommy's (2014). *Toxoplasmosis and pregnancy*. Available at: ℘ www.tommys.org/pregnancy-information/pregnancy-complications/toxoplasmosis-and-pregnancy?gclid=CN2hiNGgjs4CFQ8z0wodalMIMA.

28 Elsheikha HM (2008). Congenital toxoplasmosis: priorities for further health promotion action. *Public Health* 122: 335–53.

29 Azais-Braesco V, Pascal G (2000). Vitamin A in pregnancy: requirements and safety limits. *Am J Nutr* 71: 13255–335.

30  Department of Health (1991). *Report on Health and Social Subjects 41. Dietary Reference Values for Food Energy and Nutrients for the United Kingdom. Dietary Reference Values for the United Kingdom*. London: HMSO.

31  Jordan S (2002). *Pharmacology for Midwives: The Evidence Base for Safe Practice*. Hampshire: Palgrave, p. 18.

32  Cnattingius S, Signorello LB, Anneren G, *et al.* (2000). Caffeine intake and the risk of first-trimester spontaneous abortion. *N Engl J Med* **343**: 1839–45.

33  Food Standards Agency (2008). *Food Standards Agency publishes new caffeine advice for pregnant women*. Available at: ♫ www.food.gov.uk/news/pressreleases/2008/nov/caffeineadvice.

# Folic acid

Folic acid is a water-soluble B vitamin that is necessary for DNA synthesis and has a key role in cell division and development. Folates are folic acid derivatives found naturally in foods. The richest sources are green leafy vegetables, potatoes, and other vegetables and pulses.

Liver is one of the richest sources of folate but should not be consumed in pregnancy due to high levels of vitamin A (➔ see Food safety, p. 99). A diet that is rich in other B vitamins and vitamin C is usually rich in folates. Folates are rapidly destroyed by heat and dissolve readily in water; therefore, considerable losses can occur during cooking, keeping foods warm, and prolonged storage. Deficiency of folate can result in a megaloblastic or macrocytic anaemia, either through inadequate intake, malabsorption, or increased requirements, as in pregnancy, or through drug treatments with anticonvulsants and oral contraceptives. Requirements are increased in pregnancy due to increased cell turnover and are particularly important around the time of conception and during early pregnancy.

The RNI for folate is 200 micrograms/day for both males and females from the age of 11 years onwards. The Expert Advisory Group on folic acid and NTDs[34] recommended that to reduce the risk of first occurrence of NTDs, women should increase their daily folate and folic acid intake by an additional 400 micrograms (making a total of 600 micrograms/day) prior to conception, or from the time they stop using contraception, and during the first 12 weeks of pregnancy.

This can be achieved by:
• Eating more folate-rich foods
• Eating more fortified foods such as bread and breakfast cereals
• Taking a daily folic acid supplement of 400 micrograms.

These 400-microgram supplements are available on prescription and are easily obtainable from pharmacies and health food shops. For women who have had a previously affected baby, a 5mg supplement is prescribed.

Some countries, e.g. the United States (USA), have introduced mandatory fortification of flour used in food production with folic acid, in an effort to reduce the risk of NTDs even further. Such a strategy has been widely debated in the UK but so far has been rejected on the grounds of masking the symptoms of vitamin $B_{12}$ deficiency, issues for older people, technical aspects, and consumer choice.

## Reference

34  Department of Health (1992). *Folic Acid and the Prevention of Neural Tube Defects: Report from an Expert Advisory Group*. London: Department of Health.

# Iron

Iron (Fe) is an essential mineral that has several important functions in the body. As an important component of the proteins Hb and myoglobin, it carries oxygen to the tissues from the lungs; it is also a necessary component of some enzyme reactions. It is stored in the body in the form of the protein ferritin and haemosiderin; the amount of ferritin in serum is a useful indicator of body iron stores. Transferrin is an important protein involved in transporting iron within the body and delivering it to cells.

About 0.5–1mg/day is shed from the body in urine, faeces, sweat, and cells shed from the skin and gastrointestinal tract. High menstrual losses and increased requirements of pregnancy contribute to a higher incidence of iron deficiency in women of reproductive age. The body usually maintains iron balance by controlling the amount of iron absorbed from food.

There are two forms of iron in the diet: haem iron and non-haem iron. Haem iron in meat, fish, and poultry is absorbed very efficiently; this is not influenced by iron status. Non-haem iron, in cereals and pulses, is not as well absorbed as haem iron, but absorption is influenced by iron status and several other dietary factors. Approximately 10–15% of dietary iron is absorbed. Iron absorption follows a log linear response, in that, when iron stores are high, absorption decreases, protecting against iron overload, and conversely absorption increases when iron stores are low. Absorption is favoured by factors, such as the acidity of the stomach, which maintains iron in a soluble form in the upper gut (in the ferrous form $Fe^{2+}$, rather than the ferric form, $Fe^{3+}$). Non-haem iron absorption is improved significantly when meat proteins and vitamin C are present in the diet. Factors that can significantly inhibit iron absorption include calcium, phenolic compounds in tea, coffee, cocoa and some herbs, phytates in seeds, nuts, vegetables and fruit, and soya protein.

Demand for iron is increased during pregnancy because of the increased RBC mass and fetal growth. The need for iron is minimal in the first trimester but increases throughout pregnancy, with a substantial increase during the third trimester. The absence of menstruation, body stores, and increased absorption are believed to compensate for the increased demand.[35] Routine iron supplementation is no longer advocated, but supplementation may be necessary for women with low levels at the beginning of pregnancy.[36]

Iron deficiency results in a microcytic anaemia, and maternal anaemia during pregnancy is associated with an increased risk of preterm delivery.[37] The physiological changes in plasma volume and RBC mass make measurements of Hb concentration unreliable in pregnancy; therefore, for the purposes of screening, serum ferritin is the best single indicator of storage iron, provided a cut-off point of 30 micrograms/L is used.[38]

# References

35 Food Standards Agency (2003). *Safe upper levels for vitamins and minerals. Expert Group on Vitamins and Minerals*. Available at: ℗ cot.food.gov.uk/sites/default/files/vitmin2003.pdf.

36 Department of Health (1991). *Dietary Reference Values for Food Energy and Nutrients for the United Kingdom. Report on Health and Social Subjects 41*. London: HMSO.

37 Scholl T, Reilly T (2000). Anemia, iron and pregnancy outcome. *J Nutr* 130: 443S–7S.

38 Van den Broek NR, Letsky EA, White SA, Shenkin A (1998). Iron status in pregnant women: which measurements are valid? *Br J Haematol* 103: 817–24.

# Further reading

Evans M (2008). Iron deficiency through the female life cycle—who should care? *MIDIRS Midwifery Digest* 18: 404–8.

Webster-Gandy J, Madden A, Holdsworth M (2006). *Oxford Handbook of Nutrition and Dietetics*. Oxford: Oxford University Press.

## Peanut allergy

Peanut allergy is a serious adverse reaction to the proteins found in peanuts. The symptoms of peanut allergy vary from a mild, itchy rash or tingling around the mouth to a severe, life-threatening situation that can include breathing difficulties and collapse. The number of individuals affected with peanut allergy is increasing, and it is suggested that the prevalence is around 1:200. Peanut allergy appears to be a lifelong condition, although the severity and nature of the symptoms may change, and approximately 25% of children with peanut allergy will grow out of it.

Peanuts (also called groundnuts or monkey nuts) are classified as a vegetable as they belong to the legume family (and are thus related to peas, beans, and lentils). They were introduced into the UK around the time of the Second World War and are now used in the manufacture of a wide range of foods. Cooking or roasting peanuts does not alter the allergenicity of these proteins; therefore, both fresh and roasted peanuts may evoke a reaction. Many people have multiple allergies; therefore, reactions to other legume proteins may occur, although this is less common. However, individuals allergic to peanuts do react more commonly to tree nuts such as brazil, almond, and hazel.

The development of an allergy or allergic disease is hereditary and known to occur more commonly in people who have other atopic conditions, such as eczema, asthma, or hay fever, or who have at least one close relative with such conditions.

### Pregnancy, breastfeeding, and weaning

Although the research is inconclusive, it has been suggested that sensitization can occur *in utero* or through breastfeeding, as peanut protein has been detected in breast milk. However, the Department of Health's Committee on Toxicity of Chemicals in Food, Consumer Products and the Environment has recently completed a review and has concluded that there is no evidence that eating or refraining from eating peanuts has any bearing on a child acquiring peanut allergy.

Therefore, the revised advice is as follows.

- Pregnant or breastfeeding women who wish to consume peanuts as part of a healthy diet may do so, irrespective of any family history of allergies.[39]
- There is no reason for pregnant or nursing mothers who do not fall into this category of familial allergy to avoid eating peanuts, unless they themselves have a peanut allergy.
- The Department of Health recommends that all infants be exclusively breastfed for 6 months. If a mother decides to introduce solid food before this time, she should avoid peanuts or other allergic-type foods such as nuts, seeds, milk, eggs, wheat, and fish. When introduced, these foods should be given one at a time so that any allergic reaction is more easily identified.[40]

- If an infant has a known allergy or has been diagnosed with conditions such as eczema or there is a history of peanut allergy in the immediate family, the risk of developing an allergy is higher. For these infants, it is advised that parents consult their GP or health visitor before giving peanuts or peanut-containing foods to their baby for the first time. There is no evidence to suggest that avoiding peanut consumption until 3 years of age will prevent peanut allergy.[30,40]

## References

39 Department of Health (2009). *Revised Government Advice on Consumption of Peanut during Pregnancy, Breastfeeding and Early Life and Development of Peanut Allergy*. London: Department of Health.

40 Committee on Toxicity (2009). *Statement on the review of the 1998 COT recommendations on peanut avoidance*. London: Food Standards Agency. Available at: ℘ cot.food.gov.uk/cotstatements/cotstatementsyrs/cotstatements2008/cot200807peanut.

# Exercise

There are many benefits to be gained from taking exercise such as brisk walking, swimming, and gentle aerobic exercise during pregnancy:

- A more positive, healthy outlook during pregnancy
- Greater ability to cope with the discomfort of pregnancy and labour
- Less need for induction of labour, epidural analgesia, and Caesarean section
- An improvement in muscle tone, strength, and endurance resulting from regular exercise can prepare the woman for the physical stresses of labour and caring for the baby afterwards
- After delivery, regaining the normal pre-pregnancy weight is easier.

## Limiting factors

Certain situations that arise in pregnancy may limit the amount of exercise that is safe to take or may make exercise contraindicated. The woman should seek medical advice prior to exercising if she has any of the following:

- Preterm rupture of the membranes
- PIH
- APH
- History of premature labour or several miscarriages
- Muscle or joint problems
- Multiple pregnancy
- Low back pain
- Medical conditions such as existing heart disease.

## Advice

Reassure women that being active in pregnancy is safe for both them and their baby, even for women who were not active before.

However, women with gestational diabetes should monitor blood glucose, regulate mealtimes, schedule rest periods and carefully track the fetal activity and uterine contractions.

Provided there are no other problems and the woman is otherwise healthy, the following advice should be given regarding safe exercise during pregnancy.

*For all women*

- Drink water before, during, and after exercise.
- Do not undertake any exercise that results in becoming overheated. Symptoms of overheating are headache, dizziness, muscle cramps, and nausea. The fetus does not cool down as quickly as the mother and its oxygen requirements remain raised for longer.
- Avoid exercises lying on the back, due to lower maternal cardiac output and symptomatic hypotension after 16 weeks of gestation.
- Avoid activities with an increased risk of falling or excessive joint stress (e.g. horse riding, cycling, and skiing) and physical contact sports, as hormonal changes lead to raised joint laxity and hypermobility.

- Avoid any exercise causing a loss of balance and sports with a high risk of falling. Avoid bouncing and jerking movements and deep knee bends that put a strain on the hip and leg joints.
- Stop immediately if any exercise causes dizziness, faintness, shortness of breath, nausea, contractions, vaginal bleeding, or fluid leakage.

*For women who are used to regular exercise*
- Exercise should be to maintain fitness, rather than trying to reach peak fitness level or train for athletic events.
- Do not scuba-dive, as the fetus is not protected from decompression sickness and gas embolism.

*If the mother is new to regular exercise*
- Start very slowly, with a 10–15min period of gentle exercise.
- Gradually increase this to 30min as she becomes more familiar with the routine.
- Start exercise gradually, as the body rapidly shifts oxygen and energy towards the working muscles. Lower the intensity of aerobic exercise to 60% of the maximum heart rate for her age, and monitor the heart rate regularly throughout the exercise period.

Most gyms and fitness clubs have trained attendants who can devise a programme for the pregnant and newly postnatal woman. It is safe to exercise for 30–40min, three times per week.

# Employment

Many women want to continue to work during their pregnancy and there is legal protection for women who wish to do so.

A woman is not legally obliged to inform her employer of her pregnancy until she gives notice of the date she intends to start her maternity leave. That notification must be given by 15 weeks before the expected week of childbirth at the latest, i.e. when the woman is approximately 6 months pregnant.

It is advisable for the woman to inform her employer of her pregnancy, as she is entitled to certain rights:

• Protection under the Sex Discrimination Act against less favourable treatment
• Protection against being subjected to adverse working conditions and discrimination or being dismissed for a reason connected to pregnancy
• A right to paid time off for antenatal care
• Protection against being treated less favourably for taking time off for antenatal care
• A right to health and safety protection.

These rights are important, as adverse working conditions can affect the health of the mother and fetus.

There is a significant association between preterm births, SGA infants, maternal hypertension, pre-eclampsia, and working conditions.

Advise women who work during pregnancy that the following may limit their ability to stay at work for the full pregnancy, unless their employer can rearrange their workload or responsibilities:

• Physically demanding work
• Long working hours
• Shift work
• Prolonged standing
• Heavy or repetitive lifting.

All employees are entitled to 52 weeks' maternity leave, regardless of the length of service or the number of hours worked. Maternity leave is divided into 26 weeks of ordinary maternity leave and 26 weeks of additional maternity leave. Factsheets are available from Working Families (available at: ℘ www.workingfamilies.org.uk).

# Minor disorders of pregnancy

## Introduction

Minor disorders of pregnancy are a series of commonly experienced symptoms related to the effects of pregnancy hormones and the consequences of enlargement of the uterus as the fetus grows during pregnancy.

The conditions themselves pose no serious risk to the mother, but they are unpleasant and can affect her enjoyment of the pregnancy overall.

Close questioning of the mother is necessary to ascertain that the symptoms are not masking a more serious problem, and a sympathetic and helpful approach with prompt advice and treatment is needed.

# Backache

Up to 90% of women may experience backache during their pregnancy, making this the most common of the minor disorders of pregnancy. Obesity, a history of back problems, and greater parity increase the likelihood of backache occurring.

- During pregnancy, ligaments become softer under the influence of relaxin and stretch to prepare the body for labour.
- This is particularly focused on the pelvic joints and ligaments which become more supple to accommodate the baby at delivery.
- The effects can put a strain on the joints of the lower back and pelvis, which can cause backache.
- As the baby grows, the curve in the lumbar spine may increase as the abdomen is thrust forward, and this may also cause backache.

The following advice can be given to the woman to alleviate backache.

- Avoid heavy lifting, and use a safe lifting technique when lifting or picking something up from the floor. Hold the load close to the body; maintain a wide, stable base. Bend the knees, whilst keeping the back straight. Avoid stooping, keeping the back in a neutral position by flexing at the hips.
- The woman should take particular care when picking up a heavy older child and should bend the knees to be level with the child before lifting.
- Any working surface used should be high enough to prevent stooping.
- When carrying loads, such as shopping, the weight should be equally balanced on both sides of the body.
- The woman can be shown how to sit and stand with her spine in a neutral position so that good posture is maintained.
- A firmer mattress gives better support during sleep. Using a bed board can make a soft mattress more supportive.
- Some women find relief from using pillows to support their pregnant abdomen whilst lying down.[1]
- Rest as much as possible, as the pregnancy progresses.

If the backache is very painful and debilitating, the woman can be referred to an obstetric physiotherapist for advice on lumbar support and helpful exercises.

## Reference

1 Pennick V, Young G (2007). Interventions for preventing and treating pelvic and back pain in pregnancy. *Cochrane Database Syst Rev* 2: CD001139.

# Constipation

Increased progesterone levels decrease gastrointestinal movement during pregnancy. A recent systematic review reported two studies which showed that fibre supplements in the form of bran or wheat fibre increased the frequency of defecation and led to softer stools. It appeared that stimulant laxatives were more effective than bulk-forming laxatives but may have caused more side effects.[2]

Women who were constipated prior to pregnancy may find that this condition becomes more problematic when they become pregnant.

It may be due to displacement of the bowel by the growing uterus or a side effect of oral iron therapy.

If possible, it is best to try to relieve constipation by natural means before resorting to medication during pregnancy, and the advice given by the midwife should reflect this.

Advice should include:
- Eating regular meals
- Drinking extra water, fruit juice, or herbal tea. This should be up to 2L of fluid per day, more in hot weather
- Eating five portions of fruit and vegetables per day
- Eating foods containing a high fibre content such as wholemeal bread, breakfast cereals, and prunes
- Taking gentle exercise, 20–30min, three times per week.

A mild laxative, such as lactulose (15mL twice a day), may be prescribed if the above advice does not relieve the symptoms.

## Reference

2  Jewell DJ, Young G (2007). Interventions for treating constipation in pregnancy. *Cochrane Database Syst Rev* 2: CD001142.

# Frequency of micturition

Around 60% of women develop frequency of micturition early in pregnancy. This appears to be a more common symptom for nulliparas. The urgent need to empty the bladder, even small amounts, throughout the day and night is caused by pressure from the enlarging uterus on the bladder.

• Reassure women that this is normal as urine production in the kidney increases during pregnancy.
• This generally improves by the 14th week as the uterus grows out of the pelvis.
• Advise them not to drink a large amount before going to bed.

No treatment is needed for urinary frequency alone, but if micturition becomes painful, urinary infection should be excluded.

The symptoms may return during the last 4 weeks of pregnancy, when the presenting part enters the pelvis and creates pressure on the bladder, diminishing its overall capacity.

Pregnant women are also at risk of developing stress incontinence during pregnancy, related to physiological changes, hormonal influences, and also mechanical stresses provoked by the enlarged uterus.

All pregnant women need to be taught how to perform pelvic floor exercises correctly, as improved pelvic floor tone prior to delivery can influence the return of good pelvic floor function after delivery.

• Explain how to locate the pubo-coccygeous (PC) muscle, by asking the woman to attempt to stop the urine flow whilst urinating.
• Once the PC muscle is identified, the exercises should be carried out with an empty bladder.
• The initial exercise involves squeezing and holding the PC muscle for 3–5s, relaxing, and then repeating this until the muscle tires.
• The woman should attempt three sets of five squeezes once or twice a day for a week, then build up to three sets of 8, 10, 15, and then 20 squeezes.
• Once a routine is established, maintenance is achieved by attempting three sets, four times a week.
• The exercise can be varied by including slow or rapid squeezes and by exercising at different times of the day.

## Indigestion and heartburn

During pregnancy, 30–50% of women experience indigestion or heartburn. The discomfort is caused by acid reflux from the stomach through the oesophageal sphincter as a result of the relaxing effects of progesterone. Later in pregnancy, the growing uterus displaces the stomach, increasing intragastric pressure, which makes acid reflux more likely when lying down.

A Cochrane review[3] tried to assess the best interventions for heartburn during pregnancy. The authors were unable to draw conclusions about different treatments and recommended lifestyle changes first for mild heartburn in pregnant women.

Advice should include:
- Eating several small meals a day
- Avoiding coffee, alcohol, and spicy foods
- Not to combine solid food with a drink, but take drinks separately from meals
- Sleeping with an extra pillow at night to raise the head and chest level above the level of the stomach
- Taking a calcium- or calcium–magnesium-based antacid to relieve symptoms
- Wearing loose clothing, so that there is no undue pressure on the abdominal area.

### Reference
3 Dowswell T, Neilson JP (2008). Intervention for heartburn in pregnancy. *Cochrane Database Syst Rev* 4: CD007065.

# Nausea and vomiting

Nausea and vomiting are common in pregnancy, with about 80% of pregnant women experiencing anything from mild nausea on awakening to nausea throughout the day with 50% experiencing some vomiting during the first half of pregnancy.[4]

For many women, the symptoms subside after the 12th–14th week of pregnancy, coinciding with the ability of the placenta to take over support of the growing embryo.

The reasons for nausea are not known, but it has been associated with:
- Increased levels of hCG
- Hypoglycaemia
- Increased metabolic demand
- The effects of progesterone on the digestive system.

Advice to women should include:
- Having a few mouthfuls of something before getting up
- Having a snack ready at the bedside
- Getting out of bed slowly
- Maintaining a good fluid intake and drinking small amounts frequently throughout the day
- Eating little and often, every 2–3h during the day
- Having a rest in the middle of the day
- Eating plain crackers, small pieces of fruit, dry toast, or yoghurt
- Avoiding alcohol, caffeine, and spicy or fatty foods
- Ginger, in the form of tea or tablets, relieves nausea
- Eating a small snack before going to bed at night.

A doctor should be consulted if:
- The woman is vomiting more than four times a day
- The above advice has not worked
- The woman is losing weight
- The woman is not keeping fluids down
- The woman requires antiemetics
- The woman is experiencing dehydration. Hospital admission is advised for IV feeding, correction of electrolyte imbalance, and rehydration.

## Reference

4 Matthews A, Haas DM, O'Mathúna DP, Dowswell T (2015). Interventions for nausea and vomiting in early pregnancy. *Cochrane Database Syst Rev* 9: CD007575. Available at: ℔ onlinelibrary.wiley. com/doi/10.1002/14651858.CD007575.pub4/abstract;jsessionid=BE2E4430CB6C6AB2A856 B850323DBDFC.f04t03.

# Varicose veins and haemorrhoids

Varicose veins are caused by weakening of the valves in the veins returning blood to the heart from the lower extremities, so they can occur in the legs, vulva, or rectum. Rectal varicosities are called haemorrhoids.

They can occur in any age group, but pregnant women are particularly prone if they have a family history of varicosities, are carrying twins, or have to sit or stand for long periods of time, for instance at work.

During pregnancy, the extra circulating blood volume increases pressure on the vessel walls and progesterone relaxes the blood vessel walls. The weight of the growing uterus creates back pressure in the pelvic and leg vessels. Constipation exacerbates haemorrhoids.

## Signs and symptoms
- Legs ache and feel heavy.
- Throbbing sensation in the legs or vulva.
- Dilated surface veins in the vulva or legs.
- The vulva may be swollen and painful.
- Discomfort and itching round the anus and when opening the bowels.

## Advice
- Avoid constipation and straining on the toilet.
- Ensure an adequate intake of fibre, e.g. fruit and also fluids.
- Avoid standing for prolonged periods of time.
- Wear graduated support tights to assist venous flow.
- Avoid constrictive clothing.
- Do not sit with the legs crossed.
- Take gentle exercise, such as walking, to help the circulation.
- Use vulval ice packs to reduce swelling.
- A proprietary haemorrhoid cream can be used safely during pregnancy.
- Be aware that iron supplements can cause constipation in some women and a liquid preparation may be preferable in this instance.

Teach the woman to recognize the signs and symptoms of deep vein thrombosis.

## During delivery
- Promote a spontaneous normal delivery, and use a non-directed pushing technique. Forceps or ventouse delivery may cause haemorrhoids to prolapse.
- Advise and encourage the woman to refrain from pushing during the second stage of labour until the vertex is visible, as this reduces straining efforts to a minimum.
- Avoid laceration to any vulval varicosities.

# Helping women cope with pregnancy: complementary therapies

## Introduction

The use of complementary therapies (CTs) has escalated in recent years, with approximately two-thirds of the population accessing some kind of CT or treatment. This has been attributed to a change in people's expectations and choice, resulting in a desire for less dependency on drugs and invasive treatments that often involve adverse side effects.

Almost one-third of this group are pregnant women, so therefore many women choose to use CTs during pregnancy and childbirth. It is therefore pertinent that midwives familiarize themselves with the knowledge and safety issues of CTs with regard to pregnancy and childbirth.

Complementary and alternative medicine cannot replace conventional antenatal care; pregnant women should be informed that there are very few high-quality studies into the effectiveness and safety of CTs during pregnancy and current recommendations are that CTs should be used as little as possible during pregnancy.[1,2] If women do choose to use CTs during pregnancy, they should be advised to consult a qualified practitioner dedicated to working with the special needs of pregnant women and to inform their midwife or GP of any therapies commenced.[2]

It has been argued that the randomized clinical controlled trial is not truly evaluative of some of the traditional elements of homeopathy, reflexology, acupuncture, thus making it difficult to compare their effectiveness with orthodox medicine. There is also a plethora of anecdotal evidence that supports the safe use of CTs from European and Eastern cultures—such as Chinese medicine and herbal medicine. Some midwives may therefore choose to specialize in the use of CTs, whilst others will have received in-house training to use CTs in their practice. However, caution should always be exercised with any form of treatment or therapy during pregnancy—expert advice should be sought where there are any queries regarding the use of CTs for pregnant women.

### References

1 National Institute for Health and Care Excellence (2008). *Antenatal care for uncomplicated pregnancies*. NICE guidelines CG62. Available at: ℘ www.nice.org.uk/guidance/cg62.
2 NHS Choices (2015). *Are complementary therapies safe during pregnancy?* Available at: ℘ www.nhs.uk/chq/Pages/957.aspx?CategoryID=54&SubCategoryID=129.

### Further reading

Ernst E, Pittler M, Wider B (eds.) (2006). *The Desktop Guide to Complementary and Alternative Medicine: An Evidence-based Approach*, 2nd edn. Edinburgh: Mosby.
Mantle F, Tiran D (2009). *A–Z of Complementary and Alternative Medicine: A Guide for Health Professionals*. Edinburgh: Churchill Livingstone.
Miccozzi MS (2006). *Fundamentals of Complementary and Integrated Approach to Care*, 3rd edn. London: Elsevier.
Natural Therapy Pages. Available at: ℘ www.naturaltherapypages.co.uk/therapy.

# Homeopathy

Homeopathy is a system of medicinal healing which aims to promote the body's natural tendency of self-healing by the use of plant, animal, and mineral extracts prepared specifically by homeopathic pharmacies. The House of Commons Science and Technology Committee[3] currently reputes homeopathic remedies as 'scientifically implausible'. However, homeopathic remedies may offer a gentle alternative means of relieving some of the common ailments of pregnancy. NICE recommends that pregnant women considering the use of homeopathic remedies should seek advice from a qualified homeopath and inform their midwife and GP of any treatment undertaken.[4]

## General principles and administration

- Based on the theory of 'like cures like'—whereby matching the symptoms to the correct remedy profile is crucial.
- Tablets are taken sublingually, allowed to dissolve, or chewed or sucked between meals to ensure optimum efficiency of the remedy.
- When taking homeopathic remedies, strong tastes should be avoided for at least 15min before and after taking the remedy. This applies to: smoking, alcohol, toothpaste, spicy foods, coffee, and some essential oils. These substances are said to act as an antidote to the effect of the remedies.
- Occasionally current symptoms can worsen before improvement is noted. This is usually only temporary and is an indication that the body has been stimulated into a healing response.
- Remedies should only be taken for when symptoms persist and then discontinued when they subside.
- Remedies should not be taken prophylactically.
- It is safe to use homeopathic remedies with orthodox medication; however, some drugs may have an antidotal effect.
- Homeopathic remedy dosages come in a dilution factor—the higher the dilution, the more potent the remedy.
- Homeopathic remedies are prepared by a method of dilution and succussion (vigorous shaking) to the potency required.
- Minimal handling of remedies is important as the active ingredient of the remedy is on the outside of the tablet or pilule. Ideally the tablet should be tipped into the lid and then directly into the mouth.
- An important factor is that it is the amount of times the remedy is repeated which enhances the healing effect, and not the strength of the remedy that is administered.

## Examples of treatment with homeopathy

### Constipation

Constipation is a common feature of pregnancy due to the effect of hormones in pregnancy, dietary changes, and maybe the effect of iron therapy. Attention to diet is always important to help with the underlying cause. However, homeopathic remedies have a lot to offer for the relief of symptoms—in addition to physical symptoms, the emotional disposition of the person is considered too.

*Backache*

Backache in pregnancy may be caused by physiological changes associated with the pregnant condition. Homeopathy can be of benefit alongside other supportive treatments such as physiotherapy, transcutaneous electrical nerve stimulation (TENS), chiropractic therapy, and massage.

*Heartburn*

Homeopathic remedies may provide an alternative to the conventional remedies for heartburn. Careful attention to matching individual symptoms to the most appropriate remedy is important, e.g. when the symptoms are worse (after eating, first thing in the morning, etc.), the abdominal sensations experienced (bloated, burning sensation, empty feeling, etc.).

*Arnica*

This remedy is the most commonly used homeopathic remedy for physical and emotional trauma. Excellent for soft tissue bruising, falls, concussion, and before and after surgery. It can also be applied topically to bruised areas, provided the skin is unbroken.

## References

3  House of Commons (2010). *Science and Technology Committee: Fourth Report. Evidence Check 2: Homeopathy.* Available at: ℠ www.publications.parliament.uk/pa/cm200910/cmselect/cmsctech/45/4502.htm.

4  National Institute for Health and Care Excellence (2008). *Antenatal care for uncomplicated pregnancies.* NICE guidelines CG62. Available at: ℠ www.nice.org.uk/guidance/cg62.

## Further reading

Mantle F, Tiran D (2009). *A–Z of Complementary and Alternative Medicine: A Guide for Health Professionals.* Edinburgh: Churchill Livingstone.

## Aromatherapy

Aromatherapy is a practice which uses essential oils, through massage or inhalation. The benefits of aromatherapy are claimed to come from the scent of the oils which have the power to transform emotions and heal. A practitioner will safely prepare a unique blend of essentials and cold pressed oils and apply to the skin through massage or vaporization in a vaporizer or diffuser.

Aromatherapy is a holistic treatment which is designed to significantly improve physical and psychological well-being. The use of essential oils during pregnancy and childbirth constitutes the most commonly used therapy within maternity care, possibly due to the subtle therapeutic effects of the oils themselves, together with the nurturing aspects of some of the techniques used within aromatherapy. Due respect to the potency of essential oils should be paramount at all times.

Dilution safety, and potential toxicity of essential oils is the key to safe administration in pregnancy. Some oils have diuretic and/or emmenagogic* properties which may limit the use of popular oils.

Many oils are contraindicated in pregnancy due to their strength and potential abortifacient properties, so when in doubt as to whether an oil is suitable, professional advice should be sought. Women should be encouraged to seek advice from their midwife or GP and to consult a registered aromatherapist if she wishes to use essential oils in pregnancy.[5]

### General principles

• Essential oils should never be taken internally.
• All essential oils should be diluted in some form prior to use, e.g. in a base oil or lotion, water, or vaporized, or compress.
• Store in a dark, locked cupboard away from children.
• Respect the storage and shelf life of essential oils.
• Adhere to recommended dosages for pregnancy.
• Adhere to cautions regarding pregnancy, epilepsy, hypertension, and other medical conditions.
• Use sound, respected sources of oils and carrier oils to ensure therapeutic quality.
• Always enquire about potential allergies prior to use; some oils may cause skin reactions if used neat or in high doses—therefore, exercise caution with women who have sensitive skin or a history of allergies.
• Be aware of the woman's medical and obstetric history to ensure there are no contraindications to the use of essential oils or methods of administration.

### Administration of essential oils

Debate about the essential oils that are considered safe for pregnancy and childbirth continues. Table 7.1 is not an exhaustive list of essential oils but reflects the most common oils used for pregnancy and childbirth.

### Routes of administration of essential oils

• Massage to parts of the body (head, neck, back, feet) or whole body.
• Bath: 4–6 drops suspended in milk or carrier oil and added after water has been run and then agitated to disperse oils evenly.

* Emmenagogue: an essential oil that contains properties which can induce or assist menstruation.

**Table 7.1** Oils for pregnancy and childbirth

| Essential oil | Properties | Comments |
| --- | --- | --- |
| Chamomile (Roman—*Anthemisnobilis*) (German—*Matricariachamomilla*) | Antispasmodic, antiseptic, calming, antifungal, analgesic, anti-inflammatory. Soothing for the skin, nervous, and digestive systems. Stimulates immune system | Avoid use of Roman chamomile until late pregnancy Avoid use of German chamomile in early pregnancy. German chamomile useful for sensitive skin |
| Clary sage (*Salvia sclerea*) | Antidepressant, hypnotic, antiseptic, antispasmodic, anti-inflammatory, uterine tonic—assists contractions. Mainly used as a massage or compress | Do not use in pregnancy. May cause drowsiness; care with driving and alcohol. Oestrogenic properties. Reduces panic and lowers blood pressure |
| Eucalyptus (*Eucalyptus globulus*) | Nasal decongestant, antiseptic, pain relief, urinary tract infection. Inhalation, massage, compress | Avoid in epileptics and hypertension. May cause skin irritation. Clears head and cools emotions |
| Frankincense (*Boswellia carteri*) | Hysteria, hyperventilation, depression, genitourinary tract infections, decongestant | One drop inhaled from tissue/taper to relieve hyperventilation. Slight emmenagogue—low doses during pregnancy, calming oil for labour |
| Geranium (*Perlagonium graveolens*) | Balancing, analgesic, antispasmodic, decongestant, antiseptic, diuretic | Heavy aroma, check acceptability prior to use. Regulates hormone function. Eliminates waste and congestion. Useful for nervousness, fatigue, fluid retention, varicose veins, and cystitis |
| Grapefruit (*Citrus paradisi*) | Antiseptic, analgesic. Good for massage during pregnancy | Gentle safe oil, light refreshing aroma, phototoxic. Shelf life: 3 months. Relief of stress headaches. Useful for colds and flu |
| Jasmine (*Jasminium officinale*) | Analgesic, antispasmodic, uterine tonic, pain, hormone-balancing, sedative, aphrodisiac | Emmenagogue—not to be used until term. Very expensive. Aroma is overpowering; caution with vaporizing; best used as massage in low doses. Regulates and deepens breathing |

(*Continued*)

**Table 7.1** (Contd.)

| Essential oil | Properties | Comments |
|---|---|---|
| Lavender (*Lavendula angustifolia*) | Antiseptic, analgesic, pain relief, antispasmodic hypotensive. First-aid oil | Emmenagogue, use with caution in first trimester. Care with vaporization. May cause headaches or drowsiness.[5] Not to be used in combination with epidural anaesthesia or pethidine |
| Lemon (*Citrus limon*) | Anti-anaemic, antispasmodic, bactericidal, circulatory tonic, skin tonic, immune system stimulant | Minimal phototoxic effect, short shelf life. Vaporization or in combination with other oils for massage. Headache, *Candida*, cleansing action |
| Lime (*Citrus aurantifolia*) | Antiseptic, antiviral, antispasmodic, balances immune system, appetite regulator. Useful for sickness in pregnancy | Gentle, relaxing, safe oil, phototoxic |
| Mandarin (*Citrus reticulata*) | Antiseptic, analgesic, hormone-balancing, flatulence, anxiety, nausea. Gentle uplifting effect | Good all-round oil with pleasant aroma. Special affinity for women and children. Excellent for stretch marks |
| Neroli (*Citrus aurantium* or *bigaradia*) | Antispasmodic, aphrodisiac, induces peacefulness, uterine tonic, skin tonic | Very expensive. Stretch marks, stress, depression. Hypnotic effect—care with driving |
| Sweet orange (*Citrus sinesis*) | Antiseptic, skin tonic, relaxing, digestive disorders, anxiety | Phototoxic, possible skin irritation as with most citrus oils. Gentle versatile oil. Suitable for nausea, vomiting, stress, oedema, hypertension |
| Petitgrain (*Citrus bigaradia*) | Relaxing, stress, anxiety, nervous exhaustion, antioxidant, antispasmodic, skin tonic, antiseptic | Good for fear and panic. Insomnia, skin problems, depression, digestive disorders |
| Rose (*Rosa centifolia* or *damascena*) | Antidepressant, antiseptic, antiviral aphrodisiac, vasoconstrictive, hormone-balancing. Affinity with female reproductive system | Use for anxiety, insomnia, constipation. Emmenagogue—preferably avoid until late pregnancy. Very expensive, but ideal oil for all women's needs. Ensure high-quality oil used for therapeutic purposes |
| Sandalwood (*Santalum album*) | Calming, sedative, astringent, diuretic, decongestant, antiseptic, bactericidal | Suggested use: varicose veins, cystitis, vaginal discharge, bronchitis, coughs, sore throats, heartburn, and nausea |

(Continued)

**Table 7.1** (*Contd.*)

| Essential oil | Properties | Comments |
|---|---|---|
| Tea tree (*Melaleuca alternifolia*) | Strong antiseptic, antibacterial, antiviral, antifungal, stimulates white blood cell production. Inhibits growth of many pathogenic bacteria | Effective for *Candida* infection, acne (facial sauna). Prevention of infection, natural alternative to treat colds and influenza. Also effective as first-aid treatment for mouth ulcers, bites, boils, burns, cold sores |
| Ylang ylang (*Cananga odorata*) | Aphrodisiac, sedative, tonic, antidepressant, hypotensive, antiseptic, emotionally balancing, stimulates the ovaries | Heady aroma. Use for anxiety, depression, panic, fear, and shock. Regulates heart beat and slows breathing. Regulates flow of adrenaline |

- Compress: 3–4 drops in hot or cold water. Flannel or sanitary pad is then immersed, wrung out, and applied to the skin. Repeated once the flannel cools to body temperature.
- Foot bath: 3–4 drops of essential oil added to warm water. Agitate and then soak for a minimum of 10min to gain benefit.
- Vulval wash: useful to help prevent infection; douches should not be used in the intrapartum period and postnatally. Use three drops of essential oil to 1L of warm water; agitate, and pour over the vulval area.
- Room spray: ten drops of oil to 200mL of water, preferably in a fine-nozzle spray container.
- Tissue/cotton wool: 1–2 drops of essential oil and inhale as required.
- Taper: one drop of essential oil, and waft under nostrils as required.
- Inhalation: traditional method of inhaling via a bowl containing hot water and oils, with a towel over one's head. Safety precautions need to be exercised. Two drops of oil in the bowl and inhale for 10min. This procedure is not recommended for asthmatic people. This method may also be used as a facial sauna for skin conditions.
- Vaporizer or diffuser: naked flames are prohibited within maternity units; however, electrical vaporizers are most suited and safe for institutional use. One to two drops of essential oil is used and the vaporizer switched on for no more than 10–15min per hour to prevent overintoxication of the oils chosen. Where women may wish to vaporize essential oils at home via a device with a naked flame, they should be advised of the correct usage and safety implications.

### Reference

5  National Institute for Health and Care Excellence (2008). *Antenatal care for uncomplicated pregnancies.* NICE guidelines CG62. Available at: ℅ www.nice.org.uk/guidance/cg62.

### Further reading

Price S, Price L (2003). *Aromatherapy for Health Professionals.* Edinburgh: Churchill Livingstone.

## Bach flower remedies

Bach flower remedies (BFRs) were discovered by Dr Edward Bach in the 1930s and are created from flower essences to treat emotional states that are believed to be the initiating causes of disease. BFRs are known to act gently and the Bach system is a simple self-help therapy that can be used alongside orthodox medicine. Women should, however, be advised to inform their midwife or GP and to consult a registered Bach Flower practitioner before beginning any treatment.[6]

### Using Bach flower remedies in pregnancy

For all the many emotional states that may occur, BFRs may help to bring balance and stability.
- *Walnut*: may help with adjusting to the physical, emotional, and mental changes of pregnancy.
- *Mimulus*: may help with worries about pregnancy, what people might think, fear of medical tests, or needle phobia.
- *Honeysuckle*: may help when there are regrets and fears about past birthing experiences.
- *Elm*: may help if there is a sudden, overwhelming feeling of responsibility to the prospect of motherhood.
- *Red chestnut*: may help when there is over-concern for the well-being of the fetus.
- *Olive*: may be useful for alleviating tiredness and exhaustion in early pregnancy.
- *Scleranthus*: may be helpful when there is difficulty in decision-making, e.g. whether or not to have screening tests.
- *Crab apple*: for feeling unsightly or disgust of the pregnant state.
- *Pine*: for feelings of guilt, possibly harming the fetus in some way or neglecting other family members.
- *Willow*: if there is resentment about the pregnancy and the changes that are required, e.g. work, finances, etc.

As pregnancy starts to draw to a close, the woman may again experience conflicting emotions:
- Gratitude that the pregnancy and its physical discomforts will soon be finished
- Most will hope that they do not go past their due date
- Some may feel unhappy that the pregnancy is coming to an end, due to the special relationship they have developed with the fetus
- Others may be fearful of labour looming, how they will cope, how painful it will be, whether the baby will be alright, and how their partner will cope.

As a result, many women find the final few weeks a time of anxiety and irritation.
- *Mimulus*: may be helpful for all the looming fears experienced.
- *Gentian*: may help if the woman feels despondent, particularly if she goes past her due dates.
- *White chestnut*: may be helpful if there are constant worrying thoughts.

- *Impatiens*: may help if there is irritability and impatience in the last few weeks, and especially if overdue.
- *Aspen*: for the mother who experiences a sense of uneasiness or unexplained fear.
- *Beech*: may be helpful if the woman is critical and irritated by people's company.
- *Agrimony*: for those who hide their fears and concerns behind a brave face.

## Rescue remedy

Rescue remedy is a combination of five of the 38 remedies that Dr Bach formulated, to be taken as an emotional first-aid remedy at times of stress and anxiety. Rescue remedy contains the following:

- *Star of Bethlehem*: for shock and trauma
- *Cherry plum*: for feeling out of control and irrational
- *Impatiens*: for irritability and impatience
- *Rock rose*: for extreme fear and panic
- *Clematis*: for dreaminess and detachment.

## Reference

6 National Institute for Care & Clinical Excellence (NICE) (2008). CG62: Antenatal Care. Available at: ℞ http://www.nice.org.uk/guidance/cg62/chapter/guidance.

## Further reading

Ball S (2005). *The Bach Remedies Workbook: A Study Course in the Bach Flower Remedies.* London: Random House.

# Reflexology

Reflexology is an ancient therapeutic form of foot and hand massage that activates the body's natural healing responses. The feet and hands are seen as a miniature map of the whole body and therefore can be utilized to treat various physical and emotional disorders.

## Benefits of reflexology in pregnancy

- Enhances the relaxation response, therefore reducing stress, which also has a positive effect on the fetus.
- Improves circulation, promoting the carriage of oxygen and nutrients to the cells.
- Stimulates the immune system.
- Improves nervous system function.
- Assists in the removal of toxins.
- Encourages the cooperation of all the organs in the body.

Reflexology may be used for many of the ailments experienced in pregnancy or used alongside conventional treatments to provide extra support and reduce anxiety that often exacerbates physical disorders.

Pregnant women should be treated with reflexology by either a qualified reflexology practitioner with an understanding of the pathophysiology of pregnancy or a midwife/reflexologist.

## Contraindications to the use of reflexology in pregnancy

- Habitual miscarriage or unstable pregnancy.
- Threatened abortion.
- Vaginal bleeding.
- Severe PIH.
- Deep vein thrombosis (DVT).
- Ectopic pregnancy.
- Low-lying placenta.
- Placental abruption.
- Preterm labour.

## Further reading

Mackareth PA, Tiran D (2002). *Clinical Reflexology: A Guide for Health Professionals.* London: Churchill Livingstone.
Tiran D (2009). *Reflexology for Pregnancy and Childbirth: A Definitive Guide for Health Professionals.* London: Elsevier.

# Oriental medicine

The oriental approach to health is based on a holistic view of the individual, nature, and the universe. Illness is viewed as a process of energetic dishar-mony within the body, which eventually undermines emotional, physical, and spiritual health. Various therapeutic practices are employed, including acupuncture, massage, herbal medicine, dietary reform, meditation, exer-cise, and breathing techniques.

## Acupuncture

The systematic insertion of fine needles at specific acupuncture points to stimulate or balance the flow of Qi throughout the body. This therapy is based on empirical knowledge gained from the close observation of the effects of needling specific points, dating back at least 2500 years.

• During pregnancy, acupuncture treatment should always be carried out by an acupuncturist practitioner or a midwife acupuncturist.
• Acupuncture can be used for all the common ailments associated with pregnancy, e.g. backache, carpal tunnel syndrome, nausea, constipation.
• A full medical and obstetric history should be taken prior to commencing treatment.
• It is important to work closely with health practitioners involved in the woman's care, so that underlying medical conditions or problems arising as a result of pregnancy, where intervention may be necessary, can be initiated promptly, e.g. bleeding, severe sickness, abdominal pain.
• Certain acupuncture points are forbidden during pregnancy because they create a strong stimulating downwards force in the body. However, some of these points may be used for induction/augmentation of labour or to assist with delivery of the placenta.

### Moxibustion

This is the use of heat (produced by burning moxa, the herb mugwort) to stimulate acupuncture points. Cigar-shaped sticks of dried moxa are lit and held closely to the skin over specific points. The most common use for this in pregnancy is to turn breech babies from 33/34 weeks onwards; moxa is a relatively safe, effective, and easily administered method of turning a breech presentation and could be considered as a first option prior to external cephalic version (ECV).[7] However, more research is needed to substantiate the success claims for moxibustion.

• The contraindications are the same as for ECV.
• Other therapies that may be considered for turning the breech are: hypnosis, chiropractic, yoga, homeopathy, and fetal acoustic stimulation.

## Shiatsu

Shiatsu is an ancient form of massage used to aid relaxation and healing, also known as acupressure. Shiatsu means 'finger pressure', although hands, fists, and elbows, as well as fingers, may be used to apply pressure. Shiatsu follows the same principles as acupuncture, except that manual techniques, rather than needles, are applied to the acupuncture points. No drugs or oils are used, which makes it a safe therapy to use during pregnancy. The mas-sage is undertaken over clothing.

*Benefits of shiatsu*

Shiatsu can:
- Help with the ailments of pregnancy
- Initiate a close relationship with the baby
- Help the woman tune in to her individual needs during pregnancy
- Encourage the woman to trust in the process of pregnancy and birth and foster a positive approach
- Help the fetus to maintain optimal positioning, especially for labour
- Harness a positive and rewarding relationship with her partner, encouraging involvement during the process of pregnancy and childbirth.

## Reference

7  Kanakura Y, Kometani K, Nagata T, *et al*. (2001). Moxibustion treatment of breech presentation. *Am J Chin Med* 29: 37–45.

## Further reading

Ewies A, Olah K (2002). Moxibustion in breech version—a descriptive review. *Acupunct Med* 20: 26–9.

Neri I, De Pace V, Venturini P, Facchinetti F (2007). Effects of 3 different stimulations (acupuncture, moxibustion, acupuncture plus moxibustion) of BL 67 acupoint at small toe on fetal behavior of breech presentation. *Am J Chin Med* 35: 27–33.

Tiran D (2004). Breech presentation: increasing maternal choice. *Complement Ther Nurs Midwifery* 10: 233–8.

West Z (2001). *Acupuncture in Pregnancy and Childbirth*. London: Churchill Livingstone.

Yates S (2003). *Shiatsu for Midwives*. London: Elsevier.

# Yoga

Preconception or pregnancy is the ideal time to start practising yoga, as it encompasses physical, emotional, and spiritual preparation that will be helpful for this unique time in a woman's life. Many women experience deeper, instinctual, and nurturing feelings as they embark on their pregnancy, and may find that the gentle and relaxing practice of yoga provides fulfilment for them. A woman who practises yoga throughout pregnancy builds confidence in her body's ability to cope with the many adjustments that take place and is thus more likely to work harmoniously with her body during labour and birth.

However, particular care should be taken if yoga is first commenced during pregnancy due to the increased laxity of joints and muscles; hence practitioners facilitating classes for pregnant women must have a thorough understanding of the pathophysiology of pregnancy with regard to yoga postures. Many postures are contraindicated for symphysis pubis diastasis, particularly abductor movements, whilst others will require some modification due to the physical restrictions in pregnancy of the musculoskeletal system. However, regular gentle yoga practice may bring relief for many of the physiological discomforts of pregnancy, including backache, and provides tremendous benefits to enhance the experience of birth.

## Physical benefits

- Increased suppleness, flexibility, and strength in the joints and important muscle groups that are used in labour and birth.
- Improved posture: helps the woman to cope with carrying the extra weight involved in pregnancy and encourages the adoption of a favourable position for birth by the fetus; thus engagement of the fetus into the pelvis is more efficient.
- Helps to open up the pelvic outlet by simulating squatting and upright postures (squatting can open up the pelvic outlet by up to 30%).
- Pelvic floor muscles are strengthened and toned.
- Improved breathing and circulation, thus increased oxygen supply to the fetus.
- Elimination of toxins and waste material.
- Back pain related to pregnancy responds well to regular yoga practice.
- Other aches and pains and common ailments of pregnancy may be relieved.

## Emotional/spiritual benefits

- Breathing awareness encourages relaxation, the release of tension, and better sleep patterns.
- Pregnancy is less tiring.
- The woman feels more energetic.
- The regular practice of relaxation during pregnancy enables the woman to tap into this sensation during labour, to help her cope better.
- The woman feels confident, empowered, and optimistic.
- Creates a more sensitive and receptive relationship with the fetus.
- Enhances nurturing and mothering instincts during pregnancy, in readiness for motherhood.
- Enables women to get in touch with their inner feelings and intuition.

# Herbal medicine

Herbal medicine has its roots in history and folklore and is a natural approach which uses the chemical derivatives from natural plant compounds.

The goal of herbal medicine is to provide a holistic approach to disease prevention/treatment and individuals may be prescribed a set of herbal remedies to be used as directed. Extreme caution should be used during pregnancy, as medicinal herbs are often quite potent, potentially toxic, and may interact with conventional drugs by either inhibiting or potentiating their effect.[8] Table 7.2 highlights the possible interactions of herbal medicines and conventional drugs that may be used during pregnancy.

Herbal medicines should only be prescribed by medical herbalists whose practice is subject to regulation. All herbal remedies should be discontinued at least 2 weeks prior to planned surgery, as many may potentially affect blood clotting mechanisms.

## Raspberry leaf tea

- Raspberry leaf tea is often recommended for pregnant women during pregnancy to tone the uterus and prepare for labour. It is known for its therapeutic properties as a uterine and circulatory tonic. Studies suggest that it may also have an antispasmodic effect.
- It is thought to aid ripening of the cervix, enhance uterine activity in labour, and promote involution, although this tends to be anecdotal evidence, rather than robust studies.
- It should not be taken throughout the whole of pregnancy, but commenced at about 32 weeks' gestation.
- Taken as a tea, the amount is gradually increased; a tablet form is also available.
- If Braxton Hicks contractions become strong and repetitive, the dose should be reduced or discontinued.
- Raspberry leaf is contraindicated in the following conditions:
  - Uterine scar
  - History of preterm labour
  - Placenta praevia
  - Planned lower segment Caesarean section (LSCS)
  - Bleeding from the genital tract.

Table 7.2 Interactions between herbal medicines and conventional drugs

| Drugs—reason for use in pregnancy, labour, and after the birth | Herbal remedies and dietary supplements to AVOID |
| --- | --- |
| Drugs used for severe morning sickness and for nausea in labour | Co-enzyme Q10; kava kava (withdrawn from sale in the UK) |
| Aspirin for pain relief or to prevent problems of severe pre-eclampsia | Ginger; feverfew; gingko biloba |
| Ibuprofen and similar drugs used for pain relief | Ginger; feverfew |
| Contraceptive pill | St John's wort; ginseng; liquorice; chasteberry (Vitex agnus castus) |
| Steroids—used in premature labour to mature the baby's lungs | Chromium; liquorice; ginseng |
| Drugs to treat high BP, including pre-eclampsia | Ginseng; St John's wort |
| Anaesthetic drugs—stop all herbal remedies 2 weeks before surgery, including planned Caesarean section | Ginger; gingko biloba, ginseng; liquorice |
| Antidepressants (monoamine oxidase inhibitors (MAOIs)) | St John's wort; ginseng; kava kava (withdrawn from sale in the UK) |
| Bromocriptine—may be used in infertility treatment | Chasteberry (Vitex agnus castus) |
| Blood-thinning/anticoagulant drugs (e.g. warfarin)—best to avoid herbal remedies completely, except with expert advice | Dong quai; feverfew; garlic; ginger; gingko biloba; ginseng; papaya extract |
| Drugs to treat immune system problems— best to avoid herbal remedies completely | Echinacea; garlic; ginseng; St John's wort |
| Drugs to treat epilepsy— best to avoid herbal remedies completely, except with expert advice | Grapefruit juice; echinacea; goldenseal; liquorice; St John's wort; evening primrose oil |
| Drugs used to treat diabetes—best to avoid herbal remedies completely | Gingko biloba; ginger; ginseng; co-enzyme Q10 |
| Drugs to treat heart conditions—to avoid herbal remedies completely, except with expert advice | St John's wort; ginger; motherwort; magnesium; ginseng; liquorice; black pepper essential oil; peppermint essential oil; passiflora (passion flower); co-enzyme Q10 |

MAOI, monoamine oxidase inhibitor.

Reproduced from www.expectancy.co.uk. Copyright © Tiran D (2005), reprinted by permission of the publisher.

# Reference

8 Mills S, Bone K (2005). The Essential Guide to Herbal Safety. St Louis: Elsevier.

# The need for social support

# Social support

The care that all pregnant women receive should be woman-centred where her views, beliefs, and values in relation to her care and that of her baby should be sought and respected at all times. Kindness, respect, and dignity should be pivotal within that care. This is especially important for women who have complex social factors and who may have additional needs. There are various definitions for the concept of social support, but all have similarities and relate to the person's perception of the social resources available to them and/or those that are actually provided for them both informally and formally. Most social support is provided by friends, family, and community, but social support by health professionals is important. It has been shown to have a positive impact on general health and well-being.

The three key components of social support are:[1]
• Emotional support: this may be a warm and caring relationship, a presence or companionship, or a willingness to listen
• Informational support, which is the giving of good advice or information
• Practical or tangible support which may be financial, or could be physical comfort support during labour, or practical with breastfeeding.

## How does social support work?
• It works as a buffer against stress.
• It assists the development of coping strategies.
• It can influence behaviours that impact on health.
• It can facilitate recovery from illness.

## Midwives and care provision

Midwives have a key role in supporting women through pregnancy and childbirth. This role is crucial in assisting women and their partners to come to terms with the events of birth, early child rearing, and the effects of this for their future relationship.[2] Key areas of midwifery support are:
• Good communication skills which incorporate good listening skills
• Practical support
• Knowing their carers and being known by them
• Continuity of care and carer.[3]

Social support should be integral to maternity service.

## Effects of social support

*In pregnancy*
• Reduces anxiety resulting in greater confidence, lack of nervousness, reduced fear, and positive feelings towards birth.
• Reduces psychological and physical morbidity.
• Can increase satisfaction with care and communications.
• Gives an increased sense of control.

*In labour*
It can reduce:
• Duration of labour
• The amount of pain relief required
• Operative vaginal delivery

- The 5min Apgar score of <7
- The likelihood of a Caesarean section where companions were not normally admitted.

There is also evidence of:[3]
- Greater satisfaction with birth
- Longer duration of breastfeeding
- Decrease in perineal trauma
- Less postnatal depression and less difficulty in mothering.

## Considerations

- Social support may not be adequate to counter the effects of poverty and social disadvantage on health.
- Little is known as to which elements of social support are useful or effective.
- Doulas have been found helpful in providing social support, especially in labour, although they are not commonly present at birth in England.
- A wide range of interventions has been utilized in research and all are classified as social support.

## Guidelines for care of woman with complex social factors

NICE has developed guidelines for the service provision for pregnant women with complex social factors.[4] Although the guidelines apply to all women with complex social needs they have provided exemplars for four groups: women who misuse substances (alcohol and/or drugs), women who are recent migrants, asylum seekers, or refugees or who have difficulty speaking English, young women under 20, and women who experience domestic abuse.

The general recommendations for all women with complex social factors are:
- Development of multi-agency needs assessments, including safeguarding issues so that there is a coordinated care plan
- Respect the woman's right to confidentiality and discuss her fears in a sensitive and non-judgemental manner
- Inform the woman that her information may need to be shared with other agencies
- Provide information and care for the woman that includes:
  - The need for antenatal care
  - Offering an antenatal booking appointment or referral to sexual health services if considering a termination
  - Providing one-to-one consultation to facilitate discussion of sensitive issues.

## References

1 McCourt C (2006). Becoming a parent. In: Page LA, McCandish R, ed. *The New Midwifery: Science and Sensitivity*, 2nd edn. Edinburgh: Churchill Livingstone, pp. 49–72.
2 Magill-Cuerdan J (2006). Social support in pregnancy: midwives have a crucial role to play. *Br J Midwifery* **14**: 156.
3 Hodnett ED (2005). Continuity of caregivers for care during pregnancy and childbirth. *Cochrane Library*, Issue 2. Oxford: Update Software.
4 National Institute for Health and Care Excellence (2010). *Pregnancy and complex social factors: a model for service provision for pregnant women with complex social factors*. NICE guidelines CG110. Available at: ℳ www.nice.org.uk/guidance/cg110.

# Management of substance misuse

The use of illicit substances such as cocaine and heroin during pregnancy is associated with a number of unfavourable outcomes. Early referral to a specialist midwife will provide a more efficient coordination of care. This is particularly significant in view of the contribution of substance misuse to maternal mortality.[5]

Poor outcomes associated with substance misuse can range from:
- Prematurity
- IUGR—reductions in birthweight are most marked in the infants of women who are multiple-drug users
- Premature rupture of the membranes
- Meconium-stained amniotic fluid
- Fetal distress
- Opiates increase the likelihood of APH
- Cocaine has been associated with placental abruption, particularly if taken around the time of delivery.[6]

Antenatal care is often inadequate because of late presentation, reluctance to have involvement with social services, and a chaotic lifestyle. In order to improve outcomes it is important to engage pregnant drug users early and some drug services have set up joint clinics with antenatal services and also liaise with labour wards.

The overall aim of antenatal care is to minimize harm and stabilize the woman's lifestyle. For women using opiates, substitution therapy with methadone is associated with greater success of antenatal care and better maternal and infant outcomes. Referral to an appropriate substance misuse programme should be offered along with information about relevant additional services such as drug and alcohol misuse services.[7]

It is recommended[6] that the midwife should aim to:
- Encourage the woman to attend antenatal care regularly
- Normalize the care as much as possible taking into account the social and medical problems associated with substance misuse
- Give accurate and honest advice on the risks of substance misuse
- Provide good communication between professionals so advice is consistent
- Provide an individualized multi-agency plan for each client
- Encourage the woman to use relevant additional services.

## Obtaining a history

All information disclosed is confidential and should only be recorded in the hospital notes, not the client-held notes. The following information should be documented:
- What drugs are being used with any additional substances such as alcohol or diazepam
- The amount used daily in either dosage or monetary terms
- The method of use and whether clean equipment is used
- Length of time of use and what was being used at the time of conception
- Partner's drug use if any
- What social support is available, including the involvement of any other agencies.

## Investigations

The following investigations may be performed, having first asked for consent:
- Hepatitis C
- HIV
- Drug screen.

The woman may be referred to a specialist drug liaison midwife to coordinate her antenatal care if one is available in the area and also to a medical social worker. The woman's health visitor may also be involved, especially in follow-up care.

The notes need to have a paediatric alert documented for continuing care of the baby once delivered.

## References

5 Centre for Maternal and Child Enquiries (CMACE) (2011). *Saving Mothers' Lives. Reviewing maternal deaths to make motherhood safer: 2006–2008. The Eighth Report of the Confidential Enquiries into Maternal Deaths in the United Kingdom. BJOG* 118(Suppl 1): 1–203.
6 Department of Health (England) and the devolved administrations (2007). *Drug Misuse and Dependence: UK Guidelines on Clinical Management*. London: Department of Health (England), the Scottish Government, Welsh Assembly Government, and Northern Ireland Executive.
7 National Institute for Health and Care Excellence (2010). *Pregnancy and complex social factors: a model for service provision for pregnant women with complex social factors*. NICE guidelines CG110. Available at: ℘ www.nice.org.uk/guidance/cg110.

# Screening for domestic abuse

- Domestic abuse refers to a wide range of physical, psychological, sexual, emotional, and financial abuse of people who are, or who have been, intimate partners regardless of gender or sexuality. It also covers issues that mainly concern women from minority ethnic backgrounds, i.e. forced marriage, female genital mutilation, and 'honour crimes'.
- The Confidential Enquiry into Maternal and Child Health[8] highlights that 20% of women in England and Wales say they have been physically assaulted by a partner and more than 30% of cases first started during pregnancy.
- Women may also experience an increase in the extent and nature of physical abuse during pregnancy.
- Domestic abuse impacts on maternal and perinatal mortality and morbidity.[8]
- Domestic abuse is generally underreported. It has been found that women are more likely to disclose if asked specific questions by a midwife, than if left to disclose themselves. This then enables an opportunity for women to access help.

## What do women need?

Women need to be:
- Asked
- Believed
- Treated with respect
- Given time
- Given information.

Use RADAR, a mnemonic for professionals:
R = Routine enquiry
A = Ask direct questions
D = Document findings safely
A = Assess woman's safety
R = Resources; give women information on resources available and Respect their choices.

## Routine enquiry

- Offer at a range of points throughout the childbirth experience.
- Women should be seen alone at least once during the antenatal period to enable disclosure more easily.
- Because disclosure can be difficult, asking at different times during the childbirth experience is recommended. Suggested times:
  - At booking
  - 15/16 weeks
  - 28 weeks
  - 36 weeks
  - During the postnatal period
  - At discharge
  - Or at any opportune time.

- To facilitate disclosure, the environment needs to be quiet and private and where confidentiality can be assured.
- Women whose first language is not English, or with other communication barriers, should have access to appropriately trained interpreters.
- It is important that the woman understands the limits of confidentiality with regard to the well-being and safety of any children in the household.

## Ask direct questions

- Women should always be unaccompanied when being asked about domestic abuse.[9]
- How to ask: 'Because abuse or violence is so common in women's lives, we now routinely ask about abuse in relationships so that we can give all women information about agencies that can help'.
- This can then be followed up by more specific questions, e.g.:
  - 'Have you ever been afraid of your partner's behaviour or are they verbally abusive?'
  - 'Have you ever been hurt by your partner—slapped, kicked, or punched?'
  - 'Have you ever been forced to do something sexual that you didn't want to?'

## Document findings safely

- Health-care professionals have a duty of care to record domestic abuse. The records may form part of future protection for an abused woman.
- Where to record:
  - In the hospital notes, not in the hand-held notes.
- What to record:
  - Who accompanies the woman, with information regarding their behaviour
  - Any disclosure
  - Are there any children in the household?
- Try to obtain a safe correspondence address from the woman.

## Assess the woman's safety

- Does she feel safe?
- Is it safe for her to go home?
- You may need to help her with direct referral to support services.
- Discuss safety planning.

## Resources

- Give women information and contacts for local services that provide support:
  - Wallet cards
  - Leaflets
  - Free phone National Domestic Abuse Helpline—0808 2000 247
  - Display information within the maternity unit
  - Wallet cards available in 'women only' areas, e.g. toilets.

- Routine enquiry about domestic abuse can help reduce the stigma associated with abuse and the hidden/taboo nature of domestic abuse.
- Your role within routine enquiry is to signpost the woman towards appropriate support services, rather than attempting to solve her problems. Find out how women and midwives can be supported in the area where you work; what are the local support services and how can they be accessed?

## References

8 Centre for Maternal and Child Enquiries (CMACE) (2011). *Saving Mothers' Lives. Reviewing maternal deaths to make motherhood safer; 2006–2008. The Eighth Report of the Confidential Enquiries into Maternal Deaths in the United Kingdom. BJOG* **118**(Suppl 1): 1–203.
9 Department of Health (2013). *Health visiting and school nursing programmes: supporting implementation of the new service model No.5: domestic violence and abuse—professional guidance.* Available at: ℘ www.gov.uk/government/system/uploads/attachment_data/file/211018/9576-TSO-Health_Visiting_Domestic_Violence_A3_Posters_WEB.pdf.

## Further reading

Department of Health (2005). *Responding to domestic abuse: a handbook for health professionals.* London: Department of Health. Available at: ℘ www.domesticviolencelondon.nhs.uk/uploads/downloads/DH_4126619.pdf.
Refuge and Women's Aid. Available at: ℘ www.nationaldomesticviolencehelpline.org.uk/site-services/cover-your-tracks.aspx.
Tacket A (2004). *Tackling domestic violence: the role of health professionals,* 2nd edn. Home Office Development and Practice Report. London: Home Office Publications. Available at: ℘ webarchive.nationalarchives.gov.uk/+/rds.homeoffice.gov.uk/rds/pdfs04/dpr32.pdf.

# Recognition of sexual abuse

It is important that midwives are open to the possibility that any woman they are caring for may have been sexually abused. It is difficult to estimate how many women have suffered sexual abuse, as statistics vary widely and it is often underreported. However, a third of all rapes recorded by the police are committed against children under 16 years of age.[10] This means that given the high incidence of childhood sexual abuse, midwives will, at some point, care for a survivor of sexual abuse.

## Consequences of sexual abuse for pregnancy and childbirth
- Increased risk of pregnancy.
- Increased risk of late booking.
- Increased anxiety about birth.
- Slower, more difficult birth.
- Increased risk of intervention.
- Increased difficulties with breastfeeding, bonding, and postnatal depression.

## Recognition of sexual abuse survivors
Women who have a history of sexual abuse may present with a combination of any of the following:
- Little or no prenatal care
- Multiple unplanned pregnancies, many ending in abortion
- Repeat attendance at antenatal clinics, GP, or emergency departments for minor injuries or trivial or non-existent complaints
- Drug and alcohol abuse
- History of multiple sexually transmitted diseases
- Recoiling when touched
- Obsession with cleanliness
- Scars from self-mutilation
- Unusual fear of needles
- Insistence on female carers, unless cultural
- Extreme sensitivity about body fluids on under-pads, sheets, and gowns
- Unable to labour lying down
- Extreme concerns about exposure and nakedness during labour and with breastfeeding
- Refuses catheterization
- Intense gag reflex
- Refuses the taking of the infant's temperature rectally.

## Simple steps to prevent re-traumatization
- All midwives should undergo education and/or training so that they feel equipped with the knowledge and skills to deal with a disclosure of sexual abuse.[11]
- As part of routine antenatal care, ask all women sensitively if they have been sexually abused. Reassure that this is more common than many women realize, but certain events in childbirth can trigger memories and flashbacks.

- Consider what you would say and do if a woman discloses a sexual abuse history to you.
- Never trivialize or minimize the impact of sexual abuse. It is important to adopt non-judgemental and supportive responses to women who disclose.
- Give control to the woman, by telling her about the procedures; explain what is going to happen; ask for permission to proceed, and wait until it is given, at all stages antenatally, intranatally, and postnatally.
- Be alert to signs that might indicate a sexual abuse history.
- Ensure absolute privacy.
- Be alert to non-verbal communication and listen to what is not being said.
- Reassure and affirm to the woman that her body is working for her, that the pain is natural labour pain, and explain what is happening to her body.

## References

10 Office for National Statistics (2013). Table A4. In: *Crime in England and Wales 2012/13: findings from the British Crime Survey and police recorded crime* (xls). Newport: Office for National Statistics.
11 Jackson KB, Fraser D (2009). A study exploring UK midwives' knowledge and attitudes towards caring for women who have been sexually abused. *Midwifery* 25: 253–63.

# Women from ethnic minorities or with limited understanding of English

Due to continued major demographic changes, the UK has an ethnically and culturally diverse population.[12] These changes are also reflected within the childbearing population and women who are recent migrants, asylum seekers, refugees, and women from ethnic minorities will be presenting for care within the maternity services.

Recent migrants may have entered the UK either legally or illegally. An asylum seeker is a person who has submitted an application for protection under the Geneva Convention (1951) and is awaiting their claim for asylum to be decided by the Home Office. In the UK, a person is a refugee when their asylum claim has been accepted by the UK Home Office.

Many women within these groups often fail to make full use of antenatal services. This is either because they are unfamiliar with the health service or because they may have a limited understanding of both written and spoken English, making it difficult to communicate.[13] Early access to antenatal care is important, especially as their social status can have an impact upon their health and well-being and that of their baby. The following impacts have been identified:[14]

- Ethnic origin:
  - Low birthweight
  - Increased risk of death in the first year of life
  - Maternal death.
- Asylum seekers, recent migrants, and refugees:
  - Rape
  - Poor maternal health
  - Depression
  - Poor nutrition.
- First language not English:
  - Increased Caesarean section rate.

Midwives need to support these women's uptake of antenatal services by:
- Following the general recommendations for all women with complex social factors (➔ see p. 141)
- Using a range of means to communicate with women
- Informing women of antenatal services and how to use them
- Undertaking training in the specific needs of these women, e.g. female genital mutilation or HIV, religious and psychological needs
- Providing an interpreter who can communicate with her in her preferred language. This should not be a member of the woman's family, her legal guardian, or her partner
- Ensuring the woman's understanding of any spoken information provided.

## References

12 Office for National Statistics (2012). *Ethnicity and national identity in England and Wales: 2011*. Available at: ℘ www.ons.gov.uk/peoplepopulationandcommunity/culturalidentity/ethnicity/articles/ethnicityandnationalidentityinenglandandwales/2012-12-11.

13 National Institute for Health and Care Excellence (2010). *Pregnancy and complex social factors: a model for service provision for pregnant women with complex social factors*. NICE guidelines CG110. Available at: ℘ www.nice.org.uk/guidance/cg110.

14 Raynor M, Mander R, Marshall J (2014). The social context of pregnancy childbirth and motherhood. In: Marshall JE, Raynor MD, eds. *Myles Textbook for Midwives*, 16th edn. Edinburgh: Churchill Livingstone, pp. 16–17.

# Young pregnant women aged 20 or under

For many years, the UK has had the undesirable status of having the highest rate of teenage pregnancy and teenage parenthood in Europe.

However, recent figures from the Office of National Statistics[15] have shown a decline in England and Wales for the number of pregnancies in women <18 years old, from 45 495 in 1969 when records began to 31 051 in 2011. Despite this decline, teenage pregnancy remains a major issue because most teenage pregnancies are unplanned and frequently end in poor outcomes for both the mother and baby. The poor outcomes include:[16]

- The infant mortality rate is 60% higher for teenage pregnancies
- Teenage mothers are 22% more likely to be living in poverty and are much more likely to be unemployed or living with a partner when they are 30 years old compared to a mother who gave birth aged 24 years or more
- Similarly they are 20% more likely to have no qualifications at 30 years old
- Teenage mothers are more likely to have partners who are poorly qualified and are more likely to be unemployed
- Compared to older mothers, teenage mothers have three times the rate of postnatal depression and are more likely to have poor mental health for 3 years following the birth
- They are three times more likely to smoke and 50% less likely to breastfeed
- The children of teenage mothers are 63% more likely to be born into poverty and incur a higher incidence of accidents and behavioural problems.

Teenage mothers often present late for antenatal care and are also more likely to develop complications during pregnancy, including:

- Hypertensive disorders
- Intranatal complications
- Health risks associated with poverty and smoking
- Increased mortality and morbidity among babies born to teenage mothers.

With appropriate support teenage mothers can achieve a successful outcome to their pregnancy and again with appropriate support young mothers and fathers can make a successful transition to parenthood.

Midwives should:[17]

- Follow the general recommendations for all women with complex social factors (➜ see p. 141)
- Offer age-appropriate services
- Be aware that other social problems may be present
- Provide information about assistance with transportation to and from appointments
- Offer antenatal care in the community
- With the mother's agreement, provide opportunities for the partner/father of the baby to be involved with antenatal care.

# References

15 Office of National Statistics (2013). *Conceptions in England and Wales 2011*. Available at: ℵ www.ons. gov.uk/peoplepopulationandcommunity/birthsdeathsandmarriages/conceptionandfertilityrates/ bulletins/conceptionstatistics/2013-02-26.

16 Department for Children, Schools and Families and Department of Health (2010). *Teenage pregnancy strategy: beyond 2010*. Available at: ℵ www.education.gov.uk/consultations/ downloadableDocs/4287_Teenage%20pregnancy%20strategy_aw8.pdf.

17 National Institute for Health and Care Excellence (2010). *Pregnancy and complex social factors: a model for service provision for pregnant women with complex social factors*. NICE guidelines CG110. Available at: ℵ www.nice.org.uk/guidance/cg110.

# Dealing with disability during pregnancy and beyond

Increasing numbers of women with disability are becoming users of maternity services, as they seek to live full and independent lives.[18] Often, simple measures can be taken by the midwife to enhance these women's experiences of maternity services. The Disability Discrimination Act, related to 'Access to goods, facilities, and services', came into force in December 1996, making it unlawful for service providers to discriminate against people with disabilities by:

• Offering a lower standard of services
• Offering less favourable terms
• Failing to make alterations to enable disabled access.

This includes all hospitals and health-care facilities.

## Who are the disabled?

The World Health Organization (WHO) has defined disability as an umbrella term for impairments, activity limitations, and participation restrictions, referring to the negative aspects of the interaction between an individual (with a health condition) and that individual's contextual factors (environmental and personal factors).[19]

However, the definition of disability varies widely between different social groups and cultures, as do the meanings which are attached to a person being labelled as disabled.[20] In the UK it is very difficult to measure the number of disabled because, although local authorities must keep a record, disabled individuals are not required to register. Disability is also very subjective; not all people with impairments see themselves as disabled.[21]

## Disability, sexuality, and pregnancy

The non-disabled population, inclusive of health professionals, has:

• Disputed that disabled women might have sexual desires, have sex, or wish to reproduce
• Defined sexual performance and reproduction for the disabled as a medical problem
• Disputed that the disabled are capable of being, and entitled to become, parents.[22]

Women with disabilities are expected to forgo mothering in the interest of the child, as some fears exist that:

• The disability will be handed on to the child
• The child will be psychologically harmed
• The child will be deprived
• The child will be burdened.

## Disability and the midwifery services

Disabled women have reported the following difficulties encountered with maternity services:

• Lack of physical access
• Lack of accurate information about pregnancy and childbirth, especially in relation to their disability

- Lack of effective communication
- Ignorance of maternity professionals about both the medical and practical needs of disabled mothers
- Inflexibility in maternity services
- Language and attitudes which reflect prejudice
- Doubts about a disabled woman's ability to cope with motherhood
- Staff who do not respect a disabled woman's own knowledge of her disability
- Negative attitudes from health professionals.[23]

The Royal College of Midwives (RCM)[24] supports the principle that:

*'It is important that services reflect the needs of women who have disabilities and ensure that action is taken to overcome the obstacles which confront them. While physical obstructions are of course a frustrating problem, there are other equally daunting barriers resulting from prejudice and ignorance of able bodied professionals.'*

## Midwives and disabilities

Midwives must be aware of their own values and attitudes regarding the rights and responsibilities of childbearing.

Midwives have the potential to strengthen a woman in her ability to give birth and to be a parent in a society that may not be 100% supportive of her decision to do so.

However, midwives have expressed concerns that:

- They do not always feel equipped to do this
- There is a lack of a coordinated approach by health professionals and health authorities
- Little is known about available information and resources
- They are unsure about alternative support agencies
- They feel that service provision is preventive, rather than reactive.

## General recommendations for practice

- Identify disabled clients early and ensure this information is passed on to other service providers involved.[21]
- Provide services in settings that are architecturally/physically accessible.
- Provide services that are psychologically accessible.
- Provide preconceptual care to assist the woman and her family prior to the decision to become pregnant.
- Provide pregnancy care that is sensitive, based on thorough assessment of physical and psychosocial needs, and well planned.
- Identify the woman's strengths, focusing on the social model and how needs can be met safely, rather than directly on the impairment.
- One-to-one care and continuity are important; refer to the specialist or named midwife with responsibility for disability if there is one.
- Plan for the special needs of labour and birth.
- Assist the mother to organize for the many needs of the post-partum period.

## Sensory impairment

*Recommendations for women with visual impairment*

- One-to-one care and continuity are important.
- Tactile models are helpful when describing aspects of the childbirth process, e.g. doll and pelvis, knitted uterus, cervical dilation chart which has holes representing the different stages of dilation.
- Teach and encourage the woman to palpate her own abdomen; focus in on fetal movements and listen to the fetal heart. This will enable her to know her infant antenatally.
- Familiarize the woman with the hospital prior to admission. If the woman requests the presence of her guide dog, organize this well in advance.
- All health-care workers should introduce themselves verbally by name and function.
- Give full explanations before all procedures.
- Encourage immediate skin-to-skin contact following birth, to enable the woman to know her baby.
- Perform any examination of the baby with the woman present, giving a clear explanation of the procedure.
- Describe the baby's characteristics, expressions, movements, and behaviours.

*Recommendations for women with hearing impairment*

- Determine the way in which the woman communicates most comfortably, e.g. writing, hearing aid, lip-reading, finger spelling, sign language, or interpreter.
- Provide one-to-one care or small classes for antenatal education.
- Make it clear in the records that the woman has a hearing impairment.
- If the woman is able to lip-read, obtain her attention before speaking; face the woman; do not over-mouth words; do not stand in shadows, and do not dim the room lights.
- Be patient; repeat and rephrase as required; avoid analgesia that causes drowsiness.
- Familiarize the woman with the hospital prior to admission. Choose a quiet room.
- Watch for facial expressions during procedures; the woman may not be able to communicate discomfort or concern.
- Wear a transparent mask if one is needed.
- Provide as much written literature as is available on all aspects of care.
- Provide early screening for babies at risk of either inherited or acquired deafness.
- Ensure that application for a baby alarm is made early in the antenatal period.
- Inform mothers about the Disability, Pregnancy & Parenthood International (DPPI) DVD *Pregnancy and childbirth—a guide for deaf mothers*.[24]

## Women with learning disabilities and perinatal mental health disorders

*Recommendations for women with learning disabilities*

Most parents with learning disabilities recognize that they need extra help and support. The support may be practical, emotional, or social, and most likely a combination of all three. In order to provide successful support, midwives need to:

- Recognize that these parents are individuals who may have many skills and abilities on which to build
- Ask the person who best knows the parent about the most effective ways of communicating[21]
- Recognize ways in which self-confidence and self-value can be increased
- Recognize that external influences will impact on the individual.

When teaching parenting skills, the midwife should:

- Break a task down into smaller sections, allow time, and be prepared to repeat the same information
- Avoid using long words or jargon
- Keep to the facts and avoid using abstract concepts
- Demonstrate the task alongside the parent; the parent then can watch the task and repeat the actions
- Allow the parents to complete as much of the task as they know before reminding them what comes next
- Always repeat the same prompt and the same set of instructions
- Write down training plans explicitly, showing verbal and physical prompts and at what stage of the task they occur
- Remember that the written word is not always the most effective or the best way to impart knowledge to parents. A variety of visual or audio tapes, photographs, or drawings may be more accessible, either on their own or accompanied by simple written information.

When using written information:

- Avoid abbreviations
- Use simple words that are not too long
- Use large print; ask if they prefer capitals
- Highlight the main points
- Use lists or bullet points where possible.

*Recommendations for perinatal mental health*

The term 'perinatal mental health' is a term used increasingly to relate to the various mental health disorders experienced by women during pregnancy and the postnatal period. These include a previous history of mental disorder, signs and symptoms demonstrated in the antenatal period, along with the range of disorders that appear in the postnatal period. Despite the high prevalence of postnatal depression and anxiety (15–20%) such disturbances often go undetected.[25]

It is important to recognize that the management of mental health problems during pregnancy and the postnatal period will differ from that at other times because of the nature of this life stage.[25]

Midwives have a crucial role in reducing the effects of perinatal mental health disorders on the mother, her child, and the family.[26] Midwives should:
- Provide continuity of care and carer whenever possible
- Carry out a modified psychiatric history during the booking interview[26]
- Be alert to the increased likelihood of a woman relapsing or developing postnatal mental illness if she has a personal or family history of a psychiatric illness and/or a post-partum illness[27]
- Acknowledge the woman's role in caring for her baby and support her to do so in a non-judgemental and compassionate way[25]
- Involve the woman and, with her consent, her partner, family, or carer, in all decisions about her and her baby's care[25]
- Liaise swiftly and appropriately with the multidisciplinary team.

If the woman has a previous history of mental disorders, antenatal assessment by a psychiatrist is essential, along with a management plan for after delivery and access to a perinatal mental health team.

*Post-traumatic stress disorder*
Childbirth has been identified as an event that could be psychologically traumatic, leading to the development of post-traumatic stress disorder.[28] Postnatal post-traumatic stress disorder is a condition, however, that has only been acknowledged since the 1990s. The prevalence rate varies from 1% to 6% although it is thought that it may be increasing due to further medicalization of childbirth and women's dissatisfaction with intranatal care.[29]

Midwives should be aware of:
- The trauma a woman may experience in childbirth
- The action that health professionals can take in order to prevent its occurrence
- The factors that can contribute to post-traumatic stress disorder, including:
  - Violent birth
  - Fear for the baby
  - Post-partum pain
  - Low energy levels
  - Sexual abuse before and during pregnancy
  - Excessive vomiting in pregnancy
  - Ectopic pregnancy
  - Hospital treatment for miscarriage
  - Macrosomia
  - Episodes of preterm labour although the mother gave birth at term.[28]
- Post-traumatic stress disorder can result from loss of control and a sense of powerlessness in labour, lack of trust, and inadequate information.[30]

All women should have the opportunity to discuss with their midwife the care they received during childbirth.

Referral either to a postnatal listening service or to a 'Births after thoughts' programme should be available to all mothers where they can talk to a midwife trained in this area.

## Women with physical disabilities and chronic illness

Women may present with a wide range of physical disabilities and chronic illness during pregnancy, including multiple sclerosis, spinal cord injuries, cerebral palsy, amputees, and rheumatoid arthritis, to name but a few. The general recommendations for practice identified at the start of this section should be followed, together with the following:

- Caregivers should respect the woman as the primary source of information about how to proceed with care
- Women with disabilities are very aware of their abilities and limitations, and all care should be discussed fully with them and their partners
- Assist the woman to focus on her abilities and not her disabilities
- Women with chronic illnesses will require information about the effect of their illness and drug therapy on the pregnancy, birth, post-partum period, and the newborn, as well as the possible effects of the pregnancy upon their condition
- A multidisciplinary approach to care must be adopted to include the midwife, the obstetrician, the woman's disability and/or medical consultant, the physiotherapist, and the occupational therapist, etc.
- Help the woman to manage her own care regimes as much as possible
- Take extra care to prevent skin breakdown if mobility is restricted.

## References

18 Raynor MD, Mander R, Marshall JE (2014). The midwife in context. In: Marshall JE, Raynor MD, eds. *Myles Textbook for Midwives*, 16th edn. Edinburgh: Churchill Livingstone, pp. 3–53.

19 World Health Organization (2011). *World report on disability*. Geneva: World Health Organization. Available at: ℘ www.who.int/disabilities/world_report/2011/report.pdf?ua=1.

20 Helman CG (2007). *Culture, Health and Illness*, 5th edn. London: Arnold.

21 Royal College of Nursing (2007). *Pregnancy and disability: RCN guidance for midwives and nurses*. London: Royal College of Nursing. Available at: ℘ www.rcn.org.uk/__data/assets/pdf_file/0010/78733/003113.pdf.

22 Walsh-Gallagher D, McConkey R, Sinclair M, Clarke R (2013). Normalising birth for women with disability: the challenges facing practitioners. *Midwifery* **29**: 294–9.

23 Walsh-Gallagher D, Sinclair M, McConkey R (2012). The ambiguity of disabled women's experiences of pregnancy, childbirth and motherhood: a phenomenological understanding. *Midwifery* **28**: 156–62.

24 Disability, Pregnancy & Parenthood International (2006). *A guide to pregnancy and childbirth for deaf parents*. Available at: ℘ www.dppi.org.uk/journal/5354/resources2.html#dppidvd.

25 National Institute for Health and Care Excellence (2014). *Antenatal and postnatal mental health: clinical management and service guidance*. NICE guidelines CG192. Available at: ℘ www.nice.org.uk/guidance/cg192.

26 Centre for Maternal and Child Enquiries (CMACE) (2011). *Saving Mothers' Lives. Reviewing maternal deaths to make motherhood safer: 2006–2008. The Eighth Report of the Confidential Enquiries into Maternal Deaths in the United Kingdom. BJOG* **118**(Suppl 1): 1–203.

27 Bates C, Paeglis C (2004). Motherhood and mental illness. *Midwives* **7**: 286–7.

28 Alcorn KL, O'Donovan A, Patrick JC, Creedy D, Devilly GJ (2010). A prospective longitudinal study of the prevalence of post-traumatic stress disorder resulting from childbirth events. *Psychol Med* **40**: 1849–59.

29 Peeler S, Chung MC, Stedmon J, Skirton H (2013). A review assessing the current treatment strategies for postnatal psychological morbidity with a focus on post-traumatic stress disorder. *Midwifery* **29**: 377–88.

30 Laing KG (2001). Post-traumatic stress disorder: myth or reality? *Br J Midwifery* **9**: 447–51.

# Sexuality during pregnancy and beyond

Sexuality is one of the most difficult areas of human experience to define, as it is complex, varied, and contradictory. Defined simply, it is a person's capacity for sexual feelings, and childbirth is intrinsically linked with a woman's sexuality and sexual health. The changes that occur during pregnancy, childbirth, and the transition to motherhood are some of the most fundamental changes that a woman will encounter. Pregnancy is a normal life event that involves considerable adjustment by both the woman and her partner. A first pregnancy will bring the greatest changes. There are many contradictory and confusing aspects of pregnancy and sexuality, and it is a time surrounded by myths and misconceptions. It is the role of the midwife to dispel these myths and to provide sensitive support and information for the woman at all stages of pregnancy and childbirth.

## Sexuality and pregnancy

How pregnancy affects sexuality will vary considerably from woman to woman. Women will be affected differently by physical and psychological changes that occur in pregnancy, as well as how they view their changing body image. Sexual desire may vary during pregnancy; it may decrease, increase, or remain unaltered, depending upon the stage of pregnancy and also upon other factors, which may include:

- Whether the pregnancy was planned or unplanned
- Whether the pregnancy was conceived naturally or with fertility treatment
- The response of others to the pregnancy
- Fears associated with pregnancy, e.g. harming the baby
- Stress, e.g. related to work, finances, etc.
- The woman's health and how tired she feels
- Her relationship with her partner.

Sexual intercourse is usually safe in pregnancy, provided both partners desire it and it does not cause discomfort. Sexual intercourse should be avoided in the relevant stage of pregnancy if there is:

- A history of recurrent miscarriages
- Vaginal bleeding
- Placenta praevia
- Premature dilation of the cervix
- Rupture of the membranes
- History of premature labour.

Some women may find penetrative sex uncomfortable during pregnancy and this could be due to any of the following physical factors:

- Pelvic vaso-congestion: pelvic floor exercises may help relieve this
- Vaginal congestion and reduced lubrication: lubricants may help
- Retroverted uterus: particularly in the first few week of pregnancy
- Subluxation of the symphysis pubis and sacro-iliac joints
- Weight of the partner on a gravid uterus later in pregnancy: alternative positions may be adopted
- Deep engagement of the fetal head

- Infections of the genital area: *Candida*, *Trichomonas vaginalis*, genital herpes, or warts
- Psychosocial factors may include tiredness, anxiety and fear, low self-esteem, poor body image, sexual guilt, and interpersonal problems between the woman and her partner.

## Sexuality and labour

Some of the procedures and examinations performed during labour involve the exposure of the genital area and penetrative vaginal examination by either the hand or a speculum. Many women find this very disturbing and difficult to cope with, not only because of the associated physical discomfort but also because of psychological feelings of vulnerability and power-lessness. This is especially relevant to women who have been sexually abused. There is an increased need for awareness of these factors by mid-wives and doctors, who often perform these examinations in a ritualistic manner and often without a sound rationale.

Obstetric procedures, including artificial rupture of the membranes (ARM), episiotomies, instrumental deliveries, and Caesarean sections, can also have a profound effect on a woman's sexuality. Many women find these procedures traumatic and they can have long-term consequences for sexual relationships.

The experience of seeing their significant other in childbirth can affect the partner's sexuality. It can be a very powerful and overwhelming experience, which will bond the couple together, but it may also be a traumatic experience. The partner may feel responsible for the pain and procedures their significant other may be undergoing, or their reaction could be linked with feelings of inadequacy and powerlessness. In extreme cases this experience has been known to cause impotency for male partners.

Midwives and obstetricians need to be aware of the implications of obstetric procedures and the traumatic effects they can have on the lives of couples who have been in their care.

## Sexuality postnatally

Sexuality following childbirth is a much neglected area that is inadequately addressed by many midwives and health professionals. Sexual behaviour and sexual health of women following childbirth have been shown to be influenced by profound psychological, interpersonal, social, and physical factors.[31] Many women are anxious about their bodies following the birth of a child and this is linked to perineal pain, soreness, and a decreased sense of attractiveness. Sexual activity and enjoyment following childbirth is usually diminished for up to 1 year.

### Resuming sexual relations

There is no set time when to resume sexual intercourse. It is more important that it is the right time for both of the partners. It is advisable to wait 3 weeks before having penetrative sex. It is important to avoid deliberately blowing air into the vagina during oral sex during pregnancy and in the weeks following birth, as this may cause an air embolism. Contraception needs consideration before resuming sexual intercourse, as the woman will ovulate prior to menstruating. Some women will experience dyspareunia for a while following childbirth, but if this does not resolve, they should be referred for medical advice.

Common causes of postnatal dyspareunia include:
- Decreased vaginal lubrication, associated with either breastfeeding or diminished sexual arousal
- Inflammation and infection
- Contracture and scarring of the perineum
- Sensitive hymenal or skin tags through malalignment of perineal repair.

## Breastfeeding and sexuality

Women who breastfeed may find that they and their partners have a diminished sexual desire, whilst others may find it enhanced. The physiological and psychological experiences associated with breastfeeding may reduce sexual libido for the woman and also reduce vaginal lubrication. Tenderness of the breasts and leakage of milk may inhibit women from sexual activity whilst some partners may find it off-putting.

It is normal for some women to feel sexual arousal whilst breastfeeding; this is a response to the oxytocin increase during breastfeeding.[32] Mothers will need reassurance as it may engender feelings of guilt and anxiety in the woman.

Many women will not menstruate whilst exclusively breastfeeding. Menstruation returns when the number of night-feeds declines or when the baby begins to have solid foods and breastfeeding is less frequent. Ovulation will occur before menstruation returns and the mother needs to ensure adequate contraception if another pregnancy is to be avoided.

## Maternity care for lesbian mothers

When considering sexuality in relation to childbirth, it is important to acknowledge that some mothers are choosing to have babies outside of a heterosexual relationship and some will have a female partner. Many lesbian women have negative health-care experiences and therefore it is important that midwives provide support and information in a non-judgemental, sensitive, woman-centred approach that takes into consideration the individual mother's needs. Specific considerations are:
- Lesbians want to be treated, and be treated to the same standard, as everyone else whilst having their individual differences recognized and appreciated[33]
- Disclosure of sexual orientation should be confidential and not recorded in the notes
- Other health professionals should not be informed without the woman's expressed consent
- Provision of information should be appropriate to their needs
- The lesbian partners should be acknowledged as a couple and co-parents
- Creation of an atmosphere that acknowledges sexual diversity.

# References

31 De Judicibus MA, McCabe MP (2002). Psychological factors and the sexuality of pregnant and postpartum women. *J Sex Res* 39: 94–103.

32 Convery KM, Spatz DL (2009). Sexuality and breastfeeding: what do you know? *MCN Am J Matern Child Nurs* 34: 218–23.

33 Dibley LB (2009). *Experiences of lesbian parents in the UK: interactions with midwives. Evidence-based midwifery*. Available at: &#8734; www.rcm.org.uk/learning-and-career/learning-and-research/ebm-articles/experiences-of-lesbian-parents-in-the-uk-0.

## Preparing the parents for birth

'*Antenatal education is a crucial component of antenatal care, yet practice and research demonstrate that women and men now seek far more than the traditional approach of a birth and parenting program attended in the final weeks of pregnancy*'.[34]

Many women having their first baby find themselves isolated from a social support network, having moved away from where they were brought up and working full-time, which isolates them from neighbours and the surrounding community. Through attendance at antenatal classes, parents may benefit from meeting new friends who will be going through the same experiences.

Parent education classes can also provide an opportunity to discuss fears and worries and to exchange views with other parents-to-be, as well as providing information about aspects of pregnancy, labour, birth, and the care of the baby. Special classes may be developed, for instance, for teenagers or women experiencing multiple pregnancies.

Parents attending antenatal classes need to:
• Obtain balanced, realistic information so they know what to expect
• Learn skills that will help them to cope during labour
• Know about the emotional and social aspects of birth and being a parent
• Learn about life after birth and caring for their new baby.

### Antenatal class management

Managing an antenatal class requires practice, and experience can be gained from working alongside an experienced class leader. The main points for the midwife who facilitates a class to consider are listed below.
• It is important to have received good preparation in adult learning techniques and to have gained confidence in managing and leading small interactive learning groups.
• Continuity of course leadership is essential to avoid duplication or omission of content and, more importantly, because the leader has to earn the trust of the group, in order to build relationships that enable the group to reflect on and discuss sensitive issues.
• Lectures are of limited value; it is more important to give information in short sessions that allow the learning of practical skills and subsequent discussion.
• Parents need to have the opportunity to learn about, and to try out, self-help strategies for dealing with labour.
• Topics such as labour pain, crying babies, exhaustion, and postnatal mental health issues need to be given a realistic perspective.

### Reference

34 Svensson J, Barclay L, Cooke M (2008). Effective antenatal education: strategies recommended by expectant and new parents. *J Perinat Educ* 17: 33–42.

# The birth plan

Discuss the birth plan with the woman and take opportunities to support her in her choices for the birth at any point during pregnancy. As the birth becomes imminent, record her wishes and give her the opportunity to discuss any concerns in the last few weeks of the pregnancy.

A birth plan should be flexible enough to take into account the unexpected. Enable the woman to appreciate that labour does not always go to plan. The following are some suggestions of things a woman may wish to discuss for inclusion in her plan.

• The place of birth will have been organized early in pregnancy, but this may alter if significant changes occur such as the presentation and position of the fetus or if the pregnancy goes beyond the due date by more than 1 week.
• Birth companion—name of who the woman wants to have with her in labour. This may be her partner, or a female relative, or a friend.
• Positions for labour and birth. Provide explanations of the benefits of certain positions and remaining mobile for as long as possible.
• Pain relief. Explain the risks and benefits of methods of pain relief and their effect on labour and on the fetus, so the woman makes an informed choice about her preferences.
• Eating and drinking during labour. Preference within a range of suitable easily digested foods and drinks can be expressed, provided the mother remains at low risk during her labour.
• The third stage of labour. Discuss how this is to be managed and how this may need to change if her risk of haemorrhage alters.
• The need for perineal suturing. Small first-degree tears need not be sutured if they are not actively bleeding. There is limited evidence to support non-suturing of larger tears or of second-degree tears.[35]
• The first feed, skin-to-skin contact, and breast crawl. If breast feeding, the baby will be encouraged to feed during the first hour after birth. If left in close skin-to-skin contact the baby may crawl and seek out the breast unaided. All mothers should be offered the opportunity for early skin-to-skin contact with their baby.
• Discuss the administration of prophylactic vitamin K for the prevention of haemorrhagic disease of the newborn.
• Discuss any cultural or religious customs the mother may wish to observe.

## Reference

35 Kettle C, Tohill S (2008). Perineal care: non-suturing of muscle and skin in first- and second-degree tears. *BMJ Clin Evid* 2008 pii: 1401. Available at: ℜ www.ncbi.nlm.nih.gov/pmc/articles/PMC2907946/.

# Doulas

The term 'doula' has its origins in Ancient Greece and refers to a woman that is trained and has experience in assisting a woman in pregnancy, through to birth and beyond. It is important that women recognize that a doula is there in a purely advisory and supportive capacity and is not a mid-wife, nurse, or medical practitioner. Doulas do not provide medical, nursing, midwifery, or therapeutic care, nor should they comment on, interpret, or judge the care that is provided.

During pregnancy, doulas are able to:

• Access resources and information so that women are able to make informed choices about their pregnancy, labour, and birth

• Refer women to classes such as antenatal fitness, birth preparation, lactation classes, pregnancy yoga, and also pregnancy massage services

• Assist in preparing for the birth and creating a birth plan.

Following a successful pilot study, a programme of doula training has been initiated in a large city in the north of England.[36] Doulas receive accredited training and can support vulnerable women through late pregnancy, birth, and the early postnatal period.

## Reference

36 Sheffield City Council. *Become a doula volunteer.* Available at: ℛ www.sheffield.gov.uk/caresupport/childfam/childrens-social-care/doula-project.html.

# Chapter 9

# Infections and sepsis

# Antenatal screening

The Department of Health has published standards to support the UK Antenatal Screening Programme on screening for infectious diseases in pregnancy.[1] These standards are both generic and specific and are part of a wider initiative to establish a quality-assured national screening programme. Responsibilities in the trust/strategic health authority, clinic, or laboratory are clarified in the standards. The information below concentrates on the responsibilities at clinical level.

## Generic standards for infectious diseases

All pregnant women are offered screening for syphilis, HIV, and hepatitis B as an integral part of their antenatal care during their first and all subsequent pregnancies. Repeat testing during pregnancy is not usually necessary. The women have a right to decline screening.

Pregnant women arriving in labour who have not had antenatal care elsewhere are to be offered screening, priority being given to HIV and hepatitis B, and presumptive action is taken on a preliminary positive result until such time as the result is confirmed. If an HIV test result will not be available in time, appropriate preventive measures should be offered. Use of rapid test devices may be appropriate in this context.

Screening is only performed with documented consent, though this does not require a signature from the patient and the usual standards of confidentiality apply.

## Screening for rubella antibodies

- Congenital rubella syndrome was first described in 1941.
- Rubella is now extremely rare in the UK, and tests are likely to confirm *absence* of the infection
- If the rubella virus is contracted during the first 8 weeks of pregnancy there is an 80% risk of malformations, microcephaly, and severe learning difficulties.
- If the virus is contracted after 9 weeks of gestation there is a 20% risk of deafness and brain damage. Handicap is rare after the 16th week.
- In order to prevent congenital rubella syndrome all children are offered protection from the virus with the MMR vaccine.
  - Emphasis is now ensuring a high uptake of the MMR vaccine.
  - Women are no longer screened during early pregnancy, following UK National Screening Committee advice.
- If a pregnant woman reports recent contact with an infected individual her immune status is confirmed. A titre >10IU suggests immunity.
- If the titre is <10IU the test is repeated 2–3 weeks later. A fourfold increase in the titre suggests a recent infection.
- If a woman presents >10–14 days after exposure a high IgM titre indicates viraemia in the last 4 weeks.
- If infected in early pregnancy with a high risk of abnormality, termination of pregnancy would be offered.

## Reference

1 Public Health England (2010). *Infectious diseases in pregnancy screening: programme standards.* Available at: ℡ www.gov.uk/government/publications/infectious-diseases-in-pregnancy-screening-programme-standards.

## Further reading

National Institute for Health and Care Excellence (2015). *Rubella. Scenario: Pregnant—suspected/confirmed rubella or possible exposure.* Clinical Knowledge Summaries. Available at: ℡ cks.nice.org.uk/rubella#!scenario:1.

UK National Screening Committee (2012). *The UK NSC recommendation on Rubella susceptibility screening in pregnancy.* Available at: ℡ legacy.screening.nhs.uk/rubellasusceptibility.

# Screening for syphilis

Syphilis can seriously complicate pregnancy and result in spontaneous abortion (commonly at around 18–20 weeks' gestation), stillbirth, IUGR, and perinatal death.

- Antenatal screening for syphilis is well established, forming part of the routine screening of all pregnant women during the first or early second trimester.
- The UK National Screening Committee (2013) recommends continuation of the existing screening programme.
- Women who are at risk will be retested in the late second to early third trimester, as infection acquired during pregnancy still poses a significant risk to the fetus.
- Women who screen positive for the Venereal Disease Research Laboratory (VDRL) test will have this result confirmed by retesting with a *Treponema*-specific assay (*Treponema pallidum* haemagglutination (TPHA) test) and will be treated with antibiotics such as amoxicillin.

**Further reading**

UK National Screening Committee (2013). *The UK NSC recommendation on syphilis screening in pregnancy*. Available at: ℬ legacy.screening.nhs.uk/syphilis.

## HIV screening

# HIV screening

Pregnant women should be offered screening for HIV infection early in antenatal care because appropriate antenatal interventions can reduce mother-to-child transmission of HIV infection. A system of clear referral paths should be established in each unit or department so that pregnant women who are diagnosed with an HIV infection are managed and treated by the appropriate specialist teams.[2] The Department of Health[3] has produced guidelines for the management of HIV screening during pregnancy and the following information is taken from this report.

- Most HIV-infected children in this country have acquired the infection from their mothers. There are now interventions that can reduce the risk of mother-to-child transmission of HIV from 25% to 2%. In order to take advantage of these it is vital to diagnose the infection before birth.
- HIV prevalence varies across the UK, but antenatal screening and the chance to offer treatment to affected women remain a cost-effective screening strategy.
- Information about the test is given to the woman during the booking interview. Pre- and post-test counselling should be offered. The nature of the test and how she will receive the results are explained.
- The implications of a positive result need to be explored. The woman is informed personally if the result is positive and she will be offered specialist counselling and support which is available for partners and family if requested.
- Women found to be positive are referred for specialist HIV treatment and advice about how to manage their own infection and interventions to reduce the risk of vertical and sexual transmission.
- Discussions cover the use of antiretrovirals and Caesarean section, early treatment and care for the child, and decisions about breastfeeding.
- The implications of a negative result and general sexual health are discussed. This is also an opportunity to discuss the dangers of becoming infected during pregnancy or lactation.
- Women who refuse an HIV test at booking should be re-offered a test, and should they decline again a third offer of a test should be made at 36 weeks.
- Women presenting to services for the first time in labour should be offered a point-of-care test (POCT).[4] A POCT may also be considered for the infant of a woman who refuses testing antenatally.[4]
- In areas of higher seroprevalence, or where there are other risk factors, women who are HIV-negative at booking may be offered a routine second test at 34–36 weeks' gestation as recommended in the British HIV Association (BHIVA) pregnancy guidelines.[4]

# References

2 National Institute for Health and Care Excellence (2008). *Antenatal care for uncomplicated pregnancies*. NICE guidelines CG62. Available at: ℰ www.nice.org.uk/guidance/cg62.

3 Public Health England (2010). *Infectious diseases in pregnancy screening: programme standards*. Available at: ℰ www.gov.uk/government/publications/infectious-diseases-in-pregnancy-screening-programme-standards.

4 British HIV Association (2014). *British HIV Association guidelines for the management of HIV infection in pregnant women 2012 (2014 interim review)*. Available at: ℰ www.bhiva.org/documents/Guidelines/Pregnancy/2012/BHIVA-Pregnancy-guidelines-update-2014.pdf.

# Further reading

Royal College of Obstetricians and Gynaecologists (2010). *HIV in pregnancy, management (Green-top guideline No. 39)*. Available at: ℰ www.rcog.org.uk/en/guidelines-research-services/guidelines/gtg39/.

# Group B haemolytic *Streptococcus*

Group B haemolytic *Streptococcus* (GBS) is one of a number of common bacteria found in the gut of 30% of men and women. It is estimated that 25% of women carry this organism in the vaginal tract with no ill effect. Its significance is that it can be transmitted to the baby during delivery and is the most common cause of fatal bacterial infection in the early neonatal period.

## Incidence

The incidence of early-onset GBS (EOGBS) disease in the UK in the absence of systematic screening or widespread intrapartum antibiotic prophylaxis (IAP) is 0.5/1000 births, which is similar to that seen in the USA after universal screening and IAP, despite comparable vaginal carriage rates (RCOG 2012).[5]

## Presentation

There are two ways in which the infection will present:
• 90% of the infections are early onset, and 70% of babies are symptomatic at birth
• 10% are late onset, occurring after 48h and up to 3 months after birth.

## Screening

There is little organized antenatal screening for GBS carriage in the UK at present and most maternity units rely on risk factor estimation to identify carriers and situations where the infection may be transmitted to the neonate.

*Risk factors*
• Previous baby affected by GBS.
• GBS bacteriuria detected in the present pregnancy.
• Preterm labour.
• Prolonged rupture of the membranes.
• Pyrexia during labour.

IAP is offered to women who have any of these risk factors. This approach differs from that in the USA where all pregnant women are offered bacteriological screening at 35–37 weeks' gestation. This involves taking vaginal and rectal swabs, and all women who carry GBS are offered IAP. This results in 27% of all pregnant women being offered IAP during labour and a reduction in EOGBS disease of 86%.

Antenatal screening and treatment may carry disadvantages for the mother and baby. These include anaphylaxis, increased medicalization of labour and the neonatal period, and possible infection with antibiotic-resistant organisms.

The Royal College of Obstetricians and Gynaecologists (RCOG)[6] has made the following recommendations in the absence of clinical trials and recent data on the prevalence of GBS carriage in the UK.
• Routine antenatal screening is not recommended.
• Antenatal treatment with penicillin is not recommended if GBS is detected incidentally.

- IAP should be considered if GBS is detected incidentally.
- There is no good evidence to support IAP in women who carried GBS in a previous pregnancy.
- IAP should be offered to women who had a previous baby with GBS disease.
- The argument for IAP is stronger in the presence of two or more risk factors.
- IAP should be offered, after discussion, to women with GBS bacteriuria.
- Antibiotic prophylaxis is not required for women undergoing elective Caesarean section in the absence of labour and with intact membranes.
- Antibiotic prophylaxis is unnecessary for women with preterm rupture of membranes unless they are in established labour.
- Benzylpenicillin 3g should be administered IV as soon as possible after the onset of labour, and then 1.5g 4-hourly. Clindamycin 900mg should be given IV 8-hourly in the event of penicillin allergy.

(➔ See also Chapter 3.)

## Reference

5 Royal College of Obstetricians and Gynaecologists (2012). *The prevention of early-onset neonatal group B streptococcal disease (Green-top guideline No. 36)*. Available at: ℅ www.rcog.org.uk/globalassets/documents/guidelines/gtg_36.pdf.

# Other infections

## Coughs and colds

These common infections pose little threat to the fetus and symptom relief is all that is necessary. Advise fluids, rest, and paracetamol up to normal maximum doses, e.g. 1g four times a day. Inhaled decongestants are safe but cough linctus should be avoided.

A productive cough could be a sign of bacterial infection requiring antibiotic treatment and the woman should be referred to her GP.

## Influenza

Pregnant women and their unborn children are at high risk of morbidity and mortality from influenza infection.

Flu can cause maternal intensive care admission, preterm labour, low birthweight, and other problems for the mother and baby. One in 11 maternal deaths during 2009–2012 was caused by influenza. Public Health England and the WHO therefore recommend annual influenza vaccination for all pregnant women.

The injectable vaccine is inactivated and does not contain live virus; the vaccine can be given safely during any trimester and there are no increased risks of maternal complications or poor fetal outcomes associated with inactivated influenza vaccination in pregnancy.

The most common side effect is a sore arm at the site of injection; occasionally mothers may briefly feel systemically unwell due to an immune response; the vaccine cannot cause influenza infection as it does not contain live virus.

Flu vaccination reduces the risk of prematurity and the risk of low birthweight. The vaccine provides passive immunity to the fetus, which can protect the infant for up to 6 months following birth. The vaccine reduces adverse maternal outcomes attributed to influenza infection.

Midwives should be aware of vaccination arrangements in their local area and encourage mothers to understand the risks of influenza and benefits of vaccination. Patient information leaflets are available to support these messages.

## Urinary tract infections

Women should be offered screening by mid-stream urine (MSU) culture for asymptomatic bacteriuria early in pregnancy, as identification and treatment reduce the risk of preterm birth.[6]

Around one in 25 women develop a urinary tract infection during pregnancy. The symptoms are:
- Discomfort or a burning sensation on micturition
- Pain in the bladder region/lower pelvis
- Frequency of micturition.

An ascending infection involving the kidneys or bloodstream may cause:
- Loin pain
- Vomiting
- Fever

- Uterine contractions—the symptoms of premature labour may mask a urinary tract infection and an MSU should be obtained for culture to rule this out.

Mild infections are treated with oral antibiotics, but a more serious infection requires admission to hospital for IV antibiotic therapy and rest.

## Chickenpox

This is a fairly common infection and many women are exposed during pregnancy.

If a woman has already had chickenpox, there is no risk to the fetus, but if a woman has never had chickenpox and contracts it before 20 weeks' gestation, there is a risk of the fetus developing a severe infection—chickenpox syndrome.

Women who have not had chickenpox, or are known to be seronegative for chickenpox, should be advised to avoid contact with chickenpox and shingles during pregnancy and to inform health-care workers of a potential exposure without delay

When contact occurs with chickenpox or shingles, a careful history must be taken to confirm the significance of the contact and the susceptibility of the patient.

Pregnant women with an uncertain or no previous history of chickenpox, or who come from tropical or subtropical countries, who have been exposed to infection should have a blood test to determine varicella-zoster virus (VZV) immunity or non-immunity.

If the pregnant woman is not immune to VZV and she has had a significant exposure, she should be offered varicella-zoster immunoglobulin (VZIG) as soon as possible.

VZIG is effective when given up to 10 days after contact (in the case of continuous exposures, this is defined as 10 days from the appearance of the rash in the index case). Non-immune pregnant women who have been exposed to chickenpox should be managed as potentially infectious from 8 to 28 days after exposure if they receive VZIG and from 8 to 21 days after exposure if they do not receive VZIG.

A pregnant woman who develops a chickenpox rash should be isolated from other pregnant women when she attends a GP surgery or a hospital for assessment.

Oral aciclovir should be prescribed for pregnant women with chickenpox if they present within 24h of the onset of the rash and if they are 20+0 weeks of gestation or beyond. Use of aciclovir before 20+0 weeks should also be considered. Aciclovir is not licensed for use in pregnancy and the risks and benefits of its use should be discussed with the woman. IV aciclovir should be given to all pregnant women with severe chickenpox.

If maternal infection occurs in the last 4 weeks of a woman's pregnancy, there is a significant risk of varicella infection of the newborn. A planned delivery should normally be avoided for at least 7 days after the onset of the maternal rash to allow for the passive transfer of antibodies from mother to child, provided that continuing the pregnancy does not pose any additional risks to the mother or baby.

A neonatologist should be informed of the birth of all babies born to women who have developed chickenpox at any gestation during pregnancy. Women with chickenpox should breastfeed if they wish to and are well enough to do so.

## Toxoplasmosis

Toxoplasmosis is caused by the parasite *Toxoplasma gondii*, which is found in raw meat and in cats that eat raw meat and their faeces. It rarely causes illness in an adult, although it can present as a flu-like illness with swollen lymph glands (➔ see also Food safety, p. 98).

In pregnant women it is of concern as it can lead to fetal infection and the following potential problems:

- Miscarriage
- Stillbirth
- Growth problems
- Blindness
- Brain damage
- Epilepsy
- Deafness.

Prevention is the best strategy. Women may be offered pyrimethamine or sulfadiazine to limit transmission of the infection.

Advise pregnant women to:

- Cook all meat thoroughly until there are no pink areas and the juices are clear
- Wash hands, utensils, and surface areas after preparing raw meat
- Wash soil from fruit and vegetables before eating
- Always use gloves when gardening and wash hands afterwards
- Ask someone else to clean litter trays if a cat owner, or to wear gloves and wash hands thoroughly afterwards.

## Reference

6 National Institute for Health and Care Excellence (2008). *Antenatal care for uncomplicated pregnancies*. NICE guidelines CG62. Available at: ℘ www.nice.org.uk/guidance/cg62.

## Further reading

Public Health England (2015). *Influenza vaccination in pregnancy: information for healthcare professionals*. Available at: ℘ www.gov.uk/government/uploads/system/uploads/attachment_data/file/393974/Influenza_vaccination_in_pregnancy_factsheet_v15_CT__2_.pdf.

Royal College of Obstetricians and Gynaecologists (2015). *Chickenpox in pregnancy (Green-top guideline No. 13)*. Available at: ℘ www.rcog.org.uk/globalassets/documents/guidelines/gtg13.pdf.

## Sepsis

# Sepsis

The MBRRACE Report[7] identified that 25% of UK women who died following birth had systemic sepsis (severe infection). Prompt recognition and treatment and action *can* make the difference between life and death; in many cases decline and death may be prevented if the cause is identified early and acted upon before the woman deteriorates beyond the point of reversibility.

## 'Think Sepsis'

Bacteraemia, which can be present in the absence of pyrexia or a raised white cell count, can progress rapidly to severe sepsis and septic shock, leading to collapse. The key actions for diagnosis and management of sepsis are:

- Timely recognition
- Fast administration of IV antibiotics
- Quick involvement of experts—senior review is essential.

Sepsis usually begins with pyrexia and a restless mental state with a warm, flushed complexion. Then hypotension, tachycardia, cold extremities, cyanosis, tachypnoea, jaundice, and coma may occur as late signs. Predisposing factors include pyelonephritis, prolonged rupture of membranes, pyrexia of 38°C or above, operative delivery, and manual removal of the placenta.

Organisms commonly associated with septic shock include:

- *Escherichia coli*
- *Pneumococcus*
- *Klebsiella* sp.
- *Proteus mirabilis*
- *Pseudomonas aeruginosa*
- *Staphylococcus aureus*
- *Bacteroides* sp., *Streptococcus* groups A, B, and D—haemolytic *Streptococcus*.

Repeated presentation to the GP or community midwife, or repeated self-referral to the obstetric triage or day assessment unit, should be considered a 'red flag' and warrant a thorough assessment of the woman to investigate for signs of sepsis.

When presented with an unwell pregnant, labouring, or recently pregnant woman, health professionals should take appropriate observations and act on them:

- In early stages of deterioration there are often important clinical changes in respiratory rate, oxygen saturation, BP, heart rate, temperature, and conscious/mental status which may go unrecognized if not systematically recorded.
- *Diagnosis depends on careful observation and documentation of signs by the midwife*. A 'track and trigger' system that documents continuous measurement of vital signs and 'triggers' a predetermined response of intervention/review has been shown to help trap and/or avoid deterioration early and help mitigate deterioration by initiating an early response.[8] The MEOWS (modified early obstetric warning system) chart is a simple bedside screening tool which identifies women at risk

of morbidity, whilst a diagnostic test seeks to confirm its presence definitively.

- Obtain an MSU, a high vaginal swab, and introital and rectal swabs and send for urgent culture.
- Obtain blood cultures. Take venous blood samples for FBC and platelets, C-reactive protein (CRP), clotting, urea and electrolytes (U/E), and liver function tests (LFTs) and send for screening.
- Arrange a chest X-ray.
- Senior advice should be promptly sought from a microbiologist and the administration of IV antibiotics should be initiated (e.g. piperacillin, tazobactam, netilmicin). If the woman fails to respond to the first-choice antibiotic early advice from an infectious diseases physician should be sought.
- Severe septic shock may precipitate disseminated intravascular coagulation (DIC) (➔ see Disseminated intravascular coagulation, p. 500).
- Admit to a high dependency area for observation and care by a midwife.

## References

7 Knight M, Kenyon S, Brocklehurst P, Neilson J, Shakespeare J, Kurinczuk JJ (eds.) on behalf of MBRRACE-UK (2014). *Saving Lives, Improving Mothers' Care: Lessons learned to inform future maternity care from the UK and Ireland Confidential Enquiries into Maternal Deaths and Morbidity 2009–12.* Oxford: National Perinatal Epidemiology Unit, University of Oxford. Available at: ℜ www.npeu. ox.ac.uk/mbrrace-uk/reports.

8 Singh S, McGlennan A, England A, Simons R (2012). A validation study of the CEMACH recommended modified early obstetric warning system (MEOWS). *Anaesthesia* 67: 12–18.

# Medical conditions during pregnancy

# Asthma

Asthma is the most common chronic disease in children and young adults and is on the increase; 4–8% of pregnant women have asthma. The condition is often underrecognized and suboptimally treated.[1]

### Effect of pregnancy on asthma

- Asthma tends to improve in pregnancy especially during the last 12 weeks, but it can be very variable, with some remaining stable and others worsening.
- Breathlessness due to the increasing size of the uterus is sometimes mistaken for worsening asthma.
- Many women experience a worsening of their symptoms because they stop taking their asthma medication because of concerns about the effects on the fetus.
- Women who deteriorate during pregnancy tend to have the most severe asthma.

### Effects of asthma on pregnancy

- Good control is essential for maternal and fetal well-being. Poor control is associated with PIH, pre-eclampsia, increased Caesarean section, preterm delivery, IUGR, and low birthweight.
- Asthma treatment during pregnancy is no different to that at other times and the inhaled medications are safe.
- The risk of harm to the fetus from severe or chronically undertreated asthma outweighs any small risk from the medications used to control asthma.
- Very little inhaled medication reaches the fetus.
- More harm is likely from withholding treatment than from continuing it.

### Management of asthma during pregnancy

- Objective monitoring of lung function.
- Avoiding or controlling asthma triggers.
- Patient education and individualized pharmacological therapy.
- Counsel women with asthma regarding the importance and safety of continuing their asthma medications during pregnancy to ensure good asthma control.
- Those with persistent asthma should be monitored by peak expiratory flow rate, spirometry to measure the forced expiratory volume in 1s, or both.
- For women with poorly controlled asthma during pregnancy there should be close liaison between the respiratory physician and obstetrician, with early referral to critical care physicians for women with acute severe asthma.
- The ultimate goal of asthma therapy is maintaining adequate oxygenation of the fetus by prevention of hypoxic episodes in the mother.
- Asthma exacerbations should be aggressively managed, with a goal of alleviating asthma symptoms and attaining peak expiratory flow rate or forced expiratory volume in 1s of 70% predicted or more.

- Deliver high-flow oxygen immediately to maintain saturation 94–98%.
- Continuous fetal monitoring is recommended for acute severe asthma.
- Women with asthma may safely use all forms of usual labour analgesia.
- If anaesthesia is required, regional blockade is preferable to general anaesthesia in women with asthma.
- Pregnancies complicated by moderate or severe asthma may benefit from ultrasound for fetal growth and accurate dating and antenatal assessment of fetal well-being.
- Asthma medications should be continued during labour, and the mother should be encouraged to breastfeed.

## Reference

1 British Thoracic Society and Scottish Intercollegiate Guidelines Network (2014). Treatment of acute asthma in adults. In: British Thoracic Society and Scottish Intercollegiate Guidelines Network. *British guideline on the management of asthma. A national clinical guideline*, pp. 85–90. Available at: www.brit-thoracic.org.uk/document-library/clinical-information/asthma/btssign-asthma-guideline-2014/.

# Cardiac conditions

Women with congenital heart disease are surviving to become pregnant in greater numbers due to advances in surgery and better management of care. Antenatal care is a complex issue and early referral to a specialist centre is advisable so that the specialist midwife, cardiologist, obstetrician, anaesthetist, fetal medicine specialist, haematologist, neonatologist, and cardiac nurse can meet the woman to plan her care and review her progress regularly. This appointment should take place as early as possible as she is a high-risk case and requires multidisciplinary care.

## Significance of cardiac conditions

- Congenital heart disease occurs in 0.8% of newborns.
- Advances in medical treatment and surgery have resulted in 85% survival rates.
- Cardiac disease is the leading cause of maternal death in the UK with 54 deaths in the last triennium.[2]
- Cardiac conditions have many implications for pregnancy due to the normal associated cardiovascular changes:
  - Peripheral vasodilation which is the body's initial response to pregnancy
  - Decreased peripheral resistance
  - Increase in plasma volume by 50%
  - Increase in RBCs of 20%—physiological haemodilution giving the impression of anaemia but is normal to pregnancy
  - Cardiac output increases by 50%.

## Cardiac conditions

Cardiac conditions can be congenital or acquired and are classified as:
- Low risk:
  - Uncomplicated septal defects
  - Mild/moderate pulmonary stenosis
  - Corrected anatomical defects such as transposition of the great vessels or Fallot's tetralogy.
- Medium risk:
  - Cyanosed mother with pulmonary stenosis
  - Prosthetic cardiac valves
  - Marfan's syndrome.
- High risk:
  - Pulmonary hypertension
  - Tight mitral stenosis
  - Severe aortic stenosis
  - Myocardial infarction
  - Any case where heart failure is difficult to control.

## Assessment

This can be difficult as normal pregnancy symptoms mirror the symptoms of cardiac disease. The following are all associated with normal pregnancy; however, the woman should be encouraged to report any new symptoms no matter how subtle:

- Shortness of breath—dyspnoea, at rest, or on exertion
- Raised respiratory rate—tachypnoea
- Tiredness
- Dizziness
- Fainting—syncope.

The woman should be examined at every visit for:
- Cyanosis
- Pallor
- Prominent neck veins
- Peripheral oedema
- Rapid weight gain
- BP, heart rate, and rhythm
- Auscultation of heart sounds to record type and grade of murmurs
- Auscultation of the lung bases to detect pulmonary oedema.

## Investigations
- Electrocardiogram (ECG).
- Echocardiogram.
- 12- and 20 week scans.
- Fetal growth scans every 4 weeks.
- Exclude diabetes; avoid anaemia, and treat any infection.

## Management
Drug therapy will continue during the pregnancy and may involve the use of anticoagulants in some conditions. Regimens should be monitored closely, with individual drugs considered for their likely effect on pregnancy and the fetus.

Pregnancy itself raises the risk of acute myocardial infarction by 3- to 4-fold, with the risk being 30 times higher for women over the age of 40 years, compared with women aged less than 20 years.

The key component of good management is therefore a high index of suspicion for myocardial infarction in any pregnant woman presenting with chest pain.

The possibility of an aortic dissection should also be considered. All women with chest pain in pregnancy should have an ECG interpreted by someone who is skilled at detecting signs of cardiac ischaemia and infarction and, if the pain is severe, they should have a computed tomography (CT) or a magnetic resonance imaging (MRI) scan of the chest.

Because there are so many types of cardiac disease, often with very different implications, it is important that a risk assessment of any woman with a heart murmur or a history of any cardiac defect should be carried out early in pregnancy in a joint clinic attended by a consultant obstetrician, a cardiologist, and an anaesthetist.

Cardiovascular assessment should be carried out at every antenatal clinic. BP should be measured manually with a sphygmomanometer according to the recommendations of the British Hypertension Society.

A multidisciplinary meeting should take place at 32–34 weeks of gestation to establish a plan of management for delivery. Important features of such a plan include deciding who should be involved in supervising the labour, whether a Caesarean section is appropriate, whether bearing down is advisable in the second stage, and appropriate prophylaxis against post-partum haemorrhage (PPH) (routinely used oxytocic regimes can have major cardiovascular adverse effects; a low-dose oxytocin infusion is probably the safest option, and at Caesarean section prophylactic uterine compression sutures can be considered instead of oxytocics). The plan should also include post-partum management, including whether prophylaxis against thrombosis is appropriate, the length of post-partum stay in hospital, and the timing of cardiac and obstetric review.

The general principle of intrapartum management is to minimize cardiovascular stress. In most cases, this will be achieved by the use of early slow incremental epidural anaesthesia and assisted vaginal delivery. A Caesarean section is usually necessary only for obstetric indications.

## Reference

2  Knight M, Kenyon S, Brocklehurst P, Neilson J, Shakespeare J, Kurinczuk JJ (eds.) on behalf of MBRRACE-UK (2014). *Saving Lives, Improving Mothers' Care—Lessons learned to inform future maternity care from the UK and Ireland Confidential Enquiries into Maternal Deaths and Morbidity 2009–12.* Oxford: National Perinatal Epidemiology Unit, University of Oxford.

## Further reading

Royal College of Obstetricians and Gynaecologists (2011). *Cardiac disease and pregnancy. Good practice No. 13.* Available at: www.rcog.org.uk/globalassets/documents/guidelines/goodpractice13cardiacdiseaseandpregnancy.pdf.

# Diabetes

- Diabetes during pregnancy can be classified into three forms:
  - Insulin-dependent diabetes, which is present prior to pregnancy (type 1 diabetes)
  - Non-insulin-dependent diabetes (type 2 diabetes)
  - Gestational diabetes mellitus (GDM) or impaired glucose tolerance, which arises as a result of pregnancy and then resolves after the birth. The incidence is between 3% and 12% of the pregnant population. Overt diabetes will develop in 20–30% of women with GDM within 5 years.[3]
- Non-diabetic pregnant women are offered a glucose challenge screen to detect GDM if any two of the following risk factors are present:
  - Glycosuria on two occasions on testing at an antenatal visit (early morning sample)
  - History of diabetes in a close relative
  - Obesity, BMI >27
  - Previous baby weighing >4.5kg
  - Previous unexplained perinatal death
  - Previous baby with congenital malformations
  - Unexplained severe polyhydramnios (excess amniotic fluid in the uterus).
- Maternal complications which might arise in the pregnant diabetic client are related to poorly controlled glucose levels in the maternal serum:
  - Urinary tract infection
  - Vaginal infection
  - Polyhydramnios
  - PIH
  - Fetal macrosomia leading to shoulder dystocia.

## Fetal complications

- Congenital abnormality—four times higher than in non-diabetic women.
- Prematurity associated with delayed lung maturity.
- Perinatal death (due to the above conditions).
- 1:100 risk of the child themselves becoming diabetic.

## Carbohydrate metabolism during pregnancy (non-diabetic)

- Pregnancy itself is said to be diabetogenic as a result of changes due to the action of the pregnancy hormones.
- The fetal/placental unit alters glucose metabolism in the following ways:
  - From the tenth week fasting blood sugar progressively falls from 4 to 3.6mmol/L
  - The placenta produces a hormone called human placental lactogen, which increases the maternal tissue resistance to insulin
  - Blood glucose levels therefore are higher after meals and remain so for longer than in the non-pregnant state
  - More insulin is required by the body and output of insulin in the pancreas increases by 3–4 times the normal rate.

- Extra demands on the pancreatic β cells precipitate glucose intolerance or overt diabetes in women whose capacity to produce insulin was only just adequate prior to pregnancy (GDM).
- Utilization of fat stores results in raised free fatty acid and glycerol levels, making the woman more readily ketotic.

## Management of diabetes/gestational diabetes

- Diagnose GDM[4] if the woman has either:
  - A fasting plasma glucose level of 5.6mmol/L or above *or*
  - A 2h plasma glucose level of 7.8mmol/L or above.
- Women with type 2 diabetes may form the largest population of pre-pregnancy diabetics and be exposed to the same levels of risk related to pregnancy outcomes. Their condition may indeed be diagnosed for the first time during pregnancy due to screening for GDM. Careful monitoring of glycaemic control and provision of insulin as a replacement of, or in addition to, metformin therapy could improve outcomes.
- For women who develop GDM, a careful assessment of their insulin needs is required and therapy commenced in accordance with the need to control blood glucose levels in the prescribed range.

If the mother is already diabetic, her insulin requirements will be increased during pregnancy and her pregnancy will be monitored carefully.

- Advise pregnant women with any form of diabetes to maintain their capillary plasma glucose below the following target levels, if these are achievable without causing problematic hypoglycaemia:
  - Fasting: 5.3mmol/L
  - 1h after meals: 7.8mmol/L *or*
  - 2h after meals: 6.4mmol/L.
- Women with insulin-treated diabetes should be advised of the risks of hypoglycaemia and hypoglycaemia unawareness in pregnancy, particularly in the 1st trimester. Test urgently for ketonaemia if a pregnant woman with any form of diabetes presents with hyperglycaemia or is unwell, to exclude diabetic ketoacidosis.
- During pregnancy, women with insulin-treated diabetes should be provided with a concentrated glucose solution and women with type 1 diabetes should also be given glucagon; women and their partners or other family members should be instructed in their use.

## General principles of care for women with diabetes in pregnancy

- Ensure as much as possible that pregnancies are planned.
- Early booking (before the tenth week of pregnancy).
- Joint care with an endocrinologist specializing in diabetes.
- Blood sugar profiles every 2 weeks and glycosylated Hb monthly (HbA$_{1c}$).
- Advise women with diabetes who are planning to become pregnant to aim for the same capillary plasma glucose target ranges as recommended for all people with type 1 diabetes.
- Prevention of excessive maternal weight gain.

- Health-care professionals should be aware that the rapid-acting insulin analogues (aspart and lispro) have advantages over soluble human insulin during pregnancy, and should consider their use.
- Pregnant women with pre-existing diabetes should be offered retinal assessment by digital imaging with mydriasis using tropicamide following their first antenatal clinic appointment and again at 28 weeks if the first assessment is normal. If any diabetic retinopathy is present, an additional retinal assessment should be performed at 16–20 weeks. If retinal assessment has not been performed in the preceding 12 months, it should be offered as soon as possible after the first contact in pregnancy in women with pre-existing diabetes.
- If renal assessment has not been undertaken in the preceding 12 months in women with pre-existing diabetes, it should be arranged at the first contact in pregnancy. If serum creatinine is abnormal (120micromol/L or more) or if total protein excretion exceeds 2g/day, referral to a nephrologist should be considered (estimated glomerular filtration rate (eGFR) should not be used during pregnancy). Thromboprophylaxis should be considered for women with proteinuria above 5g/day (macroalbuminuria).
- Careful screening for urinary tract and vaginal infection, with prompt treatment.
- Discuss the need for a fetal anomaly scan in light of the increased risk of malformations.
- Careful monitoring of fetal growth by regular ultrasound scans.
- Advise pregnant women with type 1 or type 2 diabetes and no other complications to have an elective birth by induction of labour, or by an elective Caesarean section if indicated, between 37+0 weeks and 38+6 weeks of pregnancy.
- Advise women with gestational diabetes to give birth no later than 40+6 weeks, and offer elective birth (by induction of labour, or by Caesarean section if indicated) to women who have not given birth by this time.
- For women who were diagnosed with GDM and whose blood glucose levels returned to normal after the birth:
  - Offer lifestyle advice (including weight control, diet, and exercise)
  - Offer a fasting plasma glucose test 6–13 weeks after the birth to exclude diabetes (for practical reasons this might take place at the 6-week postnatal check)
  - If a fasting plasma glucose test has not been performed by 13 weeks, offer a fasting plasma glucose test, or an $HbA_{1c}$ test if a fasting plasma glucose test is not possible, after 13 weeks
  - Do not routinely offer a 75g 2h oral glucose tolerance test (OGTT).
- Offer an annual $HbA_{1c}$ test to women who were diagnosed with GDM who have a negative postnatal test for diabetes.

## References

3 Bellamy L, Casas JP, Hingorani AD, Williams D (2009). Type 2 diabetes mellitus after gestational diabetes: a systematic review and meta-analysis. *Lancet* **373**: 1773–9.

4 National Institute for Health and Care Excellence (2015). *Diabetes in pregnancy: management from preconception to the postnatal period*. NICE guidelines NG3 Available at: ℬ www.nice.org.uk/guidance/ng3/chapter/Key-priorities-for-implementation.

# Epilepsy

It is estimated that one in 250 of all pregnancies in the UK are in women with epilepsy. These women face unique problems when it comes to controlling their epilepsy during a pregnancy.[5]

Women with epilepsy taking AEDs have a 2–3 times greater risk of having a child with a major congenital malformation than women without epilepsy. Nevertheless, it is still overwhelmingly likely that a woman with epilepsy will have a normal pregnancy and give birth to a healthy child.[5]

The pregnancy should be identified early so adjustments to anticonvulsive therapy can be made and a higher dose of folic acid (5mg) can commence. Some AEDs have been associated with altered concentrations of folate and an increased incidence of NTDs.

The main problems in pregnancy are related to the number of seizures experienced. During pregnancy some women notice a reduction in the number of seizures, but others may experience an increase.

Generalized convulsive seizures may cause metabolic alterations in the mother's body, increase her blood pressure, and change her circulation pattern. There is also an increased risk of injury to the fetus from falls.

An epileptic seizure presents as follows:[6]
• Presence of aura
• Generalized or focal motor movements
• Changes in respiration
• Loss of consciousness and loss of bowel/bladder function.

Symptoms following a seizure include:
• Amnesia
• Lethargy
• Headache
• Muscle aches and transient focal weakness.

## Management of epilepsy during and after pregnancy

Recommendations for management during pregnancy:[5,6]
• Continue folic acid 5mg daily until at least 12 weeks' gestation
• Adjust anticonvulsant regime if necessary on clinical grounds
• Offer serum screening at 16 weeks and a detailed anomaly scan at 18–22 weeks
• For women on enzyme-inducing anticonvulsants, prescribe oral vitamin K 20mg daily from 36 weeks until delivery. Commence earlier if judged to be at risk of preterm delivery.

Postnatal care should include advice about the likelihood of breakthrough seizure in the post-partum period. This is related to hormonal change and lack of sleep.

It is difficult to distinguish eclamptic seizures from an epileptic seizure.[6]

The initial management of patients presenting with active seizure in pregnancy should include maintenance of the airway, oxygenation, and support of adequate perfusion.

Immediate attention must also be applied to the fetus, particularly if it has reached a viable gestational age.

Whilst an ongoing evaluation is in progress to investigate the organic causes, administration of parenteral benzodiazepine, followed by IV phenytoin at conventional doses, is a reasonable approach. A CT scan of the brain is required to differentiate the central organic cause of seizures from that of eclampsia, but concern for safety of the mother and her fetus because of radiation exposure remains.

## References

5  National Institute for Health and Care Excellence (2012). Women and girls with epilepsy. In: National Institute for Health and Care Excellence. *Epilepsies: diagnosis and management*. Available at: ℘ www.nice.org.uk/guidance/cg137/chapter/1-Guidance#women-and-girls-with-epilepsy.

6  Hart L, Sibai BM (2013). Seizures in pregnancy: epilepsy, eclampsia and stroke. *Semin Perinatol* 37: 207–24. Also available at: ℘ www.sciencedirect.com/science/article/pii/S0146000513000487.

# Thromboembolic disorders

Venous thromboembolism (VTE) is the obstruction of a blood vessel, usually a large vein, with thrombotic material carried in the blood from its site of origin to block another vessel.

Several factors are associated with an increased risk of VTE during pregnancy:

- Increasing maternal age
- Increasing parity
- Operative delivery
- Immobility and bed rest
- Obesity
- Dehydration
- Thrombophilia.

According to Knight et al.[7] it is particularly important to recognize the risk of VTE in the mother with a raised BMI of 30 or above. The risks are present from the first trimester onwards. In the years 2003–2005, 41 women died of VTE and 16 of these women had a BMI of 30 or over.[7]

Thromboembolic disorders can be categorized as:

- Superficial thrombophlebitis
- DVT
- Pulmonary embolism (PE).

## Superficial thrombophlebitis

- This is caused by the formation of a clot in a superficial varicose vein as a result of stasis and the hypercoagulable state of pregnancy.
- Varicose veins commonly occur in pregnancy because of increased venous pressure in the legs and the action of progesterone.
- A red, inflamed area appears over the vein, which feels firm on palpation.

*Management*

- Encourage the woman to mobilize wearing thromboembolic deterrent stockings (TEDS).
- Instruct her to raise her leg when sitting and give her exercises to be carried out daily.
- Local warming applications may provide additional comfort.
- The inflammation should subside within a few days and the clot in the superficial vein causes no immediate hazard.
- Observe the woman closely for signs of DVT.

## Deep vein thrombosis

- A less common but more serious condition.
- A clot forms in the deep vein of the calf, or femoral or iliac veins and there is a risk that fragments may break off and travel through the circulation, causing an embolus.
- The woman will complain of pain in the leg and there may be oedema and a change in colour in the affected leg.
- The calf or leg is painful on palpation and dorsiflexion of the foot causes acute pain.

*Management*

- Commence anticoagulant therapy to prevent further clotting and reduce the risk of a PE.
- Continue IV low-molecular-weight heparin (LMWH) via an infusion pump until the acute signs have resolved.
- Elevate the leg and give analgesia as required.
- When symptoms have improved, begin mobilization with the leg well supported with TEDS.
- Continue anticoagulants for 6 weeks with self-administered subcutaneous low-dose heparin. During the postnatal period, warfarin may be used. Breastfeeding is not affected by either therapy.

## Pulmonary embolism

- This occurs when a clot becomes detached from a leg vein and is carried via the inferior vena cava through the heart and into the pulmonary artery.
- Small clots passing into the lung cause pulmonary infarction. If the artery is completely blocked, death occurs quickly. PE occurs as a result of a DVT in the ilio-femoral veins. Most cases occur in the immediate postnatal period.
- This remains the leading direct cause of maternal death in the UK.[7]
- Symptoms include:
  - Acute chest pain due to ischaemia in the lungs
  - Difficulty breathing (dyspnoea)
  - Blue discoloration of the skin (cyanosis)
  - Coughing up blood (haemoptysis)
  - Pyrexia
  - Collapse.

*Management*

- Summon urgent medical assistance.
- Sit the woman upright and administer oxygen.
- Measure vital signs every 15min.
- If resuscitation is required, commence cardiac massage and artificial ventilation.
- Give anticoagulation with IV LMWH and strong analgesia such as morphine.
- If the woman survives, continue anticoagulation therapy and administer the thrombolytic drug streptokinase to accelerate the breakdown of the clot. Patients with a minor embolus may present with less specific symptoms such as fever, cough, or pleuritic pain. Commence anticoagulant therapy and continue until symptoms resolve.

*Postnatal anticoagulation*

- Therapeutic anticoagulant therapy should be continued for the duration of the pregnancy and for at least 6 weeks postnatally and until at least 3 months of treatment have been given in total.
- Before discontinuing treatment the continuing risk of thrombosis should be assessed. Women should be offered a choice of LMWH or an oral anticoagulant for postnatal therapy after discussion about the need for regular blood tests for monitoring of warfarin, particularly during the first 10 days of treatment.

- Post-partum warfarin should be avoided until at least the fifth day and for longer in women at increased risk of PPH.
- Women should be advised that neither heparin (unfractionated or LMWH) nor warfarin is contraindicated in breastfeeding.

## Reference

7  Knight M, Kenyon S, Brocklehurst P, Neilson J, Shakespeare J, Kurinczuk JJ (eds.) on behalf of MBRRACE-UK (2014). *Saving Lives, Improving Mothers' Care—Lessons learned to inform future maternity care from the UK and Ireland Confidential Enquiries into Maternal Deaths and Morbidity 2009–12*. Oxford: National Perinatal Epidemiology Unit, University of Oxford.

## Further reading

Royal College of Obstetricians and Gynaecologists (2015). *Thromboembolic disease in pregnancy and the puerperium: active management. Green-top guideline No. 37b*. Available at: ℛ www.rcog.org.uk/globalassets/documents/guidelines/gtg-37b.pdf.

# Principles of thromboprophylaxis

Following the publication of the latest report of the Confidential Enquiries into Maternal Deaths in the UK in 2014,[8] the recommendations of the RCOG on thromboprophylaxis in the antenatal, intranatal, and postnatal periods may be followed. A summary of the recommendations appears in the report and can also be found in RCOG guidelines.[9]

VTE is uncommon in pregnancy or in the first 6 weeks postnatally, and the absolute risk is around one in 1000 pregnancies. It can occur at any stage in pregnancy, but the first 6 weeks following birth is the time of highest risk, with the risk increasing by 20-fold.

The guidance emphasizes that all women should undergo a thorough assessment for VTE in early pregnancy or pre-pregnancy and again intrapartum or immediately post-partum.

The risk factors for VTE include:[10]
• Previous VTE
• Congenital or acquired thrombophilia
• Obesity (BMI 35 or above; those with a BMI of 40 or above are at high risk)
• Parity of 4 or above
• Gross varicose veins
• Surgical procedures during pregnancy or in the postnatal period
• Hyperemesis
• Dehydration
• Severe infection
• Pre-eclampsia
• Long-haul travel
• >4 days of bed rest.

The main recommendations for thromboprophylaxis are:[9]
• All women should be screened for risk factors for VTE in early pregnancy and again if admitted to hospital or on development of other problems
• Women with a previous VTE should be screened for thrombophilia
• In all pregnant women, immobilization should be minimized and dehydration avoided
• Women with a previous VTE should be offered thromboprophylaxis with LMWH in the postnatal period
• Women with recurrent VTE, or VTE with a family history of VTE in a first-degree relative, or with previous VTE and thrombophilia should be offered LMWH antenatally and for 6 weeks post-partum
• Women with three or more persisting risk factors should be considered for LMWH for 3–5 days postnatally.

# References

8 Knight M, Kenyon S, Brocklehurst P, Neilson J, Shakespeare J, Kurinczuk JJ (eds.) on behalf of MBRRACE-UK (2014). *Saving Lives, Improving Mothers' Care—Lessons learned to inform future maternity care from the UK and Ireland Confidential Enquiries into Maternal Deaths and Morbidity 2009–12.* Oxford: National Perinatal Epidemiology Unit, University of Oxford.

9 Royal College of Obstetricians and Gynaecologists (2015). *Thromboembolic disease in pregnancy and the puerperium: active management. Green-top guideline No. 37b.* Available at: ℵ www.rcog.org.uk/globalassets/documents/guidelines/gtg-37b.pdf.

10 Royal College of Obstetricians and Gynaecologists (2015) *Revised guidelines on reducing the risk and treatment options for thromboembolic disease in pregnancy, 13th April 2015.* Available at: ℵ www.rcog.org.uk/en/news/rcog-release-revised-guidelines-on-reducing-the-risk-and-treatment-options-for-thromboembolic-disease-in-pregnancy/.

# Thyroid disorders

Pregnancy makes special demands on the thyroid gland which enlarges due to the influence of oestrogen. The hormone hCG has thyroid-stimulating properties and may even cause hyperthyroidism in excessive amounts.

There are four main disorders of the thyroid affecting pregnancy:

- Iodine deficiency
- Hypothyroidism
- Hyperthyroidism
- Postnatal thyroiditis.

## Iodine deficiency

- Leads to a condition called goitre. In mothers who have goitre and are also hypothyroid, 30% of pregnancies will result in spontaneous abortion, stillbirth, or congenital abnormalities.
- This condition is rare in the UK as iodine is present in a variety of foods such as shellfish, saltwater fish, mushrooms, and soya beans.
- When iodine deficiency occurs in the 1st trimester, this may lead to developmental failure of the CNS, resulting in severe learning difficulties, deafness, and spasticity.
- In the second and third trimesters, the iodine deficiency may lead to an infant being born with hypothyroidism. This consists of a large tongue, dry coarse skin, an umbilical hernia, and lethargy. The condition responds to iodine or thyroid hormone replacement and the prognosis is related to when the condition first started.

## Hypothyroidism

*Symptoms*

- Hypothermia and intolerance to cold.
- Decreased appetite, weight gain, and constipation.
- Dry, rough flaky skin and hair loss.
- Impaired concentration and memory.
- Extreme fatigue.

*Effects on pregnancy*

- Spontaneous abortion and stillbirth rates are higher in this group.
- Symptoms should be observed for and thyroid function measured in any pregnant woman in whom there is a suspicion of dysfunction.
- If diagnosed, treatment with replacement thyroid hormone is prescribed.

## Hyperthyroidism

*Symptoms*

- Increased temperature and heat intolerance.
- Restlessness and insomnia.
- Increased appetite, weight loss, and diarrhoea.
- Exophthalmos—protrusion of the eyeball.

*Effects on pregnancy*
- A high fetal mortality rate.
- The condition should be suspected in any pregnant woman who fails to gain weight despite a good appetite or presents with any other features of the condition.
- Anti-thyroid drugs may be used with caution as they may cause hypothyroidism in the fetus.

## Postnatal thyroiditis

Around 11–17% of women develop postnatal thyroid dysfunction between 1 and 3 months post-delivery. It resolves spontaneously in two-thirds of those with this condition. The remainder pass into a hypothyroid state and although most recover, a small number continue to be hypothyroid.

## Management

Thyroid disease can have significant effects on a woman's reproductive health and screening for women presenting with fertility problems and recurrent early pregnancy loss should be considered.

Hyperthyroidism is found in approximately 2.3% of women presenting with fertility problems, compared with 1.5% of women in the general population. The condition is linked with menstrual irregularity. Hypothyroidism affects around 0.5% of women of reproductive age.

Evidence suggests that routine screening of the general population for thyroid dysfunction at the start of pregnancy may be beneficial.

Women diagnosed with thyroid disease should continue on anti-thyroid medication throughout pregnancy and receive close monitoring.

## Further reading

Jefferys A, Vanderpump M, Yasmin E (2015). Thyroid dysfunction and reproductive health. *The Obstetrician & Gynaecologist* 17: 39–45. Available at: ℞ onlinelibrary.wiley.com/doi/10.1111/tog.12161/abstract.

# Renal conditions

There are a number of changes in the urinary tract as a result of pregnancy.
• Plasma volume expansion of 30–50% is conserved by the kidneys.
• There is an increased frequency of micturition in the first trimester due to the growing uterus compressing the bladder within the pelvis. This effect is noticed again in the 3rd trimester as the bladder displaces when the fetal head engages.
• As a result of the hormonal effect on the renal tubules, the renal threshold for glucose is lowered independently of blood glucose levels.
• There is dilation and enlargement of the ureters under the influence of progesterone, leading to an increased risk of urinary stasis, obstructed urine flow, and ascending infection.
• Pregnancy does not make renal function worsen in women who are normotensive and who have normal kidneys.
• Proteinuria, hypertension, or impaired renal function present at conception determines fetal prognosis.

Renal disorders in pregnancy can range from asymptomatic bacteriuria to end-stage renal disease requiring dialysis. Every pregnant woman with renal disease should be classed as a high-risk pregnancy, especially when impaired renal function or hypertension is present.

For optimal management, a multidisciplinary approach is essential and care should be in a facility with experience of high-risk pregnancies and a neonatal intensive care unit (NICU), and the woman's care coordinated by an obstetrician and a nephrologist from the outset.

## Glomerular nephritis

This condition can follow a streptococcal infection and occurs in response to an abnormal antibody–antigen reaction.

*Signs and symptoms*
• Oedema.
• Aching loins.
• Dyspnoea.
• Bradycardia.
• Oliguria.
• Haematuria.

*Treatment*
• Antibiotics.
• Restricted protein diet.
• Restricted fluids until diuresis begins.

Overall fetal loss is 21% with a preterm delivery rate of 19%.

## Nephrotic syndrome

This can follow glomerular nephritis or be a result of diabetes or renal vein thrombosis.

*Signs and symptoms*
- Marked proteinuria.
- Oedema.
- Anaemia.
- Decreased levels of plasma proteins.
- Decreased osmotic pressure.
- Decreased blood volume.

*Treatment*
- High-protein, low-sodium diet.
- Carefully monitor electrolytes.
- Fetal loss is high.

## Maintenance dialysis

Fertility generally decreases in women with end-stage renal disease, but improved treatment can lead to health improvement enough to restore fertility. There is, however, a low fetal survival rate; prematurity is a major problem and polyhydramnios is common.

## Renal transplant recipients

There is a greater chance of a successful pregnancy with a gap of 2 years between transplant and conception. The incidence of preterm delivery is high as is IUGR. Fetal prognosis depends on how well the allograft continues to function and hypertension, proteinuria, and renal function must be closely monitored.

## Management of renal disease in pregnancy

If progressive renal failure occurs either in early pregnancy or before fetal viability can be assured, dialysis may need to be considered.

Dialysis should be initiated when the serum creatinine level is 3.5–5.0mg/dL or the GFR is below 20mL/min. Fetal outcome is improved with longer, more frequent haemodialysis sessions, which usually involves 20h of dialysis per week. Daily dialysis is more likely to prevent hypotension and significant metabolic shifts.

Dialysis should aim to keep blood urea nitrogen levels below 50mg/dL, because controlling uraemia may avoid polyhydramnios, control hypertension, and improve the mother's nutritional status. Peritoneal dialysis with smaller volumes and frequent exchanges can also be done to achieve these same goals.

Anaemia should be treated with erythropoietin and careful attention to iron therapy. Nutritional support that allows weight gains of 0.3–0.5kg/week should be maintained in the second and third trimesters.

## Pregnancy in patients receiving dialysis

Although fertility is significantly impaired in women with end-stage renal disease, pregnancy may still occur. Most women on dialysis are anovulatory, with either irregular or no menses, which can result in significant delays in the diagnosis of pregnancy in those who do conceive. In addition, the spontaneous abortion rate for pregnant women who require dialysis is approximately 50%. For pregnancies that continue, however, the fetal survival rate is as high as 71%.

Guidelines for pregnancy in kidney transplant recipients include the following:
- Good general health for 2 years post-transplantation, with serum creatinine levels below 2.0mg/dL (preferably <1.5mg/dL)
- No recent acute rejection or ongoing rejection
- Normotension, or hypertension controlled with minimal antihypertensive agents
- No or minimal proteinuria.

The following are complication risks in kidney transplant recipients:
- Immunosuppressive agents increase the risk of hypertension during pregnancy
- Pre-eclampsia occurs in approximately one-third of kidney transplant recipients
- Almost 50% of pregnancies in these women end in preterm delivery due to hypertension
- Blood levels of calcineurin inhibitors need to be frequently monitored due to changes in volumes of distribution of extracellular volume
- There is an increased risk of cytomegalovirus, toxoplasmosis, and herpes infections, which raises concern for the fetus.

### Further reading

Krane NK (2015). *Overview of renal disease and pregnancy*. Available at: ℘ emedicine.medscape. com/article/246123-overview.

# Obesity

# The impact of obesity during pregnancy and beyond

Recent figures suggest that in the UK the rising rate of obesity within the general population will have a major impact on public health. For the child-bearing population this is already having an impact. Obesity represents one of the greatest and growing overall threats to the childbearing population of the UK.

Obesity in pregnancy is usually defined as a BMI of $30kg/m^2$ or greater at booking.[1] In the UK national statistics about the prevalence of obesity during pregnancy suggest that 50% of women of childbearing age are over-weight or obese.[2]

The predominance of obese women among those who died from thromboembolism, sepsis, and cardiac disease recorded in the latest CEMACH report[3] means that early multidisciplinary planning regarding the mode of delivery and use of thromboprophylaxis for these women is essential.

Pre-pregnancy counselling and weight loss, together with wider public health messages about optimum weight, should help to reduce the number of obese women who become pregnant.

## References

1 Centre for Maternal and Child Enquiries, Royal College of Obstetricians and Gynaecologists (2010). *Management of women with obesity during pregnancy*. Available at: ℜ www.rcog.org.uk/globalassets/documents/guidelines/cmacercogjointguidelinemanagementwomenobesitypregnancya.pdf.
2 The Information Centre, National Statistics (2008). *Health survey for England 2006: CVD and risk factors for adults, obesity and risk factors for children*. London: The Information Centre. Available at: ℜ www.hscic.gov.uk/pubs/hse06cvdandriskfactors.
3 Lewis G (ed.) (2007). *The Confidential Enquiry into Maternal and Child Health (CEMACH). Saving Mothers' Lives: reviewing maternal deaths to make motherhood safer: 2003–2005. The Seventh Report on Confidential Enquiries into Maternal Deaths in the United Kingdom*. London: CEMACH.

# Risks of obesity in pregnancy

Obesity in pregnancy is associated with increased risks of complications for both mother and baby. Women with obesity in pregnancy also have higher rates of induction of labour, Caesarean section, and PPH and there is an increased risk of post-Caesarean wound infection.[4]

There is also evidence that babies of obese women have significantly increased risks of adverse outcomes, including fetal congenital anomaly, prematurity, stillbirth, and neonatal death.[4]

## Risks for the mother
- Maternal death or severe morbidity.
- Cardiac disease.
- Spontaneous first-trimester and recurrent miscarriage.
- Pre-eclampsia.
- GDM.
- Thromboembolism.
- Post-Caesarean wound infection.
- Infection from other causes.
- PPH.
- Low breastfeeding rates.

## Risks for the baby
- Stillbirth and neonatal death.
- Congenital abnormalities.
- Macrosomia.
- Prematurity.

## Reference
4 Catalano PM (2007). Management of obesity in pregnancy. *Obstet Gynecol* **109**: 419–33.

## Pre-pregnancy care

- Women of childbearing age should have the opportunity to optimize their weight prior to pregnancy.
- Advice on weight and lifestyle plus regular monitoring of weight, BMI, and waist circumference should be offered during consultations for family planning or during pre-conception consultations.
  - Women of childbearing age with a BMI of 30kg/m² or above should receive information and advice about the risks of obesity during pregnancy and be supported to lose weight before conception.[5]

### Reference

5 National Institute for Health and Care Excellence (2010). *Weight management before, during and after pregnancy.* NICE guidelines PH27. Available at: ℜ www.nice.org.uk/guidance/ph27.

# Pregnancy care

- Women should have their BMI calculated at the booking visit and the result documented in the handheld and electronic record.
- Discuss her eating habits and how physically active she is. Find out if she has any concerns about diet and the amount of physical activity she does and try to address them.[6]
- Advise her that a healthy diet and being physically active will benefit both her and her unborn child during pregnancy and will also help her to achieve a healthy weight after giving birth. Advise her to seek information and advice on diet and activity from a reputable source.[6]
- Advise her on how to use Healthy Start vouchers to increase the fruit and vegetable intake of those eligible for the Healthy Start scheme (women <18 years and those who are receiving benefit payments).[6]
- Dispel any myths about what and how much to eat during pregnancy. For example, advise that there is no need to 'eat for two' or to drink full-fat milk. Explain that energy needs do not change in the first 6 months of pregnancy and increase only slightly in the last 3 months (and then only by around 200cal/day).[6]
- Advise her that moderate-intensity physical activity will not harm her or her unborn child. At least 30min per day of moderate-intensity activity is recommended.[6] Swimming or brisk walking is ideal and this should start slowly and build up for those who are not used to this level of activity.
- Pregnant women with a BMI of 40kg/m² or above should be referred for a consultation with an obstetric anaesthetist, so that difficulties with venous access or regional or general anaesthesia can be identified. A management plan for labour should be discussed and documented.
- An appropriate-sized arm cuff should be used to measure BP at antenatal visits and the cuff size recorded in the antenatal notes.
- Women with a BMI of 30kg/m² or above should be screened for GDM.
- Pregnant women with a BMI of 40kg/m² or above should have a third-trimester assessment of their manual handling requirements.
- A risk assessment for thromboembolism should be carried out and both antenatal and post-delivery thromboprophylaxis considered.

## Reference

6 National Institute for Health and Care Excellence (2010). *Weight management before, during and after pregnancy*. NICE guidelines PH27. Available at: ℛ www.nice.org.uk/guidance/ph27.

# Care during labour

- Women with a BMI of $35kg/m^2$ or above should give birth in a consultant-led obstetric unit.
- An obstetrician and anaesthetist of appropriate seniority should be informed and available for care of a woman in labour with a BMI of $40kg/m^2$ or above.
- Women with a BMI of $40kg/m^2$ or above should have venous access established in early labour. These women should receive continuous midwifery care.
- Operating department staff should be informed early of any woman weighing >120kg who requires operative delivery.
- Women with a BMI of $30kg/m^2$ or above should have an actively managed third stage of labour.

# Postnatal care

- Obesity is associated with low breastfeeding initiation and maintenance rates, so specialist advice and support should be offered both antenatally and postnatally.
- Early mobilization should be encouraged.
- Women with a BMI of $30kg/m^2$ or above should continue to receive nutritional and physical activity advice with a view to weight reduction. The 6- to 8-week postnatal assessment can be a useful time to offer further support. This can continue to be followed up at 6-monthly intervals by the GP or other appropriate health professional.[7]
- Women with a BMI of $30kg/m^2$ should have regular follow-up by their GP for the development of type 2 diabetes.
- Women who develop GDM should receive annual screening for cardio-metabolic risk factors and receive advice on nutrition and weight management.

### Reference

7 National Institute for Health and Care Excellence (2010). *Weight management before, during and after pregnancy*. NICE guidelines PH27. Available at: ℠ www.nice.org.uk/guidance/ph27.

# Practical considerations

Maternity units should have guidelines in place to facilitate the care of women with a BMI of $30kg/m^2$ or above with respect to referral criteria, facilities, and equipment.

The following are required:
- Large BP cuffs
- Sit-on weighing scale
- Large chairs and wheelchairs
- Ultrasound scan couches and ward and delivery beds
- Theatre trolleys and operating theatre tables
- Lifting and lateral transfer equipment.

# Pregnancy complications

# Bleeding in early pregnancy

Once a pregnancy has been confirmed, any vaginal bleeding should be reported as it could signal a potential complication.

Around 15% of women experience bleeding early in pregnancy. This could be related to events such as:

- *Implantation bleed*—a small amount of blood escapes as the fertilized ovum embeds in the lining of the uterus
- *Decidual bleed*—bleeding from the decidual lining at the time a menstrual period would be expected, before the enlarging gestation sac completely fills the uterine cavity.

There may be other causes of bleeding not related to the uterus, such as:

- Cervical erosion that bleeds on contact
- Vaginitis
- Cervical polyp
- Ectopic pregnancy—a pregnancy implanted outside the cavity of the uterus, commonly in the Fallopian tubes
- Hydatidiform mole
- Cervical erosion that bleeds on contact—post-coital bleed.

The most significant cause of bleeding is spontaneous miscarriage, 80% of which occur in the first trimester. Spontaneous miscarriage can be classified as:

- *Threatened*: bleeding with no uterine contraction or pain and the cervix does not dilate
- *Inevitable*: when the cervix dilates or the membranes rupture
- *Complete*: the cervix closes and bleeding stops after the expulsion of the gestation sac
- *Incomplete*: retained placental tissue causes persistent bleeding and uterine contractions; requires evacuation of the uterus under anaesthetic to prevent the development of infection
- *Missed*: the retention of a dead pregnancy; chorionic tissue may survive and produce hCG which enables the pregnancy to be retained in the uterus
- *Miscarriage with infection*: infection following expulsion of the gestation sac, commonly after incomplete abortion
- *Recurrent*: loss of three or more early pregnancies
- *Induced*: surgical or medical method.

The woman does not require any specific treatment if bleeding is minimal and resolves spontaneously, although she may wish to confirm that the pregnancy is still viable.

Advise a woman with vaginal bleeding and a confirmed intrauterine pregnancy with a fetal heartbeat that:

- If her bleeding gets worse or persists beyond 14 days, she should return for further assessment
- If the bleeding stops, she should start or continue routine antenatal care.

Use expectant management for 7–14 days as the first-line management strategy for women with a confirmed diagnosis of miscarriage. Explore management options other than expectant management if:

- The woman is at increased risk of haemorrhage (e.g. she is in the late first trimester) *or*
- She has previous adverse and/or traumatic experience associated with pregnancy (e.g. stillbirth, miscarriage, or APH) *or*
- She is at increased risk from the effects of haemorrhage (e.g. if she has coagulopathies or is unable to have a blood transfusion) *or*
- There is evidence of infection.

The National Service Framework (Department of Health, 2004) recommends provision of early pregnancy assessment units (EPAUs) where a woman may be referred for a further pregnancy test and an ultrasound scan to confirm whether or not the pregnancy is continuing.

- Persistent bleeding with pain requires admission to hospital for assessment and management.
- Post-miscarriage bleeding may require further treatment.
- Occasionally, if no infection is present and the uterus is empty, bleeding will settle after administration of ergometrine.

## Further reading

National Institute for Health and Care Excellence (2012). Management of miscarriage. In: National Institute for Health and Care Excellence. *Ectopic pregnancy and miscarriage: diagnosis and initial management*. Available at: ℰ www.nice.org.uk/guidance/cg154/chapter/1-recommendations#management-of-miscarriage.

# Hyperemesis gravidarum

Hyperemesis means excessive vomiting and this condition can occur in 3–20% of pregnancies. It is an extremely unpleasant condition and sufferers can become depressed and demoralized that the early stage of pregnancy makes them feel so ill.

Hyperemesis gravidarum should be considered when all other causes of persistent nausea and vomiting have been ruled out.

Pyelonephritis, pancreatitis, cholecystitis, hepatitis, appendicitis, gastroenteritis, peptic ulcer disease, thyrotoxicosis, and hyperthyroidism can present in similar fashions, with intractable nausea and vomiting, and are treatable conditions. Late presenters need also to be ruled out for HELLP syndrome and other causes of hepatic and CNS dysfunction.

It usually lasts any time from the 6th to the 16th week of pregnancy and is characterized by:
• Vomiting several times a day
• Persistent nausea
• Dehydration
• Reduced urine output
• The appearance of ketones in the urine.

It can be a potentially life-threatening condition, especially if the electrolyte or acid–base balance becomes disordered.
• In severe cases hospitalization becomes necessary in order to provide rest.
• IV fluid, up to 5–6L per day using the appropriate amounts of sodium, potassium, chloride, lactate or bicarbonate, glucose, and water, is primarily used in correcting hypovolaemia, electrolyte and acid–base imbalances, and ketosis.
• Antiemetics can be prescribed in the short term, usually promethazine.
• Fluids and diet are gradually reintroduced until a normal diet is tolerated. There are usually no ill effects on the pregnancy and once the condition improves pregnancy proceeds normally.
• Special consideration must be given to the risk of thromboembolism in women with this condition. If hospitalized women require bed rest, the application of TEDS is recommended.

### Further reading

National Institute for Health and Care Excellence (2013). *Nausea/vomiting in pregnancy*. Clinical Knowledge Summaries. Available at: ℘ cks.nice.org.uk/nauseavomiting-in-pregnancy.

# Antepartum haemorrhage

*Definition*: bleeding from the genital tract after the 24th week of pregnancy and before the onset of labour.

APH complicates 2–5% of all pregnancies and is responsible for significant maternal mortality and morbidity. In the latest MBRRACE-UK (Mothers and Babies: Reducing Risk through Audits and Confidential Enquiries across the UK) report,[1] four women died from APH.

The most common causes are placenta praevia with an incidence of 31% and placental abruption with an incidence of 22%.[2]

## Placenta praevia

As the placenta encroaches on the lower uterine segment, bleeding occurs as the uterus stretches and grows. The lower uterine segment forms from 28 weeks.

- Bleeding is painless and presents as a fresh loss. There is often persistent malpresentation of the fetal presenting part.
- There is a further risk of PPH as the retractive power of the lower segment is poor.

*Risk factors for placenta praevia*

- Previous placenta praevia.
- Previous Caesarean section.
- Previous termination of pregnancy.
- Multiparity.
- Advanced maternal age (>40 years).
- Multiple pregnancies.
- Smoking.
- Assisted conception.

There are four grades of placenta praevia:

- *Grade 1*: the placental edge encroaches on the lower uterine segment but does not reach the internal cervical os. Blood loss is usually minimal so the mother and fetus remain in good condition and vaginal delivery is possible
- *Grade 2*: the placenta is partially in the lower uterine segment and reaches, but does not cover, the internal cervical os. Blood loss is moderate and fetal hypoxia is more likely to be present than maternal shock. Vaginal delivery is possible if the placenta is anterior
- *Grade 3*: the placenta partially covers the internal cervical os but not in a central position. Bleeding is likely to be severe, particularly in late pregnancy when the cervix starts to efface and dilate. Vaginal delivery is not possible as the placenta precedes the fetus
- *Grade 4*: the placenta completely covers the internal cervical os and the risk of a torrential haemorrhage makes a Caesarean section essential to save the mother and the fetus.

Management depends on the amount of bleeding and the gestation. Admit the mother to a consultant unit for her condition to be assessed.

*Mild to moderate bleeding*
- Abdominal examination.
- CTG to monitor fetal condition.
- Commence IV infusion.
- FBC and cross-match units of blood as per protocol.
- Ultrasound to confirm fetal well-being and position of the placental border.
- Timing and mode of delivery will depend on the general condition of the woman, the extent of bleeding, and the gestation.

*Profuse bleeding*
- Commence IV fluid immediately and transfuse blood as soon as it becomes available.
- Once the woman's condition is stable, prepare her for emergency Caesarean section.

## Placental abruption

*Causes*
- Multiparity.
- Pre-eclampsia and eclampsia.
- Hypertension.
- Abdominal trauma.
- Multiple pregnancy.
- Polyhydramnios.
- Previous abruption.
- Folate deficiency.

Presents as continuous abdominal pain, sometimes with uterine contractions superimposed, with or without vaginal bleeding. Bleeding may be concealed inside the uterus, apparent as vaginal loss or both.

There may be symptoms of severe shock, disproportionate to the amount of blood lost. The pain may be localized if the abruption is small, and is felt over the site of the abruption. The uterus is very tender on palpation and hard ridges may be felt. The fetal heartbeat may be absent.

Pain is caused by:
- Intrauterine pressure
- Stretching of the peritoneum
- Tearing of the myometrium as blood is pushed back into the muscle layers of the uterus.

*Management*
Depends on the degree of maternal shock and the condition of the fetus:
- Mild abruption may be treated conservatively with rest and careful monitoring of the fetal and maternal condition. An ultrasound scan will confirm the diagnosis and an FBC and Kleihauer's test will assess the amount of bleeding.
- The mother may return to community care once the bleeding has stopped and if maternal and fetal condition is good. Follow-up antenatal care will be consultant-led with more frequent attendance.

For a more severe abruption:
- Commence IV infusion
- FBC, coagulation screen, and cross-match 4 units of whole blood or as per protocol. U/E and LFTs should be taken
- Commence blood transfusion as soon as blood is available
- Provide pain relief
- Perform Kleihauer's test in Rh D-negative women
- CTG to monitor the status of the fetus
- Prepare for induction of labour or Caesarean section as the fetal and maternal condition dictates.

Complications due to placental abruption are:
- DIC
- Acute renal failure
- Anaemia
- Sepsis
- Fetal death
- Fetal hypoxia
- Prematurity.

## References

1 Knight M, Kenyon S, Brocklehurst P, Neilson J, Shakespeare J, Kurinczuk JJ (eds.) on behalf of MBRRACE-UK (2014). *Saving Lives, Improving Mothers' Care—Lessons learned to inform future maternity care from the UK and Ireland Confidential Enquiries into Maternal Deaths and Morbidity 2009–12*. Oxford: National Perinatal Epidemiology Unit, University of Oxford.

2 Royal College of Obstetricians and Gynaecologists (2011). *Antepartum haemorrhage*. Green-top guideline No. 63. Available at: ℅ www.rcog.org.uk/globalassets/documents/guidelines/gtg_63.pdf.

# Recognition and management of breech presentation

In this presentation the fetus is in a longitudinal lie with the buttocks entering the pelvis first.

## Incidence
- At 20 weeks: 40%.
- At 28 weeks: 15%.
- At 34 weeks: 6%.
- At 40 weeks: 3%.

## Classification
- *Breech with extended legs*: 70%. The legs are straight and the feet may lie on either side of the head, acting as a splint and making it difficult to ballot the head.
- *Complete or flexed breech*: 25–29%. The knees are bent and the ankles crossed so the feet lie close to the buttocks.
- *Footling breech*: rare. From the flexed breech, one foot falls downwards to present over the cervical os. The foot may slip through as the cervix dilates in labour.
- *Knee presentation*: very rare. From the flexed breech, one knee falls downwards over the cervical os.

## Causes
- Preterm labour.
- Polyhydramnios.
- Multiple pregnancy—the second twin is often a breech presentation.
- Placenta praevia—the placenta takes up room in the lower uterus, leaving less space for the fetal head to present.
- Contracted pelvis—not enough room for the fetal head to engage in the pelvis.
- Multiparity.
- Fetal or uterine abnormality.

## Antenatal diagnosis
- On abdominal palpation the head is felt at the top of the uterus and it ballots easily unless splinted by extended legs.
- The breech is smaller, softer, and more irregular than the hard, smooth, rounded head.
- Fetal heart sounds are heard above the level of the maternal umbilicus.

## Management
- If breech presentation is suspected at the 36-week antenatal visit, offer the mother a confirmatory ultrasound assessment.[3,4]
- If uncomplicated breech presentation is confirmed, offer ECV at 36 weeks' gestation or up to when labour begins, to convert the breech to head-presenting.
- A 50% success rate has been reported for the procedure, depending on the skill and experience of the operator.[5]

- ECV should be performed by an obstetrician or a specialist trained midwife in a hospital setting.
- The procedure should be explained to the mother with reasons and possible risks, so that she can give informed consent.
- Perform an ultrasound scan prior to the procedure to confirm the fetus is not compromised, locate the placenta, and confirm fetal position, and afterwards monitor the fetal heart and the placenta, in case of accidental bleeding.
- Some hospitals use tocolysis to relax the uterus prior to, and during, the procedure.
- The mother should have an empty bladder, and it is sometimes helpful to elevate the foot of the bed.
- The obstetrician disengages the breech from the pelvis, locates the fetal head, and attempts to manoeuvre the fetus through a forward somersault towards the iliac fossa until the head is presenting. (Be careful not to pinch the mother's skin!)
- The procedure should be abandoned if the fetus does not turn easily.
- A CTG is used to monitor the fetal heart throughout the procedure.
- The woman stays in hospital for about 2h after the procedure and will be seen a week later to confirm the presentation.
- Anti-D Ig is offered if the woman is Rh-negative.
- If the procedure fails, or the presentation re-converts to breech, the woman has the option of attempted vaginal delivery or an elective Caesarean section at 39 weeks.

## Contraindications
- Previous Caesarean section.
- APH.
- Placenta praevia.
- Multiple pregnancy.
- SGA fetus.
- Hypertension.
- Pre-eclampsia due to increased risk of placental separation.
- Oligohydramnios.
- Ruptured membranes.

## References

3  Royal College of Obstetricians and Gynaecologists (2006). *The management of breech presenta-tion*. Guideline No. 20b. Available at: &#x1F52E; www.rcog.org.uk/globalassets/documents/guidelines/gtg-no-20b-breech-presentation.pdf.
4  National Institute for Health and Care Excellence (2012). Quality statement 11: Fetal wellbeing—external cephalic version. In: National Institute for Health and Care Excellence. *Antenatal care. Quality standard*. NICE quality standard QS 22. Available at: &#x1F52E; www.nice.org.uk/guidance/qs22/chapter/Quality-statement-11-Fetal-wellbeing-external-cephalic-version.
5  Royal College of Obstetricians and Gynaecologists (2006). *External cephalic version and reducing the incidence of breech presentation*. Guideline No. 20a. Available at: &#x1F52E; www.rcog.org.uk/globalassets/documents/guidelines/gt20aexternalcephalicversion.pdf.

# Management of the small-for-gestational-age fetus

Small-for-gestational age (SGA) refers to an infant born with a birthweight less than the tenth centile.

## Causes of small-for-gestational-age

*Maternal factors which might influence fetal growth*

- Age >35 years.
- Alcohol abuse.
- Smoking.
- Substance misuse.
- Poor nutrition.
- Previous SGA infant.
- Hypertensive disorders.
- Maternal cardiac or renal disease.
- Diabetes.
- Antiphospholipid syndrome.

*Pregnancy factors which might influence fetal growth*

- Multiple pregnancies (twins, triplets, etc.).
- Placenta problems.
- Pre-eclampsia or eclampsia.
- Intrauterine infection.
- Unexplained APH.
- Low maternal weight gain.

## Monitoring growth

- In the third trimester, ultrasound scans can be used to measure growth of the fetus if the clinical findings give cause for concern.
- It is important to recognize large-for-gestational-age as well as growth-restricted fetuses.
- The two most common measurements used in monitoring growth are the head and abdominal circumferences.
- The abdominal circumference is useful when assessing growth, because of fat deposition in the fetal liver. This is reduced in growth-restricted fetuses and increased in macrosomic fetuses. The ratio between the head and abdominal circumferences helps distinguish between the two types of growth restriction:
  - Asymmetrical growth restriction
  - Symmetrical growth restriction.

## Asymmetrical growth restriction

- This is characterized by falling abdominal circumference measurements, but the head circumference stays within normal limits.
- This is referred to as 'brain-sparing', as the brain continues to receive nutrients and continues to develop whilst the fat and glycogen deposits in the liver dwindle as the fetus is compromised.

- It is usually apparent in the later stages of pregnancy and is due to placental insufficiency.
- This is a sign that the oxygen supply to the fetus will slow down in the near future.

## Symmetrical growth restriction

- The fetus may be genetically small but otherwise normal, or may be suffering from such poor nutrition that both the brain and other organs are affected.
- The head and abdominal circumferences have a close ratio and both measurements are reduced.
- The genetically small fetus will be apparent from the first scan, but this may also be due to external influences, such as maternal malnutrition, infection, or substance misuse, or to a congenital anomaly.

## Diagnosis and management

It is often difficult to distinguish between the growth-restricted and the merely small fetus. The cause may be attributed to incorrect dates and the woman given a revised date of delivery. Measurements taken from the early pregnancy scan are therefore essential to avoid induction of labour that is either too early or too late.

- All women should be assessed at booking for risk factors for an SGA fetus/neonate to identify those who require increased surveillance.
- Women who have a major risk factor [odds ratio (OR) >2.0] should be referred for serial ultrasound measurements of fetal size and assessment of well-being with umbilical artery Doppler from 26–28 weeks of pregnancy
- Women who have three or more minor risk factors should be referred for uterine artery Doppler at 20–24 weeks of gestation.

## Clinical examination

- Abdominal palpation has limited accuracy for the prediction of an SGA neonate and thus should not be routinely performed in this context.
- Serial measurements of the SFH are recommended at each antenatal appointment from 24 weeks of pregnancy as this improves prediction of an SGA neonate.
- The SFH should be plotted on a customized chart rather than a population-based chart as this may improve prediction of an SGA neonate.
- Women with a single SFH which plots below the tenth centile or with serial measurements which demonstrate slow or static growth by crossing centiles should be referred for ultrasound measurement of the fetal size.
- Women in whom measurement of the SFH is inaccurate (e.g. BMI >35, large fibroids, hydramnios) should be referred for serial assessments of the fetal size using ultrasound.

## Investigations

- Offer a referral for a detailed fetal anatomical survey and uterine artery Doppler by a fetal medicine specialist if severe SGA is identified at the 18- to 20-week scan.
- Interpretation of amniotic fluid volume should be based on a single deepest vertical pocket.
- Karyotyping should be offered in severely SGA fetuses with structural anomalies and in those detected before 23 weeks of gestation, especially if uterine artery Doppler is normal.
- Serological screening for congenital CMV and toxoplasmosis infection should be offered in severe SGA.
- Testing for syphilis and malaria should be considered in high-risk populations.

## Further reading

Royal College of Obstetricians and Gynaecologists (2014). *The investigation and management of the small-for-gestational-age fetus. Green-top guideline No. 31.* Available at: ℘ www.rcog.org.uk/globalassets/documents/guidelines/gtg_31.pdf.

# Multiple pregnancy

### Incidence
In natural conceptions, one in 80 results in twin pregnancy. One in 6400 conceptions results in triplets, and 1 in 512 000 results in quadruplets. The incidence of multiple pregnancies overall is on the increase due to the impact of successful infertility treatment.

Where an average incidence of triplets in a maternity unit delivering 3000 babies a year might result in a triplet birth every 2 years, it is becoming more common to see 2–3 such births in a year.

Twin pregnancy has the highest incidence and can be divided into two types.

#### Monozygotic
Sometimes referred to as identical twins. The incidence is 2.5–4 per 1000 births.
- Results from one ovum and one spermatozoon.
- There is one chorion membrane and one placenta.
- There are two amnions, one for each twin.
- The babies are always the same sex, blood group, eye colour, etc.

#### Dizygotic or non-identical twins
The incidence is more frequent with hereditary factors from both the mother and father affecting the frequency.[6]
- Results from two ova and two spermatozoa.
- There are two chorions and two placentas, though these may be so closely joined that they look like one.
- There are two amnions, one for each twin.
- The babies may be the same sex or one of each, and no more alike than any other family members.

Diagnosis is invariably made at the time of the dating scan early in the sec-ond trimester. By 20 weeks, the uterus will be large-for-gestational age and this is obvious on palpation. If a mother is late booking or has not received antenatal care, the diagnosis may be made quite late in pregnancy. It is rare nowadays to diagnose twins only once the mother is in labour.

### Special considerations
Serum screening tests for fetal abnormality are unsuitable as the results will be unreliable. Nuchal translucency scans, placental biopsy, or amniocentesis are options the mother may wish to consider.

During pregnancy the mother has a higher risk of complications develop-ing such as:
- Miscarriage
- Exaggerated minor disorders of pregnancy
- Premature labour
- PIH
- Anaemia—due to the demands of two fetuses
- Polyhydramnios—excess amounts of amniotic fluid
- Placental abruption
- Placenta praevia
- IUGR.

## Antenatal management

- Early diagnosis so relevant information and support can be organized.
- Determination of whether the twins are identical or not (zygosity).
- All women with a twin pregnancy should be offered an ultrasound examination at 10–13 weeks of gestation to assess viability, chorionicity, major congenital malformations, and nuchal translucency. A photographic record should be retained, in the case notes, of the ultrasound appearances of the membrane attachment to the placenta.[7]
- Chorionicity—if the pregnancy has only one chorion, there is a 3- to 5-fold higher risk of perinatal mortality
- Chorionicity is better assessed by ultrasound before 14 weeks than after 14 weeks.
- A multiple pregnancy can be shorter than a single pregnancy. The average is 37 weeks for twins, 34 weeks for triplets, and 32 weeks for quads.
- Identical or monochorionic twin pregnancies should have a scan every 2 weeks from diagnosis to look for discordant growth patterns—a sign of feto-fetal transfusion syndrome.
- All monochorionic twins should have a detailed ultrasound scan which includes extended views of the fetal heart.[7]
- Fetal ultrasound assessment should take place every 2–3 weeks in uncomplicated monochorionic pregnancies from 16 weeks.[7]
- Non-identical twin pregnancies should have a scan every 4 weeks to monitor growth.
- Regular measurement of maternal Hb levels and iron supplements if needed.
- The mother needs additional support both to prepare her for the birth and also for the care and feeding of the babies.
- The mother will need to pay particular attention to her dietary needs, the need for rest, and the possibility that she may have to stop work earlier than intended.
- Women with monochorionic twin pregnancies should be asked to report sudden increases in abdominal size or breathlessness, as this may be a manifestation of twin-to-twin transfusion syndrome (TTTS).[7]
- Advise women with twin and triplet pregnancies that they should take 75mg of aspirin daily from 10 weeks until the birth of the babies if they have one or more risk factors for hypertension:[8]
  - First pregnancy
  - Age 40 years or older
  - Pregnancy interval of >10 years
  - BMI of 35 kg/m$^2$ or more at first visit
  - Family history of pre-eclampsia.

## References

6 Nair M, Kumar G (2009). Uncomplicated monochorionic diamniotic twin pregnancy. *J Obstet Gynaecol* 29: 90–3.

7 Royal College of Obstetricians and Gynaecologists (2008). *Management of monochorionic twin pregnancy*. Green-top guideline No. 51. Available at: ℗ www.rcog.org.uk/globalassets/documents/guidelines/t51managementmonochorionictwinpregnancy2008a.pdf.

8 National Institute for Health and Care Excellence (2011). Determining gestational age and chorionicity. In: National Institute for Health and Care Excellence. *Multiple pregnancy: antenatal care for twin and triplet pregnancies*. NICE guidelines CG129. Available at: ℗ www.nice.org.uk/guidance/cg129/chapter/1-Guidance#determining-gestational-age-and-chorionicity.

# Hypertensive disorders of pregnancy

## Introduction

Hypertension is elevation of the arterial BP above the normal range for that expected in a particular group. In pregnancy, the normal range for BP is 100–140/60–90mmHg.

Hypertensive disorders can affect 6–7% of pregnancies and it is essential to monitor the BP regularly in accordance with the NICE guidelines for antenatal care (2008).[1] The mother should be in a seated position or supine with a left lateral tilt to avoid aorto-caval compression. The correct cuff size should be selected to avoid incorrect readings. The diastolic BP should be measured at Korotkoff V. If the sounds are heard down to zero, use Korotkoff IV.

### Reference

1 National Institute for Health and Care Excellence (2008). *Antenatal care for uncomplicated pregnancies*. NICE guidelines CG62. Available at: &#8472; www.nice.org.uk/guidance/cg62.

## Essential hypertension

- Permanently raised BP, often with no apparent cause; also associated with renal disease; phaeochromocytoma or coarctation of the aorta.
- Familial.
- Complicates 2–5% of pregnancies.
- 15–20% of these go on to develop pre-eclampsia.
- Diagnosed before the 20th week of pregnancy.
- Does not resolve postnatally.
- A mid-trimester fall in BP may mask hypertension.
- Consider as a high-risk pregnancy.
- Advise about lifestyle, weight, smoking, etc.
- Close fetal surveillance.
- Antihypertensive medication if diastolic BP >100mmHg.

# Pregnancy-induced hypertension

- Raised BP after 20 weeks' gestation in the absence of proteinuria.
- Sometimes called gestational hypertension.
- No other signs or symptoms, but increased risk of developing pre-eclampsia (15–26%)
- Aim is to give birth at the time of the EDD.
- BP usually returns to normal within 6 weeks of birth.

Midwives play a critical role in the screening and identification of women who are developing PIH. During each antenatal care appointment the midwife measures the BP, tests the woman's urine for protein, and observes for signs of excessive oedema.

If the midwife detects mild hypertension without proteinuria, an increased level of surveillance will be required and the woman asked to attend more frequently to have her BP and urine monitored. Collaborative care provides the most effective management and after referral to the consultant for investigation the woman can often resume her care in the community, provided her condition does not deteriorate.

# Pre-eclampsia

- Unique to human pregnancy.
- Definition inexact.
- Multi-system disorder thought to arise in the placenta.
- Variable severity.
- Variable mode of presentation.
- Retrospective diagnosis.
- Affects 5–10% of pregnancies.
- May show predisposition for increased BP in later life.
- Diagnosis: systolic BP >30mmHg over baseline reading, diastolic BP >15mmHg over baseline reading.
- Changes persist over two readings 6h apart.
- A single reading of >140/90mmHg after 20 weeks' gestation.
- Proteinuria >300mg in 24h.

Most women with pre-eclampsia are asymptomatic, but the following symptoms may be described:
- Headache
- Visual disturbances
- Epigastric pain
- Nausea and vomiting
- Rapidly occurring oedema.

Severe signs and symptoms which warrant admission to a high dependency facility include:
- Severe hypertension >160/110
- Hyperreflexia
- Thrombocytopenia
- Pulmonary oedema
- Fetal growth restriction <5th centile
- Oligohydramnios
- Worsening proteinuria.

## Investigations

- Urinalysis—protein (24h collection).
- Haematocrit (percentage of blood volume made up of red cells)—higher.
- Platelet count—lower.
- Coagulation can be disordered.
- Renal function—U/E, uric acid.
- Hepatic chemistry.

## Management

- Increased antenatal surveillance is required to provide more frequent maternal and fetal monitoring and a multidisciplinary approach with early senior obstetric input.
- High dependency care where appropriate if severe signs and symptoms develop.

- Plan the birth at or before the EDD if the maternal or fetal condition warrants this.
- The BP may be stabilized with an antihypertensive such as nifedipine 10mg orally 30min apart. If this is not successful, an IV infusion of labetalol is titrated in increasing amounts until the BP is under control.
- These medications do not cure the condition but prevent complications of pre-eclampsia.

# Eclampsia

Eclampsia is the occurrence of a tonic–clonic seizure in association with a diagnosis of pre-eclampsia. It signifies a worsening of the condition and can be thought of as the end-stage of the disease process. Prior management is directed to its prevention, but it can occur before the appearance of either hypertension or proteinuria.

Fits may occur antenatally (38%), intrapartum (18%), or postnatally within the first 48h (44%).

Eclampsia is an obstetric emergency.

(➔ See Chapter 22 for emergency management of eclampsia.)

# HELLP syndrome (haemolysis, elevated liver enzymes, and low platelets)

This is a severe variant of pre-eclampsia. It occurs in up to 20% of pre-eclamptic pregnancies. The syndrome is self-limiting with end-organs such as liver or kidneys recovering after the birth.

It is an indication for urgent birth.

Signs and symptoms are:
• Epigastric pain (beware of this sign in any pregnant or immediately postnatal women. Always check the BP, urine, and liver enzymes)
• Nausea and vomiting
• Dark-coloured urine
• Increased BP and other features of pre-eclampsia.

Treatment is supportive and as for eclampsia (magnesium sulfate ($MgSO_4$) indicated).

Although platelet levels may fall, platelet transfusion is only required should bleeding occur or if surgery is necessary.

### Further reading

National Institute for Health and Care Excellence (2008). *Antenatal care for uncomplicated pregnancies.* NICE guidelines CG62. Available at: ℛ www.nice.org.uk/guidance/cg62.

National Institute for Health and Care Excellence (2010). *Hypertension in pregnancy: diagnosis and management.* NICE guidelines CG107. Available at: ℛ www.nice.org.uk/guidance/cg107.

# Part 2

# Normal labour

# Normal labour: first stage

# Physiology of the first stage of labour

### Definition of labour

The physiological process by which the fetus, placenta, and membranes are expelled through the birth canal. The first stage of labour is from the onset of regular uterine contractions until full dilatation of the cervix.

### Normal labour

- Is spontaneous, occurs between 37 and 42 weeks' gestation.
- Culminates in the normal birth of a live, healthy infant.
- Is completed within 24h and there are no maternal complications.

The two main physiological changes that take place in the first stage are effacement and dilatation of the cervical os. These are initiated by the action of various hormones and prostaglandins, and the contraction and retraction of the uterine muscle. The mechanism by which labour is initiated is still not fully understood. Some theories suggest that it involves a very complex interaction between the mother, the fetus, and their environment.

### Physiology of the initiation of labour

Increasing levels of prostaglandins, oxytocin, and progesterone are thought to contribute to the initiation of the onset of labour. The levels then rise progressively, reaching highest levels at the birth of the head and after placental separation.

#### The myometrium

Individual cells within the myometrium are able to depolarize their cell membranes, allowing the movement of ions, primarily calcium, which together with ATPase (an enzyme that catalyses the hydrolysis of adenosine triphosphate into adenosine diphosphate and a free phosphate ion) initiates the contraction of myosin fibres within the cell. The cells are able to communicate their activity via gap junctions. At term, muscle fibres are present in compact bundles, reducing the gap size; therefore, the number of gap junctions increases and the potential to stimulate contractility is increased. When these processes occur together, this results in a harmonized contraction, which can spread across the uterus.

#### The cervix

The cervix consists of collagen fibres alternating with circular and longitudinal muscle fibres. Normally the cervix is firm and resistant to downward activity from the uterus and its contents. Towards term the percentage of water in the collagen fibres increases, which decreases their stability and therefore results in a softer, more compliant cervix.

#### Hormonal influences

Oestrogen enhances myometrial activity by increasing oxytocin and prostaglandin receptors, which in turn assists with the formation of gap junctions.

Prostaglandins are produced in the placenta, membranes, and decidua. Prostaglandin (PGF2a) and prostaglandin E (PGE) facilitate the production of calcium ions, which thus increases their availability for binding to the myosin receptors. This enhances contractile action and results in harmonized contractions. The presence of prostaglandins in the cervix encourages the production of the enzymes elastase and collagenase (MMP-8) which actively break down collagen fibres, leading to cervical ripening (softening).

Oxytocin acts as a hormone and neurotransmitter and is produced by the hypothalamus; it is a powerful uterotonic. An increase in oxytocin receptors, due to the action of oestrogen, dramatically increases uterine sensitivity to oxytocin at term. This facilitates the onset and maintenance of contractions by depolarization and stimulating the production of prostaglandins. Animal studies suggest that the hormone relaxin is instrumental in stimulating oxytocin-synthesizing neurons in the hypothalamus just before the onset of labour.

## Physiological changes in the first stage

It should be remembered that the onset of labour is a process, not one event. The latent phase of the first stage is considered to be during cervical dilatation of up to 3–4cm, whilst the active phase is from 3–4cm to 10cm.[1]

- *Cervical ripening*: takes place from 36 weeks' gestation.
- *Contraction and retraction*: shortening of the uterine muscles occurs with every contraction, mainly in the upper segment. Progressive pull on the weaker lower segment results in effacement and dilatation of the cervix.
- *Retraction ring*: a normal occurrence in all labours. Ridge formation occurs between the thick, retracted muscles of the upper segment and the thin, distended aspect of the lower segment. Only visible in obstructed labour, when a transverse ridge across the abdomen forms—known as Bandl's ring—indicating an imminent rupture of the uterus.
- *Fundal dominance*: contractions commence from the cornua and pass in waves in an inwards and downwards direction. Intensity of uterine action is greater in the upper segment.
- *Upper active segment/lower passive segment*: shortening of the upper segment exerts pull on the passive lower segment. This initiates a reflex, releasing oxytocin via the posterior pituitary, and assists with effacement and dilatation.
- *Polarity of the uterus*: coordination between upper and lower segments; a balanced, harmonious, and rhythmical process. The upper segment contracts powerfully and the lower contracts slightly and dilates.
- *Resting tone*: during a contraction the blood flow to the placenta is impaired, so that oxygen and carbon dioxide exchange in the intervillous spaces is reduced. The resting tone is the relaxation period between contractions, which enables placental blood flow to resume to normal levels, to ensure adequate fetal oxygenation. The uterus is never completely relaxed; the measurement of the resting tone is 4–10mmHg.
- *Intensity of contractions*: contractions cause a rise in intrauterine pressure (amplitude) which can be recorded. Contractions rise rapidly to a peak, then slowly diminish (resting tone):
  - Early labour: >20mmHg, 20–30s every 20min
  - Established labour: >60mmHg, 45–60s every 2–3min.

- *Formation of forewaters and hindwaters*: the result of the descent of the fetal head on to the cervix, which separates a small bag of amniotic fluid in front of the presenting part. The forewaters assist effacement of the cervix and early dilatation. The hindwaters fill the remainder of the uterine cavity; they help to equalize pressure in the uterus during contractions, thus providing protection to the fetus and placenta.
- *Rupture of the membranes*: is thought to occur as a result of increased production of prostaglandin E2 (PGE2) by the amnion during labour, together with the force of the contractions. In a normal labour without intervention, the membranes usually rupture between 2cm and 3cm,[2] around full dilatation, or in the second stage.[3]
- *Show*: displacement of the operculum as a result of effacement and dilatation of the cervix. This can occur at any time during labour, but more commonly towards the end of the first stage or at full dilatation. Sometimes a show may occur before the onset of labour and hence is not always an indication that labour is imminent.
- *Fetal axis pressure*: this is the force transmitted by the uterine contractions down the fetal spine to the fetal head.

## References

1 National Institute for Health and Care Excellence (2014). *Intrapartum care for healthy women and babies*. NICE guidelines CG190. Available at: ℛ www.nice.org.uk/guidance/cg190.
2 Fraser DM, Cooper MA (2009). *Myles Textbook for Midwives*, 15th edn. Edinburgh: Churchill Livingstone.
3 National Childbirth Trust (1989). *Rupture of the Membranes in Labour: Women's Views*. London: National Childbirth Trust.

## Further reading

Charles C, Chapman V (2013). *The Midwife's Labour and Birth Handbook*, 3rd edn. Chichester: Wiley-Blackwell.
Walsh D (2007). *Evidence-Based Care for Normal Labour and Birth. A Guide for Midwives*. London: Routledge.

# High- and low-risk labour

Determining whether a woman falls into a high- or low-risk category for labour is dependent on her previous BMI, and her social, medical, mental, and obstetric history. This will have been recorded in her notes at the booking visit and recommendations made for her care in labour. For a list of these, ➔ see Screening for risk in pregnancy, p. 66.

A low-risk labour may be viewed as one where the woman commences labour having experienced an uneventful pregnancy, is in good physical health, and has no known risk factors that would interfere with the normal physiological course of labour and birth.

Sometimes a woman may have had a theoretical risk factor during pregnancy which may have been resolved, e.g. a fetal abnormality which has been investigated and found normal, or a woman with active herpes which has been treated and is not active when she presents in labour. Therefore, there may be overlapping situations where decisions are not verified until a woman commences labour.

## Risk assessment in labour

The midwife should take a full and detailed account of the woman's current social, obstetric, medical, and mental health when she presents in labour. In addition to the antenatal risk factors, circumstances may occur in the current pregnancy and early labour stage that will require referral to high-risk obstetric care:

This is not a definitive list, but some key factors include:[4]

- Late or unbooked pregnancy
- Maternal mental health issues; psychiatric disorder requiring current inpatient care
- Raised BMI
- APH
- Placenta praevia
- Cord presentation or prolapse
- Breech or shoulder presentation
- Malpresentation of the fetal head
- Preterm labour
- Premature rupture of the membranes
- Multiple pregnancy
- Asthma requiring an increase in treatment or hospital treatment
- Haemoglobinopathies—SCD, β-thalassaemia major
- History of thromboembolic disorders
- von Willebrand's disease; bleeding disorder in the woman or unborn baby
- Hyperthyroidism
- Diabetes
- Cardiac conditions
- Epilepsy
- Cystic fibrosis
- Pre-eclampsia
- PIH
- Severe anaemia

- Blood group/atypical antibodies which carry a risk of HDN
- Systemic lupus erythematosus
- Risk factors associated with GBS, whereby antibiotics in labour would be recommended
- Hepatitis B/C with abnormal LFTs
- Carrier of/infected with HIV
- Toxoplasmosis—women receiving treatment
- Current active infection of chickenpox/rubella/genital herpes in the woman or baby
- Tuberculosis under treatment
- Liver disease associated with current abnormal LFTs
- Renal conditions associated with pregnancy such as pyelonephritis
- Abnormalities of the genital tract such as bicornuate uterus and female genital mutilation (FGM)
- Intrauterine growth retardation
- Acute fetal heart anomalies.

*Health professionals should always discuss, and take into account, the woman's individual needs and choices before making decisions about her care in labour.*

## Reference

4  National Institute for Health and Care Excellence (2014). *Intrapartum care for healthy women and babies.* NICE guidelines CG190. Available at: ℜ www.nice.org.uk/guidance/cg190.

# Principles of labour care for low-risk women

Since the inception of medically managed care for labour and birth, there has been a steep rise in intervention and assisted birth among a population of women who invariably have uncomplicated pregnancies. The midwife needs to assess suitability for low-risk care based on individual needs and predisposing conditions. She should not offer or advise clinical intervention if labour is progressing normally and the woman and baby are well. In view of the evidence to support midwives managing low-risk women in labour,[5] it is important that the midwife is confident in all aspects of midwifery care, to support women's choices and to enhance normal physiological principles.[6] In all stages of labour, the midwife should remember that women who have left the normal care pathway because of the development of complications should return to it if/when the complication is resolved.[7]

## Assessment

- No predisposing social, mental health, medical, or obstetric conditions.
- No antenatal pathology present.
- Maternal choice.
- Review of case notes, reports, ultrasound scan, and birth plan.
- Discussion with the woman and her birthing partner/s.

## Principles

- Consider home birth as an option.[7]
- If the woman is having a hospital birth, assessment at home in early labour is an option to avoid hospitalization too soon and the potential for unnecessary noise, distraction, and intervention.
- If the woman is having a hospital birth, she should ideally be cared for on admission in a separate or alongside a midwife-led unit.[5,7]
- Where possible, provide a home-like environment with low lighting, privacy, birthing aids, and hidden equipment.
- Inform the woman that she may eat a light diet in established labour unless she has received opioids or she develops risk factors that make a general anaesthetic more likely.[7]
- An admission CTG is *not* required if low risk. There should be no CTG equipment within the immediate area.
- Auscultation of the fetal heart should be conducted at least every 15min with a fetal stethoscope (Pinard) or a Sonicaid® immediately after a contraction for at least 1min. Always palpate the maternal pulse to differentiate between the two heart rates. The fetal heart rate (FHR) should be recorded as a single rate. Record accelerations and decelerations, if heard. If an FHR abnormality is suspected, commence a continuous CTG.[7]
- If continuous CTG has been used because of concerns arising from intermittent auscultation, but there are no non-reassuring or abnormal features on the CTG trace after 20min, remove the CTG equipment and return to intermittent auscultation.[7]

- Work towards the lower boundaries for interventions. NICE[7] suggests a cervical dilatation of <2cm in 4h for first labours, or of <2cm in 4h *or* a slowing in the progress of labour for second or subsequent labours. The midwife should also record descent and rotation of the baby's head and note changes in the strength, duration, and frequency of uterine contractions.
- Provide support and enhance confidence by encouraging relaxation and breathing techniques, mobility, and change of position. Consider the possible use of complementary therapies to help with coping strategies.

## References

5 Royal College of Midwives (2005). *Evidence-based Guidelines for Midwifery-led Care in Labour*. London: Royal College of Midwives.

6 Sandall J, Soltani H, Gates S, Shennan A, Devane D (2016). *Midwife-led continuity models of care compared with other models of care for women during pregnancy, birth and early parenting*. A Cochrane review. Available at: www.cochrane.org/CD004667/PREG_midwife-led-continuity-models-versus-other-models-of-care-for-childbearing-women.

7 National Institute for Health and Care Excellence (2014). *Intrapartum care for healthy women and babies*. NICE guidelines CG190. Available at: www.nice.org.uk/guidance/cg190.

## Further reading

Charles C, Chapman V (2013). *The Midwife's Labour and Birth Handbook*, 3rd edn. Chichester: Wiley-Blackwell.

Enkin M, Kierse M, Neilson J, et al. (2000). *A Guide to Effective Care in Pregnancy and Childbirth*. Oxford: Oxford University Press.

Lavender T, Alfrevic Z, Walkinshaw S (2006). Effects of different partogram action lines on birth outcomes: a randomized controlled trial. *Obstet Gynecol* 108: 295–302.

## Home birth

NICE[8] recommends that all women with a low risk of complications in child-birth should be encouraged to either give birth at home or in a midwife-led unit (free-standing or alongside a hospital). When pregnancy is straightfor-ward, there is no evidence to suggest any difference in mortality or morbidity between a hospital or home birth.[8] Studies have highlighted that, in low-risk women, there are: fewer Caesarean births, fewer assisted births, fewer inductions, fewer episiotomies and severe tears, and less PPH.[9] The outcomes for the baby are no different compared with an obstetric unit,[8] with fewer low Apgar scores, less fetal distress, fewer neonatal respiratory problems, and less birth trauma. They also show no difference in perinatal mortality rates, often cited as the reason for hospital birth.[9] Where women had given birth at home, they were also very satisfied with their experience and care.

In order for women to make an informed choice as to where they would like to give birth, they require unbiased and realistic information about their choices. In some areas there may be the option for low-risk women to give birth in a midwife-led 'birth centre', or these women may feel more com-fortable giving birth at home.

### Planning and preparation

- *During the first contact with the pregnant woman, discuss where she would like to give birth.* Women should not feel pressurized to go into hospital. The woman needs plenty of time to think over her options; therefore, the decision to opt for a home birth can be taken at any time during pregnancy, or even delayed until the commencement of labour, provided this has been discussed and appropriate plans made for a home birth.
- Explain to both multiparous and nulliparous women who are at low risk of complications that giving birth is generally very safe for both the woman and her baby.[8]
- Advise low-risk multiparous women that planning to give birth at home or in a midwifery-led unit (free-standing or alongside) is particularly suitable for them, because the rate of interventions is lower and the outcome for the baby is no different compared with an obstetric unit.[8]
- Advise low-risk nulliparous women that planning to give birth in a midwifery-led unit (free-standing or alongside) is particularly suitable for them, because the rate of interventions is lower and the outcome for the baby is no different compared with an obstetric unit. Explain that if they plan birth at home there is a small increase in the risk of an adverse outcome for the baby.[8]
- *If deemed to be high-risk,* discuss the risk factors thoroughly with the woman (➜ see Exclusion criteria for home birth, p. 251) and advise her to consider giving birth in a consultant obstetric unit. Discuss the additional care that can be provided in the obstetric unit with the woman, so that she can make an informed choice about a planned place of birth.[8]
- Inform the SoM when a home booking is made.
- Assess the home environment for suitability for a home birth. This includes:
  - The location of the home and ease of access, should an ambulance need to be called
  - Heating and water supply (hot and cold)

- A hygienic environment for the birth, with adequate towels, blankets, and clothing for the baby
- Adequate provision for telephone communication.
- The woman's family and birth partner need to be included in discussion of the woman's choices.
- Care of any other children should be considered, preferably with an adult identified to look after them.
- *The named midwife should ensure that working colleagues are informed of a planned home birth* and any relevant information, should they be on duty to assist or conduct the birth. Ideally colleagues who may be involved in the woman's care should be introduced to her in the antenatal period.
- A birth plan is advisable, outlining the woman's care options. Emphasize that if there are concerns antenatally or in labour regarding the welfare of the mother or the fetus, you will discuss the situation with your superiors and, if necessary, transfer to hospital care.
- *Antenatal care should be based on the guidelines for low-risk women.*[8] If there is any deviation from the normal, you may wish to refer to consultant care with the agreement of the pregnant woman.

## Exclusion criteria for home birth

This is not an exhaustive list, but NICE[8] recommends consideration of the criteria in Tables 14.1, 14.2, and 14.3.

Table 14.1 Current pregnancy

| Factor | Additional information |
|---|---|
| Current pregnancy | • Para 4 or more<br>• Age over 35 at booking<br>• Multiple pregnancy<br>• Late or unbooked pregnancy<br>• Recreational drug use<br>• Alcohol dependency requiring assessment or treatment<br>• Under current outpatient psychiatric care<br>• Antepartum bleeding of unknown origin (single episode after 24 weeks of gestation)<br>• BMI at booking of 30–35kg/m²<br>• Anaemia—Hb <85g/L at onset of labour<br>• BP of 140mmHg systolic or 90mmHg diastolic or more on two occasions<br>• Pre-eclampsia<br>• Clinical or ultrasound suspicion of macrosomia<br>• SGA in this pregnancy (<5th centile or reduced growth velocity on ultrasound)<br>• Placenta praevia<br>• Ultrasound diagnosis of oligo-/polyhydramnios<br>• Preterm labour or preterm pre-labour rupture of membranes<br>• Risk factors associated with group B *Streptococcus* whereby antibiotics in labour would be recommended<br>• Induction of labour<br>• Onset of GDM<br>• Malpresentation—breech or transverse lie |
| Fetal indications | • Fetal abnormality<br>• Abnormal FHR/Doppler studies<br>• Confirmed intrauterine death |

Table 14.2 Previous medical history

| Disease area | Medical condition |
|---|---|
| Cardiovascular | • Confirmed cardiac disease<br>• Hypertensive disorders |
| Respiratory | • Asthma requiring an increase in treatment or hospital treatment<br>• Cystic fibrosis |
| Haematological | • Haemoglobinopathies—SCD, β-thalassaemia major<br>• History of thromboembolic disorders<br>• Immune thrombocytopenia purpura or other platelet disorder or platelet count below $100 \times 10^9$/L<br>• Von Willebrand's disease<br>• Bleeding disorder in the woman or unborn baby<br>• Atypical antibodies which carry a risk of haemolytic disease of the newborn |
| Endocrine | • Hyperthyroidism<br>• Diabetes |
| Infective | • Risk factors associated with GBS whereby antibiotics in labour would be recommended<br>• Hepatitis B/C with abnormal LFTs<br>• Carrier of/infected with HIV<br>• Toxoplasmosis—women receiving treatment<br>• Current active infection of chickenpox/rubella/genital herpes in the woman or baby<br>• Tuberculosis under treatment |
| Immune | • Systemic lupus erythematosus<br>• Scleroderma |
| Renal | • Abnormal renal function<br>• Renal disease requiring supervision by a renal specialist |
| Neurological | • Epilepsy<br>• Myasthenia gravis<br>• Previous cerebrovascular accident |
| Gastrointestinal | • Liver disease associated with current abnormal LFTs |
| Psychiatric | • Psychiatric disorder requiring current inpatient care |

*Previous gynaecological history*
• Infertility.
• Major surgery.
• Myomectomy.
• Uterine anomaly (congenital or fibroids).
• Major gynaecological surgery.
• Cone biopsy or large loop excision of the transformation zone.
• Fibroids.

Table 14.3 Previous obstetric history

| Factor | Additional information |
|---|---|
| Previous complications | • Pre-eclampsia requiring preterm birth<br>• Placental abruption with adverse outcome<br>• Eclampsia<br>• Uterine rupture<br>• Primary PPH requiring additional treatment or blood transfusion<br>• Retained placenta requiring manual removal in theatre<br>• Caesarean section<br>• Shoulder dystocia<br>• History of previous baby >4.5kg<br>• Extensive vaginal, cervical, or third- or fourth-degree perineal trauma<br>• Previous term baby with jaundice requiring exchange transfusion<br>• Unexplained stillbirth/neonatal death or previous death related to intrapartum difficulty<br>• Previous baby with neonatal encephalopathy |

*Intrapartum factors indicating transfer to an obstetric consultant unit*
- Malpresentation.
- Preterm labour.
- Abnormal progress in labour.
- FHR abnormalities.
- Meconium-stained liquor.
- Maternal distress.
- Mother's request.

## Basic equipment for a planned home birth

The following basic equipment is suggested:
- Delivery pack
- Protection and safe disposal:
  - Maternity pads
  - Inco pads
  - Non-sterile gloves
  - Sterile gloves
  - Plastic aprons
  - Disposal bags
  - Clinical waste disposal bags
  - Venflon and IV therapy fluid (for cannulation in case of PPH)
  - Sharps disposal container.
- Supplementary equipment:
  - Lubricating jelly
  - Amnihook
  - Pinard and fetal Doppler
  - Syringes and needles
  - Specimen bottles and request forms
  - Oxytocic drugs
  - Naloxone
  - Urinary catheter.

- Equipment for mother's comfort:
  - Bean bag
  - Birthing ball
  - Floor mattress
  - Hot water bottle.
- Requirements for the baby:
  - Tape measure
  - Cord clamp
  - Mucus extractor
  - Name bands (only if transfer is necessary)
  - Vitamin K
  - Scales.
- For perineal repair:
  - Lidocaine
  - Suture pack
  - Suture material
  - Torch.
- Gases:
  - Inhalational analgesia (Entonox®), two full cylinders, plus mouth and mask attachments
  - Oxygen, together with adult and neonatal masks
  - Portable suction equipment.
- *Appropriate documentation* to include mother's notes, baby's notes, and birth notification.

## Principles of labour care at a home birth

- Ensure that all equipment for the birth is delivered to the woman's home at 37 weeks, or as soon as possible after a decision is made, should it be later than this. Inhalational analgesia and oxygen should be stored at the home, adhering to health and safety regulations.
- Collect resuscitation equipment from the maternity unit as soon as possible, or make arrangements to transfer the equipment in readiness for the birth. Local policies vary.
- On receipt of a labour call, the named midwife, or midwife on call, will attend the woman. Other working colleagues and the labour ward must be informed.
- A second midwife will be required to attend for the birth.
- Follow the NMC and NICE guidelines[8] for low-risk intrapartum care.
- Adhere to guidelines for the safe administration of drugs.
- The woman should have a bag packed, in case urgent transfer to hospital is necessary.
- If transfer to hospital is necessary, an emergency call for a paramedic ambulance is made. The midwife must accompany the woman in the ambulance and provide details of the woman's labour to the attending hospital staff.
- If the woman does not agree with the decision to transfer, then the supervisor of midwives must be informed.

## After the birth
- The woman's GP should be informed of the birth and asked to carry out the neonatal examination, unless the midwife has been trained to do this.
- Complete and maintain all records of the birth, according to the guidelines for records and record-keeping.
- Dispose of clinical waste and sharps in a safe manner, with reference to the local trust policy. Return inhalational analgesia, oxygen, and drugs to the hospital.
- Undertake immediate postnatal care to ensure the well-being of both mother and baby before leaving their home.

## References
8  National Institute for Health and Care Excellence (2014). *Intrapartum care for healthy women and babies*. NICE guidelines CG190. Available at: ℅ www.nice.org.uk/guidance/cg190.
9  Sandall J, Soltani H, Gates S, Shennan A, Devane D (2016). *Midwife-led continuity models of care compared with other models of care for women during pregnancy, birth and early parenting*. A Cochrane review. Available at: ℅ www.cochrane.org/CD004667/PREG_midwife-led-continuity-models-versus-other-models-of-care-for-childbearing-women.

## Further reading
Charles C, Chapman V (2013). *The Midwife's Labour and Birth Handbook*, 3rd edn. Chichester: Wiley-Blackwell.

# Hospital birth

A hospital is by far the most common place to give birth in the UK. This has been the result of government legislation arising from the 1970s (the Peel Report)[10] which advocated that all women should have the opportunity to give birth in hospital, where it was considered to be safer. This led to a radical change in the role of the midwife and maternity care, whilst increased intervention has brought a staggering rise in the rate of complications associated with pregnancy, labour and the incidence of LSCS. Advanced technology and screening have contributed greatly towards better outcomes for high-risk women. However, in recent years, there has been much opposition to these practices and interventions. The evidence for hospitalization of all women for birth is now recognized to be unfounded.[11] Women should be involved in deciding where to give birth following initial assessment in early pregnancy, to identify any risk factors, to be aware of their options and be able to make an informed choice.

## Reasons for hospital birth

- Maternal illness or pre-existing medical condition.
- Obstetric history or present obstetric condition that warrants high-risk management.
- Maternal choice: feels safer in hospital, request for epidural analgesia.
- Unsupported mother: without partner, family, or friends who can provide immediate and ongoing care.
- Social circumstances, e.g. drug misuse, poor housing/living conditions.
- Emergency admission.
- Concealed pregnancy.
- Concerns over the well-being of the fetus.

Invariably the length of stay in hospital is relatively short unless there are complications.
- *Same-day discharge*: the woman spends the latter part of labour and birth in hospital, followed by a short 2–6h recovery period prior to being discharged home to community care.
- 12–24h stay: this is most common for women who have had a normal birth and there are no complications.
- 24–48h stay: very often primiparous women, or women who have had a forceps or ventouse birth, may stay a little longer.
- 1–4 days: mainly women who have had an LSCS or where there are complications.

## Admission

- Hospital environments tend to put labour and birth into the illness mode, which equates with disease, or that something is wrong.
- The woman may be anxious about hospital admission for labour. She may not have been in hospital before and have preconceived ideas or had a previous bad experience.
- Build-up of tension will produce stress hormones that interfere with the normal physiology of labour and slow the process down. Consequently the chances of intervention are increased.

- The hospital environment may be very daunting and impersonal; care should be taken to make the woman feel comfortable and relaxed. Provision of a home-from-home environment, with low lights, music facilities, and non-clinical furnishings should be standard.
- Hospital routines and unnecessary medical terminology should be kept to a minimum.
- Women should be encouraged to make a birth plan, regardless of their parity, obstetric status, or mode of delivery, to ensure that their individual wishes are taken into account.
- Hospital birth may take place in a consultant-based unit, a midwifery-led birth suite, or a birth centre near to a hospital base.
- All maternity units should have a policy for the care of low-risk women within the hospital environment.

## References

10 Peel Report (1970). *Domiciliary Midwifery and Maternity Bed Needs. Report of the Standing Maternity and Midwifery Advisory Committee (Chairman Sir John Peel)*. London: HMSO.
11 National Institute for Health and Care Excellence (2014). *Intrapartum care for healthy women and babies*. NICE guidelines CG190. Available at: ℛ www.nice.org.uk/guidance/cg190.

# Diagnosis of the onset of labour

Although the three cardinal signs listed below (➔ see Onset of active labour, p. 258) indicate the onset of labour, each woman will be individual in her response and adaptation to labour, dependent on her parity, expectations, and pain threshold. Therefore, it is recommended that individualized care is undertaken at all times[12] to detract from rigid routine and impersonal care.

## Pre-labour signs

• Nesting instinct and spurts of energy.
• Feeling generally unwell: flu-like symptoms or a cold.
• Diarrhoea or loose stools.
• Frequency of micturition.
• Heavy sensation/discomfort in the upper thighs and pelvic area.
• Lower backache as the fetus nestles deeply into the pelvis.
• Increase in Braxton Hicks contractions in the final few weeks of pregnancy. Braxton Hicks contractions (also known as prodromal labour contractions) are sporadic, incoordinate uterine contractions that start at around 6 weeks into pregnancy. However, they are not usually felt until the second or third trimester of pregnancy.
• Feeling different, distant, and restless prior to going into labour.
• Mucoid loss per vaginum, a show (loss of the operculum).
• Intermittent leakage of liquor.
• Pre-labour rupture of the membranes—most women will proceed into labour spontaneously within 24h.

## Onset of active labour

• *Show.* The mucoid, bloodstained loss that is passed per vaginum, known as the operculum, seals the cervical canal. Dislodgement of this mucoid plug is an early sign of uterine activity and cervical ripening, but not necessarily an indication of the onset of labour.
• *Contractions.* The most important sign, as cervical dilatation is not possible without regular contractions of the uterus. They may commence as tightenings but become longer, stronger, and more regular as labour progresses. The contractions coincide with abdominal tightenings that can be felt on abdominal palpation. The contractions may commence at 20–30min intervals, lasting for 20–30s.
• *Rupture of the membranes.* This can occur at any time during or before labour. More commonly, in a normal spontaneous labour without intervention, they will rupture at a cervical dilatation of 9cm or more. Occasionally they do not rupture until the advanced second stage at birth. The amount of amniotic fluid that is lost depends on the effectiveness of the fetal presentation to aid the formation of the forewaters. With a well-fitting head that is sufficiently engaged in the pelvis, there will be little loss of fluid, with further small leaks. If the head is poorly engaged, then the loss of fluid may well be substantial.

## Latent phase of labour

Labour should always be seen as a dynamic event, not a mechanical process. NICE[12] defines the latent phase of labour as a period where there are painful contractions and there is some cervical change, including cervical effacement and dilatation of up to 4cm. The active phase of labour is therefore defined as commencing when there are regular painful contractions and there is progressive cervical dilatation from 4cm. Many women may experience a long latent phase prior to established labour. Suggested management should thus consider the individual needs and responses of the woman, as there is huge variation in experience.

- The latent phase is the 'warming up' phase prior to established labour.
- Evidence suggests that labouring at home during early labour is preferable to early admission to the delivery suite.[13]
- Admission for normal labour should be at home, or in assessment areas sited away from the delivery suite.[13]
- The environment for assessment will affect progress, depending on certain inhibiting factors such as medical procedures, clinical apparatus, bright lights, language, and being observed. Women tend to be subjected to more labour intervention as a result.[14]
- Provide psychological support, information, and clear explanations of the role of the latent phase. This will depend on the pain response and expectations of the individual.
- Utilize all your observational, clinical, and intuitive skills.
- A vaginal examination is not necessary if all observations, history, and findings are satisfactory.
- It may be advisable for the woman to return home to await the onset of established labour, i.e. when the contractions are occurring every 5–6min and of 60–90s duration.
- Provide an efficient communication network, so that the woman can phone and obtain advice regarding her progress and concerns during this phase.
- In some areas, vaginal examination to assess progress may initially be undertaken at home by the community midwife, so that unnecessary visits to the hospital are minimized and the woman remains in a non-threatening environment.
- Provide antenatal health promotion that focuses on clear explanations of the latent phase and spurious labour, so that women adopt a more realistic notion of what labour involves.

## Diagnosis of the active phase of labour

- *Uterine activity*: abdominal palpation, degree of discomfort or pain, observation of contractions—their regularity, strength, and length.
- *History so far*: when contractions started, evidence of a show or ruptured membranes.
- Observation of vital signs, urinalysis, and general examination.
- Vaginal examination if clinically indicated.
- Observation of non-verbal behaviour, and visual and auditory signs.
- All observations, clinical findings, and history of the labour so far should be clearly recorded in the maternal notes.

The above information should form the basis for a plan of care to be discussed and agreed with the woman, which should be recorded in the maternity notes.

## Differential diagnosis

Sometimes it may be difficult to ascertain the true onset of active labour, due to compounding factors such as Braxton Hicks (practice) contractions. The only way to manage this situation is to adopt a 'wait and see' policy, and it is only in retrospect that a definite diagnosis can be made.

Generally, regular contractions will cease after a few hours, with no dilatation of the cervical os. This is sometimes referred to as 'false labour' and can be a very distressing and tiring time for the woman.

In this case:
- Provide extra moral support and sound explanations to ease the woman through this difficult time
- Promote coping tactics and utilize non-pharmacological means to relieve discomfort and anxiety
- Some women may require pharmacological pain relief.

## References

12 National Institute for Health and Care Excellence (2014). *Intrapartum care for healthy women and babies*. NICE guidelines CG190. Available at: ℘ www.nice.org.uk/guidance/cg190.
13 Lauzon L, Hodnett E (2006). Labour assessment programs to delay admission to labour wards (Cochrane review). In: *Cochrane Library*, Issue 1. Chichester: John Wiley and Sons Ltd.
14 Rahnama P, Ziaei S, Faghihzadeh S (2006). Impact of early admission in labour on method of delivery. *Int J Gynaecol Obstet* 92: 217–20.

## Further reading

Charles C, Chapman V (2013). *The Midwife's Labour and Birth Handbook*, 3rd edn. Chichester: Wiley-Blackwell.
Gurewitsch E, Diament P, Fong J, et al. (2002). The labour curve of the grand multipara: does progress of labour continue to improve with additional childbearing? *Am J Obstet Gynecol* 186: 1331–8.

# Support for women in the first stage of labour

# Support for women in the first stage of labour

Research has shown that where women are supported through their birth experience by midwives in birth units or midwife-led areas,[15] there is:

- Less intervention—induction of labour, Caesarean section, forceps, ventouse, and ARM[16]
- Less pharmacological analgesia
- Fewer episiotomies
- Less immobility during birthing and labour
- Less external fetal monitoring
- Fewer fetal heart abnormalities.

In addition:

- There are more normal, spontaneous births
- Women experience greater satisfaction with their care
- Midwives express greater job satisfaction
- There is no difference in perinatal mortality or morbidity rates compared with births in other units.

These outcomes rely on the following aspects relating to care:

- *Informational support*: full, accurate, and individualized information is provided about progress and procedures. There is a two-way process of information giving and communication between mother and partner and midwife
- *Physical support*: physical activity is encouraged; tactile support is provided for some women; non-pharmacological means are provided to help women to cope better, e.g. warm baths, massage, freedom of movement, optimal positioning.[17] Reassurance is provided about physical changes and symptoms that occur during labour, e.g. show, rupture of membranes, feeling nauseated
- *Emotional support*: it is important that the midwife appreciates the range of emotional feelings and behaviour that may be expressed during labour and birth:
  - Fear: of failure, pain, the unknown; perhaps influenced by a previous negative obstetric experience
  - Hostility: due to poor previous relationships with health professionals; a defence mechanism for unexpressed anxiety; unwanted pregnancy
  - Resentment: due to personal circumstances and difficult relationships
  - Positive emotions: excitement, confidence, fulfilment, etc.
  - Unrealistic expectations
  - Awareness of fears and anxieties of partner.

Unrealistic expectations are addressed with sensitivity. Relaxation techniques, breathing awareness, and dialogue are encouraged to help allay fears.

- *Advocacy and empowerment*:
  - Birth and labour are viewed as a partnership within a social, cultural, and biophysical model of care

- The midwife acts as an intermediary for the woman when she may feel undermined by the environment of a hospital and experience loss of personal identity, or loss of assertiveness to express her needs and anxieties
  - Empowerment is encouraged by assisting women with decision-making that reflects their needs and care plans
  - Facilitate choice and control for women
  - Respect is shown for women's ability to verbalize their wishes and requirements freely.
- *Environment*: known to have a huge impact on the release of endorphins, which will enhance the physiological process of labour.[18]
  - Women are encouraged to adopt upright/alternative positions and freedom of movement.
  - Appropriate props are provided: birthing balls, beanbags, easy chairs, stools, music, etc.
  - Low lights and low noise levels.
  - Creation of a home-from-home environment within a hospital setting—medical apparatus is removed or hidden, pleasant furnishings are provided, etc.
  - Complementary therapies are used, e.g. massage, aromatherapy.
  - Privacy is provided.
  - Key carers only are involved in care—continuous support from a midwife has been shown to be associated with less use of pharmacological analgesia and epidurals. Attendance of a birth supporter (partner, friend, sister, mother) has been shown to result in shorter labours and less intervention.[16,17]
- *Individualized care*: the ability to accommodate and appreciate the woman's personal needs, expectations, and views; to achieve a meaningful experience with respect to her social and cultural background, and her emotional, mental, and physical attributes; providing the opportunity to discuss the woman's labour afterwards, to clear up any concerns or confusion.

## References

15 Sandall J, Soltani H, Gates S, Shennan A, Devane D (2016). *Midwife-led continuity models of care compared with other models of care for women during pregnancy, birth and early parenting*. A Cochrane review. Available at: ℬ www.cochrane.org/CD004667/PREG_midwife-led-continuity-models-versus-other-models-of-care-for-childbearing-women.

16 Hodnett ED, Gates S, Hofmeyr GJ, Sakala C (2003). Continuous support for women during childbirth. *Cochrane Database Syst Rev* 3: CD003766.

17 Simkin P, O'Hara M (2002). Non-pharmacological relief of pain during labour: systematic review of five methods. *Am J Obstet Gynaecol* 186: S131–59.

18 Walsh D (2006). Subverting assembly-line childbirth: childbirth in a free-standing birth centre. *Soc Sci Med* 26: 1330–40.

## Further reading

Charles C, Chapman V (2013). *The Midwife's Labour and Birth Handbook*, 3rd edn. Chichester: Wiley-Blackwell.

National Institute for Health and Care Excellence (2014). *Intrapartum care for healthy women and babies*. NICE guidelines CG190. Available at: ℬ www.nice.org.uk/guidance/cg190.

# Routine care in the first stage of labour

The first stage of labour is primarily a stage of preparation, both physically and emotionally. The cervix has to undergo radical anatomical changes in order for birth to be possible, whilst the mother has to quickly adjust to the demands of labour. As it is the longest stage of labour, its duration may place a great deal of strain on the woman and therefore be challenging in terms of care provision. However, it is always important to give individual-ized care, based on the woman's choices and her progress in labour.

It is important when taking over care from a colleague, admitting a woman in labour, or visiting for a home birth that the midwife familiarizes herself with all the necessary information about the woman.

- Be aware of previous medical or obstetric history that is relevant to the labour and birth.
- Be aware of any risk factors or possible problems that may necessitate potential referral to consultant care.
- Essential information that should be available:
  - Blood group, antibodies, and Hb result
  - Allergies and drug reactions
  - The ultrasound report confirming the location of the placenta
  - Confirmation of the woman's correct gestation.
- *Familiarize with the birth plan* and discuss any preferences the woman may have.
- *Check any information about the history of the labour so far*—whether membranes are intact, onset of contractions, loss per vaginum (PV), and so on.

The midwife should then carry out an assessment of the woman's physical condition, the degree of comfort/pain, and how she is coping emotionally with the labour so far. This will involve observation, abdominal palpation, recording vital signs, direct questioning, and possibly a vaginal examination, if indicated.

- Discuss options of care with the woman. One may need to raise questions such as:
  - How far advanced in labour is she?
  - Does she want to mobilize?
  - Does she want a bath or any other analgesia?
  - What about food and drink?
  - Is the environment how she wishes?
- Assess the woman's progress regularly whilst also being flexible in responding to her individual needs.
- If the woman is not in established labour, give her a realistic and reassuring explanation of early labour and that this could last for several hours and sometimes days before established labour begins in earnest.
- *Encourage and assist with positions of comfort and hygiene.* A shower or bath in early labour is often relaxing and refreshing.
- *Encourage her to adopt an upright position, to change position regularly, and to mobilize to assist the progress of her labour.* These measures are known to result in shorter labours, less demand for analgesia and epidural anaesthesia, and less need for augmentation of labour.[19]

- *Encourage the woman to empty her bladder every 2h* to prevent trauma and delay in labour. Test the urine for protein, glucose, and ketones.
- *Encourage the woman to maintain an adequate fluid balance and nutrition during labour.* (For further information regarding food intake in labour, ⊋ see Nutrition in labour, p. 272.)
- *Carry out regular observations of the woman's physical condition by monitoring the vital signs:* 2- to 4-hourly in early labour, progressing to hourly and half hourly as appropriate, and record on the partogram.
- *Observe for vaginal loss*—a minimal bloodstained mucoid loss indicates a show. A copious show may coincide with full dilatation.
- *Record the time of rupture of the membranes in the notes.* When the amnion and the chorion rupture, the amniotic fluid should be clear, pale, or straw-coloured; a greenish/yellowish/brownish appearance indicates the presence of meconium, the first stool of the fetus. A copious amount of thick meconium present in the liquor is associated with poor fetal outcome.
- *Observe the woman for signs of pretibial, finger, and/or facial oedema* which may be associated with a developing or worsening hypertensive state.
- *Palpate for uterine activity regularly*—the timing, strength, regularity, and duration of contractions—to assess progress. Encourage the woman to relax between contractions.
- *Carry out abdominal palpation prior to a vaginal examination* to assess position, progress, and descent of the fetal head.
- *Monitor the effect of analgesia* or other measures that may have been initiated, e.g. encouraging breathing, massage, complementary therapies such as aromatherapy.
- *Carry out a vaginal examination when appropriate* and only if clinically necessary (⊋ see Vaginal examination, p. 278).
- *Reassure the mother regarding her progress* and ability to cope. In their excitement, women (particularly primigravidae) often overestimate their progress. You will need to provide a realistic picture whilst acknowledging their excitement as well as their fears.
- *Encourage the woman's coping skills* by giving reassurance and emotional support. Encourage her to utilize breathing and relaxation techniques. Provide practical measures such as fans, birthing balls, back massage, positions of comfort, TENS, etc.
- *Support the birthing partner* and encourage their involvement.
- *Ensure that the woman's physical environment is private* and conducive to her needs.
- *Monitor the fetal heart regularly* either by intermittent auscultation via a Pinard stethoscope or a Sonicaid®.

## Reference

19 National Institute for Health and Care Excellence (2014). *Intrapartum care for healthy women and babies.* NICE guidelines CG190. Available at: ⌂ www.nice.org.uk/guidance/cg190.

## Water birth

Labouring in water is recognized as an appropriate method of assisting pain relief and relaxation, by the release of natural endorphins, raising oxytocin levels, and reducing catecholamine secretion.[20] Water provides a secure, peaceful environment and aids buoyancy, which enables the woman to adopt positions of comfort and freedom more easily. Women should therefore be offered the opportunity to labour in water for pain relief.[21]

There have, however, been several controversies regarding the use of water for giving birth and women should thus be informed that there is currently insufficient high-quality evidence to either support or discourage giving birth in water.[21] Adverse outcomes evaluated have included the risk of fetal drowning, fetal hyperthermia, length of labour, genital tract trauma, use of analgesia, low Apgar score, and blood loss.[22] However, birthing in water is also associated with fewer third- and fourth-degree tears; however, labial tears associated with naturally occurring trauma are more likely to occur.[23] Studies have found that there is no difference in the length of labour, blood loss, Apgar scores, or risk of infection,[22,23,24] or of poor perinatal outcomes such as stillbirth after the start of care in labour, early neonatal death, neonatal encephalopathy, meconium aspiration syndrome, brachial plexus injury, fractured humerus, or fractured clavicle[25] when using a birth pool.

Most maternity units have specific guidelines to ensure safe practice regarding water birth, whilst also considering the individual needs of the woman. Midwives should familiarize themselves with this mode of birth to ensure their competency when a woman chooses to labour, or give birth, in water.

### Inclusion criteria for birth in water

- Single cephalic presentation.
- Uncomplicated term pregnancy from 37 weeks until term +9–14 days, dependent on hospital policy.
- Woman's informed choice.
- Spontaneous rupture of the membranes (SROM) of <24h.
- It may be appropriate for the mother to use the pool for the first stage only—maternal choice or anticipation of possible problems in the second stage, e.g. previous shoulder dystocia or previous PPH.

### Exclusion criteria for birth in water

- Intrauterine growth retardation.
- Meconium-stained liquor.
- Following the administration of narcotics (pethidine, diamorphine), midwives need to use their discretion and professional judgement and refer to their local guidelines, regarding re-entry to the pool. A minimum of 3–12h for diamorphine has been suggested.
- IV infusion.
- Previous LSCS—not a universal exclusion; depends on the reasons for the LSCS; a risk assessment is advisable.
- APH.
- Multiple pregnancy.

- BMI at booking of 30–35kg/m². Women should be able to enter and leave the pool independently—this may result in exclusion of some women with disabilities or poor physical mobility on safety grounds. A risk assessment is advisable.
- Prolonged rupture of membranes of over 24h.
- Risk factors associated with GBS whereby antibiotics in labour would be recommended.
- Grand multiparity.
- Maternal pyrexia—37.5 or above.
- Epilepsy.
- FHR abnormalities—bradycardia, tachycardia, decelerations.
- Any fetal or maternal finding during the course of labour and birth that deviates from normal, or where continuous CTG is required.

## Preparation for water birth
- There will be local policies in place for effective cleaning and preparation of the pool. Decontamination should involve the use of a chlorine-releasing agent which is effective against HIV, hepatitis B, and hepatitis C.
- If the pool has not been used for some time, leave the water to run for a minimum of 5min before filling.
- Use a previously disinfected hose for each woman using the pool.
- Fill the pool to about two-thirds deep, approximately to the woman's breast level and sufficient to cover the uterus when in a sitting position.
- Maintain a temperature of between 35 and 37°C[21] in the first stage of labour to avoid fetal hyperthermia; frequent observation of the pool temperature is therefore crucial. You may need to add hot water every 30min to achieve this.
- The following equipment should be available:
  - Thermometer to check the water temperature
  - Waterproof Sonicaid®
  - Towels
  - Sieve for the pool to remove debris
  - Patient hoist to be placed outside the pool room door
  - Sample bottles for microbiology checks on the pool water—refer to local guidelines
  - Portable Entonox® or extended tubing for the woman to use whilst in the pool.
- Wear loose, comfortable clothing and gauntlet gloves (or half a size smaller gloves) for the birth.
- Encourage involvement of the birth partner. If the partner wishes to enter the pool, then suitable swimwear should be used.
- Adhere to health and safety principles whilst caring for a woman in the pool.

## Care in the first stage of labour for a water birth
- Allow the woman to enter and leave the pool as she wishes.
- The woman should be in established labour prior to entering the pool, i.e. 4–5cm dilated. Entering the pool too early is associated with slowing progress during labour.[22]

- Check the woman's temperature hourly, to help prevent fetal hyperthermia. A rise of 1°C above the baseline should indicate possible termination of pool use.[25]
- Check the pool water temperature half-hourly and top up to maintain the pool temperature as appropriate. Record the pool temperature on the partogram and in specified paperwork for pool use. *Pool temperature should not be above 37.5°C.*[21]
- Assist the woman in adopting a comfortable position.
- *Avoid dehydration* by encouraging the woman to drink freely. Diuresis is increased when immersed in water.
- Rehearse with the woman and her birth partner the principles of vacating the pool in the event of an emergency, with regard to health and safety.
- Amniotomy and SROM are not contraindicated if all other observations, progress, and criteria are satisfactory.
- *It is possible to perform a vaginal examination whilst the woman is in the pool*; however, this needs to be discussed with the woman and will depend on individual preferences.
- There are differences of opinion regarding the use of essential oils, generally they are not added to the pool—refer to local guidelines and information on administration of oils (➔ see Aromatherapy during labour, p. 300).
- *Adhere to the guidelines for low-risk care* during labour.

## References

20 Da Silva FMB, de Oliveira SMJV, Nobre MRC (2009). A randomized controlled trial evaluating the effect of immersion bath on labour pain. *Midwifery* 25: 286–94.
21 Cluett ER, Burns E (2009). Immersion in water in labour and birth. *Cochrane Database Syst Rev* 2: CD000111.
22 National Institute for Health and Care Excellence (2014). *Intrapartum care for healthy women and babies*. NICE guidelines CG190. Available at: ℘ www.nice.org.uk/guidance/cg190.
23 Garland D (2006). On the crest of a wave. Completion of a collaborative audit. *MIDIRS Midwifery Digest* 16: 81–5.
24 Lim SK (1994). *A study to compare midwives' visual estimation of blood loss in 'water' and on 'land'*. MSc Dissertation. Guildford: University of Surrey.
25 Birthplace in England Collaborative Group, Brocklehurst P, Hardy P, Hollowell J, et al. (2011). Perinatal and maternal outcomes by planned place of birth for healthy women with low risk pregnancies: the Birthplace in England national prospective cohort study. *BMJ* 343: d7400.

## Mobility and positioning in labour

Women should be encouraged to adopt an upright position in labour. This works with the laws of gravity to assist labour and facilitate birth and has been shown to have the following physiological advantages:[26,27,28]

- A shorter labour
- Less need to augment up the labour with IV oxytocin
- Less intervention in labour
- A shorter second stage with easier bearing down
- Fewer assisted births, fewer episiotomies (but more second-degree perineal tears)
- Increased risk of an estimated blood loss of over 500mL (although this may be due to overestimation)[29]
- Fewer reports of severe pain and reduced analgesia requirements
- Fewer FHR abnormalities
- Higher Apgar scores at 1 and 5min.

### Suggested positions

- Upright, walking freely—support during contraction from partner, wall, table, or other furniture.
- Sitting in a chair, either forward or astride, supported by pillows.
- Use of beanbags/wedges/pillows.
- Use of a birthing ball (pelvic rocking aids rotation).
- Left lateral position.

### References

26 Royal College of Midwives (2013). *Evidence based guidelines for midwifery-led care in labour: positions for labour and birth*. Available at: &#8505; www.rcm.org.uk/sites/default/files/Positions%20for%20Labour%20and%20Birth.pdf.

27 National Institute for Health and Care Excellence (2014). *Intrapartum care for healthy women and babies*. NICE guidelines CG190. Available at: &#8505; www.nice.org.uk/guidance/cg190.

28 Gupta J, Hofmeyr G (2006). Position for women during second stage of labour (Cochrane review). In: *Cochrane Library*, Issue 4. Chichester: John Wiley and Sons Ltd.

29 Lim SK (1994). *A study to compare midwives' visual estimation of blood loss in 'water' and on 'land'*. MSc Dissertation. Guildford: University of Surrey.

### Further reading

Boyle M (2000). Childbirth in bed—the historical perspective. *Pract Midwife* 3: 21–4.

Charles C, Chapman V (2013). *The Midwife's Labour and Birth Handbook*, 3rd edn. Chichester: Wiley-Blackwell.

Royal College Of Midwives (2011). *Campaign for Normal Birth: Getting off the Bed*. London: Royal College of Midwives.

Walsh D (2007). *Evidence-based Care for Normal Labour and Birth*. London: Taylor and Francis Group.

## Nutrition in labour

Studies regarding nutrition in labour are sourced primarily from anaesthetic research into delayed gastric emptying.[30]

Whenever a general anaesthetic is administered, there is a high risk of regurgitation and inhalation of stomach contents. During pregnancy, the lower oesophageal sphincter is often impaired and intragastric pressure is raised due to the gravid uterus. There is some debate regarding the more common use of spinal anaesthesia for a Caesarean section and the reduced risk of regurgitation, however. The factors below should also be considered in the overall assessment and management of eating and drinking in labour.

- *Delayed gastric emptying* may be influenced by pain, anxiety, and, most significantly, the use of narcotics.
- *There is insufficient evidence to support the practice of fasting in labour* in order to lessen the risk of gastric acid aspiration.[31]
- *There is insufficient evidence to support increasing the calorie intake during labour.* A recent study has highlighted that consumption of a light diet during labour did not appear to influence obstetric or neonatal outcomes.[32]
- *The body stores fat during pregnancy* which can be used as fuel in labour if required.[33] The smooth muscle of the uterus metabolizes fatty acids/ketones as fuel. Therefore, mild acidosis is considered to be a normal, and probably beneficial, physiological state of labour.[31]
- *In normal labour, there is little evidence to suggest that fluid balance needs correcting*; however, there has been recent caution regarding a possible risk of fluid overload where women are overzealous to drink copious amounts of water during labour.[34] The usual practice of sipping water between contractions should not pose a risk.
- *IV infusions of glucose should be used sparingly* due to the risks of rebound hypoglycaemia in the newborn infant.

In order to achieve safety and comfort for women, and not to impose a strict, unreasonable regimen for the majority, it is important to consider the risk factors and to recognize those women who may need a Caesarean section. As there is scant evidence of improved outcomes for the baby and mother regarding fasting in labour, women should be informed of the choices they have, taking into account their individual situation during labour.[31] Management will therefore depend on the risk factors present and maternal choice.

### Management

- *Self-regulation of food intake during normal labour* has been recommended. Eating and drinking may help to make a woman feel healthy and normal.
- *No restrictions of food intake* after induction, prior to the onset of labour, and beyond if the labour proceeds normally.[31]
- *Drinks and a light diet during early labour*, established normal labour without narcotics, and uncomplicated labour with an epidural.[31]

- *Non-fizzy isotonic drinks* can increase a woman's energy levels whilst providing a relatively small calorific intake. They may be more beneficial than water.[31]
- *Alcohol and fatty foods* should be avoided at all times.
- *Small amounts of clear fluids only* if labour is established with one or more of the following factors:
  - Narcotics used for pain relief[35]
  - Suspicious CTG recording
  - Trial of labour, breech, twins, etc.
  - Severe pre-eclampsia
  - APH.
- *No food or drink should be permitted if an operation is likely* to ensure the woman's safety due to the increased risk of regurgitation and delayed gastric emptying.[30]

## References

30  Sleutal M, Golden S (1999). Fasting in labour: relic or requirement. *J Obstet Gynaecol Neonatal Nurs* **28**: 507–12.
31  National Institute for Health and Care Excellence (2014) *Intrapartum care for healthy women and babies*. NICE guidelines CG190. Available at: ℘ www.nice.org.uk/guidance/cg190.
32  O'Sullivan G, Liu B, Hart D, Seed P, Shennan A (2009). Effect of food intake during labour on obstetric outcome: randomized controlled trial. *BMJ* **338**: b784.
33  Odent M (1998). Labouring women are not marathon runners. *Pract Midwife* **1**: 16–18.
34  Ophir E, Solt I, Odeh M, Bornstein J (2007). Water intoxication—a dangerous condition in labour and delivery rooms. *Obstet Gynecol Surv* **62**: 731–8.
35  Royal College of Midwives (2012). *Evidence-based guidelines for midwifery-led care: nutrition in labour*. Available at: ℘ www.rcm.org.uk/sites/default/files/Nutrition%20in%20Labour.pdf.

## Further reading

Campion P, McCormick C (2002). *Eating and Drinking in Labour*. Cheshire: Books for Midwives Press.
Young D (2007). Eating in labour: the issue deserves revisiting. *Birth* **34**: 279–81.

## Assessing progress of labour

The means by which the midwife evaluates and assesses the progress being made will influence the care and responses she gives, based on the individual needs and choices of women in her care. When performing an initial assessment of a woman in labour, the midwife should listen to her story and take into account her preferences and her emotional and psychological needs.[36]

Assessing progress during labour should not just involve monitoring the vital signs and assessing cervical dilatation and the intensity of uterine contractions.[37] The midwife should also use her hands-on skills such as abdominal palpation, observation of the mother's changing physical and emotional behaviour, vocalizations, and positioning.[37] Assessment of progress does not rely on just one set of parameters; consideration of all of the previous pointers makes for a holistic assessment.

### First stage of labour

*Latent phase*

The latent phase of labour can be defined as the period before established labour begins when there is some cervical change, including cervical effacement and dilatation of up to 4cm.[36] It can vary in duration and the mother may experience irregular, painful contractions.

- Definition of onset of the first stage varies considerably; labour is a dynamic process; therefore individualized care is important.
- There is evidence to support: minimizing early admission to a labour ward, maximizing assessment at home or in assessment areas, and encouraging women to stay at home during the early stages.[36]

*Active phase*

The active phase of labour is established when the cervix is fully effaced and 4cm or more dilated in the presence of regular painful contractions.[36]

- No differences in outcome or LSCS rate have been reported with an action line; this describes the timing of intervention/augmentation that is considered during labour of 2 or 4h. Reduced intervention has been reported with a 4h action line.[38]
- Assuming a baseline rate of 0.5cm/h, as opposed to 1cm/h, reduces unnecessary interventions and accounts for the slower labours of primigravidas.[36]
- Other means of assessing progress: pattern of contractions, women's behaviour, auditory/visual cues, and intuitive skills.

### First-stage labour care and management

- Verbal and observational history from the woman at onset and throughout labour.
- General examination and vital signs.
- Abdominal palpation and inspection (initially to give a baseline for future care), uterine activity; establish position and descent.
- Psychological and emotional aspects, coping strategies, and support from birth attendants.
- Loss per vaginum: show, colour of amniotic fluid, rupture of membranes, meconium.

- Vaginal examination: the midwife should ensure that sound clinical reasons are indicated prior to the procedure, to safeguard against unnecessary intervention, exposure, and distress for the mother.[37]
- Record all ongoing assessments, examinations, and overview of care on a partogram.

Assessment in labour is based on a medical environment and perspective; therefore, the commonly used baselines, such as length of labour/latent phase of the first stage/action curves, etc., may not reflect the normal physiology of labour. Some would suggest that this has led to increased intervention and ultimately a rise in LSCS rates.

## References

36 National Institute for Health and Care Excellence (2014). *Intrapartum care for healthy women and babies*. NICE guidelines CG190. Available at: ℜ www.nice.org.uk/guidance/cg190.
37 Charles C, Chapman V (2013). *The Midwife's Labour and Birth Handbook*, 3rd edn. Chichester: Wiley-Blackwell.
38 Lavender T, Wallymahmed A, Walkinshaw S (1999). Managing labour using partograms with different action lines: a prospective study of women's views. *Birth* 26: 89–96.

## Further reading

Walsh D (2007). *Evidence-based Care for Normal Labour and Birth*. London: Taylor and Francis Group.

## Abdominal examination

Abdominal palpation in labour is one of the key clinical skills that the midwife uses to assess progress and determine the position of the fetus. At the first contact with the woman in labour, the midwife will carry out a detailed abdominal examination to establish the progress and individual status of the woman's labour so far. This information will enable the midwife to plan care and discuss care with the mother and her partner. The examination should be carried out between contractions if they are present, avoiding any discomfort to the woman whilst facilitating a more accurate assessment. The midwife will then need to palpate the fundus during a contraction to determine the strength and length of the contractions.

In normal labour, the findings should be:

- *Lie*: longitudinal, oblique or transverse lie should be detected early and the woman referred.
- *Presentation*: should be cephalic, any other presentation should be reported immediately.
- *Position* should be established (Fig. 14.1).
- *Engagement of the fetal head* should be determined in fifths above the brim of the pelvis. In primiparous women, this is usually engaged prior to labour. When the head is engaged, the occipital protuberance is barely felt.
- *Auscultation of the fetal heart* for a minimum of 1min immediately after a contraction. Palpate the woman's pulse to differentiate between the heart rate of the woman and that of the baby. The fetal heart rate should be between 110 and 160 beats per minute (bpm).
- *Abdominal palpation*: for information on how to perform, ➔ see Abdominal examination, p. 78. During labour, an abdominal palpation is repeated at regular intervals as above to assess the position, lie, and descent of the fetal head. In addition, palpation of uterine contractions throughout labour is important:
- *Palpation of the fundus* of the uterus with the palm of the hand during contractions provides valuable information on the progress of labour.
- *The frequency of contractions*—if they are occurring very close together and are strong, this may cause fetal hypoxia; therefore, careful monitoring of the fetal heart is advised. Hyperstimulation with oxytocics may be one of the reasons for this, in which case the infusion should be stopped and a review of progress should be made. Contractions may be weaker and less frequent, which will indicate slow progress, or fatigue of the mother. Encouraging ambulation and/or repositioning may re-establish uterine activity.
- *The strength and length of the contractions*—assessing the strength of contractions may be subjective, as the midwife cannot relate to the intensity of the pain the woman may be experiencing in relation to what is felt abdominally. This will depend on the individual's pain threshold and perception.

Left occipito-anterior          Right occipito-posterior

Right occipito-anterior          Left occipito-posterior

**Fig. 14.1** Cephalic presentations prior to labour.

- *Contractions* are described and recorded in three ways:
    - *Mild*—the fundus feels tense throughout the contraction but can be easily indented with the fingertips
    - *Moderate*—the fundus feels more tense throughout the contraction and it is difficult to indent it with the fingertips
    - *Strong*—the fundus feels tense, hard, and rigid during the contraction.
- The uterus should return to feeling soft between contractions.
- *Duration*: contractions may last from 30s up to 90s. The midwife notes the time of the start of the contraction and how long it lasts.
- Uterine contractions are not felt by the woman at their beginning and end. However, the midwife can detect the start of the contraction by palpation before the woman. This may well be useful for using pain relief such as inhalational analgesia, or for encouraging coping mechanisms in labour such as breathing and relaxation techniques.

## Vaginal examination

In normal labour, vaginal examination is performed at the discretion of the midwife, dependent on the individual needs of the woman, consent, and her progress through labour. If there is uncertainty about whether the woman is in established labour, a vaginal examination may be helpful after a period of assessment but is not always necessary. If the woman appears to be in established labour, then offer a vaginal examination. Sensitivity should be employed at all times, as many women find vaginal examinations uncomfortable and traumatic. Where possible, vaginal examinations should be kept to a minimum (only when clinically indicated) and ideally should be performed by the same person.

### Indications

Vaginal examination may be undertaken to:

• Confirm the establishment of labour
• Provide a baseline for subsequent progress
• Assess progress in labour and detect abnormal indices
• Assess the presenting part/position if in doubt (Fig. 14.2)
• Confirm progress to the second stage of labour
• Determine the position and station of the presenting part
• Determine the cause of delay/lack of progress in the second stage
• Rupture membranes if indicated
• Apply a fetal electrode
• Exclude cord prolapse following rupture of the membranes when ill-fitting, or non-engagement of the presenting part, or polyhydramnios is encountered.

Left occipito-anterior (LOA)          Right occipito-anterior (ROA)

Left occipito-posterior (LOP)          Right occipito-posterior (ROP)

Fig. 14.2 Occipito-anterior and occipito-posterior positions.

## Method of undertaking a vaginal examination

Discussion with the woman is essential before examination, to explain the procedure, reassure, and gain consent. Encourage the woman to empty her bladder. Assist in making her comfortable. Carry out an abdominal examination and auscultation of the fetal heart prior to examination.

- *Clean* the surrounding labial area/apply gloves (dependent on local policy).
- *Assess the external genitalia* (lesions, scars, varicose veins, discharge).
- *Assess the cervix*: consistency, position, effacement, and dilatation.
- *Assess the membranes*: absent or intact, observation of liquor.
- *Auscultate the fetal heart* after the procedure.
- *Explain your findings* to the woman.

# The partogram

Use of a partogram in established labour is recommended by NICE.[39] The partogram is a graphical overview of the physical elements and events that take place in an individual woman's labour. This has proved to be an invaluable at-a-glance visual aid and a reference for midwives during their care of women in labour. It is especially useful when handing over the woman's care to a colleague, as it provides an instant summary of the woman's progress to date. The partogram is usually commenced when the woman is in established labour.

Details recorded on the partogram are:
- Hospital number, name of woman, age, parity, date of birth, and expected date of confinement
- The FHR, plotted at regular intervals (for NICE guidelines on the frequency of auscultation of the FHR, ➔ see Electronic fetal monitoring, p. 282)
- Observation of the liquor and what time the membranes ruptured
- Cervical dilatation and descent of the presenting part, plotted diagrammatically
- Oxytocic agents if used during labour
- Uterine activity: the length and strength of the contractions per 10min
- Drugs, inhalational analgesia, and non-pharmacological interventions used
- Urinalysis
- BP and pulse.

Legally, the partogram provides a complete and comprehensive record of care and should include the following information:
- Time of birth, gender of baby, and weight
- Any abnormalities noted at birth
- Mode of birth
- Apgar score and any resuscitation/intervention/drugs given to the baby
- Length of the first, second, and third stages of labour
- Blood loss
- Perineal repair or status of the perineum
- Whether meconium or urine passed during or post-birth
- Feeding intention and summary of feeding/skin-to-skin contact.

Most research on the first stage of labour is based on a medical model of care, where interventions are commonplace, and may not reflect normal labour and physiology. Originally, routine use of the partogram was introduced to allow the prompt recognition of cases of prolonged labour, so that appropriate action/intervention could be taken. However, this also tends to create a structured and rigid approach to care, which some midwives find restrictive, whilst not addressing the woman's individual needs. The following points should be considered:
- The duration of labour may well be much longer than anticipated, particularly in primigravid women.

- Provided progress in labour is steady and the fetus is uncompromised, more flexibility in care and less rigid action lines result in less intervention and the promotion of more spontaneous births.
- A 4h action line, as opposed to a 2h action line, is associated with less use of oxytocin.[40] There is no significant difference in Caesarean section rates or neonatal outcomes between these two options.[40] However, interestingly women in the 2h action line group appeared less likely to report a negative childbirth experience.[40]
- More recently, it has been suggested that a cervical dilatation rate of 0.5cm/h is more realistic than 1cm/h, or equally a slowing in the overall progress of labour for second or subsequent labours.[39]

Debate about the effectiveness and use of the partogram for normal, uncomplicated labour should not detract from the keeping of contemporaneous records during labour and birth.

## References

39 National Institute for Health and Care Excellence (2014). *Intrapartum care for healthy women and babies*. NICE guidelines CG190. Available at: ✒ www.nice.org.uk/guidance/cg190.
40 Lavender T, Hart A, Smyth R (2013). Effect of partogram use on outcomes for women in spontaneous labour at term. *Cochrane Database Syst Rev* 7: CD005461. Also available at: ✒ onlinelibrary.wiley.com/doi/10.1002/14651858.CD005461.pub4/full.

# Monitoring fetal well-being in labour

The fetal response to coping with the stress of labour can be assessed by the observational skills of the midwife and by clinical means, as follows:

- Fetal movements are always an indication of fetal well-being, particularly during a contraction. Fetal activity may be felt abdominally or the woman questioned about the movements she is feeling.
- Auscultation of the fetal heart using a Pinard fetal stethoscope, Sonicaid®, or electronic fetal monitor.
- Intrapartum events, such as augmentation with oxytocin, epidural anaesthesia, bleeding, etc. Electronic fetal monitoring (EFM) needs to be commenced if the woman develops risk factors during labour.
- Condition of the amniotic fluid: noting the presence of meconium in the amniotic fluid is of some value, but not always predictive of fetal distress. However, thick fresh meconium may be indicative of fetal compromise and it is recommended that continuous electronic monitoring is commenced, to establish any changes in the normal pattern of the fetal heart. Potential morbidity due to inhalation of meconium at birth must be prepared for. However, morbid inhalation of meconium is more likely to occur *in utero* when severe hypoxia causes agonal respirations prior to terminal apnoea.
- Because of the very close relationship between a mother and her fetus, a mother's anxiety regarding fetal well-being may be taken as a cue to start continuous monitoring.

## Electronic fetal monitoring

EFM was introduced initially to reduce perinatal mortality and cerebral palsy. Whilst a fall in the incidence of these conditions has not been demonstrated clinically, there has been a steep rise in interventions during labour. This has led to much debate about the value of continuous EFM in normal, low-risk labours.[41]

- The NICE guidelines[42] recommend that in normal labour the admission trace should be abandoned and auscultation of the fetal heart should be carried out intermittently, with a Pinard stethoscope or Sonicaid®, for up to 60s after a contraction, every 15min in the first stage of labour, and every 5min in the second stage of labour, unless the woman develops any risk factors. However, the timings selected are not based on sound research evidence. Certainly during the early stages of normal labour, women are encouraged to remain at home and this amount of monitoring could be regarded as extremely intrusive.
- On admission, the maternal pulse should be recorded at the same time as the FHR, to differentiate between the two.
- Intrapartum hypoxia is a relatively rare occurrence. Therefore, the risk of acidaemia is negligible if the pattern of the FHR falls into the reassuring classification.
- EFM affects the birth environment, changes relationships, and increases anxiety for the woman, birth supporters, and clinicians.[43]

- With intermittent auscultation, the fetus is protected from recurrent, transient, and mild hypoxic episodes during labour. Therefore, individual variation in the fetal response to cope with labour is unmeasurable.[44] Due to high levels of stress hormones, the fetus is able to cope with prolonged periods of hypoxia and lowering of the heart rate during contractions.
- Intermittent auscultation provides more flexible one-to-one care, which is more personalized.
- Ideally, low-risk women should be cared for in separate areas to high-risk women.
- Ideally, no EFM machines should be housed in normal birth areas.[45]
- Several randomized controlled trials have been carried out indicating that EFM results in a negative labour and birth experience for many low-risk women, due to restriction of movement and concern centred on the monitoring procedure, rather than the standard of care given.[46] However, informed consent about EFM is important and some women may not share these views.
- It is important to weigh up the risks/benefits of using technology in low-risk labours before using them. Establishing the boundaries of normal labour is key.[43]

## Documentation

When electronic CTG monitoring is commenced, it is important to maintain a continuous tracing of FHR and maternal uterine activity (contraction frequency and strength). A typical CTG reading is printed on paper and/or stored on a computer for later reference; however, a variety of systems for centralized viewing of CTG has been installed in many maternity hospitals, allowing simultaneous monitoring of multiple tracings in one or more locations. Display of maternal vital signs, contraction strength, and an electronic partogram are available in the majority of these systems. A few also have incorporated computer analysis of CTG signals or combined CTG and contraction strength data analysis. The use of wireless telemetry is now also becoming more commonplace and this can enable women requiring continuous monitoring to remain upright and mobile.

Maintain the CTG machine in good working order to ensure a satisfactory and accurate recording. Record the following information on the CTG:
- Date and time of commencing the CTG
- Name of the woman
- The woman's hospital number
- The woman's pulse rate—to establish that the tracing is the FHR
- Significant events, such as vaginal examination, siting of an epidural and epidural top-ups, augmentation with oxytocin, rupture of the membranes, and fetal blood sampling (FBS)
- The CTG should be signed and dated, and the time noted
- When the birth is complete, the date, time, and mode of birth should be recorded, and the end of the trace marked clearly to verify that the whole of the trace has been retained.

**Fetal heart rate patterns**

When reviewing the CTG trace, assess and document the baseline FHR, baseline variability, presence or absence of accelerations, and presence or absence of decelerations.

• *Baseline rate*: the normal baseline rate is between 110 and 160bpm. This is defined as the mean level of the FHR when it is stable, which excludes periods of accelerations and decelerations.

• *Tachycardia*: the baseline FHR exceeds 160bpm. A baseline rate of between 160 and 180bpm is regarded as within normal limits, provided there are no other abnormal indices.

• *Bradycardia*: the baseline FHR falls below 110bpm. A baseline rate of between 100 and 110bpm is regarded as normal, provided no other abnormal indices are present. A baseline rate below 100 suggests fetal hypoxia. Care should be taken to ensure that the maternal pulse rate is not being monitored instead of the FHR.

• *Baseline variability*: is the variation in the baseline rate over 1min, excluding accelerations and decelerations? Normal baseline variability is greater than, or equal to, a minimum of 5bpm between contractions. Good variability is an important sign of fetal well-being.

• *Accelerations*: the presence of FHR accelerations is generally a sign that the unborn baby is healthy. In labour, an acceleration is interpreted as a rise in the FHR of at least 15 beats for a minimum of 15s.

• *Decelerations*: a transient fall in the baseline rate of at least 15 beats for at least 15s. Decelerations are defined depending on their depth, shape, duration, and time lag:

  • *Early*: these are usually a repetitive and consistent pattern. There is a slowing of the FHR with the onset of the contraction, returning to the baseline at the end of the contraction

  • *Variable*: these are intermittent and variable in their timing, frequency, and shape. The FHR slows down rapidly at the onset and the decelerations are of short duration. May not occur with contraction cycle

  • *Late*: a uniform and repetitive slowing of the FHR which commences at the mid to end of the contraction. The lowest point of the deceleration may be >20s past the peak of the contraction and finishing after the contraction

  • *Isolated prolonged*: an abrupt decrease in the FHR to levels below the baseline that last at least 60–90s.

The most common abnormalities of the FHR pattern during labour are decelerations, baseline tachycardia, and loss of baseline variability. Of these, the most worrying is loss of baseline variability together with shallow decelerations occurring after the peak of contractions.

A useful mnemonic to use for interpretation of the CTG trace is shown in Table 14.4.

The overall impression is determined by how many of the CTG features were either reassuring, non-reassuring, or abnormal (Table 14.5). The NICE guideline[42] demonstrates how to decide which category a CTG falls into (Table 14.6).

**Table 14.4** DR C BRAVADO to indicate

| | | |
|---|---|---|
| DR | = | Document risk |
| C | = | Contractions |
| BR | = | Baseline rate |
| A | = | Accelerations |
| VA | = | Variability |
| D | = | Decelerations |
| O | = | Overall plan—this will involve some kind of decision-making, e.g. maintain observation, discontinue monitoring, or stop an oxytocin infusion |

**Table 14.5** Classification of fetal heart rate features

| Feature | Baseline (bpm) | Variability (bpm) | Decelerations | Accelerations |
|---|---|---|---|---|
| Reassuring | 110–160 | ≥5 | None | Present |
| Non-reassuring | 100–109 161–180 | <5 for 40–90min | Typical variable decelerations with over 50% of contractions for over 90min Single prolonged deceleration lasting <3min | Absence with otherwise normal trace of uncertain significance |
| Abnormal | <100 >180 Sinusoidal for ≥10 min | <5 for 90min | Atypical variable decelerations with over 50% of contractions or late decelerations both for over 30min Single prolonged deceleration lasting >3 min | |

**Table 14.6** Definition of normal, suspicious, and pathological FHR traces

| Category | Definition |
|---|---|
| Normal | All four features are classified as reassuring |
| Suspicious | One feature is classified as non-reassuring and the remaining features classified as reassuring |
| Pathological | Two or more features are classified as non-reassuring or one or more classified as abnormal |

## References

41 Thacker S, Stroup D, Peterson H (2003). Continuous electronic fetal monitoring during labour (Cochrane review). In: *Cochrane Library*, Issue 1. Oxford: Update Software.

42 National Institute for Health and Care Excellence (2014). *Intrapartum care for healthy women and babies*. NICE guidelines CG190. Available at: ℰ www.nice.org.uk/guidance/cg190.

43 Walsh D (2001). Midwives and birth technology: the debate that's overdue. *MIDIRS Midwifery Digest* 11: S3–6.

44 Royal College of Midwives (2012). *Evidence-based guidelines for midwifery-led care in labour: intermittent auscultation*. Available at: ℰ www.rcm.org.uk/sites/default/files/Intermittent%20Auscultation%20 %28IA%29_0.pdf.

45 Walsh D (2007). *Evidence-based Care for Normal Labour and Birth*. London: Routledge.

46 Alfrevic Z, Devane D, Gyte G (2006). Continuous cardiotocography (CTG) as a form of electronic fetal monitoring (EFM) for fetal assessment during labour. *Cochrane Database Syst Rev* 3: CD006066.

# Pain relief in labour: non-pharmacological

## Positions, mobility, and yoga

Women should be encouraged to mobilize and to adopt upright positions in labour. The midwife should therefore help the woman to move and adopt whatever positions she finds most comfortable. This not only works with the laws of gravity to assist labour and facilitate birth, but has also been shown to provide psychological advantages in terms of coping and managing during labour.[1,2]

Women should be encouraged to change position regularly, use a birth ball, furniture, wall bars, birth stool, birth mats, hanging ropes, etc. to assist them[3] and also to:

• Sway
• Rock or wiggle their hips
• Walk
• Go up and down stairs.

The woman should also be encouraged to utilize support at this time from birth companion(s) of her choice.[2]

### The use of yoga

Studies have revealed a lower level of pain intensity in the latent phase in women who had received yoga training compared with women who received standard care.[4] They also found a higher level of satisfaction with pain relief, a higher satisfaction with the childbirth experience, and a shorter labour in women who received yoga training compared with women who received standard care. No difference was found for the use of pharmacological pain relief or augmentation with oxytocin; however, one review has linked participation in yoga classes with an increased incidence of postpartum/intrapartum haemorrhage.[5]

### References

1 Royal College of Midwives (2013). *Evidence based guidelines for midwifery-led care: positions for labour and birth*. Available at: ℘ www.rcm.org.uk/sites/default/files/Positions%20for%20 Labour%20and%20Birth.pdf.
2 National Institute for Health and Care Excellence (2014). *Intrapartum care for healthy women and babies*. NICE guidelines CG190. Available at: ℘ www.nice.org.uk/guidance/cg190.
3 Lawrence A, Lewis L, Hofmeyr GJ, Styles C (2013). Maternal positions and mobility during first stage labour. *Cochrane Database Syst Rev* 10: CD003934.
4 Smith CA, Collins CT, Cyna AM, Crowther CA (2006). *Complementary and alternative therapies for pain management in labour*. Available at: ℘ www.cochrane.org/CD003521/PREG_ complementary-and-alternative-therapies-for-pain-management-in-labour.
5 Steel A, Adams J, Sibbritt D, Broom A, Frawley J, Gallois C (2014). Relationship between complementary and alternative medicine use and incidence of adverse birth outcomes: an examination of a nationally representative sample of 1835 Australian women. *Midwifery* 30: 1157–65.

# Water immersion and intracutaneous sterile water injections

## Water immersion

Immersion in water during labour is claimed to increase maternal relaxation and reduce analgesic requirements and is thus supported for healthy women with uncomplicated pregnancies.[6]

The benefits include:
- To increase uterine perfusion, which may promote endorphin and oxytocin release
- To provide buoyancy and facilitate maternal position and movement in first-/second-stage labour
- To facilitate the neurohormonal interactions of labour—thought to alleviate pain and potentially optimize labour progress
- Increased maternal satisfaction and sense of control.

Concerns that there may be greater harm to women and/or their babies, e.g. a perceived risk associated with neonatal inhalation of water and maternal/neonatal infection, have been raised. However, the most recent Cochrane review found that water immersion during the first stage of labour reduced the use of analgesia and the incidence of reported maternal pain, without adverse effects on labour duration, operative delivery, or neonatal outcome.[7] Women should therefore be offered the opportunity to labour in water for pain relief.[8]

## Intracutaneous sterile water injections

Injection of 0.1–0.5mL of sterile water into the skin over the sacrum in the points along the Michaelis' rhomboid appears to be a simple, effective, and harmless technique for relieving back pain in labour.[9] The stimulation of the skin during administration of sterile water gives rise to a similar 'gate control' effect and/or a stimulation of the endogenous opioid system as TENS and acupuncture (i.e. to block the transmission of pain by stimulating the afferent nerve fibres).[9] Studies have demonstrated that mean pain reduction scores were significantly greater in the treatment group compared to the placebo group at 30min, 1h, and 2h after injections. There was also no difference between the two groups with regard to time to delivery and rate of instrumental and Caesarean delivery.[9] A Cochrane review concluded, however, that there is insufficient evidence to make judgements on whether sterile water injections are more effective than placebo, or other interventions, for pain management in labour.[10] NICE therefore recommends that women do not use intracutaneously injected water papules during labour and birth.[8]

## References

6 Royal College of Obstetricians and Gynaecologists, Royal College of Midwives (2006). *Immersion in Water during Labour and Birth. Royal College of Obstetricians and Gynaecologists/Royal College of Midwives Joint Statement No.1.* London: RCOG; RCM.
7 Cluett ER, Burns E (2009). Immersion in water in labour and birth. *Cochrane Database Syst Rev* 2: CD000111.
8 National Institute for Health and Care Excellence (2014). *Intrapartum care for healthy women and babies.* NICE guidelines CG190. Available at: www.nice.org.uk/guidance/cg190.
9 Wiruchpongsanon P (2006). Relief of low back labor pain by using intracutaneous injections of sterile water: a randomized clinical trial. *J Med Assoc Thai* 89: 571–6.
10 Jones L, Othman M, Dowswell T, et al. (2012). Pain management for women in labour: an overview of systematic reviews. *Cochrane Database Syst Rev* 3: CD009234.

# Massage

The basis of massage is touch and regular massage from 36 weeks and during labour has been shown to reduce levels of stress hormones in women.[11] Thus, if a woman chooses to use massage techniques that have been taught to birth companions in pregnancy and labour, the midwife should support her in this choice.[12] Midwives with professional experience/a qualification in massage may also choose to perform massage as part of their intrapartum care, if a woman requests this.

There is currently minimal evidence about the benefits of massage and no evidence about the proven effectiveness of massage.[12] There is some evidence to suggest massage may reduce pain during the early latent stage of labour.[13] Studies of massage versus 'usual care' found lower reported anxiety and pain intensity in the first stage of labour in women who received massage compared with women who received standard care. No difference was found for satisfaction with pain relief used during labour, use of pharmacological pain relief, and augmentation of labour between women who received massage compared with women who received standard care. No difference was found between the two groups for pain intensity reported in the second and third stages of labour. The evidence for these outcomes was of moderate to very low quality.[13]

Essential oils may be added to enhance the therapeutic effect of massage. Care should be taken to ensure that the use of essential oils is not contraindicated and that the midwife is trained in their use and is familiar with safety precautions (➔ see Aromatherapy, p. 124 and ➔ Aromatherapy during labour, p. 300).

## Physiological and psychological benefits of massage

- Improves the circulation
- Relaxes the muscular system
- Stimulates diuresis and reduces oedema
- Stimulates the lymphatic system
- Speeds up the elimination of waste products
- Encourages the production of endorphins
- Aids digestion
- Aids sleep
- Enhances mental and physical relaxation
- Encourages release of emotional tension
- Encourages communication.

However, precautions do need to be taken prior to a massage session, to address general and pregnancy-specific contraindications. Awareness of the woman's medical and obstetric history should always be considered and consent needs to be obtained beforehand.

## General contraindications for massage

Massage should not be given, or caution should be taken, under the following circumstances:

- After a meal or alcohol; allow at least 1–2h before massage
- If there is infection, pyrexia, or inflammation

- If there has been recent injury or surgery
- Varicose veins: work very gently over these areas
- Thrombophlebitis
- Carcinoma: exert no direct pressure over the diseased site
- Sciatica: take extreme caution in the affected area
- Burns, bruising, and open wounds
- Sensitive skin: take care with these patients.

## Pregnancy-specific contraindications for massage

*Women should be advised to avoid:*

- Suprapubic or sacral massage during the first trimester
- Deep massage to the calves if the woman has a history of thrombosis
- Vigorous massage around the heel—this relates to the pelvic zone in reflexology
- Shiatsu points that are contraindicated in pregnancy
- Massage of women with hypotension or a tendency to faint; monitor the BP
- Abdominal massage if the woman has a history of APH
- In cases where a health-care practitioner expresses any uncertainty.

## References

11  Smith CA, Collins CT, Cyna AM, Crowther CA (2006). *Complementary and alternative therapies for pain management in labour.* Available at: ℜ www.cochrane.org/CD003521/PREG_complementary-and-alternative-therapies-for-pain-management-in-labour.
12  National Institute for Health and Care Excellence (2014). *Intrapartum care for healthy women and babies.* NICE guidelines CG190. Available at: ℜ www.nice.org.uk/guidance/cg190.
13  Nabb MT, Kimber L, Haines H, McCourt C (2006). Does regular massage from late pregnancy to birth decrease pain perception during labour and birth? – A feasibility study to investigate a programme of massage, controlled breathing and visualization, from 36 weeks of pregnancy until birth. *Complement Ther Clin Pract* 12: 222–31.

## Further reading

Charles C, Chapman V (2013). *The Midwife's Labour and Birth Handbook*, 3rd edn. Chichester: Wiley-Blackwell.

# Breathing awareness

If a woman chooses to use breathing and relaxation techniques in labour, the midwife should support her in this choice.[14] However, there is currently insufficient evidence about the benefits of such techniques in labour and birth.[15] One study found a lower level of pain intensity in the latent phase in women who received breathing technique and massage training compared with women who received standard care and this difference continued during the active phase of labour, including the transition phase. The same study also found women who received breathing technique and massage training had a higher level of satisfaction with pain relief than women who received standard care. Women who received training in breathing and massage technique were also found to have longer labours compared with those who received standard care.[15]

Women are encouraged to become aware of their own breathing patterns and how adjustments can be made during labour and birth to help relieve tension and aid coping skills. A non-directive approach to breathing awareness ensures that the mother follows instinctual cues for working with her contractions. This prevents hyperventilation and enables a more efficient exchange of oxygen and carbon dioxide. Care should be taken to prevent hyperventilation and light-headedness.

## Music

Studies have not found a statistically significant difference in pain intensity, use of pharmacological pain relief, anxiety, or length of labour in women who listened to music compared with women who did not.[15]

## Valsalva's manoeuvre

Involves a fixed diaphragm, a closed epiglottis, and breath-holding, usually commenced at the beginning of contraction. The continued use of this technique is no longer recommended as it leads to increased intrathoracic pressure, decreased venous blood return to the heart, reduced cardiac output, less oxygen from the lungs, lowered arterial pressure, and reduced oxygen to the placenta.[16]

## References

14 National Institute for Health and Care Excellence (2014). *Intrapartum care for healthy women and babies.* NICE guidelines CG190. Available at: 🔗 www.nice.org.uk/guidance/cg190.

15 Smith CA, Collins CT, Cyna AM, Crowther CA (2006). *Complementary and alternative therapies for pain management in labour.* Available at: 🔗 www.cochrane.org/CD003521/PREG_complementary-and-alternative-therapies-for-pain-management-in-labour.

16 Bosomworth A, Bettany-Saltikov J (2006). Just take a deep breath. *MIDIRS Midwifery Digest* 16: 157–65.

## Hypnosis and visualization

Hypnosis techniques allow women to adopt a redirected focus similar to daydreaming or being absorbed in a book, as opposed to entering a deep, trance-like state. The mind and body are relaxed whilst remaining in control and conversant with the surrounding environment. In labour and birth, hypnosis is often used to focus attention on feelings of comfort or numbness, as well as to enhance women's feelings of relaxation and sense of safety.

Hypnosis may help relieve pain in labour, but research conducted to date has not conclusively shown any proven benefit.[17] Hypnosis is an altered state of conscious awareness that involves, in part, a focus of attention to reduce awareness of the external environment. The increased responsiveness of individuals in hypnosis to communications (known as suggestions) can facilitate useful changes in perception and behaviour. Women can be guided into hypnosis by a practitioner during labour, or individuals can learn self-hypnosis during pregnancy, for subsequent use during labour. This antenatal training is sometimes supplemented using an audio recording of hypnotic suggestions.

The aim of hypnosis and visualization is to equip the woman with supportive techniques that will help her prepare and cope with labour and birth. These techniques consist of self-hypnosis, guided visualization, and breathing methods. The philosophy of hypnosis maintains that when fear, stress, and tension are absent, then the woman can utilize her natural instincts more effectively, resulting in a more calm and fulfilling birth experience.[18]

### Potential benefits of hypnosis and visualization

- Inspires confidence and optimism.
- Promotes relaxation and inner peace.
- Eliminates the fear–tension–pain cycle during labour.
- Enhances a calm, peaceful birth environment.
- Reduces fatigue during labour.
- Enhances the production of natural endorphins.
- Eliminates the risk of hyperventilation from shallow breathing.
- Enhances natural birthing instincts and behaviours.
- Fewer complications during labour and birth.
- A fulfilling and meaningful experience of childbirth.
- A dedicated role for the birth partner.
- Promotes mother, baby, and partner relationships.
- Quicker postnatal recovery.

Studies have compared women using hypnosis with controls using traditional breathing and relaxation techniques.[19] It was found that those in the hypnotically prepared group experienced:

- Reduced pain
- Shorter first-stage labours
- Less medication
- Higher Apgar scores
- Higher incidence of spontaneous deliveries.

# References

17 Madden K, Middleton P, Cyna AM, Matthewson M, Jones L (2016). *Hypnosis for pain management during labour and childbirth.* Available at: ℅ www.cochrane.org/CD009356/PREG_hypnosis-for-pain-management-during-labour-and-childbirth.

18 Melh-Madrona LE (2004). Hypnosis to facilitate uncomplicated birth. *Am J Clin Hypn* 46: 299–312.

19 Cyna AM, Andrew MI, McAucliffe GL (2006). Antenatal self-hypnosis for labour and childbirth: a pilot study. *Anaesth Intensive Care* 34: 464–9.

# Transcutaneous electrical nerve stimulation

Transcutaneous electrical nerve stimulation (TENS) is a self-administered form of non-pharmacological pain relief. NICE[20] currently recommends that TENS is not offered to women in *established* labour; however, this therapy remains a popular choice among women.

Pain relief is thought to be activated by the passage of a mild electrical stimulus across the nerves of the spine at the level which transmits pain impulses from the uterus and cervix.[21] This aims to influence the pain gate mechanism and stimulate naturally occurring endorphins. Effectiveness varies and is thought to be enhanced if the device is used from the earliest contractions onwards, before the labour becomes established. This enables the initial build-up of endorphins to take effect, e.g. 40min, thus allowing the mother to gain benefit before strong contractions commence.

The equipment can be hired or loaned by the pregnant woman for use at home before transfer to the labour ward. Electrodes in the form of adhesive pads are placed on either side of the spine and these are attached to a small control device by coated wires. Hand control buttons allow the user to select the power level required; as labour progresses a more intense level of stimulation can be selected as the contractions become longer, stronger, and more frequent. The device has a booster feature which can be operated throughout a contraction to obtain more pain relief and then a return to the selected programme once the contraction has subsided.

Instructions need to be given to the woman and her birth partner regarding the placement of electrodes:

- One on both sides of the spine just below the bra line, vertebral level T10–L1, and placed 3cm apart
- One on both sides of the spine, over the sacral dimples, vertebral level S2–S4, and placed 3cm apart.

## Advantages

- TENS appears to be safe to use alongside other methods of pain relief such as nitrous oxide and oxygen, opiates, and complementary therapies.[22]
- The mother is in control.
- Non-invasive.
- No adverse effect on the fetus.
- May reduce the need for pharmacological analgesia.

## Disadvantages

- TENS cannot be used submerged in water or alongside epidural analgesia.
- There have been occasional reports of TENS possibly disrupting CTG tracings which midwives ought to be aware of.

## References

20 National Institute for Health and Care Excellence (2014). *Intrapartum care for healthy women and babies.* NICE guidelines CG190. Available at: ℘ www.nice.org.uk/guidance/cg190.

21 Trout KK (2004). The neuromatrix theory of pain: implications for selected non-pharmacological methods of pain relief for labor. *J Midwifery Women's Health* 49: 482–8. Reprinted in: *MIDIRS Midwifery Digest* 15: 73–8.

22 Dowswell T, Bedwell C, Lavender T, Neilson JP (2009). Transcutaneous electrical nerve stimulation (TENS) for pain relief in labour. *Cochrane Database Syst Rev* 2:CD007214.

# Complementary therapies

The safety of a woman during pregnancy and birth is reliant upon the ability of the midwifery and medical team to provide evidence-based clinical care. Few complementary therapies have been subjected to scientific study; hence, there is currently insufficient evidence about the benefits of complementary therapies in labour and birth.[23] The importance of ensuring that complementary therapies and medicines are only utilized when appropriate cannot be overstated. This is not, however, to say health-care teams should not be supportive of women interested in utilizing alternative therapies, and it is essential health-care staff have a clear understanding of the underlying principles, indications, and contraindications of each treatment modality.

## Reference

23 Smith CA, Collins CT, Cyna AM, Crowther CA (2006). *Complementary and alternative therapies for pain management in labour*. Available at: &#8478; www.cochrane.org/CD003521/PREG_complementary-and-alternative-therapies-for-pain-management-in-labour.

# Homeopathic remedies for labour and birth

Homeopathic remedies can support women physically and emotionally throughout labour and birth; they enable a woman to feel empowered to progress through this physiological event without resort to chemical drugs and unnecessary interventions. It is important that health-care workers have an understanding of these techniques in order to inform women and facilitate choice of pain relief; women who are considering whether to use homeopathy should be advised to seek advice from a registered health practitioner. An informed woman may wish to self-medicate during her pregnancy, and comprehensive birth kits are now available for this use. Alternatively, a woman may choose to be attended at the birth by either a homeopath (who has gained permission prior to labour) or a midwife with the appropriate qualifications. (➔ See Homeopathy, p. 122.)

## Arnica

The most commonly used remedy for childbirth is arnica. This remedy is used extensively for emotional and physical trauma, so therefore it is an invaluable remedy for labour and the early postnatal period. It can be taken during labour and immediately following birth (preferably before the cord is cut) to minimize the general effects of trauma and to assist with pain relief. Taken for a few days after the birth, arnica will aid healing and help with afterpains.

## Other common remedies

- *Aconite*: for anxiety and fearfulness at any time during labour, but especially before labour and afterwards where there has been a sudden or traumatic birth.
- *Belladonna*: for severe, distressing, and spasmodic pains. The woman feels like she wants to escape. The face is hot, red, and flushed, often accompanied by a headache.
- *Caulophyllum*: for exhaustion and slow progress in labour. Helps to establish regular and effective contractions.
    - ❶ This should not be taken during pregnancy as it is a powerful uterine tonic and may initiate premature labour.
- *Chamomilla*: for unbearable pain and extreme irritability.
- *Cimicifuga*: for sharp, shooting pains in all directions and failure to progress. A feeling of wanting to give up, accompanied by anxiety and possibly hysteria.
- *Gelsemium*: the uterus feels heavy, sore, and squeezed, with pains radiating to the back. There may be fear, trembling, and weakness, especially in the transition stage.
- *Pulsatilla*: for an erratic, changeable, and tearful emotional state. The pains tend to be cutting and tearing, and move around. The remedy helps to establish regular contractions and restores emotional balance.

- *Sepia*: a sensation of the uterus being dragged down and heavy. Experienced by women in the second stage of labour at the crowning of the head. The overwhelming urge to bear down feels like the muscles of the pelvic floor are stretched beyond their limits. The woman is usually irritable, indifferent, and self-absorbed.
- *Nux vomica*: for irritability, chilliness, and finding fault with carers.

# Aromatherapy during labour

Aromatherapy draws on the healing power of plants with the use of essential oils to enhance physical and mental well-being. The oils may be massaged into the skin, used in a bath, or inhaled using a steam infusion or burner. Overall, there is insufficient evidence from randomized controlled trials about the benefits of aromatherapy on pain management in labour. A recent review of trials found no difference between groups for pain intensity, assisted vaginal birth, Caesarean section, or the use of epidural anaesthesia.[24]

However, women should be supported in their choices and the use of essential oils in labour may enhance the individual woman's coping strategies when used alone, or in conjunction with other complementary therapies, other coping mechanisms, such as breathing and relaxation techniques, or conventional methods of pain relief.

The main contributions of essential oils during labour and childbirth are to:
- Assist with pain relief
- Relieve stress and anxiety
- Assist with efficient functioning of the uterus
- Prevent fatigue.

For details of the safe administration and therapeutic properties of essential oils, → see Aromatherapy, p. 124.

The following oils are some of the most commonly used essential oils for labour and delivery.[25,26] Some aromatherapy practitioners/midwives may wish to use other oils not listed here.
- *Lavender*: is a very versatile oil, with relaxing, antispasmodic, and pain-relieving properties. It is therefore useful to help ease the pain of contractions and as a general, all-round, helpful oil throughout labour. It is best avoided by people with hay fever and asthma. Take care with vaporizing the oil, as some women find the aroma unpleasant and overpowering; it may also cause headaches in some people.
  - *Women should not* use lavender in conjunction with epidurals because it has hypotensive properties. It may also possibly interact with narcotics, so care should be taken in conjunction with pethidine or diamorphine.
- *Chamomile*: is calming and relaxing during labour. It has significant anti-inflammatory and antispasmodic properties. Chamomile should not be used until late pregnancy because it has emmenagogic properties, which theoretically may induce menstruation, and therefore bleeding.
- *Clary sage*: a uterine tonic and euphoric oil, it is useful for stimulating contractions and pain relief. Clary sage has emmenagogic properties so should not be used in pregnancy until near term and if overused may cause drowsiness and headaches.
  - Driving is not recommended if exposed to Clary sage for lengthy periods, and it should not be combined with alcoholic drinks.

- *Frankincense*: is a very useful oil for calming anxiety and panic, especially where this is associated with hyperventilation. This may not be suitable for asthmatic women, however, due to its strong aroma and previous conflicting evidence against its safe use.[24]
- *Jasmine*: is a uterine tonic that has been used traditionally as an aid to childbirth. It helps to strengthen contractions, whilst also having pain-relieving and antispasmodic properties. It is reputed to be useful as a compress, placed on the lower abdomen, to help expel a retained placenta. Emotionally it has energizing and antidepressant qualities.
  - *Women should not* use jasmine until the onset of labour.
- *Lemon*: is an antiseptic and astringent, also reputed to be a circulatory tonic. A gentle, uplifting oil with a pleasant, fresh aroma. Often mixed with other oils to minimize pungent aromas, this makes it a versatile oil to use at any time during labour and birth. Lemon has phototoxic properties, therefore after use care should be taken to reduce exposure to sunlight, as with most citrus oils.
- *Mandarin*: a refreshing and gently uplifting oil, with a delicate aroma. Helpful for nausea and anxiety. Has antispasmodic properties and helps to balance the metabolic rate. This makes mandarin a safe, all-round oil for use in labour. Slightly phototoxic.
- *Rose*: aids uterine action due to its hormone-like action. It stimulates the pituitary gland and releases dopamine. It also possesses antispasmodic properties and is a general circulatory tonic. Rose is said to have a strong affinity for the female reproductive system, making it a special oil for labour and childbirth.
- *Petitgrain*: a useful oil for the transition phase, as it helps to soothe emotions, especially where there is panic and loss of control.

Other oils that are beneficial during labour and birth include grapefruit, lime, sweet orange, neroli, sandalwood, geranium, eucalyptus, and ylang ylang.

## References

24 Smith CA, Collins CT, Crowther CA (2011). *Aromatherapy for pain management in labour.* Available at: ℞ www.cochrane.org/CD009215/PREG_aromatherapy-for-pain-management-in-labour.
25 Pallivalapila AR, Stewart D, Shetty A, Pande B, Singh R, McLay JS (2015). Use of complementary and alternative medicines during the third trimester. *Obstet Gynecol* 125: 204–11.
26 Kaviani M, Azima S, Alavi N, Tabaei MH (2014). The effect of lavender aromatherapy on pain perception and intrapartum outcome in primiparous women. *Br J Midwifery* 22: 125–8.

## Further reading

Lawless J (1992). *The Encyclopaedia of Essential Oils.* Shaftesbury: Element Books Ltd.

## Bach flower remedies during labour

Childbirth presents an enormous physical and emotional challenge; consequently emotional reserves of strength and staying power may well be put to the test. Bach flower remedies are thought to help by assisting the mother to stay calm and work with her body, resulting in the release of endorphins and encephalins which greatly assist in the process of labour. However, one recent review found that women who used flower essences during labour exhibited a higher incidence of emotional distress.[27]

Rescue remedy is the most widely utilized remedy and is sipped between contractions for the duration of labour. For dosages and administration, ➔ see Bach flower remedies, p. 128. Other remedies that may prove useful at this time are:

- *Olive*: may be useful when the woman is emotionally and physically exhausted, perhaps due to a long labour
- *Gorse*: may help when there is a feeling of wanting to give up and cannot go on any longer
- *Beech*: may help when there are feelings of intolerance towards birth partners and carers
- *Red chestnut*: may be useful for overanxiety for the baby during labour and birth
- *Cherry plum*: may help when there is fear of losing control or behaving in an irrational way
- *Aspen*: may help when apprehension or fear of the unknown is experienced
- *Clematis*: for when there is too much detachment and distance from the process of birthing, possibly causing delay/disruption to progress
- *Impatiens*: for feeling impatient and irritable with those around her or with the slow pace/progress of labour
- *White chestnut*: may assist to relieve constant anxiety and worrying
- *Mimulus*: for fear of pain, procedures, or the hospital environment
- *Walnut*: may help in adjusting to the changes occurring during labour and birth, and extra protection to be able to cope better
- *Gentian*: may help when there are feelings of despondency, perhaps because of slow progress or setbacks during labour
- *Willow*: for feelings of self-pity and resentment.

If the mother uses up less energy on anxiety and stress related to labour, she can then retain more energy to cope physically with labour. During labour, the calming effect of the remedies may also impact on the fetus in adjusting and coping with the stress of birth.

To enable the provision of accurate information to women in their care, and to assist in safely supporting women to assist with pregnancy, labour, and birth, health professionals need to be aware of the potential birth outcomes associated with complementary therapy use.

### Reference

27 Steel A, Adams J, Sibbritt D, Broom A, Frawley J, Gallois C (2014). Relationship between complementary and alternative medicine use and incidence of adverse birth outcomes: an examination of a nationally representative sample of 1835 Australian women. *Midwifery* 30: 1157–65.

# Reflexology during labour

Reflexology involves the application of deep pressure to specific areas of the feet using the thumb and forefinger. It is believed there are reflex points on the feet corresponding to organs and structures of the body, and that pain may be reduced by gentle manipulation or pressing certain parts of the foot. It is claimed that the application of pressure to these reflex 'zones' promotes the reabsorption of energy-blocking agents, such as calcium, lactate, or uric acid crystals, which are then later eliminated. Reflexology may also reduce stress and tension and maintain balance or homeostasis; however, this complementary therapy has not yet been the subject of rigorous scientific study.[28,29]

Only midwives who have received training should perform techniques in reflexology relating to labour care. The woman may be attended by a midwife/reflexologist, or have arranged for an independent reflexology practitioner to attend her during labour. However, the overall care of the woman rests with the midwife or doctor in charge and, in the event of complications, this complementary therapy may not always be appropriate.

Encourage the woman to adopt a comfortable, well-supported position appropriate to labour, to prevent postural hypotension whilst maintaining good eye contact and communication. Adjust your posture to accommodate the mother's varying positions throughout labour.

- Familiarize yourself with the woman's relevant medical and obstetric history and present labour circumstances.
- Obtain consent from the woman.
- Adhere to the local policy for treatment using complementary therapies.

## Uses in labour

- General relaxation.
- Relief of stress and anxiety.
- Helps to relieve the pain of contractions and backache.
- Minimizes nausea and vomiting.
- Relief of cold feet in labour.
- Encourages strong rhythmic contractions—may assist with augmentation. It is important to work within local policy and liaise with medical staff if used as a measure to augment labour.
- Induction of labour should not be undertaken by a midwife or practitioner unless there is a local policy clearly stating the conditions when complementary therapies can be used for induction of labour, or with the agreement of the woman's consultant.
- For the third stage of labour, reflexology may be used in uncomplicated retained placenta.
- Treatments may consist of general reflexology massage for relaxation or shorter, more specific treatments focusing on a particular area, e.g. the ankles pertaining to the pelvic area or the pad of the thumb pertaining to the pituitary gland.
- Treatments should be recorded in the woman's notes.

- Reflexology *may* also be useful in the postnatal period. Some of the conditions that *may* respond to treatment are:
  - Retention of urine
  - Painful perineum
  - Breast engorgement
  - Constipation
  - Inadequate lactation
  - Oedema.

## References

28 Jones L, Othman M, Dowswell T, et al. (2012). Pain management for women in labour: an overview of systematic reviews. *Cochrane Database Syst Rev* 3: CD009234.

29 Smith CA, Levett KM, Collins CT, Jones L (2012). *Massage, reflexology and other manual methods for managing labour.* Available at: ✆ www.cochrane.org/CD009290/PREG_massage-reflexology-and-other-manual-methods-for-managing-pain-in-labour.

## Further reading

Tiran D (2009). *Reflexology for Pregnancy: A Definitive Guide for Healthcare Professionals.* London: Elsevier.

# Acupuncture in labour

Acupuncture may be beneficial for the management of pain during labour; however, the number of women studied has been small.[30] Some midwives may be qualified acupuncturists, or an acupuncturist practitioner may attend a woman; however, it is important that the practitioner has in-depth knowledge of the appropriate points to use in labour and how to needle them effectively. Insight into a woman's behavioural patterns and emotional needs will also influence the choice of points used to maximize effective treatment for the individual.

Acupuncture is believed to help release endorphins which enhance relaxation, aid pain relief, and assist with coping mechanisms. A variety of techniques may be used, from traditional needling of the points, moxibustion, electro acupuncture, and ear acupuncture; shiatsu techniques may also be utilized. However, a systematic review found no benefit of acupuncture compared to sham acupuncture (where acupuncture needles are inserted into non-acupuncture points) in reducing labour pain at 1 or 2h of labour. Acupuncture did, however, reduce pain by 11% compared with placebo for the first 30min of labour.[31]

Four patterns of disharmony that may be manifested in labour have been identified:[32]

- *Deficiency of Qi and blood*: this may be due to premature rupture of membranes to labour or it can be the result of heavy periods or blood loss following previous deliveries.
- *Kidney deficiency*: this may be due to multiple pregnancies or *in vitro* fertilization (IVF) pregnancies; short gaps between pregnancies deplete the kidney energy.
- *Spleen and stomach deficiency*: this may be due to a lack of proper nourishment prior to labour.
- *Ki and blood stagnation (liver Qi stagnation)*: this is due to emotional problems or bad premenstrual tension prior to pregnancy.

## First stage of labour

- In early labour, the points used are to facilitate uterine action and help with general pain relief.
- As labour progresses, acupuncture may be used to augment weak or irregular contractions.
- Specific pain relief, as in posterior position and backache.
- Boost and maintain energy levels.
- May help to dispel fear and anxiety at any stage.
- May support with the difficulties of the transition stage.

## Second stage of labour

- Helps to alleviate exhaustion.
- Helps to dispel fear and anxiety, which blocks the mother's energy network.
- Augments contractions if they are becoming too far apart.
- Many of the points forbidden in pregnancy will be used during labour as they generally have a strong downwards movement of energy in the body, which greatly enhances the birthing process.

## Third stage of labour

- Chinese philosophy dictates that vessels are depleted of blood following birth and therefore are vulnerable to attack from external pathogens. Very often tonifying treatment to build up the blood is commenced soon after birth.
- Retained placenta: points that have a strong downwards movement will be used to initiate uterine action.
- Other points may be used to help to regulate uterine action and stimulate the movement of blood.

The main disadvantage of acupuncture treatment in labour is that it cannot be used in conjunction with water birth. Some women may find needling slightly painful, and some points may not be accessible due to the variety of positions and restlessness of the woman at times.

## References

30 Jones L, Othman M, Dowswell T, et al. (2012). Pain management for women in labour: an over-view of systematic reviews. Cochrane Database Syst Rev 3: CD009234.
31 Cho SH, Lee H, Ernst E (2010). Acupuncture for pain relief in labour: a systematic review and meta-analysis. BJOG 117: 907–20.
32 West Z (2001). Acupuncture in Pregnancy and Childbirth. London: Churchill Livingstone.

# Shiatsu in labour

Shiatsu may help the woman to tune into the powerful and changeable energy patterns associated with labour, which makes it an ideal therapy to complement normal midwifery practice and provide individual and woman-centred care. The main focus is to help the woman's energies to flow freely from the onset of labour, rather than waiting until the energies become blocked. Various techniques may be used to move or balance energy such as strong pressure and holding of key points along the meridian lines, knuckling, hooking, stroking, and massage to selected areas or acupoints. Shiatsu *may* be used throughout the whole of labour if the woman wishes and *may* be particularly beneficial if used in this way.

Working on the meridians located in the back is key. The Governing Vessel (GV) is considered the main source of Yang energy, which is required for labour to proceed effectively. By working on the GV, the therapist can tap into and balance all of the energy sources in the body. The Bladder (BL) meridian located in the back is worked on in the first stage of labour to try and help relieve fear and anxiety. Sacral work aims to relieve pain and tension, particularly on the sacral grooves, which may help release energy to the uterus, perineum, and vagina. If the woman feels comfortable for the therapist to work in the abdominal area, it is believed to be directly linked with the uterus and represents earth energy, which may help the woman ground herself. The Kidney (K) meridian is located on the underside of the foot, being the lowest point of the body; this point links to earth energy and is considered very grounding and calming.

## Benefits in labour

Shiatsu shares the same benefits as previously mentioned in the acupuncture section; it is a manual form of acupuncture, accessing the key meridian lines and points without needles. This makes it less invasive and *more* easily combined with normal midwifery care given by the midwife. Shiatsu *is believed* to provide the following benefits:

• Emotionally releasing—tension and emotional stasis may block the process of birth
• Relieves headaches and assists concentration
• Helps to calm the baby. Helps the woman to connect and focus her energy on her baby rather than on the pain.

Encouraging the birth partner to assist with some of the techniques provides a key role for involvement of the partner.

# Pain relief in labour: pharmacological

# Nitrous oxide and oxygen administration

NICE[1] suggests that Entonox® (a 50:50 mixture of oxygen and nitrous oxide) is made available to women in all birth settings, as it may reduce pain in labour. Entonox® is a very good method to use in practice as:

- It is easily available to all midwives in all birth settings
- The woman controls it herself
- It works quickly, usually within 3–4 breaths, and reaches maximum effect after 2min
- It wears off quickly when administration stops
- It is safe to use in conjunction with other methods of pain relief
- It is useful as an aid to enhance coping strategies over 'a rough patch' or whilst waiting for other forms of pain relief to be effective
- Entonox® is known to cross the placenta, but has no known negative effects on the fetus. In fact the oxygen component will increase the levels of circulating oxygen which will benefit the fetus during uterine contractions.[2]

## Method

A mixture of nitrous oxide 50% and oxygen 50% is delivered from a cylinder via an Entonox® apparatus. The *Midwives Rules and Standards*[3] outline the midwife's responsibilities in the administration of pain relief.

*How to advise women to use it*

- Start use as soon as a contraction begins—to achieve maximum relief at the height of the contraction.
- A mask should cover the nose and mouth with a good seal. Listen to ensure that the valve is delivering the gas mixture correctly.
- The gas mixture should be inhaled throughout the contraction. The midwife may also palpate contractions and warn the woman to start breathing through the mask or mouthpiece (ask her preference!).
- It may take up to three contractions before good pain relief is experienced.
- Once started, onset of relief is usually within 20s.
- Recovery takes place between contractions. If the woman is too drowsy to operate the apparatus effectively, then no gas will be delivered and she will quickly recover. It is very unlikely to cause sleep or loss of consciousness.
- The midwife may need to remind the woman that she does not need to inhale the gas mixture when there is no contraction.

## Disadvantages

- It may cause drowsiness, dizziness, and nausea.[1]
- Some women do not like the odour.

- The nitrous oxide constituent of Entonox® causes inactivation of vitamin $B_{12}$ which is a co-factor of methionine synthase. Folate metabolism is consequently interfered with and DNA synthesis impaired. These disturbances may result in megaloblastic bone marrow changes. Continuous Entonox® use of >8h is thus not recommended.[4]
- Some concern regarding the possibility of cross-infection and staff safety has arisen; however, it is still considered a safe and simple method of pain relief for women.[2]

## References

1  National Institute for Health and Care Excellence (2014). *Intrapartum care for healthy women and babies*. NICE guidelines CG190. Available at: ℞ www.nice.org.uk/guidance/cg190.
2  Rosen MA (2002). Nitrous oxide for relief of labor pain: a systematic review. *Am J Obstet Gynecol* 186: S110–26.
3  Nursing and Midwifery Council (2012). *Midwives Rules and Standards 2012*, p. 19. Available at: ℞ www.nmc.org.uk/globalassets/sitedocuments/standards/nmc-midwives-rules-and-standards.pdf.
4  Royal College of Midwives. *RCM Entonox Guidance*. Available at: ℞ www.rcm.org.uk/content/entonox.

# Opiates

### Considerations for the use of opiates during labour

The use of opiates for the relief of pain during labour has been some-what superseded by the growing popularity of epidural analgesia. There does remain a place for an alternative to epidurals, and NICE[5] recommends that pethidine, diamorphine, or other opioids are made available in all birth settings. Midwives need to be able to advise women about their range of choices but should also inform them that these drugs will provide limited pain relief during labour and may have significant side effects for both her and her baby.[5]

In discussion, clients need to be made aware of the following issues:
- The efficacy of the analgesic effect.[6,7]
- The effect upon the FHR and features of the CTG trace if this is in progress.
- The effect on labour.
- The potential depressant effects on the neonate following birth with respect to the initiation of respiration and establishment of breast feeding.[5,8,9]

The commonly used opiates are pethidine and morphine derivatives, e.g. diamorphine.

### Pethidine
- Usual dosage: 50–100mg via IM injection.
- Narcotic—respiratory depressant, can cause drowsiness. Women should not enter water (a birthing pool or bath) within 2h of administration or if they feel drowsy.[5]
- Antispasmodic.
- Can cause nausea and vomiting—administer an antiemetic.[5]
- Reduces gastrointestinal motility.
- Crosses the placenta—causes short term neonatal respiratory depression and drowsiness which may last several days. Action reversed by IM Naloxone Hydrochloride 60 mcg/kg neonatal body weight i.e. for a term infant, 0.5mls (200mcg) of a 400mcg/ml solution.[10]

### Diamorphine
- Usual dosage: 10mg via IM injection.
- Strongly narcotic—respiratory depressant, drowsiness. Women should not enter water (a birthing pool or bath) within 2h of administration or if they feel drowsy.[5]
- Can cause nausea and vomiting—administer an antiemetic.[5]
- Reduces gastrointestinal motility.
- Crosses the placenta—causes short term neonatal respiratory depression and drowsiness which may last several days. Action reversed by IM Naloxone Hydrochloride 60 mcg/kg neonatal body weight i.e. for a term infant, 0.5mls (200mcg) of a 400mcg/ml solution.[10]

# References

5 National Institute for Health and Care Excellence (2014). *Intrapartum care for healthy women and babies.* NICE guidelines CG190. Available at: ℅ www.nice.org.uk/guidance/cg190.
6 Tsui MHY, Kee WDN, Ng FF (2004). A double blinded randomized placebo-controlled study of intra-muscular pethidine for pain relief in the first stage of labour. *BJOG* 111: 648–55.
7 Wood C, Soltani H (2005). Does pethidine relieve pain? *Pract Midwife* 8: 16, 18–20, 22–5.
8 Hunt S (2002). Pethidine: love it or hate it? *MIDIRS Midwifery Digest* 12: 363–5.
9 Sosa CG, Buekens P, Hughes JM, et al. (2006). Effect of pethidine administered during the first stage of labor on the acid-base status at birth. *Eur J Obstet Gynecol Reprod Biol* 129: 135–9.
10 British National Formulary (2016) Naloxone Hydrochloride available at: https://www.evidence.nhs.uk/formulary/bnf/current/15-anaesthesia/151-general-anaesthesia/1517-antagonists-for-central-and-respiratory-depression/naloxone-hydrochloride.

# Lumbar epidural analgesia

This is a very effective method of pain relief which has gained in popularity since its use in obstetrics became more widespread in the 1970s.

A senior anaesthetist must be present to administer lumbar epidural anaesthesia; thus, it is only available in obstetric units.

## What is an epidural?

- A local anaesthetic, usually bupivacaine hydrochloride, is injected into the epidural space between the second and third lumbar vertebrae.
- This drug acts on the spinal nerves at this level to produce a sensory and partial motor block.
- The sensory block produces excellent pain relief, as it affects the uterine and cervical nerve plexuses, which are the main transmitters of pain sensation during uterine contractions.
- The partial motor block leaves the woman unable to walk around, so she is cared for in bed.
- There is a reflex relaxation of the blood vessels in the lower body, leading to increased warmth and a feeling of heaviness in the lower limbs.
- This haemodynamic shift results in rebound hypotension, improved circulation in the lower body, and relaxation of the pelvic floor.
- As labour advances, contraction pain is centred on the rectum and pelvic floor, and the sacral nerve plexus is then involved in the transmission of pain. A stronger dose of bupivacaine can be administered with the woman in a more upright position to give effective pain relief at this time (referred to as a second-stage top-up).

## Types of epidural

An epidural anaesthetic can be administered in several ways:

- *Standard*: 10mL of bupivacaine 0.25–0.5% via an epidural cannula. Each dose lasts 1–2h; therefore, the drug is re-administered as required (epidural top-up).
- *Combined epi-spinal*: a combination of low-dose bupivacaine (0.15%) into the epidural space, with a small dose of opiate (3 micrograms of fentanyl) into the subarachnoid space, is used to produce a less dense motor block, allowing the woman more mobility. This is sometimes referred to as a mobile epidural, but it does not mean the woman can walk about! She will have improved motor control so she will be able to move around in bed more easily. Regular injections every 1–2h of bupivacaine into the epidural space will still be required.
- *Continuous lumbar epidural infusion*: once the epidural block is established, 10–15mg/h of a 0.1% or 0.125% solution of bupivacaine (with or without opiate) is administered via an infusion pump attached to the epidural cannula. This can be combined with a patient-controlled device that allows the woman to top up the dose, within a strict limit (a very popular option with mothers and midwives!).

The choice between the above methods depends on availability (midwives to administer the top-ups), unit protocol, and the mother's preference.

If a woman is contemplating regional analgesia, before asking for consent the midwife/anaesthetist should talk with her about the risks and benefits and the implications for her labour.[10] Women should be told that regional analgesia:

- Provides more effective pain relief than opioids.
- Is not associated with long-term backache.
- Is not associated with a longer first stage of labour or an increased chance of a Caesarean birth.
- Is associated with a longer second stage of labour and an increased chance of vaginal instrumental birth.
- Will be accompanied by a more intensive level of monitoring and IV access, and so mobility may be reduced.

## Indications

- *If an instrumental or operative delivery is necessary*, epidural analgesia provides excellent pain control during operative procedures, avoiding the risks of general anaesthesia
- *Malpresentations or malpositions* (e.g. breech, occipito-posterior) where there is a higher risk of slow progress and intervention. The advantages of epidural analgesia have to be balanced against the loss of pushing sensations and failure of the presenting part to rotate and descend, which are crucial to achieve a vaginal delivery.
- *Multiple pregnancy* where there is a higher than normal risk of delivery problems with the second twin.
- *Women with breech presentations or multiple pregnancy* who aim to give birth vaginally may refuse an epidural and their wishes should be respected.
- *PIH.* Lowered BP induced by an epidural anaesthetic offsets the increased BP due to the response to painful contractions, making the BP easier to control during labour.
- *Induction of labour.* The drugs used to induce labour create artificially high levels of uterine contraction for a longer period of time. The length of labour is often extended, so adequate pain relief becomes more problematic.
- *Maternal request.* This is not a good option for low-risk deliveries in normal spontaneous labour, as the side effects often outweigh the benefits. Women need good preparation, midwifery support, and encouragement to try other pain relief options first. However, if a woman has understood and given careful consideration to the information given, then her choice should be respected.

## Contraindications

- Abnormalities of the spine: refer to an anaesthetist during pregnancy if the woman is keen to have epidural analgesia during labour.
- Systemic infection: because of the added risk of spread into the epidural site.
- Bleeding/clotting disorders: because of the risk of haematoma formation in the epidural space.

- Maternal reluctance: if the woman is not keen, she has not given proper consent!
- Absence of adequate levels of midwifery staff/anaesthetic staff to ensure safe care.

## Complications

- *Impaired descent and rotation of the presenting part*: this can sometimes be countered by the use of IV oxytocin during the second stage. This is the main cause of the increase in instrumental delivery associated with epidural analgesia.
- *Sudden profound hypotension* can be prevented by adequate loading of the maternal circulation throughout. Emergency resuscitation drugs should be available in the room at all times.
- *Dural tap*: the spinal needle or cannula pierces the dura mater, allowing the cerebrospinal fluid (CSF) to escape and causing severe headache. Pushing efforts may need to be restricted. Following delivery, the mother must be nursed flat for 24h. A blood patch may be performed to seal the dura mater.
- *Infection at the site of introduction.*
- *Fetal hyperthermia* due to the increased warming effect in the woman's lower body. This increases as the length of labour increases. Continuous electronic monitoring of the fetal heart is thus required throughout. This can be offset by delaying the commencement of epidural analgesia by using other methods, such as an opiate or inhalational analgesia, during early labour and then by using the lowest doses possible to achieve maternal comfort.
- *Neurological problems*: injury/trauma to the spinal cord caused by drug or operator errors.

## Care of the woman during epidural analgesia

*How is the lumbar epidural commenced?*
- Perform continuous CTG for at least 30min during establishment of regional analgesia and after administration of each further bolus of 10mL or more.[10]
- Before inserting the epidural, 500mL of IV normal saline (or equivalent) is used to preload the maternal circulation, to offset the hypotensive effects of the epidural. This infusion must be maintained throughout labour until the epidural analgesic is no longer required (approximately 1h following delivery).
- A senior anaesthetist sites the epidural cannula, and the first dose is administered at this time.
- The cannula is inserted through a spinal needle, which is used to locate the epidural space. The woman's position during insertion is critical—she must sit up with her legs over the edge of the bed, feet supported, or lie flat, on her left side with her spine curved outwards and legs flexed, and lie completely still until the cannula is in place.
- This position is very difficult to achieve and maintain during frequent painful contractions. The midwife must assist the woman and remain with her until the procedure is completed.
- If the anaesthetist needs assistance, a second midwife should be present.

- During insertion, it is very important to have a clear record of the fetal heart, and the midwife may need to use a hand-held ultrasound transducer to achieve this.
- The cannula is secured firmly with adhesive dressings and the filter on the distal end is left easily accessible.
- The anaesthetist ensures that the woman has an adequate block before leaving her in the care of the midwife. The anaesthetist also leaves precise instructions about the dosage and frequency of any top-ups, and the dosage during the second stage of labour and for instrumental vaginal delivery.

*Care as labour progresses*
- After the initial and subsequent doses, measure maternal BP, pulse, and the FHR every 5min for 15min. Medical staff should be alerted if the readings give any cause for concern, e.g. if the FHR is below 110bpm or the maternal systolic BP below 100mmHg.
- If the woman is not pain-free 30min after each administration of the local anaesthetic/opioid solution, recall the anaesthetist.
- Thereafter, measure pulse, BP, and contractions half-hourly, and monitor the fetal heart continuously.
- Assess the level of the sensory block hourly using a cooling alcohol spray.[10]
- Help the woman to change position frequently, Encourage women with regional analgesia to move and adopt whatever upright positions they find comfortable throughout labour,[10] both to facilitate progress and to avoid pressure sores.
- Absence of sensation in the bladder is a feature of this method of pain relief and the woman will not be aware of the need to pass urine. Help her to empty her bladder every 2h, by a urinary catheter if necessary. This prevents injury to the urinary tract and obstruction of labour due to a full bladder.
- Do not allow the woman to lie supine. This may reduce blood flow to the placental sit, leading to fetal bradycardia. Avoid aorto-caval compression by positioning the woman on her side or with a small wedge/pillow under her side, to tilt her abdomen.
- The fetus ejection or pushing reflex is often lost as a result of epidural analgesia. Thus, upon confirmation of full cervical dilatation in a woman with regional analgesia, unless the woman has an urge to push, pushing should be delayed for at least 1h (or longer if the woman wishes), after which actively encourage her to push during contractions.[10] Ideally, the presenting part should be either visible or below the ischial spines before you encourage the woman to push.
- After diagnosis of full dilatation in a woman with regional analgesia, agree a plan with the woman in order to ensure that birth will have occurred within 4h, regardless of parity.[10]
- Do not routinely use oxytocin in the second stage of labour for women with regional analgesia.[10]

## Reference

10 National Institute for Health and Care Excellence (2014). *Intrapartum care for healthy women and babies.* NICE guidelines CG190. Available at: ◌ www.nice.org.uk/guidance/cg190.

# Normal labour: second stage

# Recognition of the second stage of labour

The second stage of labour is defined as the period of time from full dilatation of the cervix until the birth of the fetus. NICE[1] provides two further useful definitions:

## 1. Passive second stage of labour

The finding of full dilatation of the cervix before, or in the absence of, involuntary expulsive contractions.

## 2. Active second stage of labour

The woman is experiencing expulsive contractions with a finding of full dilatation of the cervix on vaginal examination, or with other signs of full dilatation of the cervix such as pouting of the anal sphincter or the presenting part being visible at the introitus.

Routine vaginal examination is not recommended.[2,3] The sometimes difficult transition between the first and second stages of labour is usually an indicator of the changes and readjustments that are made physically and emotionally, in order for labour to continue successfully.

Changes in the woman's behaviour and physical demeanour provide the midwife with visual and auditory clues, which are characteristic of the end of the first stage of labour and the onset of the second stage. During this time, the stress hormones associated with labour are at their peak, suggesting a favourable physiological response to labour.

## Visual, auditory, and physical signs

Women may:
- Experience contractions that come very close together, feeling more intense and painful (due to the action of stretch receptors and the effect of oxytocin).
- Feel a sensation of wanting to bear down, although the cervix is not quite fully dilated—there is no rationale for preventing women from bearing down if they so desire.
- Rest or sleep for periods: sometimes women enter a sleepy phase where contractions are weaker and less frequent.
- Appear to be in trance-like state, distant and withdrawn from carers, difficulty in concentrating; the focus is mainly on giving birth.

This is thought to be the result of the maternal release of β-endorphins during labour, which peak at birth. In a drug-free and non-interventionist labour, the woman (and the baby) will be impregnated with opiates which also contribute to the early dependency (attachment) of mother and baby following birth.

Women may:
- Lose control or feel unable to cope
- Strongly vocalize their needs by:
  - Distressed statements such as 'Get me an epidural', 'I can't do this', 'I am going home', 'Get this baby out!'
  - Swearing or using language that is uncharacteristic
  - Shouting and groaning

- Feel strange, shaky, and trembling
- Feel nauseated or actually vomit
- Experience extremes of hot and cold
- Express body language of restlessness and irritability.

## Passive phase of the second stage: physiology

The anatomical recognition of the second stage is full dilatation of the cervix, but this does not necessarily coincide with expulsive contractions.

- The contractions may subside for a period of 10–12min, or up to 2h; women often take this opportunity to sleep or doze. Often referred to as the 'rest and be thankful' phase.
- Contractions and the urge to push may be absent or weak.
- Once the presenting part has passed through the cervix, some adjustment due to decreased uterine volume may be needed. This requires the muscle fibres of the upper segment of the uterus to shorten and thicken further; only when the 'slack' has been taken up can progress be made to expulsive contractions and descent down the birth canal.
- Stretch receptors in the vagina, rectum, and perineum communicate changes in volume, tension, and tone, possibly accounting for the complexity of symptoms experienced at the transition stage.
- Passive descent should be allowed until the fetal head becomes visible.

There is scant evidence to suggest that active pushing in the latent phase of the second stage achieves much, other than exhausting and discouraging the mother.

## Active phase of the second stage: physiology

- The urge to push allows the presenting part to descend to compress the tissues of the pelvic floor.
- Approximately 1cm above the ischial spines, pressure from the fetal presentation stimulates nerve receptors in the pelvic floor (Ferguson's reflex) and an uncontrollable urge to bear down is experienced.
- During expulsive contractions, muscle fibres of the vagina and uterus draw up and tighten the lining of the birth canal, providing a taut surface against which the presenting part can slide down.
- Beynon's (coat/sleeve) analogy: when an arm is quickly put in a coat sleeve, the lining is dragged out with the hand; if the lining is held at the top, everything stays in place. In childbirth, when told to push immediately at the beginning of a contraction, the pulling up mechanism may be diminished or prevented, leading to delay, or damage.
- Odent[4] identifies the 'fetal ejection reflex' when there is a steep rise in the release of catecholamines during the last few contractions before birth. This is recognized by the woman suddenly becoming more alert and energized. She may need to drink a glass of water and perhaps hold on to someone. This ensures that the woman is alert and therefore protective for when the baby is born. The fetus also releases its own catecholamines at this time resulting in the wide eyed, alert baby who gazes at its mother directly after birth.

*Contractions of the second stage*

$$\text{Contraction alone} = 70\text{–}80\text{mmHg}$$
$$+$$
$$\text{Extra surges at peak of contraction} = 70\text{–}80\text{mmHg}$$
$$\text{Therefore, total effort} = 140\text{–}160\text{mmHg}$$

*Stretch receptors and pushing*

Stretch receptors are activated in the wall of the vagina, rectum, and perineum, especially during the surges of the contractions:

Uterine surges + abdominal pressure + receptors = overwhelming desire to push

## Early physical and auditory signs of the active second stage

- As dilatation progresses, the gap between the fundus and the breast bone becomes smaller—at full dilatation, one can no longer palpate a gap between the two.
- If the membranes are intact, they commonly rupture at full dilatation.
- The woman has a sensation of wanting to have her bowels open during a contraction.
- A bright red PV loss may be observed.
- The woman shows renewed strength and excitement, and the ability to work with her contractions.
- A purple line may gradually appear, extending from the anus to the nape of the buttocks. This is not recognizable in all women, due to obesity or upright positions. Although the cause is not known, it has been suggested that the appearance of the purple line may be due to vasocongestion at the base of the sacrum.[5]
- The woman may grunt at the height of a contraction and show facial congestion during pushing efforts.
- Involuntary curling of toes during contractions, even when the rest of the body is loose and relaxed.
- If standing, instead of curling her toes, the woman may stand on her toes.
- The smell of birth:[6] as the woman enters transition, the smell in the room changes (hard to notice in hospital settings).
- Angle of the body during a contraction: as a woman progresses in labour, if she is standing, she will lean further forward than before; by transition she may be nearly bent in two at the waist.
- Goose bumps may appear on the buttocks and upper thighs.

## Advanced signs of the second stage

- Vulval and perineal areas bulge and gape.
- The anus pouts and then flattens. The woman may empty her bowels during a contraction.
- The Rhombus of Michaelis:[7] the lowest three lumbar vertebrae and the sacrum move backwards and the ilia fan outwards, increasing the pelvic capacity. This only happens in the second stage if the woman is upright or on all fours. If the woman is naked, it is visible; if clothed, a caregiver may palpate a 'lump' (diamond-shaped) on the lower back.

## References

1 National Institute for Health and Care Excellence (2014). *Intrapartum care for healthy women and babies.* NICE guidelines CG190. Available at: ℵ www.nice.org.uk/guidance/cg190.
2 Downe S, Gyte GML, Dahlen HG, Singata M (2012). Routine vaginal examinations for assessing progress of labour to improve outcomes for women and babies at term (Protocol). *Cochrane Database of Syst Rev* 9: CD010088.
3 Royal College of Midwives (2012). *Evidence based guidelines for midwifery-led care in labour: assessing progress in labour.* Available at: ℵ www.rcm.org.uk/sites/default/files/Assessing%20Progress%20in%20Labour.pdf.
4 Odent M (2001). New reasons and new ways to study birth physiology. *Int J Gynecol Obstet* 75(Suppl 1): S39–45.
5 Shepherd A, Cheyne H, Kennedy S, McIntosh C, Styles M, Niven C (2010). The purple line as a measure of labour progress: a longitudinal study. *BMC Pregnancy Childbirth* 10: 54.
6 Wickham S, Roberts K, Howard J, Waters S (2004). Body wisdom: detecting birth by smell. *Pract Midwife* 7: 30–1.
7 Wickham S, Sutton J (2002). The Rhombus of Michaelis: a key to normal birth, or the poor cousin of the RCT? *Pract Midwife* 5: 22–3.

## Further reading

Lemay G (2005). To push or not? *Midwifery Today* 74: 7.
Sutton J (2003). Birth without active pushing and a physiological second stage of labour. In: Wickham S, ed. *Midwifery Best Practice.* Edinburgh: Books for Midwives, pp. 90–2.

# Mechanism of labour

During labour, the fetus makes a series of passive movements, collectively known as the mechanism of labour (Figs. 17.1–17.5). These enable the fetus to adapt to the changes of the pelvis and birth canal, making use of the best space available. It is important to have a sound understanding of this mechanism, so that the normal manoeuvres of the fetus at birth are anticipated and situations when assistance may be necessary recognized. This is best depicted diagrammatically.

- *Descent* commences before labour begins in the primigravida; in the multigravida, this may not occur until labour is established. Further descent is facilitated during labour, particularly during the second stage, when auxiliary muscles (diaphragm and abdominals) are employed to aid expulsion.
- *Flexion* is the natural attitude of the fetal head at commencement of labour. Flexion becomes more marked as labour progresses. Resistance of the birth canal exerts pressure through the occiput.
- *Internal rotation* occurs when the occiput (or whichever denominator meets the pelvic floor first) meets the resistance of the pelvic floor, rotating through one-eighth of a circle. The contour of the pelvic floor assists by presenting the longest diameter of the pelvic outlet (antero-posterior diameter). The occiput is then able to escape under the pubic arch and crowning takes place.
- *Crowning* of the head occurs when it has emerged under the pubic arch and does not recede between contractions. The widest diameter of the head (biparietal) is apparent.
- *Extension* of the head takes place to facilitate the bregma, forehead, face, and chin to sweep the perineum and accommodate the changed contour of the pelvis.

Fig. 17.1 First stage of labour. The cervix dilates. After full dilatation, the head flexes further and descends further into the pelvis.

**Fig. 17.2** During the early second stage, the head rotates at the levels of the ischial spine so the occiput lies in the anterior part of pelvis. In late second stage, the head broaches the vulval ring (crowning) and the perineum stretches over the head.

**Fig. 17.3** The head is born. The shoulders still lie transversely in the mid pelvis.

- Following the birth of the head, *restitution* (untwisting of the fetal head) takes place to enable realignment of the head and shoulders, in preparation for birth of the shoulders and body.
- The shoulders then undergo *internal rotation*, lying in the antero-posterior diameter of the outlet, to follow the direction of restitution.

The anterior shoulder is then born by applying gentle axial traction. The posterior shoulder and trunk are then born by lateral flexion. If traction is not applied, it is not uncommon for the posterior shoulder to be born first.

**Fig. 17.4** Birth of the anterior shoulder. The shoulders rotate to lie in the anteroposterior diameter of the pelvic outlet. The head rotates externally and 'restitutes' to its direction at onset of labour.

**Fig. 17.5** Birth of the posterior shoulder.

# Principles of care in the second stage of labour

The second stage of labour places extra emotional and physical demands on the woman. Extra vigilance is required in terms of midwifery care and support.

## Second stage principles

- Close observation of the woman's subtle behaviour, vocalizations, and emotional responses provides the midwife with key information about her progress, e.g. a quiet restful time prior to strong pushing urges, changing position, pelvic rocking, renewed strength, grunting during a contraction, etc.
- Observation of the physical signs of descent of the presenting part (➔ see also Mechanism of labour, p. 324). If all observations are satisfactory and progress of the vertex is not apparent after a reasonable period of time, then obstetric review or possibly augmentation/intervention may need to be considered.
- Be mindful that progress may be affected by maternal and fetal conditions.
- Women's choice for care should be taken into consideration, regarding position, care of the perineum, and monitoring the fetal heart.
- Time restrictions for the second stage should be reconsidered, and a holistic approach taken, based upon individual progress.
- Encourage the woman to adopt a comfortable position to aid progress; upright postures tend to shorten the duration of the second stage.[8]
- Encourage the woman to push spontaneously with the surges of her contractions, to help her assist with descent and progress of the presenting part.

## Second stage management

- *Vital signs.* In normal labour, unnecessary recordings of the BP and pulse will hinder the woman's concentration and focus. Women may be affected by pain, anxiety, fear, and contractions; therefore, taking the BP is of minimal value when the woman is actively pushing. However, hourly BP and 4-hourly temperature should be documented.[8]
- *Fetal heart.* Auscultate the fetal heart every 5min and between contractions in the latter part of the second stage.
- *Contractions.* Note frequency, strength, and length. Identify the different phases of the second stage—strong expulsive contractions indicate the active phase. Document the frequency of contractions half-hourly.[8]
- *Examination.* Offer an abdominal palpation and a vaginal examination hourly in the active second stage or in response to the woman's wishes.[8]
- *Vaginal loss.* Observe amniotic fluid or blood loss. Be aware of any abnormalities.
- *Bladder.* Document the frequency of passing urine.[8] Encourage the woman to empty her bladder at commencement of the second stage. Failure to do this can lead to delay and trauma to the bladder at birth.

- *Cleanliness and comfort.* Due to the woman's extra physical efforts and emotional strain, it may help to:
  - Sponge her face or use a fine water spray/mister
  - Sponge her hands, neck, and arms
  - Give her sips of iced water or mouthwash between contractions
  - Have a fan in the room if it is hot
  - Give her simple massage, particularly if she is prone to cramp
  - Give her physical support during contractions
  - Clean/swab her vulval area and provide a clean pad as frequently as required
  - Use complementary therapies if she wishes
  - Explore positions for comfort and to assist with the birth—an upright position will aid descent of the fetus and give the woman more control over the process
  - Play music if she wishes
  - Encourage her to use breathing awareness
  - Encourage the involvement of her birth partner.
- *Emotional support*:
  - Give verbal and non-verbal encouragement
  - Appreciate the woman's individuality and needs
  - Be informative and gain consent for procedures
  - Be aware of birth plan choices
  - Communicate and give reassurance
  - Understand, appreciate, and be tolerant of her vocalizations, behaviour, and expressions during the second stage
  - Prepare her to welcome the baby into the world.

## Conduct of normal vaginal birth

If a woman and her birthing partner have established a good rapport with their midwife, the environment is peaceful and unhurried, there is low lighting and privacy, with good communication and information, then the woman is likely to have a positive and empowering experience of birth.

## Positions for the second stage of labour

Positions adopted in the second stage have the potential to maximize the pelvic outlet by up to 20–30% and to influence favourably stretching of the perineum.[9] The woman should be enabled to adopt a position for birth that she feels comfortable with, and should be relaxed enough to verbal-ize (shouting, grunting, etc.) to relieve tension and anxiety and to prevent breath-holding.[8]

- *The traditional semi-recumbent position*: even when well supported with pillows, there is a tendency to slide down the bed, leading to compression of the vena cava. The perineum is stretched adversely sideways when the legs are bent and the knees flopped open, thus substantially reducing the pelvic outlet. Therefore, this position is not recommended in current midwifery practice.
- *Left lateral position on a bed or mattress on the floor*—particularly useful for when women require some temporary relief from an upright position or during a restful phase.
- *Kneeling* on the floor or a bed.

- *Squatting* (this is difficult to maintain without support).
- *Supported squatting* (partner, chair, parallel bars, furniture). Squatting positions open up the pelvic outlet, whereas the sacrum is fixed when lying flat.
- *On all fours*: the perineum is stretched favourably lengthways to form a continuation of the birth canal, maintaining flexion of the fetal head.
- *Birthing chair or stool* (linked to a higher incidence of haemorrhage).[9]

The laws of physics and gravity can improve the intravaginal pressures in upright and sitting positions. Sitting is 30% more effective than the lateral or supine positions.[10,11]

The choice of analgesia, EFM, and IV infusions will impair a woman's mobility, and to make an informed choice, women need to be made aware of these restrictions. However, for women who escalate to the need for EFM, wireless telemetry can enable them to remain upright and mobile.[8] Interventions and procedures may also interfere with use of postural coping strategies in labour. Support should be given to continue, or resume, the use of postural strategies if these have been interrupted by care procedures.[8]

### Preparation for the birth

- When birth is anticipated, put on protective glasses or visor (in case of blood spillages).
- Wash hands thoroughly; put on protective wear and gloves, and prepare the necessary equipment. A sterile area for equipment will need to be organized and accessible.
- The immediate birthing area should be prepared, e.g. mattress, birthing chair, etc.
- Prior to the birth, wash the vulva with water/lotion; drape sterile towels around the immediate area, and place a sterile pad over the anus to prevent faecal contamination.
- If the woman is in an upright position, the anal area will need to be kept free from faecal material.
- Encourage the woman to work with her contractions as before.
- At crowning, encourage her to breathe gently and/or to pant her baby's head out in a slow and controlled way. This helps to minimize perineal trauma, empowers the mother's experience, and prevents the need for too much hands-on intervention. A reported increase in anal sphincter damage has recently stimulated hypotheses that midwifery practice had moved to a 'hands-off' approach which had led to the increase in perineal injury.[12] However, this hypothesis has recently been invalidated with the majority of midwives shown to still use 'hands-on' techniques during the birth of the baby's head, dependent upon the mother's position and the place of birth—these techniques are of course not required if the woman is upright and/or in a birth pool.[13]
- Be ready to prevent sudden birth of the head. There is no physiological rationale for the application of firm pressure and resistance to maintain flexion, which serves only to increase the diameters of the fetal skull (➔ see Flexion technique, p. 337).

- Encourage the mother, both verbally and by non-verbal communication. This is crucial in helping to maintain her efforts and confidence. Make plenty of eye contact and give her praise, using a quietly spoken and supportive tone throughout.
- The Ritgen manoeuvre is generally not required if the birth is proceeding normally. Grasping the parietal eminences to overextend the head serves only to increase the diameters of the fetal skull (➔ see Care of the perineum, p. 336).
- Checking for the cord around the neck of the baby can cause considerable discomfort for the woman, and opinions are mixed as to whether this procedure is routinely necessary.
  - If the cord is around the neck, it can usually be untangled following birth.
  - If the cord is very tight, some suggest cutting the cord—two pairs of artery forceps are applied 2.5cm apart and the cord cut between them, using cord scissors, and then unwound. However, this can often be a difficult procedure and if delivery is delayed may result in lower Apgar scores.
  - Others suggest that cutting a nuchal cord is unnecessary, as the baby will be born through the loops of cord.
- The mother may wish to touch or watch the baby's head as it births; she may wish to assist with the birth of the trunk.
- Following restitution (after the head is born, it realigns itself with the shoulders), observe for external rotation of the head. If the mother is in an upright position, it may be difficult to see the baby, but be ready to receive the baby's head and body and assist if necessary. Upright positions maximize the diameters of the pelvic outlet and therefore the need for manoeuvres is less likely. If necessary, assist in delivery of the shoulders by placing a hand on either side of the baby's head and applying gentle traction with the next contraction to free the anterior shoulder, and then further gentle traction to deliver the posterior shoulder and trunk by lateral flexion.
- Place the baby directly on to the mother's abdomen/chest/arms to encourage immediate bonding. Cover the baby and keep him/her warm by maintaining skin-to-skin contact with the mother.
- Note the time of birth.
- Use delayed cord clamping, unless there are specific reasons not to (➔ see Active management of the third stage, p. 356).
- Keep contemporaneous records of the labour and birth.

## Directed sustained versus spontaneous physiological pushing

Breath-holding, closed glottis, and fixed diaphragm—commonly known as Valsalva's manoeuvre—is no longer recommended due to its negative effects (➔ see Breathing awareness, p. 292).[12,14] At the peak of a contraction, the utero-placental blood flow ceases—a physiological factor that the fetus can cope with for short periods.

This technique is said to reduce the length of the second stage; however, a technique for pushing infers that something needs to be done in place of the body's own efforts, which undermines the mother's ability and instincts.[10,12,13,14]

## Spontaneous physiological pushing

This allows the woman's body to tell her what to do. If she is left to push spontaneously, she will do so 3–5 times within a contraction, to coincide with extra surges. The length of pushing may be significantly reduced, but it is more intense and productive if the woman tunes into this natural pattern.[10]

*Disadvantages*
• It can be challenging for the woman to work with her own body and its intense sensations.

*Advantages*
• All fetal and maternal complications are minimized.
• Spiritual and psychological fulfilment/empowerment.
• Breathing awareness will automatically become easier and therefore assist with coping abilities.
• The woman can save her strength for the active/perineal phase.

## Length of the second stage

Limited quality of evidence makes it difficult to assess the significance of a prolonged second stage hence there is little ground for intervention whilst maternal and fetal conditions are satisfactory and there is clear progress with the descent of the presenting part.[11] Any perceived increase in risk needs to be weighed against the risks of instrumental delivery. However, the following may be used as a guide.[8]

• *For a nulliparous woman*: suspect delay if rotation and/or descent of the presenting part is inadequate after 1h of the active second stage. At this point the midwife may offer a vaginal examination and then offer amniotomy if the membranes are intact.[8] Birth would be expected to take place within 3h of the start of the active second stage in most nulliparous women. NICE recommends a diagnosis of delay in the active second stage when it has lasted 2h and suggests referral of the woman to a health-care professional trained to undertake an operative vaginal birth if birth is not imminent.[8]

• *For a multiparous woman*: suspect delay if rotation and/or descent of the presenting part is inadequate after 30min of the active second stage. At this point the midwife may offer a vaginal examination and then offer amniotomy if the membranes are intact.[8] Birth would be expected to take place within 2h of the start of the active second stage in most multiparous women. NICE recommends a diagnosis of delay in the active second stage when it has lasted 1h and suggests referral of the woman to a health-care professional trained to undertake an operative vaginal birth if birth is not imminent.[8]

• *If there is delay in the second stage of labour*, an obstetrician should assess a woman before contemplating the use of oxytocin. After initial obstetric assessment of a woman with delay in the second stage, there should be ongoing obstetric review every 15–30min.[8] If the woman is excessively distressed, support and sensitive encouragement and the woman's need for analgesia/anaesthesia are particularly important at this time.

# References

8 National Institute for Health and Care Excellence (2014). *Intrapartum care for healthy women and babies*. NICE guidelines CG190. Available at: ℘ www.nice.org.uk/guidance/cg190.
9 Downe S, Gerrett D, Renfrew M (2004). A prospective randomised controlled trial on the effect of position in the passive second stage of labour on birth outcomes in nulliparous women using epidural anaesthesia. *Midwifery* 20: 157–68.
10 Perez-Botella M, Downe S (2006). Stories as evidence: why do midwives still use directed pushing? *Br J Midwifery* 14: 596–9.
11 Royal College of Midwives (2012). *Evidence based guidelines for midwifery-led care in labour: second stage of labour*. Available at: ℘ www.rcm.org.uk/sites/default/files/Second%20Stage%20of%20Labour.pdf.
12 Bosomworth A, Bettany-Saltikov J (2006). Just take a deep breath. A review to compare the effects of spontaneous versus directed Valsalva pushing in the second stage of labour on maternal and fetal wellbeing. *MIDIRS Midwifery Digest* 16: 157–65.
13 Davies L (2006). Maternal pushing: to coach or not to coach. *Pract Midwife* 9: 38–40.
14 Byrom A, Downe S (2005). Second stage of labour: challenging the use of directed pushing. *Midwives* 8: 168–9.

# Care in the second stage of labour for a water birth

- Continue with low-risk care as recommended on ➔ p. 328.
- Adjust the water temperature to 37°C and check the pool temperature every 15min if birth in the pool is anticipated.
- Adopt a hands-off approach for the birth—touching the head is thought to stimulate the breathing response.[15]
- A pool birth should be facilitated completely under water, to avoid premature cessation of the breathing response. No increase in perinatal morbidity or mortality has been found when comparing births in water and conventional vaginal births in low-risk women.[16,17]
- If at any time during birth the baby is exposed to air, then the baby must be born out of water.
- Once the head is born, it is usually visible as a dark shadow under the water. Do not check for the cord routinely. If the baby is not birthed with the next contraction and the cord does require clamping and cutting, the woman should be eased out of the water on to the pool edge to undertake the procedure. The baby must then be born out of water.
- Allow the remainder of the body to birth spontaneously; it may be appropriate to assist/encourage the woman to bring the baby to the surface herself, with the baby's face uppermost. Assistance to birth the shoulders can be utilized in the same way as a birth out of water.
- If episiotomy is required, assist the mother to sit on the ledge or to get out of the pool for the procedure.
- Due to the more gentle birth, babies born in water often do not cry or appear to breathe instantaneously. The usual checks of the baby's colour, respiration, and heart rate should be observed. If there is any cause for concern, then the baby may be rubbed with a towel or lifted into the cooler air out of the water and this will usually result in a crying response.
- The vasoconstriction action of the cord may be delayed whilst in the water, thus the midwife should cut and clamp the cord (to avoid the risk of neonatal polycythaemia) before the mother leaves the pool.
- Keep the mother and baby warm by submerging the baby's body under the water and draping a towel over the woman's shoulders.
- The midwife should recognize that the time immediately after the birth is when the woman and her birth companion(s) are meeting and getting to know the baby. Ensure that any care or interventions are sensitive to this and minimize separation or disruption of the mother and baby. Usually women choose to vacate the pool for the third stage of labour.

# References

15 Royal College of Midwives (2014). *Report of a survey exploring the position of midwives' hands during the birth of the baby's head*. Available at: ℀ www.rcm.org.uk/sites/default/files/Perineal%20 Audit%20Report%202014_0.pdf.
16 National Institute for Health and Care Excellence (2014). *Intrapartum care for healthy women and babies*. NICE guidelines CG190. Available at: ℀ www.nice.org.uk/guidance/cg190.
17 Laine K, Skjeldestad FE, Sandvik L, Staff AC (2012). Incidence of obstetric anal sphincter injuries after training to protect the perineum: cohort study. *BMJ Open* 2: pii: e001649.

# Care of the perineum

Care of the perineum is an important part of the birthing process, both for the midwife and the mother. Perineal trauma can have far-reaching effects, influencing the woman's physical, emotional, and sexual relationships for the rest of her life. Perineal trauma is associated with:

- Urinary incontinence
- Faecal/flatus incontinence
- Dyspareunia
- Psychosocial factors as a result of the above
- A negative experience of motherhood.

Much of the routine care of the perineum is based on custom and practice; however, recent studies have shown how changes in management can help to enhance perineal integrity and minimize trauma.

## Management

- Keeping the perineal area clean and free from faecal contamination is universally recognized.
- Conduct of the second stage of labour and perineal management should be discussed with the woman, to ensure informed choice and consideration of her birth plan.
- There is no evidence to suggest that applying hot flannels and pads to the perineum is beneficial; however, it may provide some temporary comfort for the woman if there are no objections to this practice.
- Antenatal massage of the perineum appears to be advantageous; however, there is no evidence to support massage of the perineum in the second stage of labour.
- Women may be offered the application of warm compresses to the perineum as this may reduce perineal trauma and the severity of pain.[18]
- Upright positions for birth generally enhance perineal integrity.
- Either the 'hands-on' (guarding the perineum and flexing the baby's head) or the 'hands-poised' (with hands off the perineum and baby's head but in readiness) technique can be used to facilitate spontaneous birth.[19] There is no evidence to suggest that guarding the perineum is beneficial as opposed to hands-free management; however, there is a correlation between hands-free management and fewer episiotomies and third-degree tears.[18]
- Women's participation and confidence to breathe or pant the baby's head out slowly, to gradually stretch the perineum, is beneficial.
- The midwife's rapport and relationship with the woman and her birthing partner during labour is crucial, leading to less intervention in management of the perineum.
- Episiotomy should be reserved for fetal reasons only.[20]

There has been much debate about whether applying pressure on the fetal head to maintain flexion, and the Ritgen manoeuvre to assist extension, are of value. Review of the key physiological principles would suggest that intervention using these techniques interferes with normal birthing mechanisms, by increasing the diameter of the fetal skull, thus inevitably leading to potential perineal trauma rather than preventing it. This is best highlighted diagrammatically (Figs. 17.6–17.8).

## Flexion technique

**Fig. 17.6** The smallest diameter of the fetal head is maintained by an attitude of flexion. Further flexion applied by the birth attendant changes the position of the head to a larger diameter. This puts unnecessary pressure on the perineum, instead of its important role as a pivotal mechanism. Flexibility of the neck ensures the smallest diameter is maintained throughout the whole of the birth process.

**Fig. 17.7** The presenting part is halfway through the 90% curve of the birth canal. Partial extension occurs to maintain the smallest diameter (suboccipito-bregmatic). Extension of the head already occurs before it is visible; therefore, flexion at this point only maintains a larger diameter. As the birth canal is not straight, there is no rationale for this technique.

**Ritgen manoeuvre**

Fig. 17.8 The Ritgen manoeuvre. As the fetal head emerges from the introitus, if over-extension is applied, this results in the occipito-frontal diameter presenting a considerably larger diameter. In an unassisted mechanism, the head increasingly extends through the 90° curve so that it is able to utilize the resistance and pivotal force of the perineum and the pubic bone. This maintains the smallest diameter at the vaginal orifice.

## References

18 Aasheim V, Nilsen ABV, Lukasse M, Reinar LM (2011). Perineal techniques during the second stage of labour for reducing perineal trauma. *Cochrane Database Syst Rev* **12**: CD006672.
19 National Institute for Health and Care Excellence (2014). *Intrapartum care for healthy women and babies.* NICE guidelines CG190. Available at: ℳ www.nice.org.uk/guidance/cg190.
20 Royal College of Midwives (2012). *Evidence based guidelines for midwifery-led care in labour: care of the perineum.* Available at: ℳ www.rcm.org.uk/sites/default/files/Care%20of%20the%20Perineum.pdf.

# Female genital mutilation

Female genital mutilation (FGM), also known as female circumcision, is deeply rooted in the traditions and religion of about 30 countries. In the UK, it is most commonly seen among immigrants from Somalia, Eritrea, Mali, Sudan, Ethiopia, Sierra Leone, and Nigeria. The practice is illegal in the UK. It is also illegal to arrange for a child to be taken abroad for FGM. If caught, offenders face a large fine and a prison sentence of up to 14 years.[21] If FGM is confirmed in a girl under 18 years of age (either on examination or because the patient or parent says it has been done), reporting to the police is mandatory and this must be within 1 month of confirmation.[22]

## Definition

FGM involves a variety of invasive procedures that result in partial or total removal of the external female genitalia and/or other injury to the female genital organs, for cultural or any other non-therapeutic reason.

## Classification

- Type 1: excision of the prepuce, with or without excision of part or all of the clitoris.
- Type 2: excision of the prepuce and clitoris, together with partial or total excision of the labia minora.
- Type 3: excision of part or all of the external genitalia and stitching/narrowing of the vaginal opening (infibulation).
- Type 4: unclassified—includes pricking, piercing, or incision of the clitoris and/or labia; stretching of the clitoris and/or labia; cauterization by burning the clitoris and surrounding tissues; scraping of the vaginal orifice or cutting the vagina; introduction of corrosive substances to the vagina to cause bleeding, or herbs placed in the vagina to cause tightening or narrowing of the vagina; any other procedure that falls under the above definition.

## Cultural and historical background

- Most parents believe they are 'doing their best for their daughters' and that they are adhering to sound cultural practices.
- A circumcised woman is regarded as spiritually pure and clean. An uncircumcised woman is regarded as shameful and unnatural by society and therefore not fit to marry or have children.
- It is believed a woman must undergo this procedure in order for her to identify with the everyday hardships of being a woman.
- Religious reasons—some women see it as a religious obligation. There are no references in the Bible or the Koran to FGM.
- It is claimed to promote chastity and virginity.
- It negates sexual pleasure.
- It is advocated as improving fertility and preventing maternal and infant mortality. The opposite is true—FGM puts the health of the woman and the baby at great risk during pregnancy and childbirth.
- It is claimed to ensure that a woman is faithful to her husband, thereby preventing promiscuity.
- It is believed to promote cleanliness.
- Parents believe that FGM ensures a good marriage for their daughters.

## Prevalence

FGM is commonly performed on girls between the ages of 4 and 10 years but may also be performed soon after birth, at adolescence, at the time of marriage, or during the first pregnancy. The procedure is usually carried out by a traditional midwife or a woman within the local community. FGM is practised widely on the African continent, with countries such as Somalia and Sudan performing infibulation on 90–98% of girls. The WHO estimates that over 120 million women from 30 different countries have undergone FGM. It has been estimated that over 20 000 girls under the age of 15 are at risk of FGM in the UK each year, and that 66 000 women in the UK are living with the consequences of FGM.[21] However, the true extent is unknown, due to the 'hidden' nature of the crime.

## Complications

Following FGM, immediate complications are haemorrhage, pain, shock, infection, urine retention, injury to surrounding tissue, ulceration of the genital area, and death. Long-term complications include:
- Delayed wound healing, keloid formation, and severe scarring
- Pelvic infection, recurrent urinary tract infection
- Formation of epidermoid cysts and abscesses
- Neuromata
- Haematocolpos—vaginal closure leading to scarring can impair the flow of menstrual blood and exacerbate dysmenorrhoea
- Trauma and fears during childbirth
- Painful coitus
- Infertility
- Psychological trauma.

## Complications during labour and birth

- Prolonged obstructed labour, due to tough scar tissue formation commonly found in type 3 FGM. Clitoridectomy does not cause obstructed labour.
- Perineal laceration.
- Uterine inertia, due to prolonged labour.
- Fetal distress caused by obstructed labour; may lead to fetal death (a common occurrence in Africa).
- Post-partum wound infections.
- Re-infibulation is commonly practised in Africa but is illegal in the UK; there is no clinical justification for re-infibulation and it should not be undertaken under any circumstances.[22] The health professional must explain the UK law on FGM; women should be informed that re-infibulation will not be undertaken under any circumstances.

Where possible, it is important to identify women who may have been subjected to FGM early in pregnancy, by asking sensitive but leading questions. In an area with a high ratio of African residents, there may well be a specialist midwife. Women identified as having FGM should be referred to the designated consultant obstetrician or midwife with responsibility for FGM patients. Screening for hepatitis C should be offered in addition to the other routine antenatal screening tests (hepatitis B, HIV, and syphilis).[22] Although it is mandatory to report all pregnant women to social services or the police, an individual risk assessment should be made by a member of the clinical team (midwife or obstetrician) using an FGM safeguarding risk assessment tool (an example of such a tool can be found at: ℗ www.gov.uk/government/ publications/safeguarding-women-and-girls-at-risk-of-fgm). If the unborn child, or any related child, is considered at risk, then a report should be made.[22]

Reversal of infibulation can be carried out from 20 weeks to allow for complete healing prior to labour, in the first stage of labour, or at the time of birth.[22] It can usually be performed under local anaesthetic in a delivery suite room. It can also be performed perioperatively after a Caesarean section.[22] A woman whose planned de-infibulation is not performed because of delivery by a Caesarean section should have follow-up in a gynaecology outpatient or FGM clinic, so that de-infibulation can be offered before a subsequent pregnancy.[22]

Adequate pain relief is crucial so that the woman is not further traumatized by the procedure. With the woman's consent, an anterior midline incision that exposes the urethra and clitoris (which is often buried under scar tissue) is performed during labour. Prompt assessment of suturing requirements following birth should be attended to, and sensitive follow-up care of the woman's physical and psychological welfare should be ongoing. Referral for psychological assessment and treatment should be offered.[22]

## References

21 HM Government (2015). *Statement opposing female genital mutilation*. London Crown Copyright 2015. Available at: ℗ www.nhs.uk/Conditions/female-genital-mutilation/Documents/FGM_ June_2015_v10.pdf.

22 Royal College of Obstetricians and Gynaecologists (2015). *Female genital mutilation and its management*. Green-top guideline No. 53. Available at: ℗ www.rcog.org.uk/globalassets/documents/ guidelines/gtg-53-fgm.pdf.

## Further reading

Momoh C (ed.) (2005). *Female Genital Mutilation*. Abingdon: Radcliffe Publishing Ltd.

# Episiotomy

The majority of women who have a vaginal birth will sustain perineal trauma from a spontaneous perineal tear.[23] However, there is no evidence of short-term or long-term maternal benefit to support the use of routine episiotomy.[23,24] The only real indication for an episiotomy should be if the fetus is compromised in the second stage of labour and birth needs to be facilitated quickly. In rare cases, a rigid perineum that is unquestionably obstructing the process of birth may require an episiotomy.

Evidence suggests that:
- Women who receive midwifery-led care are less likely to have an episiotomy[23]
- Protection against anal sphincter damage is unfounded[24]
- Episiotomy is more likely to cause unnecessary perineal trauma and may predispose to third-degree tears[23]
- There is no difference between tears and episiotomies in terms of pain and dyspareunia[23]
- There is a risk of healing complications[23,24]
- Episiotomy is contraindicated for third-degree tears, except in the event of shoulder dystocia, to prevent extensive perineal damage when undertaking internal manoeuvres to release the impacted fetal shoulder.

Awareness of anatomical structures is important, especially the location of the external sphincter muscle, which extends 2.5cm around the anus (Fig. 17.9). A medio-lateral incision is used, as opposed to the midline incision, which is associated with an increased incidence of third-degree tears.[24]

## Performing an episiotomy
- Obtain consent after explaining the rationale determining the procedure.
- Prepare the necessary equipment:
  - Sterile swabs
  - Lidocaine 0.5% (10mL) or 1% (5mL)
  - 10mL syringe
  - Gauge 21 needle.
- Clean the skin with antiseptic using aseptic technique.
- Insert the first and second fingers of a gloved hand into the vagina to protect the fetal skull from injury and anaesthetic.
- An episiotomy is usually performed on the maternal right. Insert the needle via the fourchette and direct it at a 45° angle from the midline for 4–5cm, to ensure a medio-lateral incision (Fig. 17.9).
- Withdraw the piston before infiltrating the anaesthetic, to check that the needle is not in a blood vessel. If so, the needle must be withdrawn and repositioned.
- Lidocaine can be injected slowly as the needle is withdrawn. However, it is considered to be more effective if 3–4mL are injected initially and then, before removing the needle, the remaining lidocaine is injected on either side of the initial injection, in a fan shape.
- At least 4–5min must be given for the analgesic to be effective prior to incision (Fig. 17.9).
- Use blunt-ended scissors.

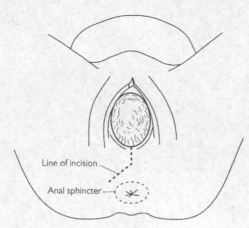

Fig. 17.9 Right medio-lateral episiotomy.

- Insert two fingers of a gloved hand into the vagina, as before.
- Open the blades of the scissors; insert the blade accessing the vagina flat over the fingers, and then rotate into the cutting position with the outer blade.
- Make a cut of approximately 4cm within the anaesthetized area.
- Cut concisely and deliberately at the height of a contraction, when the perineum is maximally stretched, to minimize bleeding and pain.
- A medio-lateral incision is commonly used, or sometimes a 'J'-shaped incision. Both methods help to prevent extension of the incision to the anal sphincter.
- Preparation for an imminent birth is important. It is vital to deliver the head carefully and prevent the shoulders from being expelled before restitution has occurred.
- If the birth is delayed, control bleeding by applying pressure to the episiotomy.

### References

23 Royal College of Midwives (2012). *Evidence based guidelines for midwifery-led care in labour: care of the perineum.* Available at: ℘ www.rcm.org.uk/sites/default/files/Care%20of%20the%20 Perineum.pdf.
24 Carroli G, Mignini L (2009). Episiotomy for vaginal birth. *Cochrane Database Syst Rev* 1: CD000081.

# Normal labour: third stage

# Care during the third stage of labour

Women who have midwifery-led care and whose pregnancies are low risk for PPH should be aware of the choices available to them for the third stage of labour. Women should receive information both antenatally and again at the initial assessment in labour, to ensure they are able to make an informed choice between physiological care and an actively managed third stage of labour.[1]

## Definition of primary post-partum haemorrhage

Globally, obstetric haemorrhage is the leading cause of maternal morbidity and accounts for up to 50% of maternal deaths worldwide.[2] In the UK, this figure is approximately 10% of all direct maternal deaths which equates to 0.49 per 100 000 maternities.[3] Primary PPH (within the first 24h) is the most common form of major obstetric haemorrhage. The traditional definition of primary PPH is the loss of 500mL or more of blood from the genital tract within 24h of the birth of a baby. However, consideration needs to be given to women who may be symptomatic of haemorrhage, even with a blood loss of <500mL, particularly if her Hb levels were low antenatally. PPH can be minor (500–1000mL) or major (>1000mL). Major PPH can be further divided into moderate (1000–2000mL) or severe (>2000mL).[4]

## Causes and risk factors associated with primary post-partum haemorrhage

*History*
- Previous PPH or previous retained placenta.
- Previous precipitate, prolonged, or traumatic labour.
- Previous APH.
- Uterine scar.
- Uterine fibroids or other anomalies.

*Pregnancy*
- High parity (parity 4 or more).
- Multiple pregnancy.
- Polyhydramnios.
- Coagulation disorders.
- Maternal Hb level below 85g/L at the onset of labour.
- BMI >35kg/m$^2$.
- Placenta praevia.
- Maternal age of 35 years or older.
- APH.
- Over-distension of the uterus (i.e. multiple pregnancy, polyhydramnios, or macrosomia).
- Existing uterine abnormalities.
- Pre-eclampsia.

*Labour*
- Precipitate labour.
- Prolonged labour (first, second, or third stage of labour).
- Induction of labour or augmentation of labour.
- Operative birth or Caesarean section.
- Large doses of narcotics and/or epidural analgesia.
- General anaesthesia.
- Tocolytic drugs (used to suppress uterine activity in preterm labour).
- Infection—chorioamnionitis.
- Ketoacidosis.

*Third stage*
- Incomplete separation of the placenta.
- Full bladder.
- Retained cotyledon, placental tissue, or membranes.
- Mismanagement of the third stage, disrupting the rhythm of myometrial activity.
- Inversion of the uterus.

## Expectant or physiological management of the third stage

There are two ways in which the third stage of labour may be managed—either by active management or by physiological management. Ambiguity remains around the most appropriate management of the third stage of labour for women with low-risk pregnancies. Due to this uncertainty within the midwifery profession, there are concerns as to whether low-risk women are really offered informed choice at all.[5] It has been suggested that the third stage should not be managed at all and that attention to creating the right environment to enhance physiological efficiency is far more important, therefore preventing intervention that is likely to lead to complications.[6] This suggestion is at odds with most clinical guidelines which strongly recommend active management, in order to reduce the risk of bleeding.[1]

The most recent Cochrane review which has informed much of the national guidance around active management over physiological management concluded that for all women, irrespective of their risk of bleeding, active management reduced severe bleeding and anaemia.[7] However, it also reported an increase in the mother's BP, afterpains, vomiting, and the number of women returning to hospital with a secondary PPH.[7] It is important to note that criticism has been levelled in some of the five studies used within this review, i.e. that some women involved had pre-existing risk factors for PPH and that many midwives in the studies were not used to providing physiological care, resulting in a mixed approach.[8]

Current guidance for intrapartum care suggests that the midwife should inform the woman of the following information when assisting her to make an informed choice for the third stage of labour.[1]

*Active management*
- Shortens the third stage compared with physiological management.
- Is associated with nausea and vomiting in 100 in 1000 women.
- Is associated with an approximate risk of 13 in 1000 of a haemorrhage of >1L.
- Is associated with an approximate risk of 14 in 1000 of requiring a blood transfusion.

*Physiological management*
- Is associated with nausea and vomiting in about 50 in 1000 women.
- Is associated with an approximate risk of 29 in 1000 of haemorrhage of >1L.
- Is associated with an approximate risk of 40 in 1000 of requiring a blood transfusion.

## General care
- The midwife should be proficient with the proposed management of the third stage of labour, including for mothers who choose to give birth in a birthing pool.
- The latest Hb results and BP recordings in pregnancy should be noted by the midwife. Review BP recordings and any complications arising in labour before the third-stage management is determined.
- Ensure that the woman is fully conversant with, and understands, the process of the third stage and her involvement.
- Maintain positions of comfort and dignity throughout.
- Careful observation of blood loss, and arrange for assistance to be available should abnormal bleeding occur.
- Blood loss >500mL is considered to be significant. Generally, blood loss tends to be underestimated, especially the greater the blood loss.
- Some schools of thought suggest that healthy women can cope with a blood loss of up to 1000mL.[3] However, accurate estimation of blood loss is crucial for both active and physiological management.
- If blood loss is significant, do not delay; proceed immediately to providing care following local major obstetric haemorrhage guidance.
- Check the placenta and membranes thoroughly following delivery, to ensure there are no abnormalities and that they are complete. Retained products can result in sepsis and secondary PPH. Any suspicion of ragged membranes or missing placental tissue should be recorded in the notes and the information passed on to the receiving midwife taking over the woman's care.
- The woman should be alerted to monitor her lochia and report any abnormally heavy bleeding or clots.

## Pool birth: the third stage of labour
- Usually women choose to vacate the pool for the third stage of labour. We should recognize that the time immediately after the birth is when the woman and her birth companion(s) are meeting and getting to know the baby. Ensure that any care or interventions are sensitive to this and minimize separation or disruption of the mother and baby.[1]
- Keep the mother and baby warm by submerging the baby's body under the water and draping a towel over the woman's shoulders.
- If active management of the third stage is chosen, then this should be undertaken out of the pool.[1] If the woman chooses to stay in the pool, then a physiological third stage is the only option. Ensure that the woman is aware of this before she makes the decision to stay in the pool.

- Blood loss may not be easy to assess. Normal amounts of bleeding associated with separation of the placenta will sink to the bottom of the pool. However, if the bleeding appears to be diffusing very quickly through the water, and there is any doubt, it is best to ask the woman to vacate the pool so that more accurate assessment of bleeding can be established.
- In the event of bleeding, administer an oxytocic drug when the mother has vacated the pool.
- Carry out an examination of vaginal trauma as in normal labour.
- After use, empty the pool and decontaminate according to local policy. Thorough cleaning of the pool after use is essential.[9] Some units use a disposable pool liner for each woman.

## References

1 National Institute for Health and Care Excellence (2014). Third stage of labour. In: National Institute for Health and Care Excellence. *Intrapartum care for healthy women and babies.* NICE guidelines CG190. Available at: ℜ www.nice.org.uk/guidance/cg190/chapter/1-recommendations#third-stage-of-labour.

2 Lale S, Chou D, Gemmill A, et al. (2014). Global causes of maternal death: a WHO systematic analysis. *Lancet Glob Health* 2: e323–33. Available at: ℜ www.sciencedirect.com/science/article/pii/S2214109X1470227X

3 Knight M, Kenyon S, Brocklehurst P, Neilson J, Shakespeare J, Kurinczuk JJ (eds.) on behalf of MBRRACE-UK (2014). *Saving Lives, Improving Mothers' Care: Lessons learned to inform future maternity care from the UK and Ireland Confidential Enquiries into Maternal Deaths and Morbidity 2009–12.* Oxford: National Perinatal Epidemiology Unit, University of Oxford. Available at: ℜ www.npeu.ox.ac.uk/mbrrace uk/reports.

4 Royal College of Obstetricians and Gynaecologists (2011). *Prevention and management of postpartum haemorrhage.* Green-top guideline No. 52. Available at: ℜ www.rcog.org.uk/globalassets/documents/guidelines/gt52postpartumhaemorrhage0411.pdf.

5 Selfe K, Walsh D (2015). The third stage of labour: are low risk women really offered an informed choice? *Midwifery Digest* 25: 1.

6 Odent M (1998). Don't manage the third stage of labour! *Pract Midwife* 1: 31–3.

7 Begley CM, Gyte GML, Devane D, McGuire W, Weeks A (2011). Active versus expectant management for women in the third stage of labour (review). *Cochrane Database Syst Rev* 11: CD007412. Available at: ℜ onlinelibrary.wiley.com/doi/10.1002/14651858.CD007412.pub3/pdf/standard;jsessionid=1ECFA907668981B79A4D626709E16627.f02t02.

8 Walsh D (2012). *Evidence and Skills for Normal Labour and Birth: A Guide for Midwives,* 2nd edn. London: Routledge.

9 Garland D (2006). On the crest of a wave. Completion of a collaborative audit. *MIDIRS Midwifery Digest* 16: 81–5.

# Physiological management of the third stage

A physiological third stage of labour may be the choice for women who prefer to avoid intervention during childbirth. Placental separation occurs physiologically without resorting to oxytocic drugs, and expulsion of the placenta is achieved by maternal effort. The average length of the third stage is 15–60min, although in some cases, provided there are no abnormal signs, it may occasionally last up to 120min. Physiological management is suitable if the woman has had a physiological labour and birth.

## Physiology of the third stage

- Detachment of the placenta commences with contractions that deliver the baby's trunk.
- Once the baby is born, the uterus is greatly reduced in size due to the powerful contraction and retraction of the uterine muscles.
- Consequently, the placental site is also greatly reduced. When the placental site is reduced by one-half it becomes puckered and starts to peel away from the uterine wall.
- This is assisted by the tightly compressed and contracted uterus. As a result, fetal blood is pumped into the baby's circulation. Maternal blood is driven back into the spongy layer of the decidua.
- The congested veins are then forced to rupture. The effused blood from the congested veins results in detachment of the placenta. The veins are caused to rupture as the blood in these veins cannot return to the maternal circulation.
- Bleeding is controlled by the presence of 'living ligatures'. Plain muscle fibres of the uterus entangle around the exposed bleeding blood vessel site, preventing further blood loss.
- When separation of the placenta is complete (usually 3–5min), the upper segment of the uterus contracts strongly, forcing the placenta into the lower segment and then the vagina.
- Detachment of the membranes commences in the first stage of labour; when the membranes rupture they are shorn from the internal os. This is then completed in the third stage, when the weight of the descending placenta allows them to peel away from the wall of the uterus.

## Methods of detachment

### Schultze method

Approximately 80% of cases detach by this method. The placenta starts to detach from the centre and leads its descent down the vagina. The fetal surface of the placenta therefore appears first at the vulva, with the membranes trailing behind. The retroplacental clot is situated inside the membrane sac. Minimal visible blood loss is the result.

### Matthews Duncan method

Separation of the placenta commences at the lower edge, which allows the placenta to slide down sideways, exposing the maternal surface. This usually results in increased bleeding due to the slower rate of separation and no retroplacental clot being formed.

## Management

- Do not give oxytocic prophylaxis.
- Leave the cord unclamped until completion of the third stage. This practice allows the physiological action of contraction and retraction of the uterus to proceed naturally and is thought to minimize any delay in separation and to prevent excessive bleeding.
- If planning on cutting and clamping the cord, wait until it has stopped pulsating. This allows for the transfer of maternal blood to the neonate; once cord clamping and cutting occur, it immediately suspends the transfer of blood, resulting in a decrease of circulating blood volume of the newborn.[10] The volume of blood if clamped prior to the end of pulsation can deplete as much as 100mL of oxygenated blood from the neonate. It has been suggested that this could potentially lead to neonatal complications.[11]
- Ideally, the baby should be put to the breast to suckle, as this ensures the continued release of oxytocin to assist the separation and expulsion of the placenta. (Nipple stimulation could be considered if breastfeeding is not an option the mother chooses.)
- Ensure that the bladder is empty; failure to do this may cause delay in the third stage and possibly predispose to bleeding.
- A 'hands off the abdomen' approach is crucial, as any manipulation of the uterus disturbs the rhythmical coordination of the uterine muscles and will negate the physiological process.
- Observe vaginal loss to ensure that bleeding is not excessive. A gush of blood indicates the beginning of separation.
- A squatting position is most beneficial to aid expulsion of the placenta as this works with gravity and gives increased intra-abdominal pressure.
- Await the onset of expulsive contractions—this is usually an indication that the placenta has separated and descended into the lower segment. The weight of the placenta causes stimulation and pressure in the vagina, which triggers off expulsive contractions. Often the woman will involuntarily bear down and push the placenta out.
- Advise the woman that expulsive contractions are similar to, but often not as strong as, the contractions experienced in the second stage, and may easily be missed.
- As the uterus descends, it becomes rounder and smaller; the fundus rises and becomes harder and more mobile.
- The cord lengthens—this is another indication that the placenta has descended into the lower segment and is ready to be expelled.
- If you are sure that the placenta has separated and the woman does not experience contractions, encourage the woman to push down in a similar way to the second stage of labour to expel the placenta.
- Once the placenta is delivered, assist with easing the membranes out of the vagina. Either attach artery forceps or hold the placenta in both hands, rotating it so that the membranes form a rope-like appearance; then use very gentle traction to avoid tearing and retention of membranous material.
- Finally palpate for contraction of the uterus and observe for any signs of abnormal bleeding. Document all findings.

## References

10 Hutchon DJ (2013). Early versus delayed cord clamping at birth: in sickness and in health. *Fetal and Maternal Medicine Review* 24: 185–93.

11 Raju T, Singhal N (2012). Optimal timing for clamping the umbilical cord after birth. *Clin Perinatol* 39: 889–900.

## Further reading

Rabe H, Diaz-Rossello JL, Duley L, Dowswell T (2012). Effect of timing of umbilical cord clamping and other strategies to influence placental transfusion at preterm birth on maternal and infant outcomes. *Cochrane Database Syst Rev* 8: CD003248. Available at: ℘ onlinelibrary.wiley.com/doi/10.1002/14651858.CD003248.pub3/abstract.

# Active management of the third stage

The third stage of labour, if managed actively, will usually be a short, passive stage for the woman, lasting no more than 10min, whilst she will be focused on her baby. However, this is also the most dangerous stage of labour as the risk of haemorrhage is at its greatest. Therefore, sound physiological knowledge and the expertise of the midwife are essential to ensure a safe outcome for the woman.

Active management for the third stage has been the routine for many decades; however, in recent years women and midwives have increasingly been returning to a physiologically managed third stage. In order for women to be fully informed about their care in the third stage, discuss the options prior to labour, so that they can make an informed, unhurried choice.

Active management is associated with less blood loss, shorter duration, fewer blood transfusions, and less need for therapeutic oxytocics.[12] However, there is debate that when the effect of oxytocic drugs wears off, women may experience heavier postnatal blood loss than those who had a physiological third stage.[12,13]

## Management

- Ensure that the woman is comfortable, whether in the dorsal or an upright position.
- Based on an earlier explanation of the third stage, reinforce what the procedure involves.
- Maintain a high standard of hygiene and aseptic technique throughout, to prevent contamination and infection.
- An oxytocic drug will have been administered at the birth of the anterior shoulder, intramuscularly into the upper lateral aspect of the thigh. Give 10IU of oxytocin to women who are thought to be at lower risk of bleeding; this drug is associated with fewer side effects than oxytocin plus ergometrine. Oxytocin acts within 2–3min.
- If the woman is at high risk of haemorrhage, or local guidelines recommend, Syntometrine® may be administered instead of oxytocin 10IU. Syntometrine® contains 5IU oxytocin and 0.5mg ergometrine. Oxytocin acts within 2–3min, whereas ergometrine acts within 6–8min, the effects lasting up to 2h.
- Ergometrine is not recommended for women with the following conditions:
  - Hypertension
  - Cardiac disease
  - Following β-agonist infusion such as salbutamol or ritodrine
  - Raynaud's disease
  - Severe asthma.
- Ergometrine can cause nausea, vomiting, and hypertension.
- Delayed cord clamping is now widely recommended even after early oxytocin administration.[13,14] Fetomaternal blood transfusion is thought to be beneficial for the neonate, even for mothers who are Rh-negative and are giving birth to Rh-positive babies.[15]

- Wait no less than 1min before clamping the cord.[13],[14] Some research into this topic is suggesting that 3min or more has been shown to reduce iron deficiency at 4 months of age with no increased risk of jaundice.[16]
- Wait for the signs of separation and descent of the placenta, i.e. the cord lengthening at the vulva, minimal fresh blood loss, and contraction of the uterus. The uterus will change from feeling broad to firm, central, and rounded at the level of the umbilicus.
- Do not manipulate the uterus in any way, in order to avoid overstimulation or incoordinate activity.
- Once you are happy that the uterus is contracted and separation has occurred, deliver the placenta and membranes by controlled cord traction.
- Place one hand (usually the left) above the level of the symphysis pubis, with the palm facing towards the umbilicus. Apply firm upwards pressure to achieve countertraction and to guard the uterus.
- With the other hand, grasp the cord firmly and wrap it around your index and middle fingers. Maintain firm, steady, and consistent traction in a downwards and backwards direction in line with the birth canal to guide the placenta and membranes into the vagina.
- If strong resistance is felt, or you feel that the membranes are breaking, then cease traction and use maternal effort instead.
- The object is to deliver the placenta in one continuous, controlled movement; however, there may need to be pauses in the process until the placenta is visible. Always reinstate your guarding hand before attempting traction after such a pause.
- Once the bulk of the placenta is visible, the direction of the traction becomes horizontal and upwards, to follow the contour of the birth canal.
- Once the whole of the placenta has become visible, cup it in both hands to gently ease it out of the vagina without causing damage to the delicate membranes.
- In order to prevent tearing of the membranes, with two hands holding the placenta, help to coax the membranes out of the vagina with an upwards and downwards movement or a twisting action, forming a rope. This action is repeated until the membranes are completely free.
- Collect the placenta and membranes in a receiver placed near the perineum.
- Consider if any bloods are needed from the placenta, i.e. whether the mother is Rh-negative, whether cord gases need to be obtained.
- Assess the blood loss as accurately as possible.
- Inspect the perineum for trauma.
- Ensure the comfort and hygiene of the woman by cleaning the immediate perineal area, applying clean sanitary towels, etc.
- Check the placenta and membranes to ensure they are complete. Report any abnormalities to a senior doctor and to the receiving midwife on the postnatal ward.

## References

12 Begley CM, Gyte GML, Devane D, McGuire W, Weeks A (2011). Active versus expectant management for women in the third stage of labour (review). *Cochrane Database Syst Rev* 11: CD007412. Available at: ஃ onlinelibrary.wiley.com/doi/10.1002/14651858.CD007412. pub3/pdf/standard;jsessionid=1ECFA907668981B79A4D626709E16627.f02t02.

13 National Institute for Health and Care Excellence (2014). Third stage of labour. In: National Institute for Health and Care Excellence. *Intrapartum care for healthy women and babies.* NICE guidelines CG190. Available at: ஃ www.nice.org.uk/guidance/cg190/chapter/1-recommendations#third-stage-of-labour.

14 World Health Organization (2014). *Delayed umbilical cord clamping for improved maternal and infant health and nutrition outcomes.* Geneva: World Health Organization. Available at: ஃ www.who.int/nutrition/publications/guidelines/cord_clamping/en/.

15 Andersson O, Hellstrom-Westas L, Andersson D, Domellof M (2011). Effects of delayed versus early cord clamping on neonatal outcomes and iron status at 4 months: a randomised controlled trial. *BMJ* 343: d7157. Available at: ஃ www.bmj.com/content/343/bmj.d7157.

16 Prendiville W, Elbourne D (2000). The third stage of labor. In: Enkin M, Keirse N, Neilson J, *et al.*, eds. *A Guide to Effective Care in Pregnancy and Childbirth*, 3rd edn. Oxford: Oxford University Press, pp. 300–10.

# Assessing and repairing the perineum

Women who require suturing to the perineum following childbirth may well experience confused and turbulent emotions, from exhilaration to tiredness and anxiety. The prospect of the repair may well prove to be daunting and stressful for her. Midwives are increasingly trained and fully supervised to carry out perineal repair, and this is now covered in midwifery training. Not only is it important for the midwife to carry out the procedure in a skilful and competent manner, but it is also important to ensure that the woman's experience is not a lonely, undignified, and threatening ordeal. This can be achieved by considering the following:

- The environment
- The comfort and position of the woman
- Presence of supportive carers
- Information and explanation about the procedure
- Consideration of the woman's birth experience
- Thorough assessment of the perineal damage and referral to an obstetrician if necessary
- Satisfactory pain relief.

Midwives involved in perineal repair should be aware of their limitations in suturing more complex trauma. It is not the midwife's responsibility to repair the following, and these should be referred to an obstetrician:

- Third-/fourth-degree tears
- Extended episiotomy
- Vulval varicosities
- Severe haemorrhoids
- Severe bruising of the perineum or a haematoma
- Labial lacerations
- Vulval warts
- Following previous third-degree tear or extensive scar tissue.

## Assessing perineal trauma

- Anterior labial tears: there is some debate about the merits of leaving these unsutured. This depends very much on the degree of bleeding. Oozing immediately following childbirth may resolve itself after a short period if a sanitary towel is placed securely between the legs; however, sometimes a single suture may be required to stabilize haemostasis.
- Posterior perineal trauma: spontaneous tears are classified by degrees of trauma relating to the anatomical structures involved.
  - *First-degree tears*: this involves the skin of the fourchette only. NICE guidance suggests that even this level of trauma should be sutured to aid healing, unless the skin edges are well opposed—discussion with the woman about her options may determine the management.[17]
  - *Second-degree tear and episiotomy*: this involves the skin of the fourchette, the perineum and perineal body. The superficial muscles affected are the bulbocavernosus and the transverse perineal muscles. Deeper muscle layer trauma may involve the pubococcygeus. (If after the muscle layer has been sutured, the skin is well opposed, there is no need to suture the skin.)[17]

- *Third-degree tear*: in addition to second-degree trauma, there is damage to the anal sphincter. This should be further classified and documented as:
  - —3a: <50% of the external anal sphincter thickness torn
  - —3b: >50% of external anal sphincter thickness torn
  - —3c: internal anal sphincter torn.
- *Fourth-degree tear*: this describes trauma that involves all of the above structures which extends into the rectal mucosa.

## Preparation for perineal repair

- Ensure the woman is in a comfortable position. To minimize the risk of DVT, do not put the woman into the lithotomy position for suturing until all preparations are in hand to commence the procedure.
- Make the environment as comfortable as possible. The mother may like to cuddle and hold her baby throughout the procedure, or even breastfeed. The procedure should not interfere with the mother–baby bonding unless the woman is bleeding and in need of emergency treatment.[17] Ensure that she is not alone—ideally she should have her partner close by to comfort and distract her.
- Give a full explanation of the trauma, what her options may be, and what the procedure involves. Reassure and relieve any anxieties she may have.
- Assess the woman's general and obstetric condition. Ensure that the uterus is well contracted, her lochia is not excessive, and her vital signs are stable.
- Gather requirements for the procedure—a perineal sterile pack, local anaesthesia, suture materials, syringes and needles, sanitary towel, incontinence pad, and sterile gloves.

## Procedure

- Ideally the wound should be sutured as soon as possible following birth. A good directional light over the perineum is essential, but dimmed lights otherwise may help to create a more relaxed environment.
- Assist the woman into the lithotomy position to ensure a clear view of the perineum. Other positions of comfort may need to be explored if the woman finds this uncomfortable.
- Prepare the trolley and sterile field.
- The midwife then scrubs to prepare for aseptic technique.
- Clean the wound; water is an acceptable solution for cleaning.[17]
- The woman is draped with sterile towels to ensure a clean sterile field.
- Inspect the perineum to assess damage and whether you can carry out the repair. If there is any doubt, an obstetrician or doctor experienced in perineal repair should be called for.
- Visual assessment of the extent of perineal trauma should include the structures involved, the apex of the injury and assessment of bleeding.
- A rectal examination to assess whether there has been any damage to the external or internal anal sphincters should be performed with informed consent. This procedure should always take place if there is any suspicion that the perineal muscles are damaged.[17]

- If it is not possible to adequately assess the degree of trauma, the woman and her baby should be transferred to obstetric-led care.[17]
- Prior to the procedure, adequate analgesia is crucial. Women report that the experience of being sutured after childbirth is highly unpleasant and that even with the use of local anesthetic, the procedure can be painful throughout:[18]
  - Infiltration of the wound with 1% lidocaine—up to 20mL maximum dose within an hour and inclusive of the amount used for infiltration prior to episiotomy
  - Epidural: if *in situ*, this can be topped up to provide analgesia for the procedure; alternatively if the woman's pain cannot be managed, she should be offered a spinal anaesthetic if necessary[17]
  - Additionally the woman may like to use inhalational analgesia to assist if she is anxious
  - Ensure that the analgesia in use is tested prior to beginning suturing; if it is found to be inadequate at any point, this should be addressed immediately.
- Infiltration: the whole of the area to be sutured should be infiltrated.
  - The needle should be inserted into the wound at the fourchette, passing superficially up the vagina; withdraw the plunger to ensure the needle is not in a blood vessel; then infiltrate as the needle is slowly withdrawn.
  - Using the same site of entry, pass the needle into the perineal body and infiltrate. The perineal skin is then infiltrated in the same way.
- Whilst waiting for the anaesthesia to take effect (ideally 15min prior to commencing suturing), check that you have everything ready for the repair and ensure the woman is comfortable and warm. This may be a good time to count all swabs, tampons, and needles to be used in the procedure. This must be performed with a colleague and recorded this in the woman's notes. This will be repeated after the procedure with the same colleague to verify that no equipment is unaccounted for.
- Suturing: repair is usually undertaken in three layers; this ensures that the repair is performed in a logical manner and nothing is missed. The layers are the vaginal epithelial layer, the perineal muscle, and the perineal skin (Fig. 18.1).
- Care should be taken to align the edges of the tissues as accurately as possible throughout the repair, to ensure a neat symmetrical result. Sutures should not be pulled too tight as oedema and bruising to the site will cause pain and slow healing. A continuous, non-locking suture technique should be used.
  - A taped vaginal tampon should be inserted into the vault of the vagina prior to the procedure to prevent blood from oozing from the uterus obscuring the operator's view. The tape of the tampon should be secured to the draped towels with a pair of forceps, so that it is removed following the procedure. On no account should loose cotton wool or gauze be used.
  - Absorbable suture material is recommended, such as polyglactin 910 (Vicryl) or Vicryl Rapide, dependent on local provision.

Vaginal epithelial layer   Muscle layer

Perineal skin

On completion

**Fig. 18.1** Repairing an episiotomy. (A) Continuous suture to the vaginal wall.
(B) Continuous suturing of the muscle layer until the skin is closer together.
(C) A continuous subcuticular suture should be used to bring the skin together.
(D) The vagina and introitus should admit two fingers. A rectal examination should
be performed to exclude sutures.

- Vaginal epithelial layer (Fig. 18.1A):
  - Visualize firstly how the tear will sit together once sutured; this can be done by gently moving the correct opposing edges back together
  - Locate the apex of the tear in the vagina; then secure the first stitch just above. Do not go too deep as the rectum is in close proximity. Proceed using a loose continuous non-locking stitch in order to achieve haemostasis and reduce any dead space, thus helping to prevent haematoma formation. The continuous suturing technique when compared to interrupted sutures is associated with less short-term pain.[19]
- Muscle layer (Fig. 18.1B):
  - Identify the torn edges of the muscles and feel with the fingertips to judge the depth of suturing required
  - Continuous suturing of the muscle layer until the skin is closer together
  - Avoid suturing the fourchette itself as this can develop into a scar which can later cause discomfort during intercourse.

- Perineal skin (Fig. 18.1C):
  - The perineal skin edges should be almost together at this stage; if the skin is well opposed after the muscle layer has been sutured, the skin may be left unsutured[17]
  - If the skin does require bringing together, a continuous subcuticular suture should be used.
- On completion (Fig. 18.1D):
  - The tampon should be removed and the vagina inspected to ensure there are no bleeding points. The vagina and introitus should admit two fingers.
- Cleanse and dry the perineal area.
- With informed consent, a rectal examination should be performed to exclude the presence of sutures. If sutures are found, medical aid should be sought as the sutures will need to be removed and resuturing performed as soon as possible.
- Offer the woman a rectal non-steroidal anti-inflammatory drug routinely after perineal repair of a first- or second-degree repair, unless contraindicated.[17]
- Place a sanitary towel over the area; remove the drapes and assist the woman into a more comfortable position.
- Make sure that all needles and swabs are accounted for with the same person who checked them initially, then document the finding.
- Explain to the woman that the sutures will dissolve and not require removal.
- Give her information on the extent of the trauma, pain relief, diet, and hygiene and discuss the importance of pelvic floor exercise.[20]
- Record an accurate detailed account covering the extent of the trauma, the method of repair, and the material used. It is also good practice to record this information pictorially.

### References

17 National Institute for Health and Care Excellence (2014). *Intrapartum care for healthy women and babies*. NICE guidelines CG190. Available at: ℘ www.nice.org.uk/guidance/cg190.

18 Saunders J, Campbell R, Peters T (2002). Effectiveness of pain relief during suturing. *BJOG* 109: 1066–8.

19 Kettle C, Hills R, Ismail K (2012). Continuous versus interrupted sutures for repair of episiotomy or second degree tears. *Cochrane Database Syst Rev* Issue 11. Chichester: John Wiley and Sons.

20 Royal College of Midwives (2012). *Evidence based guidelines for midwifery-led care in labour: suturing the perineum*. Available at: ℘ www.rcm.org.uk/sites/default/files/Suturing%20the%20 Perineum.pdf.

# Examining the placenta and membranes

## Appearance of the placenta

## Examination

# Examining the placenta and membranes

### Appearance of full-term placenta

The placenta is approximately 18–20cm in diameter, about 2.5cm thick in the centre, and progressively thinner towards the outer edges. It is round or oval in shape and weighs approximately one-sixth of the weight of the fetus. It has two surfaces—the fetal and the maternal.

The maternal surface is deep red in colour and attached to the uterine decidua; it is indented with deep grooves, or sulci, into 15–20 lobes, known as cotyledons. The fetal surface lies to one side of the fetus and is attached by the umbilical cord. From the insertion of the cord at the placental site, blood vessels radiate to the periphery, forming subdivisions of the blood vessels that burrow into the substance of the placenta. Each cotyledon has its own branch of the umbilical artery and vein. The surface is covered with the amnion.

### Examination

- Examine the placenta and membranes as soon as possible after birth to detect any abnormalities that may have a direct influence on the neonate or provide information about intrapartum events.
- Wear protective clothing and gloves.
- Retain the clots to estimate maternal blood loss.
- Hold the placenta firmly by the cord to check that the membranes are complete—there should be a single hole through which the fetus has passed.
- Separate the amnion from the chorion to ensure that both membranes are present.
- Turn the placenta over, with the fetal surface resting on the hand and with the membranes hanging down. Carefully examine the maternal surface to see whether all the lobes are complete; there should be no spaces or ragged areas.
- Note any areas of infarction on the lobes, recognized as firm, fibrous, whitish patches. 'Gritty' areas may also be seen.
- Check the edge of the placenta for signs of the blood vessels permeating the membranes, which may be indicative of a succenturiate (accessory) lobe (➔ See abnormalities of the placenta and umbilical cord, p. 367.)
- Occasionally one vessel that tracks its way back into the placenta is seen—this is known as an erratic vessel.
- Examine the umbilical cord carefully, noting its insertion into the placenta: the length, the number of vessels, and any abnormalities.
- Usually the cord is inserted centrally into the placenta and is about 50cm long and 2cm thick, covered in a jelly-like substance known as Wharton's jelly. There should be one large umbilical vein and two umbilical arteries. Occasionally only one artery may be detected; this may be indicative of fetal abnormality and the baby should thus be examined thoroughly by a paediatrician.
- Measure blood loss as accurately as possible, including the loss that may have soaked into bed linen and pads.

- Take any blood samples required from the placenta as soon as possible after the birth of the baby, particularly if cord gases are required to determine any fetal distress.
- Record all findings in the maternal notes and inform the appropriate professional if any abnormalities were noted, alongside informing the mother.
- Check before discarding the placenta that a histology report is not required—this is usually requested if the baby was SGA or after an intrauterine death. Check local policy for a list of conditions requiring further investigation.
- Other areas to consider, although rare, may be the parents' wish to perform a stem cell harvest, or to take the placenta home, or keep the placenta after a home delivery. In these instances, refer to local trust guidance.

*Abnormalities of the placenta and umbilical cord*

- *Succenturiate lobe*: a small accessory placenta that has developed away from the main body of the placenta and is attached by blood vessels permeating the membranes. If blood vessels are detected leading to a tear in the membranes at the distal end, this would indicate that the missing cotyledon has been retained in the uterus. Consequently, cautions regarding blood loss and the passage of the products of conception need to be recorded in the woman's notes and explained to the mother. An obstetrician also needs to be informed of these findings.
- *Bipartite placenta*: the placenta is divided into two distinct lobes.
- *Circumvallate placenta*: the chorion, instead of being attached to the edge of the placenta, forms on the fetal surface, some distance from the edge of the placenta.
- *Placenta accreta*: the placenta is abnormally adherent to the uterine muscle surface, either partially or totally. Although extremely rare, there appears to be an increased risk associated with repeated surgical procedures involving the uterus such as myomectomy, Caesarean section, and termination of pregnancy.
- *Infarctions*: these are red, or more commonly white, patches detected on the maternal surface, due to localized death of placental tissue. They may be seen occasionally in most placenta, but when found in substantial amounts they are often associated with pre-eclampsia.
- *Calcification*: small, whitish-grey areas that have a gritty feeling are lime salt deposits. They may be more noticeable in the post-mature placenta.
- The umbilical cord may be either too short (causing delay in delivery) or too long, predisposing to prolapse of the cord. Occasionally it may be excessively thin or thick; in either case, extra vigilance is required when clamping the cord and observing for haemorrhage.
- Knots in the umbilical cord are caused by fetal movements prior to birth, whereby the fetus is able to slip through a loop of cord. These 'true' knots may cause tightening of the cord during labour, depending on the location of the knot along the length of the cord. 'False' knots are formed by the blood vessels being longer than the cord itself, thus doubling back in the Wharton's jelly, or a similar appearance may occur due to the formation of irregularities and nodes.

- The cord may be inserted into the placenta in an irregular manner instead of centrally:
  - *Eccentric insertion*: the cord is attached to one side of the placenta.
  - *Battledore insertion*: the cord is attached to the placental margin.
  - *Velamentous insertion*: the vessels of the cord divide and run through the membranes prior to reaching the placenta. This is particularly dangerous if the vulnerable blood vessels lie over the internal os. This condition is known as *vasa praevia* and is extremely rare, but can be a cause of severe fetal hypoxia or fetal death should one of the blood vessels rupture.

# Immediate care of the newborn

# Apgar score

The Apgar score[1] is a tool for evaluating a baby's condition at birth. The test was designed to help health-care providers assess a newborn's overall physical condition so that they could quickly determine whether the baby needed immediate medical care. It is not intended to predict a baby's long-term health, behaviour, intellectual status, personality, or outcome.

It is calculated at 1 and 5min post-birth; the 1min Apgar score assesses how well the infant tolerated the birthing process. The 5min Apgar score assesses how well the newborn is adapting to the environment. If there are problems with the neonate, an additional score is given at 10min.

The score (Table 19.1) uses five vital signs to indicate the necessity for resuscitation: respiratory effort, heart rate, colour, muscle tone, and response to stimuli. Each sign is given a score of 2, 1, or 0 and then totalled to produce a score out of 10.

## Respiratory effort

Most babies will establish spontaneous regular breathing within 3min of birth, sufficient to maintain the heart rate above 100bpm and to improve the skin colour. If apnoea or gasping persists after drying, intervention is required. Failure of the baby to establish respiration at birth may be due to:

- Airway obstruction due to mucus, blood, liquor, or meconium.
- Analgesics given during labour—pethidine, diamorphine, and general anaesthesia.
- Tentorial tears, which cause pressure on the fetal cerebellum and medulla where the respiratory centre is sited.
- Congenital abnormalities, such as choanal atresia—a congenital disorder where the back of the nasal passage (choana) is blocked by abnormal bony or membranous tissue due to failed recanalization of the nasal fossae during fetal development; hypoplastic lung, diaphragmatic hernia, and anencephaly.
- Prematurity—lack of surfactant, intrauterine hypoxia, and immature respiratory centre and associated muscle structures.
- Severe intrauterine infections such as pneumonia.

Table 19.1 Calculating the Apgar score

| Respiratory effort | Absent/no attempt to breathe (0) | Slow/weak attempts to breathe (1) | Spontaneous breathing/crying (2) |
|---|---|---|---|
| Heart rate | Absent/weak (0) | Slow <100 (1) | >100 (2) |
| Colour | Blue/pale/grey (0) | Body pink/normal for ethnic group, extremities blue (1) | Completely pink/ normal for ethnic group (2) |
| Muscle tone | Limp/pupils dilated (0) | Partial flexion of extremities (1) | Active/good tone (2) |
| Reflex irritability | No response (0) | Grimace (1) | Crying/cough (2) |

## Heart rate

An initial assessment of heart rate is vital because an increase in the heart rate will be the first sign of success during resuscitation. Listening with a stethoscope at the cardiac apex is the best method to assess the heart rate. Palpation of the umbilical pulse can only be relied upon if it is >100bpm. A rate of <100bpm should be checked by auscultation if possible.

## Colour

Skin colouring can vary greatly, depending on the gestation, race or ethnic group, temperature, and whether or not the baby is crying. At birth, the skin may appear dark red to purple colour. As respiration begins, the colour changes to pink/normal for ethnicity. The hands and feet may stay bluish in colour for several days and this is a normal response to the immature blood circulation. Blue colouring of other parts of the body, however, is not normal.

## Muscle tone

Appropriate muscle tone is important because it can affect future motor development. Full-term infants are born with strong muscle tone. They move smoothly and can curl into comfortable, flexed/bent positions on their own. Preterm infants do not have the muscle tone to flex/bend their arms and legs independently; their movements are often 'jerky', and they tend to keep their arms and legs straight or stiff.

## Reflex irritability

Reflex irritability is a term describing the level of newborn irritation in response to stimuli. Reflexes are involuntary movements or actions that help identify normal brain and nerve activity. Some movements are spontaneous, occurring as part of the neonate's usual activity. Others are responses to certain actions.

A score of 10 is uncommon, due to the prevalence of transient cyanosis. A score of 8–10 indicates a baby in good condition; a score of 4–7 represents mild/moderate asphyxia, and modest resuscitative measures are usually all that is required. Transient cyanosis is common. Although initially there may be substantial cyanosis, often babies will recover spontaneously or only require tactile stimulation and light oxygen around the face and mouth via a face mask. Care should be taken not to be overzealous with intervention in this middle group, as this may worsen the situation rather than resolve it. A score of 1–3 represents severe asphyxia, requiring urgent resuscitation. (➔ See Neonatal resuscitation, p. 557.)

## Reference

1 Apgar V (1953). A proposal for a new method of evaluation of the newborn infant. *Curr Res Anesth Analg* 32: 260–7.

# Examination of the newborn

Shortly after birth, examine the baby carefully to check for obvious external abnormalities. It is also established practice for a paediatrician or NIPE (NHS Newborn and Infant Physical Examination Programme)[2]-qualified midwife to carry out a more detailed examination of the baby within 24h of birth.

Perform the examination in the mother's, and if possible father's, presence, after obtaining consent. The examination should be accompanied by a comprehensive explanation of the procedure, the reason for it, and afterwards explaining and recording the findings. This assessment should also be seen as an opportunity for parental education and health promotion.[3] Follow a logical sequence from head to toe. Throughout the examination, the baby should be naked, in warm surroundings with a good light, so that you can clearly see the baby.

## Procedure

- *Wash hands thoroughly* prior to examination to prevent infection.
- *Note any skin blemishes or abrasions*, whether any vernix caseosa (white greasy substance) is present on the skin, or lanugo (fine downy hair) normally only found abundantly in premature babies.
- *Throughout the examination*, observe and note the baby's overall muscle tone, movements, and symmetry.
- *Colour and respirations*: the term baby should be pink with slightly less colour in the hands and feet, which may not pink up for several hours following birth. If one or both nostrils are blocked with mucus, this may result in cyanosis and difficulties with breathing. The term baby should be breathing regularly, with no gasping or chest recession.
- *Head*: note the size, shape, and symmetry. Sometimes the head may be distorted by moulding or trauma caused during birth:
  - *Caput succedaneum*—this a soft, spongy oedema caused by pressure, which is present at birth and usually disappears within 24h
  - *Cephalhaematoma*—this is caused by trauma and tends to appear and to get larger following birth. Occasionally there may be a double haematoma on either side of the head. This may take 4–6 weeks to resolve; no treatment is necessary
  - Examine the formation, width, and tension of the sutures and fontanelles on the skull. A wide anterior fontanelle may be indicative of hydrocephalus or immaturity. An extra fontanelle between the anterior and posterior fontanelles may indicate Down's syndrome.
- Check the face and neck for the following:
  - *Eyes*: symmetry, that both eyeballs are present with a clear lens. Oedema or bruising that may have occurred during birth and haemorrhage under the conjunctiva can look alarming but disappear quickly and are not significant. The spacing between the eyes is usually up to 3cm. The presence of wide, slanting epicanthic folds and white spots on the iris may be associated with Down's syndrome
  - *Ears*: symmetry. Low-set ears may be associated with various syndromes. Accessory skin tags in front of the ears may be present and should be noted

- *Mouth*: the mouth should be opened and the palate inspected with a finger. The hard palate should be arched and intact, and the uvula in a central position. At the junction of the hard and soft palate, there may be small white spots known as Epstein's pearls. Occasionally teeth may be present, which are usually loose; normally these are extracted to prevent inhalation. Tongue-tie may be observed where the frenulum seems to anchor the tongue to the floor of the mouth. This rarely causes major problems, but may cause difficulties with latching onto the breast for feeding
- *Capillary naevi*: small, pink marks may be observed on the upper eyelids, midline of the forehead, the upper lip, and the nape of the neck. These are common and fade over a period of months. Capillary naevi found elsewhere may be extensive (such as port-wine stain)
- *Neck*: observation and inspection of the neck area is important to exclude webbing, a short neck, a large fold of skin at the back of the neck, and any swellings.
- **Chest**: observe breathing and symmetry of the chest wall, spacing and positioning of the nipples and any accessory nipples present.
- **Abdomen**: the shape of the abdomen should be rounded; any obvious variations should be noted such as a scaphoid or boat-shaped abdomen or swelling. The state of the cord should be observed, ensuring that it is securely clamped. The cord should have three vessels and there should be no swelling or protrusions at the base. Absence of a vessel should be brought to the paediatrician's notice immediately, as this may indicate cardiac or renal abnormalities.
- **Limbs and digits**: count carefully and open the hands fully to expose any accessory digits, webbing, or trauma. The axillae, elbows, groins, and popliteal spaces also need to be inspected. The limbs should be inspected for equal length and observed for normal movement. The feet and ankles should be inspected for talipes equinovarus (the foot, or feet, point in and down rather than in the usual position).
- **External genitalia**: in boys, observe the position of the urethral orifice; both testes should be situated in the scrotum. The foreskin should not be retracted as this is still adherent to the glans. Any obvious swelling in the inguinal area should be noted. In girls, gently inspect the labia—the urethral and vaginal orifices should be evident and a thick, white discharge may be present. Refer any discrepancy about the sex of the baby to the paediatrician promptly.
- **Back and spine**: turning the baby over into the prone position, palpate and observe the back for any unevenness, swellings, dimples, or hairy patches that may be associated with an occult spinal abnormality. A baby from Asian or African ancestry may have a bruised appearance over the sacral area; this is normal and is referred to as the Mongolian blue spot. The presence and position of the anus can be observed. It is also important to record in the notes whether the baby passes meconium at birth or shortly after, to confirm patency of the anus.
- **Hips**: the Ortolani or Barlow's test, or possibly a modification of the two, is performed routinely to check for dysplasia of the hips. Depending on local policy, this will be carried out by the midwife or the

paediatrician. Reference to local guidelines and any additional training required should be done prior to undertaking this procedure. If the paediatrician performs the test within the first day of birth, there is no reason to do it at the initial examination.

- *Measurements*: the head circumference and length may be recorded. However, different units may have differing policies. Unless calibrated equipment is available, measuring the crown-to-heel length is grossly inaccurate. If a calibrated device is used, it is essential that the baby's legs are fully extended; this may require two people to assist to ensure accuracy. Measurement of the head circumference may be deferred to the third day, by which time any swelling will have subsided. A measuring tape is used to encircle the head at the occipital protuberance and the supraorbital ridges.
- *Record the baby's temperature.*

Record findings in the baby's notes. Communicate any abnormalities to the paediatrician or GP, and pass the information on to the midwife taking over the mother's care on the postnatal ward. Inform the parents if a paediatrician needs to be notified and give the reasons why.

## References

2 Public Health England (2013). *Newborn and infant physical examination screening: programme overview*. Available at: ℘ www.gov.uk/newborn-and-infant-physical-examination-screening-programme-overview.
3 Royal College of Midwives (2012). *Evidence based guidelines for midwifery-led care in labour: immediate care of the newborn*. Available at: ℘ www.rcm.org.uk/sites/default/files/Immediate%20Care%20%20of%20the%20Newborn.pdf.

# Immediate care of the newborn

The midwife should be familiar with the transitional requirements of adaptation to external uterine life, so that she can make appropriate preparations for the newborn's arrival.

- The birthing room, whether at home or hospital, should be warm, ideally 21–25°C. Switch off fans and draw curtains to reduce heat loss within the environment.
- As the baby's head is born, wipe excess mucus from his/her mouth.
- Touching the nasal nares (nostrils) may stimulate reflex inhalation of mucus and debris into the trachea and is not recommended.
- Following the birth of the trunk, lift the baby on to the mother's abdomen or chest, unless this has been declined by the mother.
- Most babies will start to breathe and maintain a clear airway without intervention.
- Routine suction is not recommended. When suction is required, use a mucus extractor or a soft suction catheter. It is important to aspirate the oropharynx first before aspirating the nasopharynx, to prevent mucus from being drawn down the trachea when the baby gasps due to suction stimulation of the nasal passages.
- Cut the cord approximately 2–8cm from the baby's umbilicus, between two cord clamps (➔ see p. 353). Once the cord is clamped securely to prevent blood loss, cut the cord between the two clamps. Placing a gauze swab over the cord whilst cutting it will prevent blood spray over the delivery area.

Identification of the newborn is important if the baby is born within a maternity unit; however, a home birth does not require labelling, unless the baby is a twin. Individual units will have their own policy on this; however, basic principles apply:

- Apply name bands immediately following birth; in some units, this may be before the cord is cut
- Usually two bands are applied—most commonly to both ankles
- Write the name bands legibly, clearly identifying the family surname, the time and date of birth, and the baby's gender. If gender is in any doubt, explain to the parents that you need to seek further help on this matter
- The mother or father should confirm that the information is correct before applying the name bands
- Ensure that both bands are not too tight nor too loose, but fixed securely and not causing trauma to the baby's skin
- Check the bands daily and replace them if they become loose or fall off whilst the baby is in the hospital.

Preventing heat loss in the time immediately following birth is crucial. The baby has an immature heat regulatory system; therefore, provide a warm environment, as above.

- Reduce heat loss by drying the baby at delivery. Wet towels need to be replaced with warm, pre-heated towels to prevent further heat loss.
- Skin-to-skin contact with the mother helps to reduce heat loss if the remaining exposed skin of the baby is covered.
- Cover the baby's head, as substantial heat is lost through the head.

- Loose clothing and comfortable swaddling with blankets will help to conserve body heat.
- Some units may be provided with overhead heaters in the labour rooms. Care with overheating should be acknowledged. Hot water bottles used to pre-warm the cot at a home birth should be used with caution.
- Routine bathing of the baby following birth is not to be advised, unless the baby is overly soiled from the birth process or there is risk of contamination. This will not only help to maintain the neonate's temperature, but also the microbiome, an ecosystem of symbiotic microorganisms that lives on the skin and has the potential to dramatically influence lifelong health.[4] Successful microbiome acquisition at birth is a recognized determinant of early immune programming, subsequent infection, and allergy risk. It has also been associated with obesity, cancer, mental health disorders, asthma, and autism.[4]
- Observe the baby regularly for colour and skin temperature, to ensure that hypothermia is not present. Record the body temperature following birth.

The baby may require a dose of vitamin K, given as prophylaxis against bleeding disorders. This should have been discussed thoroughly with the woman prior to birth, so that she could make an informed choice regarding the risks/benefits. Depending on local policy, this may be given orally or by intramuscular injection.

The period immediately following birth should allow some time for the parents and the baby to communicate and develop the important relationship and rapport necessary for the baby's well-being. Very often the baby is very alert following birth (unless drugs used in labour have blurred this response), resulting in an active three-way process of communication between the mother, father, and baby.

## Reference

4 Madan JC, Farzan SF, Hibberd PL, Karagas MR (2012). Normal neonatal microbiome variation in relation to environmental factors, infection and allergy. Curr Opin Pediatr 24: 753–9.

## Breast crawl and skin-to-skin

Breast crawl or baby crawl are the terms used when a newborn baby is placed on the mother's abdomen immediately after birth and demonstrates their ability to find the mother's breast and initiate the first breastfeed unaided.[5] The newborn infant has instinctive or inborn abilities, including sensory, central, motor, and neuroendocrine components, which both directly or indirectly help the baby's movement and facilitate its ability to find the maternal breast unaided. Breast crawl is examined in more detail in ➔ The infant's contribution to breastfeeding, p. 784.

Although skin-to-skin is a major element that will assist baby crawl to be initiated, all mothers should be encouraged to hold their naked baby against their skin in a calm and unhurried environment immediately following birth, regardless of their feeding intention. Mothers should be given the opportunity prior to birth to discuss how this can be acceptably achieved. Cultural influences need to be considered within this discussion, as they may make implementation of skin-to-skin unacceptable.

Newborn babies find their mother's breast partly by smell, and this instinctive process can be interfered with by clothing, wrapping in hospital towels, and separation; therefore, these should be avoided whenever possible (➔ see Management of breastfeeding, p. 776).

### Benefits of skin-to-skin contact

- Babies gradually become more active, begin to root, and are at least three times more likely to suckle successfully.
- Babies demonstrate less distressed behaviour and cry less than those separated from their mothers, e.g. during suturing.
- Increased nurturing behaviour has been seen in mothers whose babies have touched their nipples and areolae within the first half hour of birth. Mothers planning to bottle-feed could still enjoy and benefit from this instinctive interaction.
- The likelihood of PPH could be reduced as early contact and suckling stimulate the uterus to contract.
- Babies are much more likely to be breastfed for longer when uninterrupted skin-to-skin contact has occurred at birth.
- Mothers will feel higher levels of satisfaction with motherhood and have more positive feelings overall if they have been able to enjoy the first hour after birth without interruption.

### Physiological effects on the baby

- Skin-to-skin contact is an effective measure against hypothermia and hypoglycaemia.
- The blood chemistry of babies who have been acidotic or had a period of 'fetal distress' rectifies itself more quickly when skin-to-skin contact has occurred.
- Skin-to-skin contact is particularly important for babies who have had a traumatic birth, who required resuscitation, and who need to be warmed. It should be initiated as soon as possible.

Routine care practices which interfere with this process should be reconsidered and abandoned unless proven to be of benefit to the infant or mother in the circumstances in which they are initiated.

❶ Hospital routine should not take priority over the needs of the mother and child.

## Reference

5  The Mother and Child Health and Education Trust (2016). *Breast crawl*. Available at: ⅍ www.breastcrawl.org/science.shtml.

# Complicated labour

# Management of malpositions and malpresentations

# Occipito-posterior position

This is a cephalic presentation where the occiput is directed towards the right or left sacro-iliac joint—right occipito-posterior (ROP) and left occipito-posterior (LOP). These positions are the most common of all causes of mechanical difficulty and non-engagement of the fetal head at term for the primigravida. The occipito-posterior position is thought to occur in approximately 10–34% of all labours in the first stage, but only 5–8% will persist to the second stage of labour and birth.[1]

## Causes
- Occasionally linked to an abnormal shape of the maternal pelvis.
- Maternal posture and lack of physical activity during pregnancy.
- Deficient flexion of the fetal head and spine.
- Anteriorly placed placenta (diagnosed by ultrasound).

## Diagnosis
*Abdominal examination*
- On inspection, the maternal abdomen is flattened below the level of the umbilicus.
- On palpation of the abdomen, the fetal head is high and deflexed; limbs are felt on both sides of the midline. The fetal back may be felt with difficulty laterally or may not be palpable.
- On auscultation of the fetal heart, sounds are audible in the flank and over the fetal back; they are also easily heard in the midline because of the proximity of the fetal chest to the maternal abdominal wall.

*Vaginal examination*
- The degree of flexion of the fetal head can be assessed during labour.
- The anterior fontanelle lies centrally or anteriorly.
- The fetal posterior fontanelle may be out of reach.
- Caput and moulding of the fetal head are common.
- When the fetal head is deflexed, the occipito-frontal diameter of 11.5cm presents.
- The presenting part is poorly applied to the cervix.
- The cervix may become oedematous as labour progresses.

*Maternal clinical features during labour*
- Continuous backache.
- Slow progress.
- Irregularly spaced contractions which tend to couple together.
- Early spontaneous rupture of the membranes.
- Increased rectal pressure towards the end of the first stage of labour, resulting in an urge to push prior to full dilatation of the os uteri.

*Fetal clinical features during labour*
- More frequent incidence of non-reassuring FHR patterns in labour.
- Slow descent of the fetal head.
- The fetal head does not engage or descend easily, with a risk of the following consequences.

## Consequences
- Prolonged labour.
- Delay in the second stage of labour.
- Greater risk of instrumental birth.
- Difficult or traumatic birth.
- Increased risk of maternal infection.
- Possible fetal hypoxia.
- Intracranial haemorrhage.

## Outcomes

*Long rotation of the occiput*
- In two-thirds of cases, following engagement the fetal head flexes.
- When the occiput meets the resistance of the pelvic floor, it makes a long rotation forwards through three-eighths of a circle.
- The fetus is then born in the occipito-anterior position.

*Deflexed head*
In one-third of cases, flexion of the head remains deficient and the mechanism of internal rotation is affected by the following:
- *Deep transverse arrest*: an attempt at long rotation fails, the head being arrested with its long diameter between the ischial spines. Instrumental rotation with forceps or ventouse is required to complete the birth. Alternatively an LSCS may be performed
- *Persistent occipito-posterior*: the sinciput lying lower than the occiput is rotated one-eighth of a circle towards the symphysis pubis and the occiput turns to the hollow of the maternal sacrum. Delay in the second stage of labour occurs, but with good contractions, the fetal head advances; the root of the nose escapes under the pubic arch and the head is born in the face-to-pubes position. When contractions are less effective, no advance occurs and instrumental birth is required.

## Midwifery care and management
- The first stage is long and tedious, and often accompanied by severe backache. If available, consider water for injection as a non-pharmaceutical method of pain relief; this can be particularly effective in back pain.
- Mobility and an upright position encourage rotation and descent.
- An all-fours position or a squatting position may assist rotation of the head.
- The squatting position may increase the sagittal diameter of the pelvic outlet, which may aid birth.
- Maternal comfort, hydration, and prevention of infection are important.
- The woman should be encouraged to empty her bladder regularly, as a full bladder may add to discomfort and delay progress.
- Once delay and fetal and/or maternal distress are recognized, the midwife should act promptly.
- Pain relief requirements may be increased.
- Consider the use of epidural analgesia carefully, as its effects may contribute to poor flexion of the fetus, lack of descent, and failure of the rotational mechanism. However, if an instrumental birth is anticipated, then epidural analgesia is the preferred method of pain relief.

- The second stage of labour is characterized by considerable dilation of the anus, whilst the fetal head may not be visible.
- Perineal trauma is common. Look for signs of central rupture.
- Occasionally an episiotomy may be needed to expedite the birth.
- Avoid language which may demoralize the woman, e.g. 'failure to progress'.
- Give continuous explanation, empathy, and support.

**Reference**

1 Guittier M, Othenin-Girard V, Boulvain M (2014). Maternal positioning to correct occipito-posterior in labour: a randomised controlled trail. *BMC Pregnancy Childbirth* 14: 83.

# Face presentation

# Face presentation

When the attitude of the fetal head is one of complete extension, the occiput of the fetus will be in contact with its spine and the face will present. The incidence of a face presentation in labour is approximately 0.14%;[2] most cases develop in labour from occipito-posterior positions (secondary face presentation). Rarely, face presentation is apparent before labour and may be associated with congenital abnormality (primary face presentation).

## Causes
- The uterus is tilted sideways (anterior obliquity).
- Contracted pelvis.
- Tight or entangled cord.
- Polyhydramnios.
- Congenital abnormality (e.g. anencephaly).
- Multiple pregnancy.

## Diagnosis
- Antenatal diagnosis is unlikely as the presentation usually develops in labour.
- On palpation: if the mentum is anterior, the presentation may not be detected. If the mentum is posterior, a deep groove may be felt between the occiput and the fetal back.
- On vaginal examination:
  - The presenting part is high and irregular
  - The orbital ridges, eyes, nose, and mouth of the fetus are palpable
  - There may be confusion between the mouth and anus; differential signs are: open, hard gums, ridged palate, and the fetus may suck the examining finger
  - To determine the position, the mentum is located
  - Vaginal examinations should be undertaken with care so as not to injure or infect the eyes.

## Course and outcomes of labour
- Prolonged labour.
- With a mentoanterior position: spontaneous birth is possible.
- With a mentoposterior position: following rotation of the mentum to the anterior, a spontaneous birth is possible.
- Persistent mentoposterior: the mentum is in the hollow of the sacrum, so no further mechanism takes place. Instrumental assisted birth or LSCS is the outcome.

## Management of labour and birth
- Labour is often prolonged; the presenting part is ill-fitting, so there is slow progress.
- Maternal comfort and support are important.
- Communication and empathy are vital as the mother may become discouraged and anxious about her abilities.
- Prior to birth, explain the risk of possible facial bruising to the face of the newborn to the parents.

- Recognize delay or complications at an early stage.
- The use of a scalp electrode should be avoided.
- The use of IV oxytocin should be avoided.
- Birth may be facilitated by supporting the extended fetal position and applying gentle pressure on the sinciput until the mentum escapes.
- An episiotomy may be indicated, before the occiput sweeps the perineum.

## Complications

*Mother*
- Obstructed labour, as the face is resistant to moulding.
- Early rupture of the membranes.
- Cord prolapse.
- Perineal lacerations and perineal trauma.

*Neonatal*
- Facial bruising and oedema.
- Cerebral haemorrhage.

## Reference

2 Tapisiz O, Aytan H, Kiykac S, et al. (2014). Face presentation at term: a forgotten issue. *J Obstet Gynaecol Res* 40: 1573–7.

# Brow presentation

When the attitude of the fetal head is one of partial extension, the frontal bone presents. Brow presentation is less common than face presentation, occurring once in approximately 650–700 births, and is usually diagnosed in the second stage of labour.[3] The causes are the same as those for face presentation.

### Diagnosis

- On abdominal palpation, the presenting part of the fetus is high and appears unduly large. A groove may be felt between the occiput and the back.
- On vaginal examination, there may be difficulty in reaching the presenting part.
- If the brow is detected, the anterior fontanelle may be felt to one side, with the orbital ridges or root of the nose felt on the other side.
- The presenting diameter is the mentovertical—13.5cm.

### Management

- The midwife should call the obstetrician.
- Vaginal birth is rare.
- Usually an LSCS is undertaken for obstructed labour.
- Occasionally the brow presentation may convert to a face presentation.
- Complications for the mother and fetus/neonate are similar to those of face presentation.

### Reference

3 Verspyck E, Bisson V, Gromez A, Resch B, Diguet A, Marpeau L (2012). Prophylactic attempt at manual rotation in brow presentation at full dilatation. *Acta Obstet Gynecol Scand* 91: 1342–5.

# Shoulder presentation

A non-longitudinal lie of the fetus may be transverse or oblique; both can result in a shoulder presentation if not corrected. A large retrospective study undertaken in Finland found that a transverse lie occurred in around 0.12% of births and all of these babies were born via a Caesarean section.[4]

## Causes

- Laxity of uterine and abdominal muscles.
- Placenta praevia.
- Multiple pregnancy.
- Polyhydramnios.
- Uterine abnormality.
- Contracted pelvis.
- Uterine fibroid.

## Diagnosis

- A transverse lie is usually detected in pregnancy by the appearance of the shape of the woman's abdomen—there is a bulge on each side of the abdomen and the fundus appears very low.
- On palpation, the fetal head and the breech lie in opposite iliac fossae.
- There is no presenting part descending into the maternal pelvis.
- Ultrasound may be used to confirm the presentation and detect any fetal abnormality.

## Management

- External version may be attempted, followed by induction of labour if successful.
- The labour should be closely monitored by EFM and diligent observation of the maternal condition.
- Provided normal progress in labour continues, the membranes may be ruptured once the fetal head enters the pelvis.
- When the midwife detects a shoulder presentation by abdominal palpation, it should be reported immediately to a doctor.
- A vaginal examination is undertaken (if placenta praevia has been previously excluded). If rupture of membranes occurs, quickly ensure that the cord has not prolapsed.
- LSCS may be the mode of birth if the lie is persistently oblique or transverse, if there are any complications, or if there is a poor obstetric history.
- In the case of a second twin in the transverse position, the lie of the fetus is corrected immediately by external version, whilst rupturing the membranes to hasten the birth and maintain the longitudinal lie.

## Reference

4 Gardberg M, Leonova Y, Laakkonen E (2011). Malpresentations—impact on mode of delivery. *Acta Obstet Gynecol Scand* 90: 540–2.

# High-risk labour

# Principles of care for high-risk labour

### Definition

A 'high-risk' pregnancy is one in which the mother, fetus, or newborn is, or will be, at an increased risk of morbidity or mortality before, during, or after delivery. The midwife is increasingly relied upon to care for women who will fall into a high-risk category. With the medicalization of the childbirth process combined with defensive practices and maternal high-risk lifestyle choices, all these factors impact on the number of pregnancies and births requiring a higher degree of surveillance. Due to this increase, it is important that the midwife possesses the appropriate level of skill and knowledge to manage the woman's care effectively and escalate concerns appropriately and in a timely manner.

The role of the midwife when reviewing the management plan of a woman's care should always look at the following criteria:

- Previous medical conditions, including an anaesthetics and psychiatric history
- Factors from previous pregnancies
- Mental health factors
- Social factors, including safeguarding and lifestyle history
- Missed antenatal appointments
- Identification of women who refuse blood and blood products
- Assessment of an appropriate place to give birth
- Thromboembolic disease—risk assessment
- Review any new anomalies of her pregnancy or birth which have previously not been apparent and act according to local guidance.

If a new risk has been identified at any time, the midwife should be aware of the local guidance of how to transfer care from midwifery-led to consultant-led. This will allow for a medical review and an appropriate management plan to be made and documented within all records. It may also be a time when the woman will need referral to the multidisciplinary team, e.g. social services, physiotherapy, or substance misuse specialist. This again must be clearly documented in all records with emphasis on discussions around information given and consent gained noted clearly.

Ensure that all patients defined as high risk:

- Are treated sensitively, recognizing that women experiencing complications in labour may be extremely stressed and anxious or have a different interpretation of their pregnancy than the clinically defined view. Give these patients:
  - Full, unbiased explanations
  - The chance to ask questions
  - Adequate support
  - Freedom to make choices in care (support from an SoM may be offered if the woman chooses to follow a care pathway which is not in line with local guidance).

- Are seen by an appropriate professional as soon as they attend the hospital or as the complication arises.
- Have a birth plan, devised in the antenatal clinic in consultation with a senior doctor, documented in the case notes. Review the notes to find plans for labour and delivery. Discuss the plan with the woman to ensure that it is up-to-date.
- Are monitored continuously for electronic FHR in labour (unless defined as high risk due to a previous postnatal complication, e.g. third-degree tear). Some instances of referral for high-risk care may require the midwife to inform the hospital clinical risk manager.
- Have the opportunity to be referred to a debriefing session with an SoM or a birth afterthoughts clinic if the pregnancy or birth included any traumatic outcomes.

# Trial of labour for vaginal birth after a Caesarean (or other uterine scar)

A planned vaginal birth after a previous Caesarean (VBAC) is appropriate for, and may be offered to, the majority of women with a singleton pregnancy of cephalic presentation at 37+0 weeks or beyond who have had a single previous lower segment Caesarean delivery, with or without a history of previous vaginal birth. Contraindications to this choice may be that the woman has a previous classical incision on her uterus or has previously suffered from a uterine rupture.[1]

A woman may request VBAC because:
- She wishes to avoid the stress of abdominal surgery and a longer hospital stay and recovery
- Vaginal deliveries have less risk of infection or haemorrhage
- She would like a satisfying experience of birth.

It is the responsibility of the obstetrician to ensure that a plan for delivery is made antenatally and that this is clearly documented within the woman's notes. It is now considered good practice for all units to have a VBAC checklist within their records as this demonstrates that information has been given and discussed in order to gain consent within the antenatal period.[1]

However, the midwife should be aware of the risks and benefits of VBAC so that she/he can support the family in their choice of care.
- The success rate of planned VBAC is 72–75%.[1]
- Women with one or more previous vaginal births should be aware that previous vaginal delivery, particularly previous VBAC, is the single best predictor of successful VBAC and is associated with a planned VBAC success rate of 85–90%. Previous vaginal delivery is also independently associated with a reduced risk of uterine rupture.[1]
- Women should be informed that by choosing an elective Caesarean section, there is a small increased risk of placenta praevia and/or accreta in future pregnancies and of pelvic adhesions complicating any future abdominopelvic surgery.[1]
- If the woman's labour requires inducing or augmentation compared with spontaneous VBAC labour, this has a 2- to 3-fold increased risk of uterine rupture and around 1.5-fold increased risk of a Caesarean delivery.[2]
- The risk of perinatal death with a repeat planned Caesarean section is extremely low, but there is a small increase in neonatal respiratory morbidity when performed before 39+0 weeks of gestation. The risk of respiratory morbidity can be reduced with a preoperative course of antenatal corticosteroids.[1]

Because of these risks, precautions are recommended for a VBAC:
- Admission to a regional unit with access to emergency Caesarean and blood transfusion should this be required
- Continuous EFM during labour
- Careful use of prostaglandins for induction.

A woman has the right to choose a home birth or water birth after a Caesarean section and needs accurate information to make a choice appropriate for her needs. Controversially the woman also has the right to choose a planned Caesarean.[2] In instances where the mother deviates from traditional guidance during the antenatal period, arrangements should be made to meet an SoM, or a referral to a birth afterthoughts session should be offered—discussion, planning, and documentation are paramount during any meetings.[3]

## Care in labour

When admitting a woman anticipating VBAC to the delivery suite:

- Recognize the psychological distress that may have been caused by a previous long labour and an emergency Caesarean. Give clear explanations and positive support, and discuss in detail the plans for the birth.
- Admit as for 'high-risk' care:
  - Inform the senior obstetrician of the woman's arrival
  - Have a management plan documented in the hospital notes
  - Be aware of signs of uterine rupture
  - Obtain consent from the woman to monitor the fetal heart continuously in established labour, ensuring the woman's comfort and being flexible about maternal position
  - Review for any CTG abnormalities and document this review at least every hour within the partogram.[4]
- Site IV access; take and dispatch blood samples from the mother for group and save (G&S) and FBC.
- Monitor maternal observations and record within the partogram as per local guidelines.
- Women should be informed that eating during labour results in larger gastric volumes; the effect on the risk of aspiration if anaesthesia is required is uncertain.[2] However, isotonic drinks during labour can prevent ketosis without the associated risks of an increased gastric volume.[2]
- Support the woman in her choice of pain relief. Epidural anaesthesia is recommended by some obstetricians in the event of a Caesarean being required, but it could mask severe pain or may have side effects that could make vaginal birth less likely.
- Give antacids regularly if prescribed (usually oral ranitidine 150mg every 6h). These encourage reduced acidity and improved emptying of stomach contents, which may reduce risks to the mother if a Caesarean is required.
- Discuss any augmentation with the obstetrician. Oxytocin and ARM may be indicated when the progress of labour appears slow. Monitor carefully the strength, frequency, and length of the uterine contractions so that hyperstimulation may be avoided.
- Support the woman during the second and third stages of labour according to her birth plan.
- Be aware that a rare complication of pregnancy following a Caesarean is placenta accreta.
- Keep the obstetrician informed of progress throughout; document key decisions and care given.

## References

1 National Institute for Health and Care Excellence (2011). Chapter 1: guidance. In: National Institute for Health and Care Excellence. *Caesarean section*. NICE guidelines CG132. Available at: ℘ www.nice.org.uk/guidance/cg132/chapter/1-recommendations.

2 Royal College of Obstetricians and Gynaecologists (2015). *Birth after previous Caesarean birth*. Green-top guideline No. 45. Available at: ℘ www.rcog.org.uk/globalassets/documents/guidelines/gtg_45.pdf.

3 Maternity Guideline Group (2014). *Guideline for vaginal birth after LSCS or other uterine scar*. Barnsley Hospital NHS Foundation Trust Maternity Guidelines.

4 National Institute for Health and Care Excellence (2014). Monitoring during labour. In: National Institute for Health and Care Excellence. *Intrapartum care for healthy women and babies*. NICE guidelines CG190. Available at: ℘ www.nice.org.uk/guidance/cg190/chapter/1-recommendations#monitoring-during-labour.

## Obstructed labour

### Causes

### Prevention

### Signs of obstructed labour

# Obstructed labour

If progress in labour is limited in the first stage (i.e. no increase in cervical dilatation in 3–4h), consider the following:
- The woman is not in established labour—proceed as for normal labour.
- Labour may be prolonged by psychological stress; support is paramount.
- The uterine contractions are not effective after being in established labour—the woman may benefit from oxytocin augmentation. Never arrange to use oxytocin to augment labour without gaining the consent of the woman and a detailed review and management plan from the obstetric registrar.
- The labour is obstructed—there is no advance of the presenting part in the presence of strong contractions.

## Causes
- Obstruction at the pelvic brim may be apparent if the fetus is large in relation to maternal size. Contracted pelvis or previous pelvic injury could be a factor.
- Obstruction at the outlet may occur, e.g. when a deep transverse arrest complicates the second stage. A fetus in the occipito-posterior position may occasionally be unable to rotate and becomes wedged at the level of the ischial spines.
- Obstruction may occasionally occur as a result of:
  - Fetal abnormalities, e.g. the hydrocephalic fetus
  - Fetal malposition
  - Fetal malpresentation—shoulder or brow presentation
  - Persistent mentoposterior position
  - Rarely, locked twins
  - Rarely, fibroids or tumour.

## Prevention
- Refer to the senior obstetrician:
  - All women with suspected malpresentation
  - Some units require referral of primigravidae with non-engagement of the fetal head at term.
- Be alert to a history of previous prolonged labour or difficult delivery.
- Monitor labour carefully to detect a slow/no descent of the presenting head.

## Signs of obstructed labour
In the first stage:
- On abdominal palpation, assess for failure of the presenting part to engage
- The cervix dilates slowly
- The presenting part remains loosely applied to the cervix
- The forewaters may rupture early or form a loose bag before the presenting part.

In later first or second stage (late signs of obstruction):
- Maternal pyrexia and rapid pulse
- Maternal pain and anxiety
- Dehydration and poor urine output, ketotic, sometimes bloodstained urine
- Non-reassuring fetal heart recording
- Tonic contractions
- Rarely the retraction ring may be seen abdominally and marks the junction between the upper and stretched lower segments (Bandl's ring)
- On vaginal examination, the vagina feels hot and dry; the presenting part is high, and caput succedaneum and/or moulding are present on the fetal skull.

## Management
- Help to relieve anxiety by giving information and explanation.
- The obstetric registrar must be contacted if:
  - There is no progress in the first stage of labour despite the administration of IV oxytocin
  - There is no progress in descent in the second stage of labour.
- Take FBC and G&S in case of need at delivery.
- An IV infusion will correct dehydration and prepare for operative delivery.
- When the woman is pyrexial (temperature 38°C), the obstetrician will request blood cultures and antibiotic therapy.
- Under instruction from the registrar, prepare the woman for an emergency Caesarean section.
- The woman may be transferred to the obstetric theatre for trial of instrumental delivery. If this is unsuccessful, a Caesarean section can be performed immediately.
- Ensure that neonatal resuscitation facilities and personnel are available at delivery.

## Complications
### Maternal
- Infection.
- Trauma to the bladder due to pressure from the fetal head, or bruising during forceps delivery.
- Severe neglect may cause rupture of the uterus, haemorrhage, morbidity, and mortality.

### Fetal
- Asphyxia.
- Trauma at delivery.
- Infection.
- Meconium aspiration.

All of the above may lead to morbidity, stillbirth, and neonatal death.

# Delivery care for twins and other multiple births

Multiple pregnancy is linked to higher risks for the mother and babies. Women with multiple pregnancies have an increased risk of miscarriage, anaemia, hypertensive disorders, haemorrhage, operative delivery, and postnatal illness. As a guide to inform mothers of the risks, it is suggested that maternal mortality associated with multiple births is 2.5 times that for singleton births.[5]

This is especially true of monochorionic twins, due to:
• Unequal growth
• Polyhydramnios
• Fetal abnormalities
• Intrauterine death of one or both twins
• Spontaneous abortion
• Pre-eclampsia (women with multiple pregnancy and additional risks of developing gestational hypertension will be advised to take 75mg of aspirin from 12 weeks of pregnancy)
• Preterm labour.

A monochorionic twin pregnancy is one in which both babies are dependent on a single, shared placenta. Around one-third of twin pregnancies in the UK have monochorionic placentas.[6] Chorionicity is usually determined using the number of placental masses, the lambda or T sign, and the membrane thickness. If there is difficulty in determining the chorionicity, the pregnancy should be managed as monochorionic until proven otherwise.[7]
• There is a higher risk of complications during labour, due to:
  • Malpresentation of either twin
  • Fetal asphyxia
  • PPH
  • Dysfunctional labour due to the over-distension of the uterus.
• As a result, the following interventions may be necessary:
  • Intrauterine manipulation
  • Episiotomy and instrumental delivery
  • Caesarean section for one or both twins.

Factors affecting the mode of delivery, making a Caesarean section more appropriate, are:
• If there is only one amniotic sac
• For multiple births (triplets and more).

A plan for delivery will be made antenatally in discussion with the parents and obstetric consultant.

## Management of labour
• The timing of the birth in uncomplicated monochorionic twin pregnancies is generally planned for after 36 weeks after a course of corticosteroids. Dichorionic twin pregnancies plan an elective birth from 37 weeks.[5]
• When the first twin is cephalic and no other complications are present, expect to deliver the babies vaginally.

- If a vaginal delivery is anticipated, encourage the woman to telephone and attend the delivery suite as soon as possible after the onset of labour, especially if she is multiparous, since labour may progress rapidly.
- On admission, inform the senior obstetrician.
- Consider the progress of the pregnancy; review the hospital records and assess maternal BP, urinalysis, pulse, and temperature, ensuring general maternal well-being. Obtain IV access and send blood samples to the laboratory for FBC and G&S.
- Confirm the growth and presentation of the fetuses by abdominal palpation and ultrasound scan.
- If the woman is in early labour and the membranes are intact, continuous monitoring of the fetal hearts, movements, and uterine contractions may provide some assurance of fetal well-being.
- During early labour, the woman may find comfort from being able to change her position and walk around, and from the use of TENS or water.
- Encourage her to follow local guidelines on diet during labour. In early labour, light snacks and fluids are usually recommended. If prescribed by the anaesthetist, give ranitidine 150mg orally, 6 hourly.

*Established first stage*

- As labour establishes, monitor the fetal hearts continuously, alongside uterine contractions. It may be advisable to use a fetal scalp electrode for the leading twin; if there are any uncertainties around either or both of the FHRs, ultrasound scans can be used.[7]
- Epidural anaesthesia is often recommended for pain relief. It provides adequate analgesia if intrauterine manipulation of the second twin, forceps delivery, or a Caesarean is necessary in the second stage. However, be sensitive to individual choice.
- Whatever the woman's choice, an infusion of normal saline may help to keep her hydrated and maintain IV access.
- Make regular assessment of the woman's BP, pulse, temperature, and fluid balance.
- Care should be taken to ensure the woman's comfort, regularly easing her position and paying attention to hygiene. Encourage her to choose lateral positions to avoid supine hypotension.
- Assess progress and keep the obstetric registrar, anaesthetist, and paediatric team informed. If possible, introduce all personnel to the parents.

*Second stage of labour*

- When delivery is imminent, call the obstetric registrar to attend and inform the consultant in case manipulation of the second twin is necessary.
- The anaesthetist on call should be immediately available outside the delivery room and theatre staff should be aware to be on standby.
- The paediatric team should be present and additional resuscitation equipment prepared to receive both babies.
- Maintain a calm environment and minimize stress for the parents.
- A portable ultrasound scanner should be ready.

- An oxytocin infusion should be prepared to run via a pump. It should be connected to the IV cannula already *in situ* by a dual tap. Initially it remains turned off (review local guidance for dose and rate of drug).
- The woman may prefer not to deliver in the lithotomy position, but the potential for this should be available. An upright position will facilitate pushing and descent of the second twin.
- Proceed with the delivery of the first twin:
  - NEVER give Syntometrine® because the second stage is not yet concluded
  - Episiotomy may not be necessary
  - Clamp and cut the cord
  - If the baby is in good condition, encourage the father and mother to hold the baby.
- Occasionally, but not usually, the first placenta may deliver next.
- The registrar should remain present whilst the midwife performs the second delivery. The midwife should:
  - Palpate the abdomen or scan to determine the lie of the second twin, which must be longitudinal
  - Monitor the heart rate continuously
  - With the woman's consent, gently perform a vaginal examination; the midwife will be able to feel the bulging membranes (unless the twins are monozygotic) and a cephalic presentation. Confirm descent
  - The membranes of the second twin should be left intact if at all possible
  - Encourage the woman to continue pushing and, if necessary, administer the oxytocin infusion to help contractions
  - When the presenting head is well engaged and progressive descent is obvious, the membranes may rupture spontaneously or the midwife may perform ARM.
  - The second twin should be delivered within approximately 30min of the first. If there is a delay or evidence of fetal distress with the second twin, review the action plan—inform the consultant and consider instrumental vaginal birth or a Caesarean section.[5]
  - Mark the cord of the second twin with an extra clamp or ligature, to distinguish it from the first.
- If the babies are well on delivery, encourage skin-to-skin contact between babies and parents. If there is concern on delivery, the paediatric team will assess the babies.
- Samples of cord blood may be taken for assessment of pH.

*Complications with the second twin*

If the second twin does not take up a longitudinal lie following the delivery of the first twin, the obstetric registrar will take over care. With the woman's consent, the following may be performed.

- A catheter will be placed *in situ*.
- ECV may be attempted.
- If not successful, but the fetal heart is reassuring, analgesia is adequate, and the second twin is no larger than the first, internal podalic version and breech extraction may be attempted.

- Internal podalic version is performed by the obstetric registrar. The ultrasound scanner is used to assess the position and locate the feet of the second twin. If the feet are easily accessible vaginally, between contractions the obstetrician should reach into the uterine cavity and grasp the foot through the membranes. At the onset of a contraction, the fetal foot is pulled downwards with one hand whilst ARM is performed with the other hand. The fetus should then be longitudinal lie and it should be possible to grasp the other foot and encourage maternal effort to push. A vaginal breech birth should ensue.
- However, because of the perceived risks of a breech birth, protocols recommend an emergency Caesarean section.

*Third stage of labour*

- Allowing the third stage to progress unaided is not usually recommended because of the risk of excessive blood loss from two placental sites.
- Obtain the mother's consent to proceed to active management of the third stage, and give 1mL of Syntometrine® IM.
- Once delivered, the placenta should be sent for histological examination; if this is the case, do so without making any attempts to strip the membranes.[7]
- An oxytocin infusion continued for 4h following delivery will help to minimize PPH.

# Rare scenarios with twin pregnancies

*Monoamniotic twins*

- Vascular anastomoses can occur between the placental vessels of the twins.
- One twin may be small, pale, and anaemic and the other large, plethoric, and polycythaemic.
- As a result of twin–twin transfusion, fetal asphyxia can occur in either twin.
- These twins are usually diagnosed prior to labour and a Caesarean section performed to avoid the complications of fetal asphyxia.

*Locked twins*

- This situation may arise when the first twin is in the breech position and the second twin is with a cephalic presentation.
- The head of the first twin can become locked above the head of the second.
- A Caesarean section is now recommended for twins with this presentation.

# References

5  National Institute for Health and Care Excellence (2011). Timing of birth. In: National Institute for Health and Care Excellence. *Multiple pregnancy: antenatal care for twin and triplet pregnancies.* NICE guidelines CG129. Available at: ℛ www.nice.org.uk/guidance/cg129/chapter/1-Guidance#timing-of-birth.

6  Royal College of Obstetricians and Gynaecologists (2008). *Management of monochorionic twin pregnancy. Green-top guideline No. 51.* Available at: ℛ www.rcog.org.uk/globalassets/documents/guidelines/t51managementmonochorionictwinpregnancy2008a.pdf.

7  Maternity Guideline Group (2015). *Guideline for the management of multiple pregnancy and birth.* Barnsley NHS Foundation Trust Maternity Guidelines.

# Hypertensive disorders

## Definitions of hypertension during pregnancy

- *Essential (or chronic) hypertension* is raised arterial BP, 140/90mmHg or more, before 20 weeks' gestation. No proteinuria is present.
- *Gestational hypertension* (PIH) is BP raised above 140/90mmHg after 20+ weeks' gestation. No proteinuria is present. It can be classified as a BP of 20–25mmHg above the baseline diastolic reading, sustained over 24h.
- *Pre-eclampsia* is a multi-system disorder. The classification of severity depends on the levels of maternal BP and proteinuria: BP, 140/90mmHg; proteinuria, a dipstick reading of 1+, or 0.3g in a 24h urine collection.
- *Eclampsia* is defined as the occurrence of convulsions alongside signs and symptoms of pre-eclampsia.

Hypertensive disorders can worsen or flare up suddenly during labour or up to 10 days postnatally.

NB. Women with pre-existing risk factors for PIH may be advised antenatally to commence 75mg daily of aspirin from 12 weeks until 36 completed weeks of pregnancy.[8]

- All affected women should be considered to be at high risk:
  - Access consultant-led care
  - Deliver at a unit with neonatal facilities
- Untreated hypertensive disorders in pregnancy can progress to pre-eclampsia, eclampsia, HELLP syndrome, DIC syndrome, and fetal/maternal death.
- Pre-eclampsia is a global health problem, which complicates 2–8% of all pregnancies and contributes to 15% of preterm births and 9–26% of maternal deaths worldwide.[9] The incidence of pre-eclampsia is likely to have increased with the global increase in maternal age, obesity, assisted reproductive techniques, and medical co-morbidities that predispose women to pre-eclampsia such as diabetes, hypertension, and renal disease.[9]
  - Death may occur from acute respiratory distress syndrome (RDS), intracerebral haemorrhage, or hepatic, renal, or cardiovascular failure.
  - Fetal death may occur from asphyxia, compromise in labour, or placental abruption.
- The only known cure for worsening pre-eclampsia is delivery of the baby. The decision to deliver depends on the condition of the mother and fetus and the length of gestation.

## Principles of midwifery care

An experienced midwife should:
- Provide continuous care to the woman and liaise with all the team
- Monitor the maternal and fetal conditions closely
- Be aware of abnormal clinical findings/complications
- Refer changes in maternal and fetal conditions immediately to the consultant/senior obstetrician for early treatment

- Carry out the obstetrician's plan of care or assist the obstetrician and multidisciplinary team to perform actions necessary to achieve the optimum outcome, considering the appropriate time and route for delivery of the fetus. Attentive intrapartum care according to a management plan by a consultant obstetrician is paramount
- Facilitate communication between all members of the multidisciplinary team, including the senior midwife, obstetrician, anaesthetist, paediatrician, neonatal intensive care, and laboratory staff
- Ensure documentation of care and management decisions
- Be sensitive to/supportive of the woman's psychological needs and attempt to minimize stress.

## Hypertensive disorder

A pregnant woman with a hypertensive disorder may be admitted labouring to the delivery suite.
- Mild 140/90–149/99mmHg; moderate hypertension 150/100–159/109mmHg; severe hypertension 160/110mmHg or higher.[10]

On admission:
- Ensure the woman is/has been transferred from midwifery-led to consultant care, and liaise with the obstetric registrar for a detailed management plan (NB. For women with severe hypertension or pre-eclampsia, the plan should include the timing and nature of future fetal monitoring, fetal indications for birth, and if and when corticosteroids should be given. Discussions with neonatal paediatricians and obstetric anaesthetists should take place).[8]
- Review the general well-being of the woman and exclude symptoms of pre-eclampsia.
- Ensure accurate BP measurements are taken and recorded (the manual sphygmomanometer gives a more accurate reading than an automated machine, which sometimes under-records hypertension). Depending on local guidance, a BP profile of readings may be required, i.e. four readings every 10min.[11]
- Hypertension >150mmHg systolic or >100mmHg diastolic requires treatment; discuss this with the obstetrician. The first-line treatment is usually with oral labetalol to keep diastolic BP between 80 and 100 mmHg and systolic BP <150mmHg.[8]
- Use an automated reagent-strip reading device or request a urinary protein:creatinine ratio (PCR) for estimating proteinuria in a secondary care setting upon admission. (If an automated reagent-strip reading device is used to detect proteinuria and a result of 1+ or more is obtained, use a spot urinary PCR or a 24h urine collection to quantify proteinuria).[8]
- Results of the urinary PCR are significant if >30mg/mmol or a validated 24h urine collection result shows >300mg protein.[8]
- Assess the temperature, pulse, respirations, and oxygen saturation. This assessment on admission may be performed using a maternity early warning scoring system.

- In severe hypertension or suspected pre-eclampsia, consider IV access with a large-bore cannula; otherwise take venous blood samples for U/E, LFTs, FBC, and G&S. The results should be reviewed by a senior obstetrician as soon as they are available and will give an indication of the severity of the condition.
- Review fetal well-being—abdominal assessment of fetal growth. Consider continuous monitoring of the fetal heart alongside uterine contractions; also assess for fetal movements. Report and record any deviations from the normal (in women with mild or moderate gestational hypertension, only carry out CTG if fetal activity is abnormal).[8]

*During established labour*
- Keep the woman and her partner informed at all times of options available for care, and consider the woman's choices for coping in labour. Try to provide a relaxed environment.
- Encourage as much position change as practical.
- When a woman diagnosed with a hypertensive disorder is immobile as in labour, she should be encouraged to wear anti-embolic stockings.
- Pain may increase the BP further. Epidural analgesia could help; it causes vasodilation which may reduce the BP. Care should be taken not to overload with fluids the woman who has severe pre-eclampsia and who is requesting an epidural.
- Observe the balance between fluid intake and output.
- Assess the urine with a reagent strip every 2h. Note that a show/blood may contaminate the sample. If proteinuria is +2, obtain a catheter specimen to confirm the reading.
- During labour, measure BP—hourly in women with mild or moderate hypertension, continually in women with severe hypertension.[8]
- The woman's usual antihypertensive treatment should be administered during labour.
- The duration of the second stage of labour should not routinely be limited in women with stable, mild, or moderate hypertension or if BP is controlled within target ranges in women with severe hypertension. If the woman's BP is not controlled with treatment, operative birth is recommended.[8]
- Avoid ergometrine/Syntometrine® for the third stage of labour. It may aggravate hypertension. Oxytocin® 10IU IM is preferred.

## Pre-eclampsia and eclampsia
Pre-eclampsia (new hypertension, presenting after 20 weeks' gestation, with significant proteinuria PCR >30mg/mmol or 24h collection >300mg of protein) can be divided into mild, moderate, and severe:
- Mild: BP systolic 140–149, diastolic 90–99mmHg
- Moderate: BP systolic 150–159, diastolic 100–109mmHg
- Severe: defined as severe hypertension (diastolic ≥110, systolic ≥160mmHg) and/or with symptoms and/or with biochemical or haematological impairment.

Symptoms can be defined as:
- Severe headache, usually frontal and occipital; worse on standing
- Problems with vision, i.e. blurred or flashing, loss of patches of the visual field (scotomata), photophobia
- Severe pain just below the ribs or vomiting
- Papilloedema
- Signs of clonus (≥3 beats)
- Liver tenderness—probably due to liver oedema, stretching of the capsule
- Irritability, on edge, occasionally drowsy—because of cerebral oedema
- Nausea, vomiting, and generally feeling unwell
- HELLP syndrome
- Platelet count of <100
- Abnormal liver enzymes (alanine aminotransferase (ALT) or aspartate aminotransferase (AST) raises to >70IU/L).

Eclampsia is diagnosed when the woman presents with the signs and symptoms discussed above with eclamptic fits.

## Labour ward management of severe pre-eclampsia

The three main objectives when caring for a woman with severe pre-eclampsia are:[11]
- Prevention of complications, i.e. placental abruption, HELLP syndrome, pulmonary oedema
- Prevention of convulsions
- The birth of a healthy neonate with minimal maternal morbidity.

Upon admission to the labour ward and diagnosis of pre-eclampsia, the consultant obstetrician should liaise with the consultant anaesthetist and paediatrician to discuss and record the management plan for the appropriate time of the birth. This decision must be taken in conjunction with the mother and birth partner in order for them to be in full receipt of all the information. The timing of birth is based on a full assessment of the woman's condition and a fetal assessment, including a CTG.[8,11]

Timing of birth with severe pre-eclampsia:
- <24+6 weeks' gestation—stabilize the woman. Discussions with the parents would need to take place in cases of the viability of the fetus
- 25–32 weeks—expectant management. However, birth may be indicated if there are maternal or fetal indicators. A Caesarean may be appropriate
- ≥33 weeks—stabilize the woman's condition and consider arranging the birth. After 34 weeks, vaginal birth can be considered.

The woman with severe pre-eclampsia must be cared for on a high dependency unit (HDU) within the labour ward. Care should be given by one designated midwife with assistance available if required.

The room should be equipped with:
- A suitable sphygmomanometer (the manual sphygmomanometer gives a more accurate reading than an automated machine, which sometimes under-records hypertension)

- Stethoscope
- Thermometer
- Critical care monitor with $SpO_2$ monitor
- HDU chart with MEOWS chart and fluid balance chart
- Patella hammer
- Ophthalmoscope
- CTG monitor
- Ultrasound scanner
- Equipment to site IV infusions and to take blood samples and MSU, and to perform vaginal examination.

Try to alleviate any stress the woman may experience. Listen to preferences; explain procedures, and answer questions.

*Maternal care*
- Commence the HDU chart with the consultant management plan clearly recorded within it.
- Commence critical care monitoring; record the BP, respirations, and pulse every 15min for a minimum of 4h. Record the temperature every 4h. Monitor $SpO_2$ continuously; if saturations decrease below 95%, inform the doctor as this may indicate pulmonary oedema. If observations recorded on the MEOWS chart begin to score once on 4-hourly observations, report to the doctor and increase the frequency.
- Observe the woman's colour and level of consciousness.
- Measure the woman's BP accurately. Use the appropriate cuff size; the standard cuff may be too small and give an overestimation. If the arm is >33cm in circumference, use a large cuff. Ensure a correct sitting position, with the machine at the level of the woman's heart. Use Korotkoff phase V (disappearance of the sound) and note the final digit. It should be recorded accurately and not rounded up or down. Note that the mean arterial pressure (MAP) is used by some obstetricians—a value >125mmHg must be reported. Study the present findings alongside the woman's previous antenatal record; 20–25mmHg above the baseline diastolic reading may be significant. A central venous pressure (CVP)/arterial line may be indicated for accurate measurements of the maternal BP.
- Obtain IV access and take bloods for:
  - FBC: this looks at a number of things such as the number of red cells, white cells, and platelets in the blood. Low platelets may alert the team to the development of HELLP syndrome
  - U/E: measures the kidney function. The healthy kidney excretes urea and it is important in maintaining the electrolyte balance of the body, the balance between such chemicals as potassium and sodium, and the acid/alkali balance
  - Urate: a uric acid blood test, also known as a serum uric acid measurement, determines how much uric acid is present in the blood. The test can help determine how well the body produces and removes uric acid
  - LFTs: a group of blood tests that detect inflammation and damage to the liver. They can also check how well the liver is working

- Coagulation: this test measures the blood's ability to clot and the amount of time it takes to do so. This is also an indicator of the development of HELLP syndrome
- G&S: a group and save is required whenever there is a possibility of a patient requiring transfusion, e.g. surgical risk, haemorrhage, and anaemia.
- Repeat bloods every 4–8h or as directed by the medical management plan.
- Catheterize the woman with consent and complete any invasive procedure paperwork. Record the urine output every hour (ideally aim for an output of ≥20mL/h or >80mL over 4 consecutive hours). Test each sample for protein.
- Monitor a strict fluid balance regime—maximum intake should be no more than 80mL/h (see local guidance).
- Monitor for any per vaginum loss and perform a vaginal examination to assess for possible induction depending on gestation.
- Apply TEDS and consider prophylactic anticoagulants.
- Request that a registrar or consultant performs chest auscultation to check for pulmonary oedema and reviews maternal reflexes for clonus regularly.
- Give ranitidine 150mg orally every 6h (according to protocol). This may be requested by the anaesthetist. It reduces the production of hydrochloric acid in the stomach and may help to avoid the patient inhaling regurgitated stomach contents (Mendelson's syndrome) which are lethal to the lung tissue and can cause chemical pneumonitis.
- Alert the paediatrician and special care baby unit (SCBU) team to ensure availability of a cot and personnel. It may be possible for the parents to visit the SCBU or for the staff to describe and explain neonatal special care to the parents prior to delivery.
- Attend to the woman's hygiene needs; ensure sheets are kept fresh and crease-free. Monitor pressure points and skin integrity. Attention to details of comfort may reduce anxiety and pain. Be sensitive to the abdominal discomfort resulting from continuous monitoring of the fetal heart. When movement is restricted, encourage changes of position (especially right or left lateral positions or sitting upright); massage the back, hands, or feet. Pay attention to patient preferences for light and sound, peace, and space for rest.

*Fetal assessment*
- Perform an abdominal assessment of fetal well-being, especially:
  - Symphysis—fundal height for growth. Record findings on the woman's customized growth chart
  - Fetal movements
  - Begin continuous fetal monitoring (CTG).
- Review antenatal notes to determine the clinical picture and assess any IUGR and placental insufficiency: previous CTG, ultrasound scans for growth, size assessment, fetal breathing movements, amniotic fluid index, and umbilical artery Doppler analysis.

*Control of BP in severe pre-eclampsia*

The following drugs may be used:

- *Labetalol orally*, may be prescribed in milder cases. Labetalol should be avoided when a woman is known to be asthmatic as it has β-blocking properties. The obstetrician may recommend 200mg oral labetalol, if there is time and no immediate risk to the woman or fetus. The woman's BP should fall by 10mmHg within 30min. If the response is positive and adequate, maintain the dose orally—200mg tds.
- *Labetalol IV infusion bolus dose* is given if oral therapy is not possible, operative delivery is indicated, or there is no response to oral therapy. A bolus dose of 20mL of labetalol (5mg/mL) 10mL/50mg should be administered via a syringe driver over 1min. Monitor BP every 5min. This bolus dose can be repeated if no reduction in diastolic BP after 5min, up to a maximum dose of 200mg/40mL.[11]
- *Labetalol IV infusion maintenance dose* is given once the bolus dose has taken effect. The infusion is again given via a syringe driver. Give 60mL/300mg labetalol (usually three ampoules); infuse this at 4mL/h (20mg/h). The rate can then be doubled every 30min to a maximum dose of 32mL/h (160mg/h). Aim to maintain a diastolic BP of <100mmHg.[11]
- *Hydralazine (IV)*—the woman's pulse must be below 120bpm prior to administration. It acts directly on smooth muscle in arteriolar walls, causing vasodilatation. Loading dose of 5–10mg of hydralazine IV given slowly—maximum dose of 20mg. Maintenance dose—100mg of hydralazine in 50mL of normal saline; infuse via a syringe pump at a rate of 2–20mg/h (1–10mL/h). Titrate against BP; aim to maintain diastolic BP to <100mmHg.[11] Side effects can be troublesome, e.g. nausea/vomiting, tachycardia, headache. Maternal and fetal conditions should be carefully monitored.
- *Nifedipine orally*—this may be used with caution if used with magnesium sulfate. Loading dose is 10–15mg (bite and swallow, not sublingual). Maintenance dose—10mg tds or 10–15mg slow-release 12-hourly oral.[11]

In all circumstances, follow the instructions of the medical staff carefully, and abide by local protocols. IV antihypertensive drugs may cause fetal compromise if the BP is reduced too rapidly. Monitor the FHR continuously. Monitor the woman's progress and report any side effects or changes in condition to the obstetrician. Note that lowering the BP may mask symptoms and does not remove the risk of eclampsia.

*Eclampsia—immediate management*

Immediate management will be to maintain the safety of the woman and her unborn child.

- Call for help—obstetric registrar, senior house officer (SHO), anaesthetist, and senior midwife.
- Maintain airway.
- If safe, place the woman in the left lateral position.
- Administer oxygen at 15L/min.
- Prevent trauma.
- IV access (large-bore cannula): take all bloods discussed earlier.

- Commence *magnesium sulfate* regime: loading dose is magnesium sulfate 20% IV given over 5–15min (20mL, 4g). Maintenance dose is magnesium sulfate 20% (200mg/mL) given IV over 24h. Administer via a syringe pump at a rate of 5mL/h.[11] Side effects of this drug may include motor paralysis, absent tendon reflexes, respiratory depression, renal impairment, and cardiac arrhythmia—all can occur but will be minimal if the drug is administered slowly.
- The antidote to the effects of magnesium sulfate is 10% *calcium gluconate* 10mL administered slowly.

The obstetric team is responsible for the assessment of the patient and must review the woman and document a management plan regularly.

Once convulsions have ended, transfer to HDU; if not already present, continue care as for pre-eclampsia management.

*Delivery*

- All pregnant women requiring IV hypotensives should be delivered as soon as the BP is sufficiently controlled. The antihypertensive therapy should be continued during labour. If possible, she should be delivered at a unit with neonatal intensive care facilities.
- An urgent Caesarean may be necessary.
- The BP can return to more normal levels soon after delivery but may rise again within 24h. It should be monitored and therapy continued as necessary.

## References

8 National Institute for Health and Care Excellence (2010). Chapter 1, guidance. In: *Hypertension in pregnancy: diagnosis and management.* NICE guidelines CG107. Available at: ℳ www.nice.org. uk/guidance/cg107/chapter/1-guidance.

9 Steegers EAP, von Dadelszen P, Duvekot JJ, Pijnenborg R (2010). Pre-eclampsia. *Lancet* 21376: 631–44.

10 Townsend R, O'Brien P, Khalil A (2015). Diagnosis and management of pre-eclampsia: a clinical perspective on recent advances in the field. *Br J Midwifery* 23: 252–8.

11 Dunning G (2015). *Guideline for the management of severe pre-eclampsia.* Barnsley NHS Foundation Trust Maternity Guideline.

## Care of the diabetic mother and fetus

Up to 5% of all pregnancies are complicated with either pre-existing diabetes or GDM; this equates to approximately 34 000 women per year.[12] It has been highlighted that women with pre-existing medical problems, such as diabetes, are more likely to die in pregnancy.[13] Women who die as a direct cause of diabetes in pregnancy have been found to have had poor glycaemic control prior to and throughout pregnancy.[13] Closer monitoring of these women is of paramount importance.

When diabetes is present during pregnancy, risks of the following complications during intrapartum care are increased:

- Preterm labour
- Unstable lie
- Cord prolapse
- PPH—may occur as a result of polyhydramnios
- PIH occurs earlier in the pregnancy than in non-diabetic women and in a more severe form; it may complicate labour
- Large baby (macrosomic)—may result in shoulder dystocia in the second stage of labour
- Fetal abnormality (usually excluded by antenatal ultrasound scan)
- Intrauterine death when diabetes is inadequately controlled.

It is recommended that women with diabetes and a fetus which is a normal size for dates and no other complications should be offered elective birth between 37+0 and 38+6 weeks' gestation; if there are metabolic or any other maternal or fetal complications, elective birth may be advised sooner.[14] This would mean induction of labour or an elective Caesarean. However, each woman should be treated individually and given information and choice. Discussion around the mode of birth should have taken place antenatally with an obstetrician; the plan should be clearly documented within the woman's notes.[15]

### Management of labour for women with gestational diabetes (diet-controlled)

- Continuous CTG to be used during labour. No other intervention required unless indicated.
- Monitor blood glucose levels every hour—aim to keep levels between 4 and 7mmol/L.
- For women whose blood glucose is unstable, the obstetrician should be informed and the sliding scale may be considered (Table 21.1).

### Management of the immediate postnatal period for gestational diabetes (diet-controlled)

- The baby should be fed as soon as possible following birth and commence the hypoglycaemia regime.
- Postnatally the woman can resume normal eating and drinking. A random monitoring of blood glucose levels can be performed prior to transfer to community care to exclude persisting hyperglycaemia.
- Advise of an increased risk of developing diabetes in future pregnancies.

Table 21.1 Insulin sliding scale

| Blood glucose (mmol/L) | Variable-rate insulin infusion (units/h) |
|---|---|
| <2 | 0 |
| 2.1–3 | 0.5 |
| 3.1–4.5 | 1 |
| 4.6–6.4 | 2 |
| 6.5–11.0 | 3 |
| 11.1–17 | 4 |
| 17+ | 6 |

From Dixon P, Jones S, Pipe-Thomas P (2015) Guideline for the Management of Diabetes in Pregnancy. Barnsley NHS Foundation Trust Maternity Guideline.

## Management of the first stage of labour for women requiring insulin

- Inform the obstetric registrar or consultant on call once the woman has been admitted onto the labour ward.
- Treat the woman as high risk and follow the plan of care documented in the notes; offer vigilant and continuous care.
- Women should not be offered food during labour and only water to drink.[15]
- Consider the progress of the pregnancy; review the hospital records, and assess the woman's BP, pulse, and temperature, ensuring general maternal well-being.
- During labour, test all urine for ketones and protein, measuring the amount as part of careful fluid balance monitoring. Dehydration and ketosis (which is dangerous to the fetus) can thus be avoided.
- Obtain IV access and send blood samples to the laboratory for FBC, haematocrit, U/E, G&S, and blood glucose.
- Review the woman's record of blood glucose readings. Ask the woman to take a capillary sample for immediate assessment. The reading should be in the range of 4–7mmol/L.[11] Then record the woman's blood glucose levels every hour and document findings.
- Gain the woman's consent to assess the fetus and her contractions by abdominal palpation and to monitor the fetus continuously by CTG. Any non-reassuring patterns should be reported to the obstetrician.
- Begin an IV sliding scale regime; this aims to keep the blood sugar level stable. The regime would need to be prescribed within the woman's treatment chart prior to its implementation, e.g.:
  - An IV infusion with 500mL of 10% glucose saline + 10mmol of potassium chloride (KCl) is set to run at 100mL/h; this should be given via an IVAC infusion pump
  - An insulin pump with soluble insulin 50IU in 49.5mL of normal saline is set to run according to a standard regime (Table 21.1)

- Assess blood sugar every hour (see local guidance). The woman or her partner may be happy to do this. Control the sugar level at 4–7mmol/L. The variable-rate insulin infusion can then be adjusted accordingly to keep the woman's blood glucose levels within the desired limits
- NB. Some women who have been extremely insulin-resistant during pregnancy may require a modification of this regime.

If the blood sugars are >11mmol/L, inform the obstetrician.
- Recommend the drinking of only clear fluids during labour, and give ranitidine 150mg QDS.
- Blood glucose levels may be more erratic in labour. The body has greater needs for energy. In addition, pain causes catecholamine release, which may make glucose control more difficult.
- Use of patient-controlled epidural anaesthesia in established labour may be recommended to the woman by the obstetrician. Mobility can be quite limited by the sliding scale infusions and the woman will have difficulty in finding comfortable positions as labour progresses. However, the midwife and obstetric team should be sensitive to the woman's choice if the diabetes is not beset by any of the complications listed earlier.
- If labour is proceeding normally, support the parents and observe progress to ensure a safe labour and delivery. No intervention is needed.
- If it is essential to aid progress, ARM may be necessary. This should be performed with caution, ensuring that the fetal head is well engaged. The colour and quantity of liquor should be noted.
- If an oxytocin regime is requested by the registrar, ensure this is diluted with normal saline and is administered via a separate line (do not give further glucose).

## Management of the second stage of labour

- Towards the end of the first stage, inform the obstetric registrar of progress.
- If the woman has an effective epidural, the fetal head may be allowed to descend and rotate in the second stage. Oxytocin may be required for a primigravida with epidural anaesthesia, as it helps to achieve a normal, rather than assisted, delivery.
- The registrar and paediatrician should be immediately available in case of fetal compromise or shoulder dystocia.

## Immediate post-birth management for women with gestational diabetes who have required insulin

- IV infusion should be reduced by half at delivery of the placenta.
- Following delivery, insulin requirements may fall dramatically. Once the woman is able to eat and drink normally, the sliding scale should be discontinued.
- Advise continued close monitoring of blood glucose levels, testing pre- and post-meals. Women should be reminded of the symptoms of hyperglycaemia. If levels remain normal, discontinue testing.
- No further treatment is required unless hyperglycaemia persists.
- The baby should be classed as high risk for hypoglycaemia; ideally aim to initiate the first feed within 30min.

## Immediate post-birth management for women with pre-existing type 1 or 2 diabetes

The care should be as for women with GDM requiring insulin, but a detailed plan should also have been documented for each woman. The diabetic specialist nurse is available for support on diabetic control for both the woman and the midwife who is giving the care. The woman may be required to recommence or continue oral hypoglycaemic agents. Metformin and glibenclamide may be used if the mother is breastfeeding. Women requiring insulin should recommence pre-pregnancy insulin doses, unless otherwise specified in the management plan.

## References

12 Confidential Enquiry into Maternal and Child Health (CEMACH) (2007). *Diabetes in Pregnancy: Are we Providing the Best Care? Findings of a National Enquiry: England, Wales and Northern Ireland.* London: CEMACH.
13 Knight M, Kenyon S, Brocklehurst P, Neilson J, Shakespeare J, Kurinczuk JJ (eds.) on behalf of MBRRACE-UK (2014). *Saving Lives, Improving Mothers' Care: Lessons learned to inform future maternity care from the UK and Ireland Confidential Enquiries into Maternal Deaths and Morbidity 2009–12.* Oxford: National Perinatal Epidemiology Unit, University of Oxford.
14 National Institute for Health and Care Excellence (2015). Intrapartum care. In: National Institute for Health and Care Excellence. *Diabetes in pregnancy: management from preconception to the postnatal period.* NICE guideline NG3. Available at: www.nice.org.uk/guidance/ng3/chapter/1-recommendations#intrapartum-care-2.
15 Dixon P, Jones S, Pipe-Thomas P (2015). *Guideline for the management of diabetes in pregnancy.* Barnsley NHS Foundation Trust Maternity Guideline.

# Drug and alcohol misuse

## Intrapartum care

- Most women who are known to be drug- or alcohol-dependent will have normal labour and deliveries. They should receive the same information and choices in labour as other women.
- Ideally the woman should be cared for by a midwife known to her.
- A comprehensive labour and birth plan should have been completed antenatally and includes birth options, immediate care of the newborn, and feeding intentions. This is often completed by a specialist substance misuse midwife.[16]
- A paediatric alert form (dependent on the trust's guidelines) may be present with special instructions regarding the care of the newborn.
- A Common Assessment Framework (CAF) plan may document an agreed care pathway.

## On admission

- Ensure that you are familiar with any plan for social care and child protection, and inform the appropriate agencies/workers involved of the client's admission to the delivery suite. Ensure that the plan is documented in the hospital notes.
- Inform the obstetrician (although if there are no complications, the obstetrician need not be present for the birth), specialist midwife for substance misuse, paediatrician, and SCBU of admission.
- If indicated, the following people may also need to be informed: named nurse/midwife for safeguarding children, social worker, and infection control team. Multidisciplinary working is essential to care for women affected by addiction.[17]
- A woman with a history of drug addiction may have veins that prove difficult to cannulate. If she is considered to be at risk of bleeding, the anaesthetist may site a cannula early in labour as a precaution.

## The methadone programme

- Women who have opted for a methadone programme to facilitate withdrawal from their habit should continue this drug according to the dose currently prescribed.
- If caring for a woman who is an addict who has withdrawn from treatment, it should be assumed that she is taking drugs. Encourage her to disclose her most recent use. Aim to achieve cooperation and involvement of the woman and partner.
- Respect confidentiality.
- Do not tolerate illicit drug use on the hospital premises.
- Symptoms of withdrawal may occur during labour.
- Pain relief needs special attention, especially as full opioid agonists, such as diamorphine and methadone, or partial agonists, such as buprenorphine, determine the choice of analgesia in the individual pregnancy. Therefore, there should be a low threshold for considering the use of an epidural, with clear local guidance on partial versus full agonist effects explained to the pregnant woman.[18]

- Women with a history of previous addiction may wish to avoid narcotics. However, they are not contraindicated for pain relief. Unless stated otherwise in the management plan, higher doses of opiates may be necessary because of tolerance.
- Epidural analgesia can be offered.
- Avoid cyclizine; it may increase the effect of methadone and is a CNS irritant. It is also a misused drug with significant street value.
- If the woman collects her methadone directly from a pharmacy, it may be necessary for methadone prescription to be cancelled once the woman is an inpatient. This would inform the pharmacy that she is unable to collect the drug at this time and that the methadone would be given as an inpatient. If the woman remains an inpatient for three days or longer it would be important to liaise with the prescribing services in advance of discharge to ensure that appropriate re-prescribing takes place. Check local guidance on how this procedure is carried out, or speak to a specialist midwife for guidance.

## Alcohol misuse

Alcohol withdrawal can be medically serious and life-threatening for a pregnant woman and the unborn child. The onset of alcohol withdrawal can occur 6–24h after the last drink where the woman regularly consumes six or more standard drinks per day. It is important for the midwife to recognize the symptoms of alcohol withdrawal and refer appropriately.[16] Mild symptoms include nausea, anxiety, trembling, and vomiting. Severe symptoms include seizures, hallucinations, tremors, tachycardia, confusion, and disorientation.

Alcohol crosses into the breast milk by diffusion, meaning that the level of alcohol which the mother is exposed to is approximately the same level which is passed to the fetus. Alcohol in very small amounts has been shown to have a serious effect on the developing brain.[19]

## Infection risk

The woman may be at risk of developing a blood borne virus because of the following:[20]
- She is injecting drugs currently or intermittently
- She is smoking heroin/crack cocaine or uses amphetamines
- She is in a personal/sexual relationship with someone who injects drugs.

The midwife also needs to consider that the woman may have a blood-borne virus, e.g. HIV or hepatitis B or C. If this is a concern, to avoid vertical transmission:
- Membranes should not be ruptured
- A fetal scalp electrode should be avoided
- FBS is contraindicated.

Where indicated, arrange for the paediatrician to administer the hepatitis B vaccination to the newborn with parental consent.[16]

### Initiation of breastfeeding with risk of infection
- *HIV-positive*—if the woman is found to be HIV-positive, the woman should be discouraged from breastfeeding her baby as transmission via breast milk is increased; this is irrespective of the viral load.[16]
- *Hepatitis B*—a mother with hepatitis B can breastfeed her baby if the baby receives a vaccine course starting at birth.
- *Hepatitis C*—there is no evidence of transmission via breast milk; breastfeeding is appropriate.

### Care of the fetus and neonate
- Placental insufficiency may have occurred in pregnancy. IUGR is common. There is a risk of fetal compromise and intrapartum asphyxia.
- Meconium staining of the liquor and meconium aspiration are sometimes present as a result of fetal compromise due to periods of intrauterine drug withdrawal.
- During established labour, monitor the fetal heart continuously via an abdominal ultrasound transducer.
- If there are concerns, alert the paediatrician and prepare for resuscitation of the neonate—sometimes breathing may be depressed at delivery.
- Avoid giving naloxone to reverse the effect of opiates during neonatal resuscitation, since this can result in rapid withdrawal which is associated with increased perinatal morbidity and death.[20]
- The baby should be carefully assessed following delivery. Alcohol-related birth defects should be excluded as far as possible.
- The baby's condition should normally be stable at delivery; if the mother chooses, encourage her to place the baby in skin-to-skin contact and initiate early breastfeeding if this is the mother's choice and there is no risk of cross-infection.
- Transfer the baby to the postnatal ward with the mother.

Postnatal ward staff should monitor the baby for signs of drug withdrawal. This can be done by regularly (usually 4-hourly) completing the Neonatal Abstinence Withdrawal Chart. Ensure that the mother recognizes and knows to report the symptoms.

### The initiation of breastfeeding and substance misuse
- *Methadone and buprenorphine*—breastfeeding is considered safe; use caution if there is suspicion of poly-drug use.[16]
- *Benzodiazepines*—breastfeeding should be discouraged.
- *Cocaine*—breastfeeding should be discouraged.
- *Cannabis*—cannabis is attracted to breast milk; therefore, breastfeeding is dependent on the amount smoked. Advice from the specialist midwife may be required.
- *Alcohol*—breastfeeding should be avoided whilst alcohol is present within the bloodstream.
- *IV drug use*—breastfeeding is contraindicated whilst the mother is using the IV route of administration due to the risk of HIV transmission and oversedation.

## References

16 Pollard J, Poskitt J, Dunning G (2013). *Guideline for the management of babies born to substance misusing mothers*. Barnsley Hospital Foundation Trust Maternity Guidelines.

17 National Institute for Health and Care Excellence (2010). Chapter 1, Guidance. In: National Institute for Health and Care Excellence. *Pregnancy and complex social factors: a model for service provision for pregnant women with complex social factors*. NICE guidelines CG110. Available at: ℰ www.nice.org.uk/guidance/cg110/chapter/1-guidance.

18 Department of Health (England) and the devolved administrations (2007). *Drug misuse and dependency: UK guidelines on clinical management*. London: Department of Health (England), the Scottish Government, Welsh Assembly Government and Northern Ireland Executive. Available at ℰ www.nta.nhs.uk/uploads/clinical_guidelines_2007.pdf.

19 FAS Aware UK. *Has anyone told you about fetal alcohol spectrum disorder?* FAS Aware UK leaflet. Available at: ℰ fasaware.co.uk/.

20 Whittaker A (2011). *The Essential Guide to Problem Substance Use during Pregnancy: A Resource Book for Professionals*. London: Drug Scope.

# Epilepsy

Epilepsy is the most common neurological condition in pregnancy and affects about 0.5–1% of pregnant women.[21] Fourteen maternal deaths as a direct result of epilepsy were reported between 2009 and 2012; poorly controlled seizures were found to be the main contributing factor.[22] Some experience an increase in fits during pregnancy. This may be because women discontinue their medication or they experience nausea/vomiting. Also, a haemodilution and an increased metabolism of anticonvulsant drugs may lead to a fall in the concentration of the drug in the plasma. Only 1–2% of women with active epilepsy will have a seizure in labour and/or in the first 24h after birth.[23]

A brief isolated fit is unlikely to be dangerous to the fetus; only occasionally will seizure cause morbidity, but status epilepticus is a cause of maternal and fetal death.

Women with epilepsy are frequently anxious and require much reassurance. Ideally they should be cared for in labour by a midwife who is known to them and they should have met the consultant overseeing care.

## Prevention of seizures

- The midwife should listen to the woman's assessment of her own needs. She will be familiar with the factors which stimulate her seizures and she may experience warnings of an attack.
- Anticonvulsant medication should be given as normal during labour. Evidence suggests that the teratogenic risks of AEDs on the unborn baby are small and are associated with the number, type, and dose.
- Anticonvulsants include:
  - Phenytoin
  - Primidone
  - Carbamazepine
  - Phenobarbital
  - Sodium valproate is not recommended due to the higher levels of congenital abnormalities.
- Major congenital malformations for women taking AEDs increases from 2% to 4%.[24] Missed doses will cause a drop in plasma levels which should be avoided. Malabsorption during labour may also increase the risk of a seizure. If excessive nausea and vomiting occur, a parenteral alternative may be necessary.
- The midwife should help the woman to achieve a good night's sleep during early labour and prolonged labour should be avoided—exhaustion may cause a seizure.
- Anxiety and stress should be minimized. The midwife can help by encouraging support from the partner and discussing the plan of care fully with the woman.
- Pain or hyperventilation related to pain or stress may cause a seizure so adequate analgesia is paramount. The midwife should offer the same range of pain relief (including epidural) as available to other women. However, diamorphine should be given in preference to pethidine.[25]

- Water birth is discouraged in women with a history of seizures in pregnancy. Women who are not on AEDs and have been seizure-free may be allowed into the pool.
- Women should have continuous fetal monitoring if they have suffered from seizures in pregnancy and/or are taking AEDs.
- The midwife should ensure adequate hydration and nutrition since dehydration or hypoglycaemia can trigger seizures.
- The midwife and/or partner should be in attendance throughout the labour.

## Signs of epileptic seizure

Epileptic seizures occur in a variety of forms. The most dangerous are tonic–clonic seizures.

- Tonic–clonic seizure: the woman may experience aura—a strange feeling, taste, or smell. She will suddenly stiffen and, if standing, fall backwards. She may cry out or bite her tongue. Her muscles will relax and tighten causing the body to convulse. She may be incontinent of urine. Her breathing may be laboured. The colour of her skin may change to blue-grey. She cannot hear. The episode may last just a few minutes.
  - Following the seizure: the colour of the woman's skin returns to normal. The woman may feel tired and confused. She may have a headache and want to sleep.
- Tonic seizure: the woman's muscles suddenly become stiff. She may fall backwards. Recovery after a tonic seizure is quick.

## In the event of an epileptic seizure

Seizures in labour should be terminated as soon as possible to avoid maternal and fetal hypoxia and fetal acidosis.

- Call for emergency help from an obstetric registrar and an anaesthetist.
- Note the time of onset.
- Turn the woman to the left lateral position if possible.
- Ensure clear airway/breathing.
- Give oxygen.
- Remove items which might cause harm.
- Wait at least 3min as most epileptic seizures are self-limiting.
- Talk reassuringly to the woman as she regains consciousness.
- Assess maternal and fetal well-being; commence CTG if not already.

*Status epilepticus* is defined as 30min of continual seizure activity or a cluster of seizures without recovery. This is a serious emergency and requires prompt action from the multidisciplinary team. If the fit continues, the anaesthetist will administer benzodiazepines. Lorazepam IV is recommended and administered as a dose of 0.1mg/kg; a further dose may be given after 10–20min. If this is not effective, further medication may be required such as diazepam 10–20mg administered rectally or phenytoin 10–15mg/kg given IV.

   If there is persistent uterine hypertonus, consider administration of a tocolytic agent. If the fetal heart does not recover within 5min or if a seizure reoccurs, the birth should be expedited via a Caesarean if vaginal birth is not imminent.

## Immediate postnatal care for the epileptic mother and her baby

- The midwife should recommend to the parents IM vitamin K (1mg) for the baby at birth since anticonvulsant drugs (carbamazepine, phenytoin, primidone, phenobarbital) are known to increase the risk of haemorrhagic disease of the newborn caused by a deficiency in the mother and fetus of vitamin K-dependent clotting factors.
- The midwife may safely encourage initiation of breastfeeding since the resulting dose of medication received by the baby is small and is unlikely to cause sedation. The baby's progress should be kept under review.
- The infant may suffer from withdrawal effects of some AEDs, in particular benzodiazepines and phenobarbital. Monitoring of the baby should be done by way of the substance misuse withdrawal chart every 4h.

## References

21 Edey S, Moran N, Nashef L (2014). SUPED and epilepsy related mortality in pregnancy. *Epilepsia* 55: 72–4.

22 Knight M, Kenyon S, Brocklehurst P, Neilson J, Shakespeare J, Kurinczuk JJ (eds.) on behalf of MBRRACE-UK (2014). *Saving Lives, Improving Mothers' Care: Lessons learned to inform future maternity care from the UK and Ireland Confidential Enquiries into Maternal Deaths and Morbidity 2009–12.* Oxford: National Perinatal Epidemiology Unit, University of Oxford.

23 Pennell P (2006). EURAP outcomes for seizure control during pregnancy: useful and encouraging data. *Epilepsy Curr* 6: 186–8.

24 Morrow J, Russell A, Guthrie E, *et al.* (2005). Malformation risks of antiepileptic drugs in pregnancy: a prospective study from the UK Epilepsy and Pregnancy Register. *J Neurol Neurosurg Psychiatry* 77: 193–8. Available at: ℧ jnnp.bmj.com/content/77/2/193.full.

25 Royal College of Obstetricians and Gynaecologists (2016). *Epilepsy in pregnancy. Green-top guideline No. 68.* Available at: ℧ www.rcog.org.uk/globalassets/documents/guidelines/green-top-guidelines/gtg68_epilepsy.pdf.

## Cardiac conditions

## Cardiac conditions

Women with cardiac conditions should have individualized plans made for their care by a team including a cardiologist, an anaesthetist, an obstetrician, and a midwife. All women should be assessed for exercise tolerance and cardiac function prior to labour and birth with the aim to reduce the risk of cardiac failure. There are a number of haemodynamic changes taking place in the cardiovascular system during labour and birth which will affect a pregnant woman with significant cardiac disease, e.g. the cardiac output is increased by 30–50% because of the increase in stroke volume and heart rate.[26] There is also a marked increase to the BP during the second-stage contractions when this is accompanied by the mother's pushing efforts.

A multidisciplinary meeting should take place at 32–34 weeks of gestation to establish a plan of management for delivery in order to avoid complications during labour. The plan should state who should be involved in supervising the labour, whether the woman should give birth at a tertiary unit, whether a Caesarean section is appropriate, whether bearing down is advisable in the second stage, and appropriate prophylaxis against PPH (routinely used oxytocic regimes can have major cardiovascular adverse effects).[27]

### First stage of labour

- Once it has been determined that the plan for a vaginal birth is safe and preferable, a Caesarean section is usually only necessary for obstetric indications.[27]
- Inform all relevant multidisciplinary team members of the woman's arrival onto the labour ward.
- Record all observations as for a low-risk woman in labour, but measurement of the pulse rate and rhythm is also recommended as it may be the first sign of volume overload.[27]
- The BP should be measured manually with a sphygmomanometer.
- Record oxygen saturations and observe for signs of cyanosis.
- An ECG may be requested to assess the health of the heart upon the commencement of labour.
- Epidural analgesia is a good option because it decreases cardiac output by increasing peripheral dilatation and reducing the need for fluid preload. Care must be exercised in those with a fixed cardiac output.
- Fluid balance requires particular attention and care must be taken not to overload as this may precipitate pulmonary oedema.
- Maternal and fetal well-being must be continuously and carefully assessed.

### Second stage of labour

- The second stage of labour can be shortened by elective instrumental delivery to minimize the dramatic rise in BP observed when the mother is pushing.
- In mild heart disease where there have been no antenatal problems, it would not be necessary to intervene if progress is rapid and a short second stage anticipated.

## Third stage of labour

- Ergometrine and Syntometrine® should be avoided as they can cause generalized vasospasm and hypertension, resulting in a 500–800mL bolus of blood returning to the venous circulation. A low-dose oxytocin infusion is probably the safest option.[27]
- Use of an oxytocin infusion avoids the problems of bolus and PPH. However, oxytocin should be used with caution in women with severe disease because it can cause profound hypotension.
- Physiological management results in a return of 200–300mL of blood to the circulation. As no oxytocic is given, this occurs over a period of minutes rather than during one contraction.
- Women with cardiac disease should be closely monitored for at least 24h following birth.

## Cardiac conditions classified into groups according to risk

*Low-risk conditions*

- Uncomplicated septal defects.[28]
- Mild or moderate pulmonary stenosis.
- Corrected tetralogy of Fallot.
- Corrected transposition without any other significant defects.
- Acyanotic Ebstein's anomaly.
- Mild mitral or aortic regurgitation.
- Hypertrophic cardiomyopathy.

*Conditions with some risk*

- Coarctation of the aorta.
- Cyanosed mother with pulmonary stenosis.
- Univentricular circulation after Fontan operation or Rastelli conduits.
- Marfan's or Ehlers–Danlos syndrome (serious threat if aortic root dilated <4cm).
- Prosthetic cardiac valves.

*High-risk conditions*

- Pulmonary hypertension (primary), in Eisenmenger's syndrome, (residual) after closure of non-restrictive ventricular septal defect.
- Tight mitral stenosis.
- Severe aortic stenosis.
- Myocardial infarction.
- Cardiomyopathies with a low ejection fraction (<35%).
- Any case where there is heart failure which is difficult to control. The fetus may be at particularly high risk when maternal cyanosis or heart failure is present.

Some cardiac conditions may require antibiotic cover prophylactically for the prevention of endocarditis, at the onset of spontaneous labour, or for obstetric procedures such as induction of labour.

## References

26 Mooney M (2007). Managing cardiac disease in pregnancy. *Br J Midwifery* 15: 2.
27 Royal College of Obstetricians and Gynaecologists (2011). *Cardiac disease and pregnancy. Good practice No. 13.* Available at: ℳ www.rcog.org.uk/globalassets/documents/guidelines/goodpractice13cardiacdiseaseandpregnancy.pdf.
28 Siu SC, Colman JM (2001). Heart disease and pregnancy. *Heart* 85: 710–15.

## Pyrexia and sepsis

Pyrexia is defined as a persistent temperature above 38°C and is often associated with coincidental maternal infection such as upper respiratory tract infection. Pyrexia is also a symptom of the more serious condition sepsis. Early recognition and appropriate escalation of the symptoms of sepsis are essential to improving the outcome for the mother and unborn child.[29] Almost a quarter of deaths of all pregnant women during 2009–2012 were found to be due to sepsis.[30] Recommendations for the improvement of care of these women include early diagnosis, rapid antibiotic administration, and review by senior doctors and midwives.

### Risk factors and symptoms of sepsis

The following factors are associated with the risk of developing sepsis in pregnancy and should alert the midwife to the increased susceptibility of maternal infection which can quickly lead to sepsis if not recognized and treated quickly:[31]

- Obesity
- Impaired glucose tolerance test
- Impaired immunity
- Anaemia
- Vaginal discharge
- History of pelvic infection
- History of GBS infection
- Amniocentesis and other invasive uterine procedures
- Cervical cerclage
- Prolonged rupture of membranes
- Water birth
- Vaginal trauma
- Caesarean section
- Wound haematoma.
- Retained products of conception post-miscarriage or post-delivery
- Amniotomy
- Multiple vaginal examinations
- Catheterization
- Maternal sore throat or upper respiratory tract infection (or family member), e.g. group A streptococcal infection (GAS)
- Gestation <24 weeks.

Other symptoms of sepsis may include one or more of the following:
- Presence of risk factors
- Fever/diarrhoea
- Vomiting
- Abdominal/pelvic pain
- Rash
- Vaginal discharge/pelvic pain
- Vaginal discharge/unexpected heavy lochia

- Wound infection (abdominal or genital tract)
- Breast abscess or sore and painful breasts
- Pain and frequency of micturition.

## Identification and management of suspected sepsis

If the woman develops a raised temperature of 38°C (or 37.5°C in two consecutive readings)[29] with one or more of the following symptoms, the Sepsis Six package should be instigated:

- Temperature of ≥38°C or ≤36°C
- Heart rate >100bpm
- Increased respiration rate >20/min
- Abnormal white cell count <4 or >12
- Acutely altered mental state
- Blood glucose level of 7.7 or above in a non-diabetic woman.

In severe sepsis or septic shock, further symptoms may develop such as hypotension, increased oxygen requirements, reduced platelet count <100, hyperbilirubinaemia, decreased urine output (<0.5mL/kg/h for 2h despite fluid resuscitation), international normalized ratio (INR) >1.5, or activated partial thromboplastin time (APTT) >60s. If these symptoms present, then immediate stabilization of the woman by an anaesthetist and obstetrician in HDU is required.

If the woman triggers for the above criteria, perform the following tasks:
- Take vital signs and record on the MEOWS chart
- Take bloods for FBC, CRP, U/E, LFTs, glucose, lactate, G&S, blood cultures (if pyrexia ≥38°C)
- Throat swab
- MSU and high vaginal swab.

Treatment of sepsis should be commenced within the first hour of diagnosis.[29]
- Administer 100% oxygen via a face mask.
- Collect blood cultures.
- Commence IV antibiotics (discuss with the microbiologist).
- Commence fluid resuscitation (IV infusion and commence a fluid balance chart).
- Measure serum lactate levels.
- Consider catheterization.
- Cooling strategies: use of a fan, paracetamol, and tepid sponging of the skin may make the mother more comfortable and reduce the pyrexia.
- Use paracetamol for analgesia as NSAIDs can impede the ability of some antibiotics to fight GAS.
- Broad-spectrum IV antibiotics will be prescribed as per unit protocol (e.g. cefuroxime 750–1500mg IV 8h and metronidazole 500mg IV 8h).

A wide variety of organisms has been implicated in septic shock during pregnancy, including *Escherichia coli*, *Staphylococcus aureus*, and β-haemolytic *Streptococcus*.

Suspected septicaemia is an indication for transfer of the woman to a high dependency care facility, and the intensive care medical team, consultant obstetrician, and anaesthetist need to be involved prior to transfer.

## References

29  Fawzy M, Dunning G (2014). *Guideline for the care of women with sepsis*. Barnsley NHS Foundation Trust Maternity Guidelines.

30  Knight M, Kenyon S, Brocklehurst P, Neilson J, Shakespeare J, Kurinczuk JJ (eds.) on behalf of MBRRACE-UK (2014). *Saving Lives, Improving Mothers' Care: Lessons learned to inform future maternity care from the UK and Ireland Confidential Enquiries into Maternal Deaths and Morbidity 2009–12*. Oxford: National Perinatal Epidemiology Unit, University of Oxford.

31  Royal College of Obstetricians and Gynaecologists (2012). *Bacterial sepsis in pregnancy*. Green-top guideline No. 64a. Available at: ℘ www.rcog.org.uk/globalassets/documents/guidelines/gtg_64a.pdf.

# Infections

Care of the mother with an infection during pregnancy, labour, and the postnatal period should be individualized according to the needs of the woman and her family. Information shared among carers should be on a need-to-know basis in order to protect the woman's confidentiality.

## Hepatitis B

A woman newly diagnosed during pregnancy should have had the opportunity to discuss her management and been given written information about the condition. The Public Health Laboratory should have been informed of the diagnosis and a full hepatitis B serology obtained. If the woman is antigen-positive, neonatal hepatitis B immunoglobulin is indicated as there is a high risk of neonatal transmission. This can be obtained in advance on a named patient basis. Mother-to-child transmission of hepatitis B can be reduced if the baby receives the immunoglobulin and vaccination. In these situations, pregnant women with hepatitis B should not be offered a planned Caesarean section because there is insufficient evidence that this reduces mother-to-child transmission of hepatitis B virus.[32]

During labour, if possible:
- Do not apply a scalp electrode
- Do not perform FBS.

Options for analgesia are the same as for the woman who is hepatitis B-negative.

## Hepatitis C

Women who are infected with hepatitis C should not be offered a planned Caesarean section because this does not reduce mother-to-child transmission of the virus. However, if the woman is co-infected with hepatitis C virus and HIV, she should be offered a planned Caesarean section because it reduces mother-to-child transmission of both hepatitis C virus and HIV.[32]

As for hepatitis B, do not perform FBS or attach a fetal scalp electrode. The neonate will need paediatric follow-up, as detection of transmission may require more than one blood test over a 6- to 12-month period.

## HIV

Make arrangements for the birth in advance and liaise with the infectious diseases specialist and pharmacy, who need to know the EDD in advance in order to ensure enough stock of antiviral therapy. As early as possible in the antenatal period, give women with HIV information about the risks and benefits for them and their child of the HIV treatment options and the mode of birth so that they can make an informed decision.[32] It is not recommended to routinely offer a Caesarean section because of the woman's HIV status. Women taking antiretroviral therapy with a low viral load can be informed that the risk of HIV transmission is the same for a Caesarean section as a vaginal birth.[32]

Women who are not taking antiretroviral drugs or have a high viral load should be offered a Caesarean section. Most transmission is known to occur at around the time of delivery, and an elective Caesarean delivery

before the membranes rupture is known to lower vertical transmission rates compared with an emergency section or a vaginal delivery.[33]
- For women who choose to have a vaginal delivery, do not apply a fetal scalp electrode or perform scalp sampling.
- Avoid ARM if possible in HIV-positive women.
- Offer the same analgesia as would be offered to other women in labour.
- Zidovudine infusion can be commenced prophylactically during labour, to help prevent maternal–fetal transmission of the virus.[33]
  - A continuous infusion of 2mg/kg over 1h, followed by 1mg/kg/h until the umbilical cord is clamped.
  - For an elective Caesarean section, the infusion can be started 4h prior to the operation at 2mg/kg for 1h, followed by 1mg/kg/h until the umbilical cord is clamped.
- Procedures at birth include obtaining blood samples from the baby, after washing, to test for antibodies and the potential effects of zidovudine treatment during pregnancy.

## Herpes

Neonatal herpes is a severe systemic viral infection with high morbidity and mortality. The risks are greatest when a woman acquires a primary infection during late pregnancy, so the baby is born before the development of protective maternal antibodies.[34] Women with primary genital HSV infection occurring in the third trimester of pregnancy should be offered a planned Caesarean section because it decreases the risk of neonatal HSV infection.[32,34]
- Consider any woman developing lesions within 6 weeks of birth for a Caesarean section, as shedding of the virus during labour is high.
- Daily suppressive aciclovir 400mg tds should be considered as treatment for herpes in pregnancy.[34]

## Primary or recurrent genital lesions at the onset of labour

There is a 41% risk of vertical transmission.[33]
- There is some evidence to suggest that the benefit of a Caesarean section reduces if the membranes have been ruptured for >4h.
- If a woman presents in labour with genital lesions, management will be based on clinical assessment as there will not be time for confirmatory laboratory testing. A history of the woman's condition must be obtained in order to ascertain whether this is a primary or recurrent episode.
- Take a viral swab from the lesion(s) as the result may influence management of the neonate.
- The neonatologist should be informed.
- If vaginal birth is unavoidable, or it is >4h since the rupture of membranes, give IV aciclovir intrapartum to the mother (5mg/kg every 8h) and subsequently to the neonate (IV aciclovir 20mg/kg every 8h).[34]
- In these cases, do not use scalp electrodes and avoid FBS, ARM, and instrumental birth.
- An alternative approach for women who develop primary lesions within 6 weeks of birth is to offer them suppression therapy with aciclovir and vaginal birth. Discuss this with a GUM physician.

## Initiation of breastfeeding with risk of infection

- *HIV-positive*—if the woman is found to be HIV-positive, the woman should be discouraged from breastfeeding her baby as transmission via breast milk is increased; this is irrespective of the viral load.[35]
- *Hepatitis B*—a mother with hepatitis B can breastfeed her baby if the baby receives a vaccine course starting at birth.
- *Hepatitis C*—there is no evidence of transmission via breast milk; breastfeeding is appropriate.

## References

32 National Institute of Health and Care Excellence (2011). Chapter 1, Guidance. In: National Institute of Health and Care Excellence. *Caesarean section*. NICE guidelines CG132. Available at: ℘ www.nice.org.uk/guidance/cg132/chapter/1-recommendations.

33 British HIV Association (2014). *British HIV Association guidelines for the management of HIV infection in pregnant women 2012 (2014 interim review)*. Available at: ℘ www.bhiva.org/documents/Guidelines/Pregnancy/2012/BHIVA-Pregnancy-guidelines-update-2014.pdf.

34 Royal College of Obstetricians and Gynaecologists (2014). *Management of genital herpes in pregnancy*. Available at: ℘ www.rcog.org.uk/globalassets/documents/guidelines/genitalherpesotherguideline.pdf.

35 Pollard J, Poskitt J, Dunning G (2013). *Guideline for the management of babies born to substance misusing mothers*. Barnsley Hospital NHS Foundation Trust Maternity Guidelines.

# Group B haemolytic streptococcus

## Group B haemolytic *Streptococcus*

Group B haemolytic *Streptococcus* (GBS) is recognized as the most frequent cause of severe early-onset (at <7 days of age) infection in newborn infants.[36] Despite this, most units in the UK do not routinely screen for GBS as this is still not recommended.[36] The vast majority of cases are found incidentally through other routine antenatal surveillance such as a liquor sample at the time of SROM or a high vaginal swab taken during an investigative speculum examination.

### Treatment

It is worth noting that whilst IAP is recommended for the treatment and prevention of early-onset GBS,[37,38] a Cochrane review concluded that it has not been shown to reduce all causes of mortality or GBS-related mortality.[39] IAP should be offered in labour to prevent early-onset neonatal infection if the woman has:

- A history of a previous infant with neonatal GBS disease
- GBS colonization, infection, or bacteriuria found in this pregnancy (if GBS is detected in pregnancy, it should be treated at the time of detection as well as offering treatment in labour).

IAP should be considered in the intrapartum period if the woman has:

- Preterm labour with pre-labour rupture of membranes of any duration
- Preterm labour with intrapartum rupture of membranes of >18h duration.

Antibiotic therapy should be given as soon as possible after the onset of labour, ideally at least 2h prior to birth. Treatment should be continued until the birth of the baby and will consist of:

- Penicillin 3g IV followed by 1.5g every 4h until birth, or clindamycin 900mg IV given 8-hourly if the woman is allergic to penicillin
- Benzylpenicillin with gentamicin is recommended for empirical treatment of suspected infection.

Antibiotic therapy is not required in the following circumstances:

- Evidence of GBS colonization in a previous pregnancy
- Planned Caesarean section (unless evidence of SROM).

NB. Antibiotics should also be considered to treat or prevent the development of chorioamnionitis and/or maternal sepsis in cases where there is:

- Maternal pyrexia ≥38°C on one occasion or ≥37.5°C twice in 1h apart
- Prolonged rupture of membranes ≥24h at term
- Evidence of actual or suspected infection from incidental testing.

### References

36 Royal College of Obstetricians and Gynaecologists (2012). *The prevention of early-onset neonatal group B streptococcal disease.* Green-top guideline No. 36, 2nd edn. Available at: ℅ www.rcog.org. uk/globalassets/documents/guidelines/gtg36_gbs.pdf.
37 National Institute of Health and Care Excellence (2012). *Neonatal infection: antibiotics for prevention and treatment.* NICE guidelines CG149. Available at: ℅ www.nice.org.uk/guidance/CG149.
38 Dunning G, Glymond B, Hamdan (2013). *Guideline for the prevention of early onset neonatal infection (including but not exclusive to GBS).* Barnsley NHS Foundation Trust Maternity Guidelines.
39 Ohlsson A, Shah VS (2009). Intrapartum antibiotics for known maternal group B streptococcal colonization. *Cochrane Database Syst Rev* 3: CD00746.

## Preterm labour

### Definitions

### Induction of preterm delivery

## Preterm labour

Preterm labour is the most important single factor of adverse infant outcomes in regard to both survival and quality of life for the neonate. The risk of death or neurosensory disability increases with decreasing gestational age.[40] With this information in mind, preterm birth is very likely to have a huge psychosocial and emotional effect on the family, as well as being costly for health services. For the midwife caring for such vulnerable families, it is important to consider the holistic needs of the woman and not just the clinical tasks in hand.

### Definitions

- *Threatened preterm labour*: pregnancy complicated by clinically significant uterine activity but without cervical change.
- *Preterm labour*: the occurrence of regular painful uterine contractions (>1 every 10min) which cause cervical effacement or dilatation prior to 37 completed weeks of pregnancy. Other signs may be rupture of membranes, a mucoid show, or a positive Actim Partus test. It should also be noted that occasionally women with a gestation below 37 weeks may present without contractions but still be dilating (silent cervical dilating).
- The WHO gives the following definitions for the different stages of preterm birth:[41]
  - Extremely preterm: <28 weeks
  - Very preterm: from 28 to <32 weeks
  - Moderate to late preterm: from 32 to <37 weeks.

### Preterm, pre-labour rupture of the membranes

Preterm, pre-labour rupture of the membranes (PPROM) complicates only 2% of pregnancies but is linked with 40% of preterm deliveries and can result in significant neonatal morbidity and mortality.[42] The three main causes of neonatal death connected with PPROM are prematurity, sepsis, and pulmonary hypoplasia.[42] There is evidence to suggest a link between lower genital tract infection and PPROM. In patients with PPROM, about one-third of pregnancies have been found to have positive amniotic fluid cultures; studies have shown that bacteria have the ability to cross intact membranes.[43]

### Incidence of preterm delivery

- 7.3% of births were preterm[44] in England and Wales in 2011/2012, and 5.9% in Scotland. Northern Ireland currently does not collect statistics of preterm births.
- The majority (92.7%) occur between 28 weeks and 36+6 weeks' gestation.
- Nearly 85% of all babies born prematurely will have a very low birthweight (under 1000g).
- Less than one-quarter of UK preterm births are <32 weeks' gestation.

## Some predisposing factors
- Pre-eclampsia, eclampsia.
- APH, placental abruption, placenta praevia.
- Intrauterine growth retardation.
- Disease or infection in the woman or fetus.
- PPROM.
- Intrauterine death.
- Multiple pregnancy.
- Polyhydramnios.
- Congenital abnormalities.
- Previous preterm labour (in selected cases, cervical suture may have been placed to reduce the risk of a second preterm delivery).
- Cervical incompetence (may be a result of cervical surgery or surgical termination of pregnancy).

## Risks of preterm delivery
- Major problems occur for babies born after 24 weeks' (when the baby is viable) and before 33 weeks' gestation.
- Fetal death may occur as a result of intraventricular haemorrhage, RDS, infection, jaundice, hypoglycaemia, or necrotizing enterocolitis.
- In cases of PPROM, survival rates for the neonate are linked to the gestation at which the membranes rupture rather than the duration of rupture. There is a high risk of chorioamnionitis.
- The prognosis for the neonate depends on the antenatal administration of steroids to the mother, the gestation and birthweight, the condition at birth, and the immediate care after birth, including the availability of a neonatal intensive care unit (NICU).

## Preterm labour before 24 weeks' gestation
If a woman gives birth before 24 weeks' gestation,[45] it is much less likely that the baby would survive. Babies who do survive after such a premature birth often have serious health problems.[46] Caring for women experiencing very early preterm labour and birth is a very sensitive issue and requires careful and considered communication from the multidisciplinary team. There is a global consensus that at 22 weeks' gestation there is no hope of survival and that up to 22+6 weeks' gestation is considered the limit of human viability.

The parents should be given every opportunity to discuss the care of their unborn child with the senior paediatrician. Discussions should be had with the parents and paediatrician about the possible prognosis, outcomes, and any decisions regarding resuscitation. All management plans should be documented in the woman's notes. The main points to consider when caring for a woman in very early preterm labour include:
- The most appropriate method of surveillance for the fetus. Each woman will have an individualized plan of care decided by the woman, the consultant obstetrician, and paediatrician. CTG is not seen to be beneficial in this situation
- Auscultation of the fetal heart during labour can be at the discretion of the midwife
- The neonatal team should be at the delivery unless an intrauterine death has been confirmed.

## Diagnosis and management of preterm labour >24 weeks' gestation

A woman may present to the delivery suite with regular painful contractions before 37 weeks' gestation.[45,47] Check local guidance for the most appropriate place to give care. It may be necessary to undertake an *in utero* transfer to a tertiary centre if the woman presents at a unit without specialist equipment/skills to deal with the very premature neonate.[45]

The midwife should:

- Inform an obstetrician. If necessary, transfer from midwifery to consultant care
- Acknowledge the woman's anxiety and explain the rationale for care
- Review and summarize her obstetric history and the history of her current pregnancy. Note her Rh status and blood grouping
- Record a history of the recent episode leading up to the admission
- Ask the woman whether she has had any recent injury or illness
- Assess her respirations, temperature, pulse, oxygen saturation, and BP; record on the MEOWS chart. Request an MSU sample and dispatch it to the laboratory for urgent culture and antibiotic sensitivity to exclude a urinary tract infection
- Perform a gentle abdominal palpation and assessment. Assess especially the fetal size, lie, and presentation. If the woman is 26 weeks' gestation or more, measure the fundal height with a disposable tape measure and record on the mother's personalized growth chart
- There is a risk of cord presentation/prolapse if the fetus is breech or the lie oblique. Listen for the fetal heart with Doppler and ask about the frequency of fetal movements
- Assess abdominal tenderness, tension, and irritability. Sit beside the woman for a while, allowing time to assess the length, strength, and frequency of uterine contractions. Regular contractions lasting 30s, at least once every 10min, may be significant
- Ask about any discharge per vaginum (blood or fluid)
- Ask about pain other than the pain from contractions (e.g. renal pain)
- Monitor the contractions and fetal heart and movements via a CTG monitor:
  - Monitoring is not indicated if the gestational age is assessed to be <25+6 weeks' gestation
  - At <34 weeks, the fetal heart is less likely to demonstrate sleep/ wake patterns; accelerations to ten beats are considered normal in this context
- Document the findings and discuss them with the obstetrician
- Careful monitoring and assessment by the midwife will assist an accurate diagnosis of preterm labour.

*Further assessment will be made by the obstetrician.*

- Perform a speculum examination (rather than a digital assessment which may introduce infection and may augment labour) to assess cervical effacement/dilatation.

- Ensure privacy for the woman; obtain consent, and explain all procedures.
  - Ask the woman to rest on the bed for 30min and to wear a sanitary pad. This is to allow the collection of any fluid, the 'pooling of liquor' in the vagina prior to the assessment.
- Diagnosis of preterm labour is made if cervical dilatation is as much as 2cm, or a change in the cervix (length and dilatation) is noted over two speculum examinations, preferably performed by the same practitioner, 2–3h apart.
- Exclude vaginal bleeding/PPROM/discharge.
- Consider performing the Actim Partus test if membranes are intact.
- Exclude infection and take swabs for culture and antibiotic sensitivity: a high vaginal swab and an endocervical swab for *Chlamydia*, a rectal and introital swab for GBS.
- If infection is suspected, send blood cultures urgently to bacteriology.
- An ultrasound scan may be necessary, e.g. to assess fetal size, presentation, breathing movements, placental localization, and liquor volume. (The early pregnancy ultrasound scan will be most accurate when establishing gestation.)

## Treatment

- An IV line should be sited. Take blood samples for FBC and U/E, and G&S if labour seems to be establishing or there is any bleeding. If the cervix is <2cm in a primigravida or <3cm in a multigravida, commence 500mL of normal saline over 4h and give oral analgesia.
- If the woman's blood group is Rh-negative, take blood for Kleihauer's test. This test detects whether any (potentially Rh-positive) fetal cells have crossed over into the maternal circulation. This may happen, for example, as a result of injury or placental bleeding. In cases of threatened preterm labour, this cannot be excluded. Anti-D 500IU (which coats and eliminates any Rh-positive fetal cells in the mother's blood and so prevents maternal sensitivity) may be prescribed.

### Corticosteroids

Treatment: IM betamethasone 12mg × 2, given 24h apart. Alternatively dexamethasone may be given, 6mg IM in four doses, 12h apart.

- Corticosteroids should be administered to all women in preterm labour from 24+0 to 34+6 weeks' gestation and to all women in threatened preterm labour with the same gestation with a positive Actim Partus.
- Corticosteroids should be considered in cases of preterm labour at 23+0 to 23+6 weeks' gestation. This decision is usually taken on a case-by-case basis.
- Corticosteroids should also be considered in women with established or threatened preterm labour at 35+0 to 35+6 weeks' gestation.
- Corticosteroids should be administered to women undergoing elective LSCS prior to 38+6 weeks' gestation.
- *Contraindication* to administering steroids antenatally is active tuberculosis.
- *Caution* should be given to the administration of steroids antenatally if there is systemic maternal sepsis, and evidence of chorioamnionitis, or GDM (types 1 and 2) as steroids can exacerbate maternal hyperglycaemia.

*Tocolytics*

The aim of administering a tocolytic agent is to delay the birth to allow the administration of corticosteroids or to expedite transfer to another unit. Indications for use include:

• Suspected or proven preterm labour between 24 and 34 weeks' gestation
• Fibronectin positive
• Cervix <4cm dilated
• Intact membranes. Where PPROM has occurred, discuss with the consultant
• Transfer to a neighbouring unit, irrespective of the gestational age and the state of the membranes.

*Relative contraindications for tocolysis*

• Fetal distress.
• Intrauterine infection.
• APH.
• Any maternal medical condition that warrants delivery (e.g. pre-eclampsia).
• Any maternal medical disorder where the chosen tocolytic drug is contraindicated.

*Administration of tocolysis*

• Prior to administering tocolysis, discussions with the consultant should be recorded, particularly if there has been SROM and/or the woman's gestation is between 22 and 24 weeks.
• Women who most benefit from the use of tocolysis are those who are still very preterm, women who need a delay in the labour in order to facilitate transfer to a unit with specialist neonatal intensive care facilities, and women who have not yet received a full course of corticosteroids.[40]
• Atosiban is the most common tocolysis drug; however, nifedipine may be used as an alternative, but this is not licensed in the UK for this medical condition.
• Atosiban is a oxytocin antagonist and is administered IV in three stages (the following is a suggestion and local guidance should be followed):
  • Initial bolus: 6.75mg over 1min
  • Preparation of IV infusion: remove 10mL from a 100mL bag of 0.9% sodium chloride. Replace this with 10mL of atosiban 7.5mg/mL concentration of solution for infusion from two 5mL vials. Infuse at 24mL/h for 3h
  • Reduce the infusion to 8mL/h (7.5mg concentration for infusion diluted in 100mL solution) × 3–48h
  • The woman should be re-assessed after 18h of treatment.

*Antibiotics*

Routine antibiotics for idiopathic preterm labour with intact membranes are not indicated. If SROM has occurred, there is evidence to suggest that erythromycin 250mg 6-hourly over 10 days may delay the birth and reduce maternal and neonatal infective morbidity. Clindamycin is an alternative antibiotic. Co-amoxiclav should not be used as there is an increased incidence of neonatal necrotizing enterocolitis. Antibiotic prophylaxis should be considered in the intrapartum period if the woman has preterm labour with pre-labour rupture of membranes of any duration or preterm labour with intrapartum rupture of membranes of >18h duration.

## Management of preterm delivery

- One-to-one midwifery care is especially recommended.
- Liaise with other members of the team. The plan of care should be discussed between obstetric, anaesthetic and theatre, neonatal, and senior midwifery staff and parents.
- Monitor documentation of the plan in the woman's notes.
- Ensure that corticosteroids and antibiotics are given if necessary.
- Arrange an ultrasound scan to:
  - Confirm the fetal lie and presentation
  - Give an estimated fetal weight
  - Exclude serious abnormality.

*If the fetus is between 22 and 26 weeks' gestation*

- When a cot is not available locally, *in utero* transfer will be considered by the obstetrician for all threatened preterm deliveries above 22 weeks' gestation. Sometimes it may be that delivery, assessment, and postnatal transfer are more appropriate.
- Before delivery, communication with parents is especially important. They need to understand, discuss, and agree what care is appropriate. They should be made aware of the morbidity and mortality risks to their baby. Survival rates are poor below 24 weeks' gestation.
  - Follow the agreed management plan when discussing the family's needs. Be a sympathetic listener and encourage the parents to seek psychological support from family, friends, and other networks.
  - Help the parents to understand how their baby may look at delivery. Discuss the approximate size, features of prematurity, and possible bruising which may be present after delivery.
  - The parents should understand the procedure that will be followed. Be prepared to repeat explanations. Distressed and anxious parents may not remember information.
  - Check that the content of the paediatrician's discussions with the parents are documented in the woman's notes.
  - If the plan is to resuscitate the baby, the parents should understand that the baby's condition will be continually assessed and care will be provided in the NICU as long as this is appropriate.
- Initial assessment of the gestational age by ultrasound is important, alongside the mother's menstrual history. It may help determine the action necessary.
- A Caesarean section is rarely appropriate below 25 weeks' gestation. There are significant risks of complications for the mother when the lower uterine segment is not formed. Each case should be considered individually. The consultant may seek a second obstetric opinion.
- Monitor the fetal heart unobtrusively and intermittently, unless requested to monitor continuously by the obstetrician. At early gestation, an abnormal fetal heart trace would not necessarily be acted

upon. It is also sometimes difficult and time-consuming to attempt to obtain a continuous trace when the fetus is very preterm.

- Once established, labour may progress quickly. The cervix may not need to dilate to the traditional 10cm before delivery. Early preparation for delivery and confirmation of availability of personnel will minimize anxiety and help the delivery run smoothly.
- Call the paediatrician to attend all births thought to be >22 weeks' gestation to assess the condition of the baby at birth and to make a decision about resuscitation.
- At >23 weeks' gestation, the paediatrician and neonatal nurse team should attend the birth to assess the baby's condition and resuscitate actively if appropriate.
- The response of the baby to resuscitation determines whether the baby is transferred to the neonatal unit for further intensive care and assessment.
- If there has been no time to discuss a plan of action with the parents, it is acceptable to offer intensive care 'provisionally', pending further assessment and discussion.
- The placenta may be sent to histology for examination.

*If the fetus is >27 weeks' gestation*
- When a diagnosis of preterm labour is made, arrange for the parents to visit a NICU and to discuss the plan of action with the paediatrician and neonatal team.
- Ensure that the parents understand what will happen at delivery.
- The environment of care is particularly important when labour is preterm. If psychological stress is reduced, the woman may labour more effectively, with better tolerance of pain. The midwife can help provide a peaceful environment by minimizing the number of staff, interruptions, intrusive noise, or light.

*During the first stage of preterm labour*
- Monitor the woman as for a normal first stage.
- Encourage the intake of light snacks and fluids. (The anaesthetist may suggest oral ranitidine 150mg 6-hourly as an antacid in the case of emergency anaesthesia.)
- Enable the woman to mobilize. This will enhance the normal descent and well-being of the fetus. The woman's comfort may be improved with mobility. Supine positions may increase the FHR.
- If possible, provide one-to-one support with a variety of coping strategies. This may enhance the woman's experience of labour and reduce her needs for analgesia.
  - Choices for analgesia include TENS, Entonox®, and patient-controlled analgesia.
  - If opiates must be used for maternal analgesia, explain possible side effects to the woman—opiates can make the baby slow to breathe at delivery, or sleepy, with limited interest in suckling.

- Monitor the fetal heart according to the obstetrician's recommendations and parents' preference. When considering continuous monitoring (CTG), remember that the preterm fetus may demonstrate a different heart pattern:
  - The baseline may be higher than 160bpm
  - The variability may be reduced
  - Bradycardia and variable decelerations may occur more frequently.
- FBS and the use of ventouse extraction should not be used in gestations ≤34 weeks. If performed, provide support for the mother during the procedure.
- Take particular care to minimize the number of vaginal examinations, which may increase the risk of infection.
- ARM should also be avoided:
  - There is a risk of infection to the fetus
  - Cord compression or prolapse may occur
  - It may precipitate variable decelerations in the fetal heart.
- The midwife's role in the first stage of preterm labour is to observe maternal and fetal progress, support the parents, coordinate care, and report deviations from normal.

*The second stage of labour*
- Prepare a warm environment, with warm towels ready. Switch off fans and close windows.
- Check that resuscitation equipment is complete and functioning and that the heater is on. Inform neonatal staff of the impending delivery, allowing time for them to be prepared.
- The unit supervisor and the obstetrician may wish to be informed.
- If the fetal condition appears satisfactory and descent is evident, there is no necessity to limit time in the second stage.
- Pushing should be spontaneous. Encourage the woman to push as she wishes. If the woman has chosen epidural anaesthesia, do not allow it to wear off in the second stage, but let the head descend to the perineum, then encourage pushing. Directed active pushing may cause fetal compromise.
- Episiotomy is only necessary as an emergency when fetal compromise is evident.
- Forceps and ventouse will be avoided by the obstetrician (especially at <34 weeks' gestation) because they may cause trauma to the fetal head.
- At delivery, the low-risk preterm baby may benefit from being wrapped in a warmed towel and held below the level of the uterus for 30s. This may allow the normal physiological changes to take place and the optimum transfusion of blood via the cord.
- Depending on the gestation of the baby, it may be necessary to keep the baby wet and place into the neonatal plastic bag which aims to maintain the neonate's body temperature during transfer or resuscitation away from the mother.
- If the baby does not require being placed into a neonatal plastic bag, gently dry the baby, then place on the mother's abdomen and encourage the mother to keep the baby in skin-to-skin contact. The baby's head and body should be well covered with warmed towels to prevent heat loss.

*The third stage of labour*
- The third stage may be managed physiologically or actively.
- Clamp and cut the cord only if the baby is in need of urgent resuscitation and this is required by the neonatal team.
- Delayed clamping and cutting may be applied even when the third stage is managed actively. It may reduce anaemia in the preterm neonate and the red cell transfusion requirements. It may also reduce the duration of the baby's need for oxygen therapy.
- The obstetrician may ask the midwife to double-clamp the cord so that venous and arterial cord blood samples can be taken for pH analysis. This provides a baseline and may aid neonatal management.
- When clamping and cutting the cord, leave approximately 6cm at the baby's end in case of a later need for umbilical catheterization.
- Although a baby may be compromised at delivery, it is important to encourage the parents to look at and touch their baby before transfer to the NICU.
- Where possible, encourage the maintenance of skin-to-skin contact, since this maintains the baby's temperature and may reduce the baby's stress response. It promotes bonding between the mother and baby. These may be important memories for the parents after the baby's transfer to the NICU. It may improve the duration of breastfeeding.
- It is the midwife's responsibility to ensure that baby identity labels are *in situ*—one on each ankle—before transfer to the NICU.
- Take surface swabs from the ear, axilla, and umbilicus of the baby if the membranes have been ruptured for longer than 72h. These will be sent for culture and determination of antibiotic sensitivity.
- Ensure that the neonatal team has access to the mother's notes.
- A photograph may be taken in the NICU and given to the parents.
- Encourage the parents to visit as soon as a mutually acceptable time can be arranged.
- The obstetrician may request histological examination of the placenta.

## References

40 Royal College of Obstetricians and Gynaecologists (2011). *Tocolysis for women in preterm labour. Green-top guideline No. 1b.* Available at: ℘ www.rcog.org.uk/globalassets/documents/guidelines/gtg_1b.pdf.
41 World Health Organization (2015). *Preterm birth.* Fact sheet No. 363. Geneva: World Health Organization. Available at: ℘ www.who.int/mediacentre/factsheets/fs363/en/.
42 Royal College of Obstetricians and Gynaecologists (2010). *Preterm prelabour rupture of membranes. Green-top guideline No. 44.* Available at: ℘ www.rcog.org.uk/globalassets/documents/guidelines/gtg_44.pdf.
43 Galask R, Varner M, Petzold C, Wilbur S (1984). Bacterial attachment to the chorionic membranes. *Am J Obstet Gynecol* 148: 915–28.
44 Office for National Statistics (2014). *Gestation-specific infant mortality, 2012.* Available at: ℘ webarchive.nationalarchives.gov.uk/20160105160709/http://www.ons.gov.uk/ons/dcp171778_379562.pdf.
45 Fawzy M, Dunning G (2015). *Guideline for women in preterm labour (including labour at a low gestational age).* Barnsley NHS Hospital Foundation Trust Maternity Guidelines.
46 Royal College of Obstetricians and Gynaecologists (2014). *Information for you: premature labour.* RCOG patient information. Available at: ℘ www.rcog.org.uk/globalassets/documents/patients/patient-information-leaflets/pregnancy/pi-premature-labour.pdf.
47 National Institute of Health and Care Excellence (2015). Maternal corticosteroids. In: National Institute of Health and Care Excellence. *Preterm labour and birth.* NICE guidelines NG25. Available at: ℘ www.nice.org.uk/guidance/ng25/chapter/1-Recommendations#maternal-corticosteroids.

## Induction of labour

*Definition*: labour is initiated using mechanical and/or pharmacological methods. The intervention is necessary when the well-being of the mother or baby may be at risk if the pregnancy is continued. The parents should be in agreement and fully informed of procedures.[48]

### Some indications

- Post-maturity.
- PROM (>37 weeks).
- PIH, pre-eclampsia.
- APH.
- Placental insufficiency and IUGR.
- Large fetus, twins.
- Diabetes, renal disease, or other underlying conditions.
- IUD.

### Method of induction

A prostaglandin pessary is used to soften/ripen the cervix. When this is achieved, the membranes are ruptured (amniotomy) and an oxytocin infusion commenced to stimulate regular uterine contractions and dilatation of the cervix. Most women are induced as inpatients; however, there is a move to provide an outpatient induction of labour service for low-risk women in some trusts. This should only take place where there is adequate support for the woman and the service is audited regularly.[49]

### Management

- If a consultant-booked woman requires induction of labour, always act under the instructions of the obstetric consultant or registrar.[49,50]
- The obstetric consultant or registrar should authorize the induction and write the indication and method in the woman's notes.
- If a low-risk midwifery-led woman attends for induction of labour, transfer her care to the consultant on call for that day.
- The woman will be admitted to the delivery suite or antenatal ward, depending on local guidance and the consultant management plan.
- Carefully explain the length of time that induction may take and the procedures involved and possible outcomes. This will help to alleviate the prospective parents' anxiety and enable them to make appropriate arrangements for hospital admission.
- Before commencing the induction, ensure that:
  - The woman and her partner understand and consent. If induction fails, a Caesarean section is indicated
  - The rationale for induction is documented and current
  - The estimated date of delivery is correct and, if possible, confirmed on an early pregnancy scan
  - The presenting part is engaged (3/5 palpable abdominally)
  - The fetal heart (CTG) has been monitored for 30min and is reassuring

- The obstetric registrar has prescribed the treatment (if the woman is being induced purely for post-maturity, the trust may have a *patient group directive* (PGD), meaning that the midwife can write up the prostaglandin on the woman's treatment card)
- The woman is comfortable and has passed urine.
- Ensure that the woman's dignity and privacy are preserved at all times.

## Bishop score

You should be experienced in assessing the state of the cervix.

- The Bishop score[50] (Table 21.2) is a frequently used system of assessing the cervix which can give a clear indication of progress. The score should be recorded in the woman's notes each time an assessment is made, i.e. at the time of administration of prostaglandin gel and amniotomy.
- The higher the initial score, the more successful the induction.

If the Bishop score is:

- 0 to 6: the cervix is unfavourable for induction and a prostaglandin pessary will be necessary to soften the cervix
- 6 and above: the cervix is very favourable and prostaglandin is not required.

Variations on this scoring include one recommended in the NICE guidelines.[49]

## Sweeping the membranes

When a woman's care during pregnancy has been midwifery-led, induction of labour should be discussed by the midwife towards term. The community midwife may arrange with the delivery ward for the induction to be planned for a mutually convenient time. Prior to induction of labour in hospital, offer the woman a vaginal examination to assess the state of the cervix and to perform a sweeping of the membranes. This has been shown to increase the possibility of labour occurring naturally within the following 48h.[51] Nulliparous women can be offered membrane sweeps at 40 and 41 weeks' gestation; multiparous women are offered this at 41 weeks' gestation.[49] If the membrane sweep is discussed at a previous appointment, the woman has the opportunity to arrange support for the visit if she wishes.

**Table 21.2** Modified Bishop (Calder) score

| Score | 0 | 1 | 2 | 3 |
|---|---|---|---|---|
| Dilatation (cm) | <1 | 1–2 | 2–4 | 5 or more |
| Cervical length (cm) | 5 or more | 2–4 | 1–2 | <1 |
| Station above spines (cm) | −3 | −2 | −1/0 | +1/+2 |
| Consistency | Firm | Average | Soft | |
| Position | Posterior | Central/anterior | | |

This procedure may be performed in the woman's home or at an ante-natal clinic visit. It may be a preferable first step to stimulate labour and sometimes may pre-empt formal induction.
- The pregnancy should be uncomplicated.
- The gestational age should be term (40 or 41 weeks for nulliparous women and 41 weeks for multiparous women).
- The membranes must be intact.
- Warn the woman that she may experience some discomfort as a result of the procedure and that she may have a mucoid/bloodstained 'show' and should wear a light sanitary pad.
- Reassure her that membrane sweeping is not associated with increased maternal or neonatal infection.
- Auscultate the FHR and perform an abdominal palpation; record the information in the maternal notes.
- Perform a vaginal examination and locate the cervix. A finger is inserted through the internal os, stretching the cervix slightly, and the membranes are palpated. Use a sweeping circular movement of the finger to separate the fetal membranes from the decidua/lower uterine segment.
- There is potential for a natural rapid increase in prostaglandin production in late pregnancy. Sweeping of the membranes is a mechanical stimulant to tissue prostaglandin release in the cervix and lower segment. This, in turn, can initiate the onset of labour.

### Prostaglandins for induction of labour

Propess®[50] is a vaginal delivery system containing 10mg of dinoprostone (PGE2). Propess® is a sustained-release preparation delivering an active agent over 24h. Each maternity unit will have their own guidance on which prostaglandins are to be used in which circumstances; below is an example.
- Obtain consent from the woman; perform abdominal palpation to assess the fetal lie, presentation, and size. Perform maternal baseline observations. Auscultate the FHR and record all findings.
- Commence CTG for 30min prior to the administration of the prostaglandin.
- Perform a vaginal examination (with informed consent) and assess the cervix using the Bishop score.
- If the woman's cervix is not favourable (Bishop score <6), or the woman is a primigravida regardless of the Bishop score with no contractions, use the Propess® vaginal delivery system to soften/ripen the cervix, as follows:
  - The Propess® should be removed from the freezer 20min prior to insertion. It should then be positioned in the posterior fornix of the vagina using only a small amount of water-soluble lubrication
  - The Propess® should lie transversely and after insertion the withdrawal tape should be cut to within 1–2 cm of the introitus. Ensure that there is sufficient tape outside the vagina to allow removal. The woman should be encouraged to remain resting on the bed for 30min after insertion.
- Record the Bishop score and time of the procedure in the notes.

- Encourage the woman to rest on the bed for an hour following the procedure, during which time the fetal heart is monitored continuously. If the recording is reassuring, the woman should mobilize and eat/drink as normal.
- Warn the woman that she may experience mild discomfort/soreness in the vagina as a result of prostaglandin, or painful uterine contractions caused by the prostaglandin prior to the onset of the regular contractions of labour. Oral or IM analgesics may be prescribed.
- Advise the woman to inform the midwife if contractions become regular (≥3 in 10min), she becomes uncomfortable and requires pain relief, or she experiences vaginal bleeding or SROM, or if the Propess® falls out or drops into the lower vagina.
- *One hour following insertion:*
  - Record maternal observations on MEOWS (PGE2 may cause mild pyrexia, due to its effect on cerebral thermoregulatory centres)
  - Auscultate the fetal heart and document
  - Determine uterine activity
  - Note and manage any adverse effects, i.e. nausea, vomiting, fever, vaginal irritation, abdominal pain, vaginal bleeding, hypertonic uterine activity, abnormal FHR.
- *Performed as a minimum every 6h* (in the absence of regular uterine activity or rupture of membranes):
  - Maternal observations
  - Auscultation of the fetal heart
  - Assessment of the strength and frequency of contractions
  - Assessment of vaginal loss
  - Monitor and discuss pain management.
- If there are no signs of labour commencing, Propess® must be removed 24h after insertion. At this point, the woman should be assessed to see if an amniotomy is possible. If this is not possible, a review by an obstetrician must occur to decide on an appropriate management plan.
- A CTG should be performed if the woman is experiencing regular contractions (≥3 in 10min). Once the CTG is assessed as normal, it can be discontinued and intermittent auscultation can be used.
- Once labour is established, follow the process for normal labour. CTG is not indicated once the onset of labour occurs in low-risk women.

*Contraindications for the use of dinoprostone*
- Labour is already established.
- Allergy to prostaglandin.
- Placenta praevia.
- Unexplained vaginal bleeding at the time of induction.
- Severe fetal growth restriction with abnormal Doppler studies.
- Parity—women with >3 full-term deliveries.
- Suspicious or pathological CTG.
- Oxytocic drugs are already being administered.
- Evidence of cephalopelvic disproportion.
- Fetal malpresentation.
- Pre-labour rupture of membranes at term.

Some women who are considered high risk can also be induced using Propess®. In each case, a clear individualized management plan must be recorded in the antenatal notes. (An example of a high-risk management plan may be that a woman who has undergone a previous LSCS may have the Propess® removed after 12h rather than the maximum 24h). All risks and possible outcomes should have been explained to the woman and her partner prior to admission to hospital. High-risk inductions should always occur on the labour ward.

## Artificial rupture of the membranes

- If the cervix is favourable (i.e. Bishop score >6), then it may be possible to perform an amniotomy for induction of labour.
- Amniotomy may be performed if:
  - The senior registrar authorizes/performs the procedure in the high-risk client
  - The woman understands the procedure and consents
  - The fetal head is engaged or 3/5 palpable abdominally
  - The CTG is reassuring.

*Management*
- The woman may value the support of a partner/friend. She should understand that she can withdraw consent to the procedure at any point if she so wishes.
- The procedure is performed using sterile pack, gloves, lubricant, amnihook, protection for couch, and clothing.
- Monitor the fetal heart continuously.
- Entonox® should be available in case the woman experiences discomfort.
- The woman should pass urine prior to the procedure.
- Perform a vaginal examination; assess the Bishop score; insert a finger through the internal os and palpate the membranes and forewaters. Introduce the amnihook along the examining fingers and perform the amniotomy.
- Address the woman's hygiene needs.
- Document the Bishop score, time of amniotomy, and colour and volume of the liquor.
- Monitor the fetal heart:
  - Continuously following the procedure
  - For 60min when the induction is in a low-risk woman; thereafter the fetal heart should be monitored intermittently (each 15min) until contractions occur regularly or IV oxytocin is commenced.
- If the woman is not experiencing regular contractions, administer an oxytocin regimen:
  - Immediately after ARM for all primigravidae and multigravidae with an urgent indication for induction such as pre-eclampsia
  - 2h after ARM if regular contractions have not commenced and if multiparous and a non-urgent indication for delivery.

*Complications*

- Prolapsed cord may occur if the fetal head is not engaged when the membranes are ruptured or if it has not been recognized that the cord is presenting prior to the procedure.
- Non-reassuring fetal heart pattern may occur following ARM. This may be due to compression of the fetal head or placenta. It should settle to normal soon after.
- Increased infection risk once the membranes have been ruptured. It is important that effective progress in labour is achieved.

## Intravenous oxytocin

- Syntocinon® is a synthetic oxytocin. It is effective in stimulating uterine activity and promoting dilatation of the cervix.
- Before commencing oxytocin, ensure that:
  - The drug is prescribed by the registrar
  - The woman understands the procedure for administration, the restriction it will place on her mobility, and the analgesia available
  - 6h have elapsed if Prostin® vaginal tablets have been administered rather than Propess®
  - SROM is certain or that ARM has been performed
  - You are fully conversant with the client's obstetric history, since extreme caution is indicated in clients with a uterine scar or grand multiparity
  - You are aware of the current state of maternal observations, contractions, and cervical dilatation as a baseline
  - The fetal heart is monitored continuously and is reassuring.
- Siting of an IV cannula is a good time to take FBC/platelets and G&S in case of later need.
- Check the medication with a colleague—it can be given via IV infusion using a pump or a syringe driver. An example of the dilution of the oxytocin can be: 5IU of oxytocin in 50mL of 0.9% sodium chloride; this would be administered via a syringe driver at a starting rate of 4 milliunits per hour (2.4mL/h). This can then be increased every 30min by 4 milliunits, up to 12 milliunits, until there are effective uterine contractions.
- Titrate the dose against uterine activity.
- The aim is to achieve three or four regular contractions in 10min. There should be 1min relaxation between each contraction. To achieve this, the dose may be increased every 30min, as shown in Table 21.3.
- Further increases should be discussed with the obstetric registrar.

*Risks/complications of oxytocin administration*

You should remain in attendance, ensuring the safety of the mother and fetus, and observe for the following.

- The uterus may be hyperstimulated. This may cause FHR irregularities. Stop the infusion temporarily and observe the FHR. If the abnormality persists, inform the registrar who may perform FBS. If the FHR becomes reassuring, the oxytocin may be restarted at half the preceding rate.

**Table 21.3** Oxytocin regime

| 2.4mL/h | 4 milliunits |
|---------|--------------|
| 4.8mL/h | 8 milliunits |
| 7.2mL/h | 12 milliunits |

Seek advice from the registrar/consultant before
increasing above 12 milliunits

- Hyperstimulation of the uterus could cause rupture. This rarely happens in primigravidae, but care is needed in multiparous women.
- PPH is more common following induction.
- Oxytocin may be ineffective on the cervical dilatation so that labour does not progress. A Caesarean section may be necessary.
- Oxytocin tends to encourage water retention. This is minimized by diluting it in normal saline. Care should be taken to monitor IV fluids infused and assess maternal observations.
- Amniotic fluid embolism is not now thought to be precipitated by oxytocin induction.

## References

48 Collins S, Arulkumaran S, Hayes K, Jackson S, Impey L (2013). *Oxford Handbook of Obstetrics and Gynaecology*. Oxford: Oxford University Press.

49 National Institute for Health and Care Excellence (2008). Chapter 1, Guidance. In: National Institute for Health and Care Excellence. *Inducing labour*. NICE guidelines CG70. Available at: ℞ www.nice.org.uk/guidance/cg70/chapter/1-recommendations.

50 Dunning G (2015). *Guideline for induction of labour, including the use of oxytocin*. Barnsley Hospital NHS Foundation Trust Maternity Guidelines.

51 Boulvain M, Stan M, Irion O (2005). Membrane sweeping for induction of labour. *Cochrane Database Syst Rev* 1: CD000451.

# Augmentation of labour: active management

A variety of protocols exist which are aimed at avoiding a long labour and maternal exhaustion and achieving delivery of the baby within 12–18h.

Augmentation of labour may be initiated if the normal progress of labour appears slow. You may consider active management in a normal labour without previous obstetric or antenatal complications if:

- The woman is definitely in established labour (changes in the cervix demonstrating progressive effacement and dilatation) but is making slow progress because the uterine activity appears limited
- The woman states that she understands the concept, interventions, and mobility restraints and prefers active management
- You have discussed the plan and obtained the agreement of the delivery suite coordinator and the obstetric registrar.

## Management

- Careful observation of maternal and fetal conditions is necessary.
- Accurate documentation of the interventions on the partogram is essential.
- Monitor the fetal heart continuously.
- Monitor the length, strength, and number of uterine contractions.
- Site an IV infusion.
- If the membranes are intact, following abdominal assessment, perform a vaginal examination and ARM. This may shorten the delivery time if used in conjunction with an oxytocin infusion. Remember, however, that hydrostatic pressure no longer cushions the placenta. There is a higher risk of fetal cardiac irregularities. There is also a risk of infection to the fetus.
- Note the current cervical dilatation, state of descent of the presenting part, and colour of the liquor.
- Some authorities suggest a cervicograph guide may be used to measure progress. Action is recommended if cervical dilatation is 2h behind the cervicograph curve. The oxytocin regimen may be commenced as for induction of labour.
- Vaginal examination (using a sterile procedure) may be performed at regular intervals, e.g. 2–3h, to ascertain progress.
- Assess the maternal BP and pulse half-hourly.
- Monitor the maternal temperature and urine output 2-hourly.
- Encourage the woman to take fluids.
- Be guided by the woman's choice for analgesia. Assist the woman to use upright positions and some non-pharmacological methods of pain relief. However, contractions augmented by oxytocin may be experienced as more painful than those of spontaneous labour.
- If a normal delivery is not achieved within the set time frame, inform the obstetric registrar.

# Measures to assist birth

It has been found that continuous support for women during childbirth can reduce the incidence of operative vaginal delivery, particularly when the carer was not a member of staff.[52] Also the use of any upright or lateral position in the second stage of labour compared with the supine or lithotomy position has been linked to a reduction in the number of assisted deliveries.[53] The midwife may be required to assist the obstetric team when an instrumental (ventouse or forceps) or a Caesarean delivery is necessary.

When caring for a woman in labour, the midwife should report the following to the obstetric registrar:

- FHR irregularities or abnormalities of the CTG occurring in the first or second stage of labour. The registrar may request FBS
- Delay in the first or second stage when the labour does not respond to oxytocin
- Deterioration in the woman's condition.

It may be necessary to deliver the baby quickly. A Caesarean section will be necessary to expedite birth in the first stage; after full dilatation, ventouse or forceps delivery may be possible. If there is doubt about achieving delivery by forceps, trial in theatre may be arranged, with the anaesthetist and theatre team present. A Caesarean section can follow immediately if forceps delivery fails.

## Instrumental delivery: forceps

The decision to deliver by forceps is made by the registrar or consultant. Indication for forceps delivery, explanation of the procedure, and possible problems should be discussed with the parents, and their consent obtained. Provide support for the woman during the delivery by further explanation, prompting her as appropriate, and monitoring her needs.

Indications for forceps delivery include:

- Delay in, or no progress during, the second stage, related to limited maternal expulsive effort and exhaustion
- Absence of the urge to 'push' because of epidural administration
- The woman has suffered a dural tap resulting in a severe headache which becomes worse when pushing
- When excessive pushing may worsen pre-eclampsia, cardiac conditions, myasthenia gravis, spinal cord injury, or proliferative retinopathy
- When CTG is non-reassuring, the fetal head is below mid cavity, and delivery can be more quickly achieved with forceps
- If there is suspected mild malposition or asynclitism which might be corrected and delivery facilitated.

The obstetric registrar will want to know the following:

- Does the fetus feel, on abdominal palpation, to be a normal size? Could there be disproportion present? Is the fetal head 'well down'? Is there <1/5 of the fetal head palpable above the pelvic brim?
- On vaginal examination, is the cervix fully dilated? Is the station of the head below the spines (+ 1cm)? Is the moulding or caput minimal? Is the position occipito-anterior (OA)? Is the liquor clear and the FHR reassuring?

- Does the woman experience strong and sustained regular uterine contractions which achieve some descent of the head with maternal 'pushing' effort?
- Does the woman have adequate pain relief? Is the epidural effective? Is a pudendal block needed?

*Preparation for the delivery*
- Discuss the procedure with the woman. A clear explanation should be given regarding the need to expedite the birth and options available. This verbal consent should be documented.
- The birthing bed needs preparation, with facility for the lithotomy position.
- Delivery pack.
- Eye protection.
- Gown and gloves.
- Instruments.
- Local anaesthetic.
- Syringes and sutures.
- Catheterization pack.
- Good light.
- Stool.
- Syntometrine® for the third stage, if appropriate.
- Protection for the birthing bed.
- Sanitary pads for the mother.

There are three different types of forceps (Table 21.4).

*Procedure*
- Determine the best place for the birth—if there are possibilities of a difficult instrumental delivery, consider transfer to theatre. Higher rates of failure are associated with: maternal BMI >30, estimated fetal weight over 4000g or clinically big baby, occipito-posterior position and/or mid-cavity delivery, or when 1/5 of the head palpable per abdomen.[54]
- If the woman has had an epidural, and there is no emergency, a top-up in the sitting position will give good perineal analgesia. Analgesia for a trial of instrumental delivery must always be adequate for an immediate Caesarean section.
- Consider the degree of urgency and inform the multidisciplinary team. Ensure the paediatrician is present for the birth.[55]
- Be prepared for other emergencies such as PPH or shoulder dystocia. Think of possible equipment required.
- Help the woman into the lithotomy position. Supine hypertension can be avoided if a cushion is placed to lift the woman slightly off her back. The partner may choose to sit beside her and give support.

Table 21.4 Types of delivery forceps

| Wrigley's | Small size, for 'lift-out' from lower cavity |
|---|---|
| Neville Barnes | Straight, mid-cavity, at least pudendal block required |
| Kielland's | Mid-cavity rotational forceps, epidural essential |

- The registrar/midwife performs the procedure as a clean/sterile technique:
  - The bladder is emptied
  - Effectiveness of analgesia is assessed
  - The appropriate forceps are applied between contractions
  - Rotation of the fetal head is attempted if needed
  - When the forceps are safely in place, traction is applied with contractions and the woman encouraged to push
  - The obstetrician may perform an episiotomy as the fetal head distends the perineum
  - The baby should be delivered within two or three contractions
  - The forceps are removed when the head is delivered and the baby can be delivered on to the mother's abdomen.

*Risks and complications*

*The baby*

- Examine the baby for bruising and/or abrasions to the skin of the scalp and face caused by the curved blades of the forceps. If bruising is severe, jaundice may develop.
- Occasionally, VIIth nerve paralysis will occur and facial palsy will be apparent. This is due to pressure on the nerve as it is compressed against the ramus of the mandible.
- Reassure the parents that these complications will usually resolve within a few days.
- In a traumatic forceps delivery, cerebral irritability may occur due to cerebral oedema or haemorrhage. Cephalhaematoma may occasionally form as a result of trauma from forceps delivery.

*The mother*

- The mother may experience vaginal tears caused by the forceps.
- Perineal bruising, oedema, and occasionally haematoma may occur.
- Perineal trauma may be caused by extended episiotomy.
- Bruising and trauma to the urethra may cause retention or dysuria, haematuria, or incontinence.

## Ventouse delivery

The application of a suction cup to the fetal scalp to facilitate delivery by traction is associated with less maternal trauma than forceps delivery. The indications for ventouse delivery are the same as for forceps. The obstetrician/midwife will need the same information before proceeding and the midwife will make similar preparations for delivery. Training is now available for specialist midwives to become ventouse practitioners.

*Selection of the ventouse extractor*

- Electric pumps are efficient at maintaining the optimum vacuum pressure and are easy to operate, with a variety of cups available.
  - The usual size is a 5cm silicon/rubber cup for a normal occipito-anterior presentation.
  - A posterior cup (which is sometimes metal and is flatter in shape) is available for occipito-transverse or posterior positions.

- Hand-operated vacuum pumps may appear less anxiety-provoking for the woman.
  - Examples are the Mityvac®, a cup for single use which can be attached to a hand-held pump, and the Kiwi Omnicup, a small and totally disposable device.

*Procedure*

- This procedure is not suitable for babies <34+0 weeks' gestation (should be used with caution between 34+0 and 36+0 weeks' gestation).
- Explain the procedure carefully to the woman and partner, and obtain consent. Keep them informed of progress.
- The maternal position used for delivery is lithotomy, as for forceps.
- Maintain an aseptic technique.
- Perform a vaginal examination and determine the position of the fetal head.
- Select an appropriate cup and apply to the fetal head at the midline, just in front of the occiput. The obstetrician will ensure that no cervix or vaginal tissue is trapped under the cup before applying suction.
- The vacuum is built up gradually from 0.5kg/cm to 0.8kg/cm.
- Once the optimum pressure is achieved, with a strong uterine contraction and maternal expulsive pushing, steady traction is exerted gently on the fetal head following the line of the pelvic axis (curve of Carus). Descent should occur and, if necessary, rotation to an anterior position may be achieved.
- An episiotomy is not usually needed. The head is controlled carefully during crowning. As soon as the head is delivered, the vacuum is released. The body is delivered as normal.
- The delivery should occur within 30min of a decision for operative vaginal delivery being made and abandon the procedure if:[55]
  - After three pulls there is no descent
  - The cup comes off three times
  - The application of suction to the fetal head is ≥12min
  - It is >30min.
- Following the birth, a vaginal and rectal assessment is required with informed consent to identify trauma. Conduct any perineal repair as necessary and ensure that analgesia is administered — consider a diclofenac suppository 100mg if appropriate.[55]

*Complications*

- The cup may slip off and the procedure may fail.
- The baby will have trauma to the scalp as a result of the suction. A chignon develops, which is an area of bruising and oedema with the approximate shape of the suction cup. This usually resolves without problem in a few days.
- Cephalhaematoma may occur and neonatal jaundice may develop.
- Retinal haemorrhage is a rare complication in the neonate.

## References

52  Hodnett ED, Gates S, Hofmeyr GJ, Sakala C (2007). Continuous support for women during childbirth. *Cochrane Database Syst Rev* 3: CD003766.
53  Gupta JK, Hofmeyr GJ, Smyth RMD (2000). Position in the second stage of labour for women without epidural anaesthesia. *Cochrane Database Syst Rev* 1: CD002006.
54  Royal College of Obstetricians and Gynaecologists (2011). *Operative vaginal delivery. Green-top guideline No. 26.* Available at: ℥ www.rcog.org.uk/globalassets/documents/guidelines/gtg26.pdf.
55  Dunning G, Fawzy M, Khanem N (2015). *Guideline for instrumental delivery (ventouse and forceps).* Barnsley NHS Foundation Trust Maternity Guidelines.

# Caesarean section

## Types of Caesarean section

### Classical Caesarean section

- This is used only in an emergency or when there is obstruction (placenta/fibroids) in the lower segment.
- It may be necessary to perform a Caesarean section prematurely when the lower segment is not fully formed (before 32 weeks' gestation).
- The incision is made longitudinally in the upper segment of the uterus. Since the upper segment has a thick muscular structure, there is a higher incidence of excessive blood loss and rupture of the scar subsequently.

### Lower segment Caesarean section

- This is the most common type of Caesarean section.
- The lower segment is thinner and not so vascular, therefore blood loss can be less, with better healing and lower infection rate. Cosmetically the 'bikini line' scar is more discrete and acceptable to women.

### Caesarean section and hysterectomy

Very occasionally, in a severe emergency, such as massive haemorrhage, uterine rupture, or an adherent placenta (placenta accreta), this might be necessary.

## Some indications for planned/elective Caesarean section

- Singleton breech presentation when ECV was ineffective or contraindicated.
- Transverse lie or malpresentation (such as brow presentation).
- Placenta praevia.
- A twin pregnancy when the first twin is not cephalic.
- Triplets.
- HIV where women are not receiving any antiretroviral therapy or have a viral load of ≥400 copies/mL, or have HIV and are co-infected with hepatitis C.
- Genital herpes is present during the third trimester of pregnancy.
- Maternal request, e.g. where there has been a previous delivery that caused physical or psychological trauma.[56,57]

### Plan of care

- Organize a consultant appointment to discuss the mode of delivery when the woman's pregnancy has reached about 36 weeks' gestation.
- The final decision should be made by a consultant obstetrician in conjunction with the parents.
- Give information clearly, in a way that can be understood by the parents.

### Difference of opinion

- If a consultant declines a request for a Caesarean section, the woman can request a second opinion and/or be referred to the local supervisory team for support in their birth choice.
- A competent pregnant woman can refuse a Caesarean section even if she puts herself and her baby at risk.[57]

*Arrangements for planned lower segment Caesarean section*

- The timing of the Caesarean section should ideally be after 39 weeks' gestation, to decrease the risks of respiratory morbidity to the baby.
- The day before the planned Caesarean section, the woman and her companion/partner may attend a clinic appointment or they may be seen on the antenatal ward.
  - At this visit, the obstetrician verifies the rationale for the operation, clearly documents this in the woman's hospital notes, and obtains written informed consent from the woman. Document the information given to the woman.
  - Assess baseline observations of BP, pulse, temperature, and urinalysis. Review fetal well-being; this may include an ultrasound scan.
  - The anaesthetist reviews the general health of the woman. The type of anaesthetic is discussed and confirmed with the woman—usually spinal/regional anaesthesia. If a spinal anaesthetic is accepted, the partner may accompany the woman in theatre to provide support. General anaesthetic may occasionally be requested by the woman or be necessary if the regional anaesthesia proves inadequate.
  - Obtain FBC and G&S and send for testing. However, NICE guidelines suggest that G&S is not necessary for a healthy woman with an uncomplicated pregnancy.[57]
  - During the Caesarean section, antibiotics should be given to the woman; therefore, carefully document any allergy.
  - LMWH (enoxaparin) will be prescribed prophylactically to help prevent DVT.
  - Ranitidine 150mg is prescribed 6-hourly. Usually two doses prior to a Caesarean section. This minimizes the amount of gastric acid produced. Ensure that the woman understands the need to take no food/drinks for at least 6h before the Caesarean section.
  - Explain the procedure, the immediate post-operative care, and the probable length of hospital stay. It should be recognized that whilst some women will feel content to experience a Caesarean section, others may miss the sense of achievement a normal delivery can afford. Be sensitive to this; listen, and answer questions. Refer to a birth afterthoughts clinic if required/available for debriefing.
  - Give the woman and her partner an appropriate time at which to attend the ward prior to the Caesarean section.
  - Women may be given an antibacterial scrub to be used prior to surgery to reduce skin colonization and promote wound healing.[56]
  - If the woman has a BMI >35, theatre staff should be made aware. Specialist equipment may be required for a very high BMI.

*On the day of the Caesarean section*

- Ideally, the woman and her partner should be welcomed by a midwife who is known to them. Throughout the procedure, the midwife should keep the couple informed of events affecting care.

- The midwife should prepare the woman for theatre. The woman may wish to have a bath. A shave of the skin area affected by the Caesarean section scar might be considered necessary. Provide a clean theatre robe, a cap, and anti-embolic stockings. Place an identity label on the woman's wrist and remove all jewellery or cover it with adhesive strapping. Re-assess maternal observations and listen to the fetal heart.
- Give sodium citrate 30mL orally prior to transfer. This neutralizes the gastric acid.
- Measure and fit anti-embolic stockings.
- Prepare documentation according to local protocol.
- Escort the woman and her partner to theatre where the theatre staff, obstetrician, and anaesthetist should welcome them.
- The anaesthetist sites an IV infusion and spinal anaesthetic. When the woman is positioned for the operation, the theatre table is tilted, or a wedge placed to facilitate a slight left lateral position, to prevent supine hypotension.
- When the woman is comfortable and the spinal anaesthetic is effective, insert an indwelling urinary catheter, since the bladder must be empty prior to the Caesarean section. This will remain in place for 24h.
- Women will be offered prophylactic antibiotics before skin incision. The woman should be informed that administering the antibiotics prior to the incision reduces the risk of maternal infection but has no detrimental effect on the fetus.[57]
- Seat the partner so that support may be given to the woman during surgery. Sensitively describe and explain the proceedings whilst preparing baby resuscitation equipment and warm towels.
- Note the time of the start of the operation along with the time of knife to uterus, birth of baby, and delivery of the placenta. The surgeon divides the skin, fat, rectus sheath, abdominal muscle, abdominal and pelvic peritoneum, and uterine muscle. Once the uterus is opened, the amniotic fluid is aspirated and the baby is quickly delivered. Occasionally it is necessary to use forceps to deliver the head.
- The operator places the baby on a sterile towel. Dry him or her well; note the time of delivery and assess the Apgar scores. If in good condition, give to the parents and support the mother to achieve skin-to-skin contact whilst establishing breastfeeding if this is the mother's wish.
- If there is concern about the baby, call the paediatrician.
- IV oxytocin is given to the woman to facilitate the delivery of the placenta and membranes. The surgeon then repairs the wound using dissolvable sutures or clips to the skin.
- Diclofenac 100mg per rectum may be given for effective analgesia when the spinal anaesthetic wears off.
- If the woman's blood group is Rh-negative, take samples from the cord and from the woman 1h following delivery, as usual.

*Immediately post-delivery*
- The midwife accompanies the family to a recovery area. One-to-one care is maintained.
- Assess maternal BP, pressure, respirations, colour, and oxygen saturation (using pulse oximetry) every 15min until stable. Take her temperature 2-hourly. MEOWS may be used.

- Every 30min, assess:
  - Is there any oozing from the wound?
  - Is the uterus well contracted?
  - Is the vaginal loss of blood excessive?
- Monitor the fluid balance. Continue the IV infusion (e.g. 1000mL of Hartmann's solution) as prescribed by the anaesthetist. Urine output from the catheter drainage should be at least 30mL hourly.
- Ensure that the woman is comfortable and give analgesia as prescribed by the anaesthetist. Women should be offered diamorphine (0.3–0.4mg intrathecally) or epidural diamorphine (2.5–5mg) could also be a suitable alternative. Some maternity units may give subcutaneous diamorphine regularly.
- Attend to the woman's hygiene needs. The woman should continue to wear anti-embolic stockings.
- The woman may take sips of water once settled onto the ward area. If her observations are within the normal limits and the woman is well with no complications, food and drink can be given as the woman feels hungry or thirsty.

## Emergency lower segment Caesarean section

Complications can occur in pregnancy and labour which may necessitate an emergency Caesarean section.

*Some indications*

In pregnancy:
- Severe pre-eclampsia
- Severe IUGR
- Haemorrhage related to placental abruption when the fetus is still alive.

In labour:
- There is no/limited progress
- Induction of labour fails
- There is apparent scar dissonance during a trial of labour after a previous Caesarean section
- There is apparent fetal compromise
- There is a prolapse of the cord.

*The urgency of the Caesarean section*
- Grade 1 (emergency): immediate threat to the life of the mother or fetus. This is to be performed within 30min.
- Grade 2 (urgent): maternal or fetal compromise which is not immediately life-threatening. To be performed within 60min.
- Grade 3 (scheduled): the mother requires early delivery, but there is no maternal or fetal compromise.
- Grade 4 (elective): delivery timed to suit the woman and staff.

A general anaesthetic may be necessary in acute emergency or when the woman requests it.

*During emergency lower segment Caesarean section, prioritize*
- Explanation to the parents of the need for a Caesarean section and informed consent.
- Communication with, and support for, the client, obstetrician, anaesthetist, theatre staff, porters, support staff, and paediatrician.
- IV access using large-bore cannula and blood for FBC/G&S or cross-match.
- Medication: sodium citrate 30mL, to neutralize stomach acid.
- Matters of hygiene, privacy, and safety.
- Catheter to the bladder.
- Call the paediatrician to attend the birth.
- Record the time of knife to skin.

*Immediate postnatal considerations*
- A cord blood sample for assessment of fetal pH post-delivery.
- Clear documentation of urgency, time of decision, and delivery.
- High-dependency support for a woman immediately following general anaesthesia.

## Complications of a Caesarean section
- Haemorrhage that could lead to shock. This may be manifest during the surgery or immediately post-delivery, or may result from a slow, initially undetected blood loss due to internal bleeding or per vaginum trickle. Occasionally retained products may cause bleeding.
- There is a risk of DVT which can result in pulmonary embolism.
- Damage/bruising during the operation is possible and may include the bladder and ureters. Urinary tract infection may occur or urinary tract trauma may cause a fistula and leaking urine.
- Trauma to the colon is possible.
- There is a risk of infection, endometritis, or breakdown of the wound.
- Complications of general anaesthesia may occur. The effects of progesterone on the gastrointestinal tract lead to delayed emptying of the stomach. During induction of general anaesthesia, silent regurgitation may occur and cause aspiration into the lungs and chemical pneumonitis. This impairs breathing and can be serious—a cause of maternal death.

## References
56 National Institute for Health and Care Excellence (2011). Chapter 1, Guidance. In: National Institute for Health and Care Excellence. *Caesarean section.* NICE guidelines CG132. Available at: ℜ www.nice.org.uk/guidance/cg132/chapter/1-recommendations.
57 Dunning G, Brindley J (2014). *Guideline for the management of Caesarean section.* Barnsley NHS Foundation Trust Maternity Guidelines.

## Breech delivery

A breech delivery will usually take place in a hospital maternity unit with experienced obstetricians and facilities for operative measures should this become necessary. It is customary for most known cases of breech to be delivered by elective LSCS; this has been a strong trend since the Term Breech Trial.[58] Due to the decline of vaginal breech births, many midwives may feel inexperienced and vulnerable when giving care to a woman who has chosen a breech birth. However, there is a growing body of literature which suggests that as long as the woman has been carefully selected and assessed, a vaginal birth can be a safe and satisfying experience. Taking into account the possible move towards supporting some breech births and that approximately one-third of breech births are undiagnosed at the start of labour,[59] midwives need to have the appropriate skills to facilitate a breech birth safely (➔ see Recognition and management of breech presentation, p. 224).

Women will be advised against opting for a planned breech birth if the baby:[60]
• Is a footling breech
• Is large (over 3800g)
• Is small (<2000g)
• Has a hyper-extended neck.

Or if the woman has:[60]
• had a previous Caesarean section
• a narrow pelvis
• a low-lying placenta
• pre-eclampsia.

### Management of labour: first stage

• The first stage often proceeds normally as with a cephalic presentation, particularly if the breech is engaged in the pelvis. Assess progress 4-hourly and document.
• On vaginal examination, the breech feels soft and irregular with no palpable sutures. This may be mistaken for a face presentation. The anus or external genitalia may be felt. In a flexed breech, a foot may be felt.
• Sometimes the breech may not be well applied to the cervix, resulting in a long latent phase.
• Augmentation of labour is not recommended. If progress during established first stage is limited, a Caesarean section might be considered.[61]
• Do not perform an ARM.
• FBS is not advised from the buttock.
• Epidural analgesia is not recommended,[61,62] but consideration to maternal choice must be given.
• With consent, IV access should be established and FBC and G&S taken.[62]
• Monitor the fetal heart continuously and observe carefully maternal condition and progress in labour.
• Encourage maternal mobility as much as possible.
• Ranitidine may be prescribed throughout labour in view of the possibility of a general anaesthetic.

- A premature urge to push is unusual in a term breech baby; if this does occur, offer assistance to achieve an alternative maternal position and the use of Entonox® to breathe through the contractions.

*Mechanism of labour*
- The lie is longitudinal.
- The attitude is one of complete flexion.
- The presentation is breech.
- The position is the right/left sacro-anterior/posterior.
- The denominator is the sacrum.
- The presenting part is the anterior buttock.
- The bitrochanteric diameter of 10cm enters the pelvis in the right or left oblique diameter of the brim.

*Movements*
- Descent occurs with compaction due to increased flexion of the limbs.
- The anterior buttock meets the resistance of the pelvic floor and undergoes internal rotation through 45° to the anterior. The bitrochanteric diameter is then in the antero-posterior of the outlet.
- With lateral flexion of the trunk, the anterior buttock escapes under the pubic arch; the posterior buttock sweeps the pelvic floor and the body is born. The shoulders are entering the brim at this stage in the same oblique diameter as the bitrochanteric diameter. The diameter of the shoulders measures approximately 11cm.
- The buttocks undergo restitution and external rotation. This is accompanied by internal rotation of the shoulders, bringing the bisacromial diameter into the antero-posterior diameter of the outlet. The anterior shoulder escapes under the pubic arch; the posterior shoulder sweeps the pelvic floor, and the shoulders are delivered.
- The head enters the pelvis in the transverse diameter and internal rotation of the occiput through 90° to the anterior is accompanied by forward rotation of the back. The occiput escapes under the pubic arch and the mentum, face, sinciput, and vertex sweep the perineum and the head is born.

## Management of the second stage
- The delivery will be performed/supervised by either a competent midwife or obstetrician.
- A 'hands-off' approach should be adopted by the practitioner unless assistance is required. Remember to watch, wait, and support the woman.
- It is crucial that full dilatation is confirmed by vaginal examination prior to allowing the woman to push. Await the descent of the presenting part. It should be visible at the perineum before active pushing begins. The fetus may well pass meconium which should be a toothpaste consistency. Meconium-stained liquor should be acted on as it would be for a cephalic presenting baby.
- Inform the obstetrician, anaesthetist, and paediatrician of the impending birth.
- In a multigravida or a small preterm fetus, the delivery may be spontaneous with minimal intervention.

- The lithotomy position may be adopted; however, if the attending practitioner is confident in undertaking a breech birth with the woman in an all-fours position, this may be considered.[62] There is currently divided opinion around the optimal positioning for the mother during a breech birth. Minimal evidence-based literature is currently available to support one particular position (➋ see Further reading, p. 474).
- An episiotomy may be required once the baby's buttocks reach the perineum if it is too tight or there is evidence of fetal distress.[61]
- Catheterization may be carried out to prevent delay and maximize the pelvic space.
- Preparation and equipment for a forceps delivery should be to hand, but intervention should only be when strictly necessary. Allow spontaneous descent and birth.
- An episiotomy should only be performed if necessary to facilitate the birth.
- The buttocks should be born spontaneously. The baby should then descend up to the umbilicus without intervention; if the legs are flexed, they will deliver quite easily. If the legs do not deliver spontaneously, apply gentle popliteal pressure to facilitate flexion of the knee.
- There is no evidence to support the practice of loosening the tension on the cord during the birth and it could cause the cord to go into spasm.
- With the next contraction, the shoulder blades appear; if the arms are flexed, they will deliver easily.
- The shoulders rotate into the antero-posterior diameter of the outlet; the body can be tilted towards the mother's sacrum to facilitate delivery of the anterior shoulder. The posterior shoulder sweeps the perineum and is aided by lifting the buttocks towards the mother's abdomen.
- It is important that the baby is held only around the pelvic girdle and handled as little as possible, to avoid trauma to internal structures.
- The head enters the pelvis in the transverse diameter; therefore, the back is in a lateral position until restitution and internal rotation take place.
- When the back has turned uppermost, allow the body to hang by its own weight; this encourages flexion of the head and rotation into the antero-posterior diameter of the outlet, when it meets the resistance of the pelvic floor.
- When the nape of the neck becomes visible, deliver the head. It is essential that the head is delivered in a controlled manner. Many obstetricians apply forceps; otherwise the following techniques may be used.

## Assisted vaginal breech techniques

### Mauriceau–Smellie–Veit manoeuvre

This technique is used when the head is extended and therefore flexion needs to be maintained (Fig. 21.1).

- The baby's body is straddled over the operator's arm; the operator's hand is passed into the vagina and a finger is placed on each malar bone.
- The middle finger of the opposite hand is placed on the baby's suboccipital region and the other fingers over the shoulders.
- Steady traction is then applied in the axis of the pelvis—first downwards and backwards, then downwards and forwards.

*The Burns–Marshall technique*

NB. Concern has been expressed about risks of the Burns–Marshall method if used incorrectly, leading to over-extension of the baby's neck (Fig. 21.2).[61]

- The baby's ankles are grasped and a steady traction is exerted as the baby's body is lifted upwards in the arc of a circle.
- When the nose and mouth are free, clear the airway.
- The perineum is supported so that the head can be delivered slowly.
- This method, if used incorrectly, may lead to over-extension of the baby's neck. Its use is therefore not recommended.

Fig. 21.1 Mauriceau–Smellie–Veit manoeuvre.

Fig. 21.2 Burns–Marshall technique.

*Extended legs*
- If the buttocks are not expelled, the operator's finger is inserted into the fold of the baby's anterior groin or both groins and slight traction applied during uterine contractions.
- When the popliteal fossae appear at the vulva, two fingers are placed along the length of one thigh, with the fingertips in the fossa.
- The leg is swept to the side of the abdomen and the knee is flexed by the pressure on its undersurface.
- This is then repeated to deliver the second leg.

*Extended arms—the Lövsett manoeuvre*
If the arms are not across the chest as the trunk is delivered, they must be extended; this complication needs to be dealt with immediately as this will prevent delivery. This manoeuvre is the technique now used for dealing with extended arms. It is based on the premise that as a result of the curvature of the birth canal, the posterior shoulder must be at a lower level than the anterior shoulder and that the subpubic arch is the shallowest part of the pelvis (Fig. 21.3).
- The fetus is grasped by two hands around the pelvic girdle, the thumbs on the back and the fingers in the groins.
- By downward traction, the anterior shoulder is brought to lie behind the symphysis pubis and the posterior shoulder will then lie below the promontory of the sacrum, and therefore below the pelvic brim.
- The fetus is rotated through 180° so that the back always remains upwards.
- Moderate traction is used during rotation and by this manoeuvre the posterior shoulder is brought to the anterior and appears beneath the pubis.
- The arm may deliver spontaneously; if not, it may be hooked out by digital pressure.
- The shoulder that was previously anterior now lies posteriorly in the hollow of the sacrum.
- The fetus is then rotated 180° in the opposite direction, the back being kept uppermost.
- The other arm is then delivered.
- Syntometrine® must not be given until the head has been delivered.

*Midwives and breech birth*
- Occasionally the midwife may experience a planned or an unexpected breech birth at home.
- Expect meconium to be present. When FHR irregularities are present, contact help from emergency obstetric services.
- Hands and knees ('all fours') position facilitates delivery. Also squatting and standing have been used according to maternal preference and comfort. Allow spontaneous pushing.
- The progress of the delivery should be observed and no touching of the breech is recommended unless there is a complication.
- Episiotomy may be performed if the midwife perceives this is needed.
- Extended legs should be allowed to birth spontaneously and the body to the umbilicus.

**Fig. 21.3** Lövsett manoeuvre.

- Let the baby's body take some of the weight and the chin will come to the perineum. After this, the head will be born.
  - Gentle support might be given to the baby, allowing the buttocks to rest on the midwife's cupped hands. This may slow the birth of the head a little and prevent sudden decompression.
  - The midwife should be familiar with the above manoeuvres.
  - A breech baby may be slower to breathe at delivery and resuscitation equipment should be ready.
  - Conduct the third stage according to maternal preference.

## Complications of breech delivery

- Increased risk of early membrane rupture.
- Head entrapment—more common with preterm breech births.
- Increased risk of cord prolapse.
- Sometimes women experience a premature urge to push.
- Hypoxia, anoxia, cord compression.
- Premature separation of the placenta.
- Intracranial haemorrhage: rapid decompression of the after-coming head.
- Fractures, nerve/muscle damage, rupture of internal organs.
- Oedema/bruising of feet and genitalia.
- Increased risk of operative delivery.
- Increased risk of perinatal morbidity and mortality

## References

58 Hannah ME, Hannah WJ, Hewson SA, et al. (2000). Planned caesarean section versus planned vaginal birth for breech presentation at term: a randomised multicentre trial. Term Breech Trial Collaborative Group. *Lancet* **356**: 1375–83.

59 Evans J (2012). The final piece of the breech birth jigsaw. *Essentially MIDIRS* **3**: 46–9.

60 Royal College of Obstetricians and Gynaecologists (2008). *A breech baby at the end of pregnancy. Information for you.* Available at: ℅ www.rcog.org.uk/globalassets/documents/patients/patient-information-leaflets/pregnancy/a-breech-baby-at-the-end-of-pregnancy.pdf.

61 Royal College of Obstetricians and Gynaecologists (2006). *The management of breech presentation. Guideline No. 20b.* Available at: ℅ www.rcog.org.uk/globalassets/documents/guidelines/gtg-no-20b-breech-presentation.pdf.

62 Dunning G (2013). *Guideline for breech delivery.* Barnsley NHS Foundation Trust Hospital Maternity Guidelines.

## Further reading

Bogner G, Strobl M, Schausberger C, Fischer T, Reisenberger K, Jacobs VR (2015). Breech delivery in the all fours position: a prospective observational comparative study with classic assistance. *J Perinat Med* **43**: 707–13. Available at: ℅ www.researchgate.net/profile/Gerhard_Bogner2/publication/265518241_Breech_delivery_in_the_all_fours_position_a_prospective_observational_comparative_study_with_classic_assistance/links/54198dd60cf2218008bf8d5c.pdf.

# Retained placenta

The third stage is concluded when the placenta is delivered complete. If bleeding is not excessive, it is reasonable to wait for delivery of the placenta. If the placenta is undelivered after 30min (active management) or 1h (physiological), a diagnosis of retained placenta is made.[63] If the woman has had a physiological management and the placenta remains undelivered after 60min, she should be offered active management to attempt to resolve the situation.[63]

## Causes

- The physiological third stage may be longer.
- During the active third stage, unless the placenta is delivered quickly by controlled cord traction, Syntometrine®/ergometrine may cause a constriction of the muscles of the lower segment and os, which prevents delivery until the action has worn off.
- The placenta may still be partially attached.
- Placenta accreta is when the placenta is morbidly adhered to the uterine wall.

## Immediate management

- If uterine exploration is necessary and the woman is not already in an obstetric unit, arrange urgent transfer.[63]
- Inform the obstetrician if there is heavy blood loss. A partially adherent placenta where there is bleeding is an obstetric emergency.
- Assess by abdominal palpation whether the uterus feels contracted. If it feels 'boggy', lacking tone on palpation, and a contraction is not easily stimulated and IM oxytocin has been given, inform the obstetrician. Otherwise:
  - Take any cord bloods required
  - Explain the problem to the mother. She may be pleased to breastfeed the baby, which will encourage oxytocin release and stimulate uterine contractions. This may expel the placenta naturally
  - Ask the woman if she is able to sit upright on a bedpan and blow sharply into her fist (causing sudden downward movement of the diaphragm) or encourage maternal effort. Avoid excessive cord traction
  - Obtain permission from the woman to ensure an empty bladder by passing an intermittent urinary catheter
  - Perform and record maternal observations every 15min after retained placenta has been confirmed.
  - Monitor and record blood loss; be aware of any possible concealed bleeding—note the fundal height
  - If oxytocin has been used for the active third stage, wait 30min and attempt controlled cord traction again
  - If this fails or the cord snaps, manual removal in theatre is usually indicated
  - It is not recommended that umbilical vein agents are used if the placenta is retained.

## Manual removal of the placenta

- Contact the registrar, theatre, and anaesthetist.
- Good analgesia is required. This means topping up an existing epidural, siting a spinal anaesthetic, or possibly a general anaesthetic. There should never be any uterine exploration or manual removal without adequate analgesia.
- Give oral sodium citrate 30mL prior to transfer to theatre and ensure that ranitidine 150mg has been given within the last 6h.[64]
- The procedure is explained to the woman and consent obtained.
- Accompany the woman during transfer to theatre.
- An IV infusion is sited using a large cannula and bloods taken for FBC and to cross-match 2 units of blood.
- The woman is placed in the lithotomy position, aseptic precautions taken, and the bladder is catheterized. The obstetrician controls the fundus with the left palm on the abdomen and the right hand is passed into the uterus. The placenta is sheared off the uterine wall and removed on the palm of the hand.
- It is carefully examined to ensure it is complete.
- Prophylactic antibiotics should be given (e.g. cefuroxime IV 1.5g and metronidazole IV 500mg if no allergies to penicillin).[64]
- An IV infusion of oxytocin 20 units in 500mL of normal saline over 4h is given.
- The woman is observed in theatre recovery until stable. Once returned to the care of the midwife, record clinical observations onto a MEOWS chart every half hour for the first 2h. If stable, reduce to hourly for 4h and then 4-hourly for 24h. Monitor blood loss and ensure adequate pain relief.[64]
- Offer the woman the chance to debrief her experiences of her birth; this may be done informally or through a birth afterthoughts session.[64]
- An indwelling catheter should be inserted and left until the woman regains feeling in the lower limbs following anaesthetic.

## Placenta accreta

Very rarely, if the placenta cannot be separated, it may be morbidly adherent.

- If it is totally adherent and bleeding has not occurred, it can be left *in situ* to absorb during the postnatal period.
- If partially adherent, there is a high risk of prolific haemorrhage.
- Operative treatment, and possibly a hysterectomy, may be unavoidable.

## References

63 National Institute for Health and Care Excellence (2015). Third stage of labour. In: National Institute for Health and Care Excellence. *Intrapartum care for healthy women and babies.* NICE guidelines CG190. Available at: www.nice.org.uk/guidance/cg190/chapter/1-recommendations#third-stage-of-labour.

64 Dunning G, Hadfield H (2015). *Guideline for retained placenta.* Barnsley Hospital NHS Foundation Trust Maternity Guidelines.

# Maternal emergencies during pregnancy, labour, and postnatally

# Blood test results during pregnancy: detecting deviations from the norm

To detect deviations from the norm, refer to Table 22.1 for haematological values and Table 22.2 for blood chemistry values. See Table 22.3 for blood chemistry values in PIH and pre-eclamptic toxaemia (PET).

Whilst it is good practice for the midwife to have an awareness of the normal ranges of blood results, it is prudent to remember that all test results must be reviewed by a medic. NB. Be aware that levels given in the above tables may differ slightly in each trust due to the various methods of producing results.

**Table 22.1** Haematological values during pregnancy: detecting deviations from normal

| Test | Non-pregnant | Pregnancy | PIH/PET | DIC | Notes | Causes of abnormal result |
|---|---|---|---|---|---|---|
| **FBC** | | | | | | |
| Hb (g/L) | 115–165 | (↓) 110 | – | – | Normal reduction in pregnancy (physiological) | Anaemia due to any cause. Haemolysis in HELLP. Also (↓) in some haemo-globinopathies |
| Packed cell volume (PCV) | 0.35–0.47 | (↓) 0.34–0.36 | – | – | (↓) PCV represents (↑) plasma-to-red cell ratio seen in pregnancy | |
| White cell count (× 10⁷/L) | 6 (4–11) | (↑) 9–11 | – | – | Normal (↑) through pregnancy. Polymor-phonuclear cells | Labour can (↑) levels to 13–15. Infection causes (↓) levels |
| Platelet count (× 10³/L) | 150–350 | 140–440 | (↓) to (↓↓) | <50 | (↓) platelet count affects blood clotting efficiency | Idiopathic (idiopathic thrombocytopenic purpura), PIH, HELLP |
| **Coagulation** | | | | | | |
| PT (s) | 10–12 | 10–12 | May (↑) | >100 | Measures II, V, VII, and X | (↑) with liver problems or anticoagulant use (warfarin) |
| Partial thrombo-plastin time (s) | 35–45 | 35–50 | May (↑) | >100 | Measures factors II, V, VIII, IX, X, and XI | (↑) in factor VII, IX, and X deficiency and heparin use |

**Table 22.1** (Contd.)

| Test | Non-pregnant | Pregnancy | PIH/PET | DIC | Notes | Causes of abnormal result |
|------|--------------|-----------|---------|-----|-------|---------------------------|
| Thrombin time (s) | 16–20 | 15–20 | May (↑) | >100 | | |
| Fibrinogen (mg/dL) | 150–400 | 450 | May (↓) | (↓) to (↓↓) | Normally (↑) in pregnancy. Hepatic dysfunction affects production | PIH/HELLP, major haemorrhage, and DIC |
| FDPs (micrograms/mL) | <5 | <16 | May (↑) | >200 | Raised levels are evidence of clot breakdown | (↑) levels are seen in thromboembolic disease (PE/DVT). Also (↑) in small APH and DIC |

**Table 22.2** Blood chemistry values in pregnancy: detecting deviations from normal

| Test | Non-pregnant | Pregnancy | PIH/PET | DIC | Notes | Causes of abnormal result |
|------|--------------|-----------|---------|-----|-------|---------------------------|
| **Biochemistry** | | | | | | |
| Sodium (mmol/L) | 132–144 | 132–144 | – | – | Fall to lower end of non-pregnant range. Body sodium (↑) in pregnancy but levels unchanged due to water retention | Low sodium in hyperemesis |
| Potassium (mmol/L) | 3.6–5.1 | 3.6–5.1 | May (↑) | – | Raised levels represent deterioration of renal function | PIH, HELLP, primary renal disease |
| Urea (mmol/L) | 4.3 (2.5–6.6) | 2.3–4.3 | (↑) | – | Normally (↓) due to (↑) renal blood flow. Raised levels represent deterioration of renal function | PIH, HELLP, primary renal disease |

(Continued)

Table 22.2 (Contd.)

| Test | Non-pregnant | Pregnancy | PIH/PET | DIC | Notes | Causes of abnormal result |
|---|---|---|---|---|---|---|
| Creatinine (micromol/L) | 73 (55–150) | 50–73 | (↑) | – | | |
| Chloride (mmol/L) | 95–107 | 95–107 | – | – | | |
| Uric acid (mmol/L) | 0.2–0.35 | 0.15–0.35 | (↑) | – | Raised levels represent deterioration of renal function | PIH, HELLP, primary renal disease |
| LFTs | | | | | | |
| Total protein (g/L) | 78 (60–80) | 70 | (↓) to (↓↓) | – | Normally just below non-pregnant reference range. (↑) loss of protein and (↓) production due to liver dysfunction in PIH/HELLP | PIH, HELLP |
| Albumin (g/L) | 45 (36–47) | 33 | (↓) to (↓↓) | – | | |
| ALT (units/L) | 10–40 | 10–40 | May (↑) | – | Raised levels indicate hepatic cellular damage | PIH, HELLP, primary liver disease. Levels slightly (↑) post-partum |
| AST (units/L) | 10–35 | 10–35 | May (↑) | – | | |
| Gamma-glutamyl transpeptidase (units/L) | 7–50 | 7–50 | – | – | No significant change | Alcohol abuse, enzyme-inducing drugs such as barbiturates and warfarin |

**Table 22.3** Blood chemistry values in PIH and pre-eclamptic toxaemia (PET)

| Test | Non-pregnant | Pregnancy | PIH/PET | DIC | Notes | Causes of abnormal result |
|------|-------------|-----------|---------|-----|-------|---------------------------|
| Bilirubin (mmol/L) | 2–17 | 2–17 | May (↑) | – | Product of red cell breakdown | PIH/HELLP |
| Lactic dehydrogenase (LDH) (units/L) | 100–300 | 100–300 | May (↑) | – | Levels may (↑) in last few weeks of pregnancy. Significant increases in PIH/HELLP | Significant increases in PIH |
| APT (units/L) | 40–125 | (↑) 2–4 times | – | – | Normal (↑) (2–4 times) due to placental production | |
| Calcium (mmol/L) | 2.12–2.62 | 2.12–2.62 | – | – | Fall to lower end of reference interval due to reduction in serum albumin. No change in ionized calcium | |
| Bile acids (micromol/L) | 0–6 | 0–14 | – | – | Measured in pruritus | (↑ to ↑↑) in cholestasis of pregnancy |
| Lactate (mmol/L) | 0.5 | 2.2 | – | – | Measure when infection is suspected. If ≥4, sepsis is indicated and requires fast treatment | |

*(Continued)*

Table 22.3 (Contd.)

| Test | Non-pregnant | Pregnancy | PIH/PET | DIC | Notes | Causes of abnormal result |
|------|--------------|-----------|---------|-----|-------|---------------------------|
| **Blood gas results** | | | | | | |
| $P_aO_2$ (kPa) | 13 (12–15) | 13.7 | May (↓) | – | May be lower in the supine position | Fall in PIH/HELLP due to fluid overload. Blood gas results may deteriorate due to respiratory disease as well as pregnancy-induced disease |
| $PaCO_2$ (kPa) | 5.3 (4.4–6.1) | 4 | – | – | Hyperventilation associated with pregnancy | |
| $HCO_3^-$ (mmol/L) | 24 (21–27.5) | 20 | – | – | Metabolic compensation for respiratory alkalosis—incomplete | |
| pH | 7.4 (36–44) | 7.44 | – | – | Reflects incomplete compensation of alkalosis | |
| Base excess (mmol/L) | –4 to +4 | –4 to +4 | – | – | Little change in pregnancy. Lower end of reference range | |
| **Other** | | | | | | |
| Glucose (mmol/L) | 3.6–5.8 | 3.6–5.8 | May (↓) | – | | Severe hepatic dysfunction in PIH/HELLP |

# Eclampsia

Eclampsia refers to the occurrence of new-onset, generalized, tonic–clonic seizures, or coma, in a woman with pre-eclampsia and may occur before, during, or after the birth. Pre-eclampsia is a recognized disorder of pregnancy in which there are large amounts of protein in the urine, accompanied by high BP and symptoms of other organ dysfunction. As pre-eclampsia fulminates into eclampsia, one or more convulsions may occur, often followed by coma and posing a threat to the health of both mother and baby; therefore, prompt treatment and control are vital.

Mild pre-eclampsia affects up to 6% of pregnancies, and severe cases develop in about 1–2% of pregnancies. Eclampsia is quite rare in the UK, with <1% of pre-eclamptic women progressing to have convulsions and an estimated one case of eclampsia for every 4000 pregnancies.[1] Cerebral oedema and spasm, clots, or haemorrhages in small arteries are thought to be the cause. Complications include: aspiration pneumonia, cerebral haemorrhage, kidney failure, and cardiac arrest. Most women make a good recovery. However, some may die or be left with permanent disability. The fetus is at risk of acute asphyxia and may die.

## Signs and symptoms

- Headache and blurred vision, epigastric pain, nausea, and vomiting, drowsiness, or confusion may precede the onset of a fit. However, sometimes these types of symptoms occur after the fit, with no forewarning.
- Eclamptic convulsions appear similar to epileptic fits—repetitive, jerky, violent muscle spasms. Loss of consciousness occurs; the woman may hold her breath, bite her tongue, or be incontinent of urine.
- Convulsions last about a minute. If the fit continues for longer, status eclampticus ensues.

## The midwife's response

- Call for a senior obstetrician, anaesthetist, midwifery, and support staff.
- Ask for emergency eclampsia drugs and resuscitation equipment. You should know the location of these in your unit.
- Note the time of onset.
- Try to maintain a private, safe physical environment.
- Turn the woman to her left side and ensure a clear airway.
- Give oxygen at 4L/min via non-rebreathe face mask.
- When possible, observe respiration, oxygen saturation, pulse and BP, and the level of consciousness (see also Table 22.4).
- Talk to the woman, reassuring her of the presence of help and support.

**Table 22.4** Eclampsia recordings

| Action or treatment | Time and recording |
| --- | --- |
| Time of seizure | |
| Time help called | |
| Time help arrived | |
| Airway—left lateral, O₂ | |
| Breathing | |
| Circulation—BP, pulse, large-bore IV infusion | |
| FBC, clotting, G&S, U/E, LFTs | |
| Eclampsia tray | |
| Drugs (state) | |
| BP and pulse: | |
| 1 | |
| 2 | |
| 3 | |
| Time of transfer to HDU | |
| Monitoring fetal heart | |

Source: The Practice Development Midwives (2009). Sheffield Teaching Hospitals NHS Trust.

### Immediate management by the obstetric team

If a fit occurs, the mother must be stabilized before urgent delivery of the baby.

- Site an IV large-bore cannula (grey 16) and take blood for FBC, clotting, G&S, U/E and urates, and LFTs.
- Seizures are controlled with a loading dose of magnesium sulfate 4g IV over 20min. Do not use diazepam, phenytoin, or a lytic cocktail as an alternative to magnesium sulfate in women with eclampsia. If these are administered in succession, there is a risk of maternal respiratory depression.[2]
- After the initial episode, transfer the woman, accompanied by the emergency team, to the HDU, to stabilize her condition further.
- The fetal heart should be monitored continuously—eclampsia and antihypertensive agents may cause abnormal fetal heart patterns.
- Give IV magnesium sulfate slowly to prevent further fitting:
  - After the initial loading dose of 4g IV, an infusion of 1g/h is commenced and maintained for 24h
  - Recurrent seizures should be treated with a further dose of 2–4g given over 5min.

- Monitor the woman for signs of magnesium toxicity:
  - Warm/flushing, slurring of speech, visual disturbance, nausea
  - Weakness, drowsiness, hypotension
  - Loss of deep tendon reflexes
  - Respiratory depression (14–16 respirations per min is a minimum)
  - Oxygen saturation reducing below 95%.
- Refer side effects to the consultant; discontinue infusion, and give oxygen. The obstetrician may wish to monitor magnesium sulfate blood levels; the therapeutic range is 1.5–2.5mmol/L.
- If the woman's diastolic BP is >100mmHg, labetalol 20mg may be given by slow IV injection. Then maintenance therapy may be given:
  - The maternal diastolic BP should be maintained at 80–100mmHg
  - If the woman is asthmatic, hydralazine may be used (➔ see Hypertensive disorders, p. 406). Consider using up to 500mL of crystalloid fluid before or at the same time as the first dose of IV hydralazine in the antenatal period[2]
  - Oral nifedipine may also be used. Follow local protocols.

Occurrence of an eclamptic fit is the end-stage of the condition and the risks to the woman and fetus are too great to justify prolonging pregnancy.
- Urgent delivery, usually by a Caesarean section, will be arranged by the consultant obstetrician as soon as the woman's condition allows. However, induction may be attempted if the woman's condition remains stable with no further fits, the cervix is favourable for induction (Bishop score >6; ➔ see Bishop score, p. 449), and delivery is likely to occur quickly—the presentation is cephalic and the CTG is reassuring.
- Make every effort to support the obstetric team in keeping the woman and family informed about care decisions.
- In women with severe pre-eclampsia, limit maintenance fluids to 80mL/h unless there are other ongoing fluid losses (e.g. haemorrhage).
- If the woman's condition deteriorates and fitting recurs or continues, the anaesthetist may sedate and ventilate the patient.

### Eclamptic seizure
See Table 22.4 for an example of a chart for emergency recordings.

### References
1 NHS Choices (2015). *Pre-eclampsia*. Available at: ℛ www.nhs.uk/Conditions/Pre-eclampsia/Pages/Introduction.aspx.
2 National Institute for Health and Care Excellence (2010). *Hypertension in pregnancy: diagnosis and management*. NICE guidelines CG107. Available at: ℛ www.nice.org.uk/guidance/cg107/resources/guidance-hypertension-in-pregnancy-pdf.

# Major obstetric haemorrhage

Obstetric haemorrhage is a major cause of maternal morbidity and mortality in the UK, with the risk of mortality of about one in 100 000 pregnancies.[3] The definition of a major haemorrhage is an estimated blood loss of >1000mL or a blood loss which causes clinical shock in the woman. Conditions that increase the risk of haemorrhage include:[4]

- Grand multiparity (parity 4 or more)
- Maternal age 35 years or older
- BMI >35 kg/m$^2$
- Pre-existing bleeding disorders (such as haemophilia)
- Factor V Leiden (weak relationship)
- Therapeutic anticoagulants
- APH
- Over-distension of the uterus (polyhydramnios, multiple pregnancy, macrosomia)
- Uterine abnormalities
- Placenta praevia or low-lying placenta
- Large or multiple uterine fibroids
- Placental abruption
- Previous retained placenta or PPH with complications
- Maternal Hb level below 85g/L at onset of labour
- Premature birth
- Precipitate labour
- Induction of labour (oxytocin use)
- Prolonged labour
- Operative birth.

Women should be assessed for these factors at each antenatal contact. This information is used to assign women to high-risk or low-risk care.[5,6] If a woman has risk factors for haemorrhage, highlight these in her notes, and discuss and document with her a care plan covering the third stage of labour.[4]

## General prevention and management

Women known to be at high risk should attend for an obstetric review in the antenatal clinic to discuss prevention.

- Antenatal anaemia should be treated.
- A well-rehearsed obstetric haemorrhage drill should be in place on the labour ward. Staff should retain a major haemorrhage pack.
- Under certain circumstances (e.g. severe placenta praevia), cross-match several specified units of blood and have them immediately available before the woman's estimated delivery date (EDD).
- Ensure that blood is available if a woman identified at high risk of bleeding has been admitted to the labour ward.
- For a patient known to be at high risk, inform the obstetric and anaesthetic team and the haematologist immediately on arrival or at the time of birth.

## References

3 Higgins JPT, Green S (2011). *Obstetric Haemorrhage. Cochrane Handbook for Systematic Reviews of Interventions*, Version 5.1.0 (updated March 2011). The Cochrane Collaboration. Available at: ✆ www.cochrane-handbook.org.

4 National Institute for Health and Care Excellence (2008). *Antenatal care for uncomplicated pregnancies*. NICE guidelines CG62. Available at: ✆ www.nice.org.uk/guidance/cg62.

5 Royal College of Obstetricians and Gynaecologists (2011). *Antepartum haemorrhage. Greentop guideline No. 63*. Available at: ✆ www.rcog.org.uk/globalassets/documents/guidelines/gtg_63.pdf.

6 Sinha P, Kuruba N (2008). Antepartum haemorrhage: an update. *J Obstet Gynaecol* **28**: 377–81.

# Major antepartum haemorrhage

Antepartum haemorrhage (APH) is bleeding from the genital tract (after 20 weeks and before delivery) of >500mL (or any volume causing deterioration in maternal and fetal condition).[7] APH complicates 3–5% of pregnancies and is a leading cause of perinatal and maternal mortality worldwide. Up to one-fifth of very preterm babies are born in association with an APH.[7]

The haemorrhage is usually from the placental site—*a placental abruption or bleeding placenta praevia*. Placental abruption is usually a sudden and unexpected obstetric emergency, not predictable by known reproductive risk factors.[7] Health professionals should be aware that domestic abuse in pregnancy may result in APH and women with repeated presentations that include APH should be asked about this.[7]

Often with an APH, the bleeding may be occult (concealed within the abdominal cavity). Assume an occult APH if, on examination of the abdomen, you find that:
• The uterus is 'woody'/hard and extremely 'touch-sensitive'.
• The woman is in continuous pain/experiencing contractions that are disproportionately strong relative to her clinical condition.

A soft, non-tender uterus may suggest a lower genital tract cause, or bleeding from the placenta or vasa praevia.[7]

Immediate care:
• Prompt action is needed to save the fetus. The aim is to resuscitate and stabilize the woman and assess fetal well-being as soon as possible.
• Call for help from colleagues and the emergency obstetric/anaesthetic team and access the prepared pack.
• Record the pulse and BP at regular intervals.
• The woman should be laid flat, in the left lateral position, or in lateral tilt, to minimize the effects of aorto-caval compression.
• Assess the airway and respiratory effort.
• Give oxygen via a non-re-breathable face mask at 10–15L/min and monitor maternal oxygenation using a pulse oximeter. If the oxygen saturation is low (<95%) in spite of oxygen given, an arterial blood sample may also be taken by the anaesthetist for blood gases.
• Site two large-bore (grey 16 gauge) cannulae (one in each arm) and take venous blood samples; urgently request FBC, U/E, LFTs, clotting screen/D-dimers, and Kleihauer (if Rh-negative), and cross-match 4–6 units.
• The aim is, over the first hour of care, to replace the fluid lost and thereafter to replace continuing loss and maintain normal vital signs. Use normal saline followed by up to 1.5L of colloid (e.g. Gelofusine® or Haemaccel®) until blood is available. Increase the speed of IV infusion using a pressure bag.
• The haematologist will be involved. It might be necessary to give ABO- and Rh-compatible blood until fully cross-matched blood is available for the woman. It should be given via warming equipment, and a pressure bag can aid speedy administration.

- DIC may complicate obstetric haemorrhage and must be corrected (➔ see Disseminated intravascular coagulation, p. 500). If blood clotting irregularities are present, fresh frozen plasma (FFP; containing fibrinogen and all clotting factors), cryoprecipitate (containing fibrinogen and factor VIII), or platelets may be indicated.
- A speculum examination may be useful to identify cervical dilatation or visualize a lower genital tract cause for the APH. Digital vaginal examination can provide information on cervical dilatation if the APH is associated with pain or uterine activity. Digital examination *should never be performed* if placenta praevia is a possible diagnosis (e.g. a previous scan shows a low placenta, there is a high presenting part on abdominal examination, or the bleed has been painless), until this cause is excluded.
- An assessment of the FHR should be performed, usually with a CTG once the mother is stable or resuscitation has commenced, to aid decision-making on the mode of delivery. At gestations of <26+0 weeks, or where active obstetric intervention in the interests of the fetus is not planned, continuous monitoring of the FHR is not advised.
- The woman should be transferred immediately to theatre and the consultant obstetrician and team, anaesthetist, and paediatrician called.

Women with a major APH and associated maternal and/or fetal compromise are required to be delivered immediately.[7] Precise management of this will depend on the gestation. The principal neonatal concern in these circumstances is anaemia, and therefore neonatal staff should be present at the time of delivery and should be informed of the extent of the blood loss, so that arrangements for early neonatal blood transfusion can be made if necessary.

### Reference

7 Royal College of Obstetricians and Gynaecologists (2011). *Antepartum haemorrhage. Green-top guideline No. 63.* Available at: ℅ www.rcog.org.uk/globalassets/documents/guidelines/gtg_63.pdf.

# Major post-partum haemorrhage

The most common type of haemorrhage[8]—primary post-partum haemorrhage (PPH)—is the loss of 500mL or more of blood from the genital tract (or *any* volume of vaginal bleeding causing maternal compromise) within 24h of the birth of a baby.

PPH can be classified as minor (500–1000mL) or major (>1000mL). Major is further divided into moderate (1000–2000mL) or severe (>2000mL). The recommendations in this guideline apply to women experiencing primary PPH of 500mL or more.

Secondary PPH is defined as abnormal or excessive bleeding from the birth canal between 24h and 12 weeks postnatally. This guideline also includes recommendations specific to the management of major secondary PPH.

The consequences of a severe PPH include death, hypovolaemic shock, DIC, renal failure, hepatic failure, and adult RDS.[9]

## Causes of post-partum haemorrhage

- TONE: uterine atony is the most common cause—the uterus is soft, the fundus difficult to palpate, or high and full of blood clots.
- TRAUMA: lacerations and uterine rupture.
- TISSUE: retained placenta/morbidly adherent placenta.
- THROMBIN: coagulation problem.
- Rarely: uterine inversion/rupture.

## Signs and symptoms

- Signs may be obvious:
  - Deterioration in the woman's condition
  - Visible copious bleeding vaginally
  - Bulky or soft, relaxed uterus (post-partum).
- Sometimes signs are less apparent:
  - The woman looks pale
  - She feels cold and clammy
  - Her pulse is gradually rising
  - Her BP is gradually falling
  - She may have nausea/fainting and become restless/drowsy
  - Blood loss vaginally could be concealed and therefore more than is visible on examination.

## Immediate care

Once a PPH has been identified, its management involves four components, all of which should be undertaken *simultaneously*:

- Communication
- Resuscitation
- Monitoring and investigation
- Arresting the bleeding.

## Communication

- Call for help from an experienced midwife and the obstetric team (anaesthetist, operating department practitioner (ODP), consultant obstetrician).

- Alert the on-call haematologist and blood bank.
- Alert porters for the transport of blood.
- Nominate a scribe to record the sequence of events
- Explain briefly to the woman and her partner. Direct relatives to a suitable waiting point. Allocate a member of the health-care team to stay with the woman and her birth companion(s); explain what is happening; answer any questions and offer support throughout the emergency situation.[10]

## Resuscitation

- Position the woman flat and keep her warm.
- Assess the airway and respiratory effort.
- Give oxygen via a non-rebreathable face mask at 10–15L/min and monitor maternal oxygenation using a pulse oximeter. If the oxygen saturation is low (<95%) in spite of oxygen given, an arterial blood sample may also be taken by the anaesthetist for blood gases.
- Site two large-bore (grey 16 gauge) cannulae (one in each arm) and take venous blood samples; urgently request FBC, U/E, LFTs, clotting screen, including fibrinogen, Kleihauer (if Rh-negative), and cross-match 4–6 units.
- Transfuse O Rh D-negative blood as soon as possible. Until this is available, infuse a maximum combination of up to 3.5L of warmed Hartmann's solution (1–2L) and/or colloid (1–2L). Increase the speed of IV infusions using a pressure bag.
- FFP, cryoprecipitate, or platelet concentrates may be given as directed by the haematologist.
- Intraoperative cell salvage may be considered if available.

## Monitoring and investigation

### Monitor

- Record the pulse, BP, respiration rate, oxygen saturation, temperature; record observations on a MEOWS chart every 5min.
- Consider an arterial line (CVP line) monitoring once appropriate vascular access staff are available.
- Catheterize the bladder with a Foley® catheter and measure all fluid intake/output. Document the fluid balance.

### Investigate the cause

The most common cause of PPH is uterine atony.

- Rub up a contraction:
  - Feel for the fundus of the uterus
  - If it is soft/relaxed, massage the fundus using a circular movement
  - A contraction should occur.
- *Deliver the placenta* and expel blood clots with gentle pressure at the fundus.
- *Examine the placenta* to assess whether there are any missing cotyledons/retained membranes.
- *Clinical examination* must be undertaken to exclude other possible causes, e.g. vaginal or cervical lacerations, broad ligament haematoma, uterine rupture.

## Arrest the bleeding

- Commence drug therapy. No particular uterotonic drug can be recommended over any other.[11] Options include:
  - Give oxytocin 5 units via slow IV injection (two doses)
  - Consider giving 250 micrograms of ergometrine IV (contraindicated in women with hypertension)
  - Prepare for, and start, an IV infusion of normal saline with oxytocin via a pump (at 10 units/h). The exact prescription may vary with local policy
  - Give Hemabate® (carboprost tromethamine—a synthetic prostaglandin $F_2$ alpha) 0.25mg by IM injection at 15min intervals up to a maximum of 2mg—eight doses (contraindicated in asthma, hypertension, cardiac disease, and impaired pulmonary, renal, or hepatic function). Side effects include pyrexia, vomiting, and hypertension
  - A direct intra-myometrial injection of carboprost 0.25mg may be given by the obstetrician (not licensed for intramyometrial use)
  - Misoprostol 800–1000 micrograms may be given rectally.
- Assess the need for adjuvant options for managing significant continuing PPH,[11] including:
  - Tranexamic acid (TXA) IV
  - Recombinant factor VIIa, in the presence of otherwise normal clotting factors, in consultation with a haematologist.
- If measures fail to arrest bleeding, consider bimanual compression of the uterus, which will apply pressure to the placental site:
  - With the fingers of the right hand bent over, they are inserted into the vagina and the hand is made into a fist at the anterior vaginal fornix
  - The palm of the left hand is placed abdominally, using the tips of the fingers to lift the uterus slightly forward, to position the hand behind the uterus
  - The uterus is compressed between the left and right hands.
- Accompany the woman with the obstetric team to theatre for exploration of the vagina, cervix, and uterus to exclude/repair genital tract trauma, uterine inversion, or retained placental tissue under anaesthetic.
- Surgical procedures that may be attempted by the consultant obstetrician include:
  - Before surgical intervention,[11] the insertion of a Rusch® balloon catheter into the uterine cavity should be considered. The balloon is filled with warm saline and packs the uterine cavity; this may arrest bleeding and is left in place for 24h
  - Haemostatic brace suturing (B-Lynch® suture)
  - Bilateral ligation of the internal iliac arteries
  - Selective arterial embolization: the obstetrician may call on a vascular radiologist to perform pelvic arterial embolization.
- An oxytocin infusion is given over 24h to maintain the uterine tone.
- Antibiotic cover is indicated.

In the most severe cases of bleeding, when other surgical techniques have been unsuccessful[8,9] and the patient is severely shocked, a hysterectomy may be the only option. A consultant obstetrician should be present for any elective or emergency surgery.

After controlling the acute situation, attention should be paid to the possibility of rebound hypercoagulation and the risk of thromboembolism. Transfer to obstetric HDU is always required once the patient is stable.[11]

## References

8  Kollmann M, Gaulhofer J, Lang U, et al. (2016). Placenta praevia: incidence, risk factors and outcome. *J Matern Fetal Neonatal Med* 29: 1395–8.

9  Sinha P, Kuruba N (2008). Ante-partum haemorrhage: an update. *J Obstet Gynaecol* 28: 377–81.

10  National Institute for Health and Care Excellence (2008). *Antenatal care for uncomplicated pregnancies.* NICE guidelines CG62. Available at: ℘ www.nice.org.uk/guidance/cg62.

11  National Institute for Health and Care Excellence (2014). *Intrapartum care for healthy women and babies.* NICE guidelines CG190. Available at: ℘ www.nice.org.uk/guidance/cg190.

## Further reading

Mousa AH, Blum J, Ghada A, Shakur H, Alfirevic Z (2014). Treatment for primary postpartum haemorrhage. *Cochrane Database Syst Rev* 2: CD003249. Available at: ℘ onlinelibrary.wiley.com/doi/10.1002/14651858.CD003249.pub3/full.

Royal College of Obstetricians and Gynaecologists (2011). *Prevention and management of postpartum haemorrhage. Green-top guideline No. 52.* Available at: ℘ www.rcog.org.uk/globalassets/documents/guidelines/gt52postpartumhaemorrhage0411.pdf.

# HELLP syndrome

(*H*, haemolysis; *EL*, elevated liver enzymes; *LP*, low platelets)

This is an uncommon but severe complication of pre-eclampsia, although it is sometimes seen when hypertension is not present. It is a manifestation of impaired liver function. It may occur during the later stages of pregnancy, and during or up to 48h after delivery. Diagnosis is confirmed by laboratory assessment of the blood coagulation pattern.

There is a risk of maternal/fetal morbidity/mortality due to:
- Impaired clotting, or bleeding
- Severe liver damage, leading to failure or rupture
- Severe kidney damage, leading to failure
- Respiratory difficulties
- Cerebral haemorrhage/convulsions
- IUGR: premature delivery may be needed and intrauterine death may occur.

Be aware of, and assess for:
- Epigastric pain (severe, not relieved by antacid; liver tenderness)
- Nausea and vomiting, headaches
- Haematuria, jaundice
- Blood slow to clot.

Discuss management plans with a consultant obstetrician.

## Diagnosis

Blood samples to send for laboratory assessment include:
- FBC/platelets
- U/E
- Clotting and DIC screen
- LFTs
- G&S and cross-match.

Laboratory reports demonstrate the altered blood pattern:
- *Haemolysis* (the breakdown of RBCs). This process begins to occur faster than it would naturally. Severe pre-eclampsia causes damage to the vascular system. Changes occur in the liver. Platelets collect as the initial step of repair and fibrin networks form. Haemolysis results from damage that occurs as the circulating red cells are pushed through the fibrin networks. A reduction in red cell numbers occurs. The haematocrit (a measure of red cell concentration) may therefore decrease; bilirubin (a by-product of red cell breakdown) may increase.
- *Elevated liver enzymes*. Intravascular fibrin deposits obstruct the flow of blood in the liver. The liver is under stress; therefore, the liver enzyme levels become raised. Liver damage is indicated by raised alkaline phosphatase (APT), ALT, and AST.
- *Low platelets* (<100 × 10⁹/L). Platelets initiate and are essential to blood coagulation. In HELLP syndrome, clotting factors are mopped up and platelet levels in the blood decrease (thrombocytopenia). This is only treated if bleeding occurs.

## Treatment

Urgent delivery may be indicated:

- Transfusion of platelets or blood may be necessary if the woman is bleeding
- A Caesarean may be performed under general anaesthesia since regional anaesthesia may be contraindicated because of low platelets; however, intubation may increase BP further.

The aim of management is to support hepatic and renal function until the condition resolves:

- IV glucose may be needed (10% glucose/500mL in 6h) to maintain blood glucose at 5+ mmol/L
- Accurate assessment of intake and output of fluids is paramount
- A CVP or an arterial line will facilitate accuracy.

Be aware that the woman may have haemorrhage during and/or post-Caesarean. Ensure an adequate local supply of suitable cross-matched blood.

# Disseminated intravascular coagulation

- DIC may occur secondary to severe pre-eclampsia and HELLP syndrome.
- Because of injury to vessel walls, blood clotting activity is abnormally increased. Fibrin is formed, resulting in a large number of small thrombi in the capillary circulation.
- As a normal reaction to clot formation, to maintain equilibrium, the body initiates a process of clot breakdown (fibrinolysis).
- In DIC, because clot formation is widespread, a large number of fibrin degradation products (FDPs) are produced. These are also anticoagulants. Clotting factors and platelets are mopped up as a large number of microthrombi form.
- As a result, uncontrolled bleeding may occur, without clot formation.

## Diagnosis

Report:
- Any unexpected bleeding from the nose or mucous membrane and oozing from a venepuncture site
- Cyanosis of the extremities (fingers/toes).

Laboratory tests of venous blood samples should demonstrate when a case of severe pre-eclampsia is beginning to be affected by DIC. Discuss the required frequency of testing with the obstetrician. It is usually daily.
- The *D-dimer test* detects fibrin derivatives and therefore breakdown. FDPs should normally be 200ng/mL but in DIC can be >2000ng/mL. This is the most specific test for DIC.
- *FBC and platelets*. Platelets are essential factors for coagulation of the blood and will be decreased in DIC (<100 × $10^9$/L).
- *Prothrombin time* (PT) measures the coagulation time of plasma (extrinsic clotting pathway). The normal range is 11–15s. In DIC, this time may be increased.
- *Activated partial thromboplastin time* (APTT) measures plasma coagulation (intrinsic clotting pathway). The normal range is 29–37s. This time may also be increased in DIC.
- *Fibrinogen levels* detect the coagulation capacity of the blood. Fibrinogen is a protein formed in the liver. Thrombin activates fibrinogen to form fibrin. The normal range is 0–40g/L. It may be decreased in DIC.

## Treatment

This is aimed at prevention and correcting the underlying problem, and therefore removing the trigger mechanism for DIC. If the blood pattern demonstrates rising FDPs, this would form part of the rationale for a speedy delivery.
- Unless FDP levels are very high, the presence of some clotting factors should stop bleeding.
- If treatment is considered necessary, for instance to prepare a woman for a Caesarean, a senior haematologist should be consulted.
- Treatment involves replacement of clotting factors in order to restore equilibrium.

# Emboli

An embolus (plural emboli) is any detached, travelling intravascular mass (solid, liquid, or gaseous) carried by circulation, which is capable of clogging arterial capillary beds (creating an arterial occlusion) at a site distant from its point of origin.

## Thromboembolism

A thrombus (blood clot) from a blood vessel is completely or partially detached from the site of thrombosis (clot). The blood flow carries the embolus (via blood vessels) to various parts of the body where it can block the lumen (vessel cavity) and cause vessel obstruction or occlusion.

*Deep vein thrombosis* (DVT) resulting in a *pulmonary embolism* (PE) is common in pregnancy and the postnatal period. Incidence and management are discussed in Chapter 10.

## Amniotic fluid embolism

Amniotic fluid embolism (AFE) is a rare condition where an embolus of amniotic fluid enters the maternal circulation. It affects pregnant women, typically occurring during labour but can occur antenatally and up to 48h post-partum. Estimates of incidence vary between one in 8000 and one in 80 000 pregnancies.[12] It carries a high maternal mortality rate; estimates of death from this condition vary widely, from as much as 86% to as little as 16–30%.[12]

AFE may happen at amniocentesis, termination of pregnancy, or a Caesarean section.[13] Fetal skin cells or meconium in the amniotic fluid cause platelet thrombi to form, blocking the pulmonary vessels. Pulmonary hypertension ensues, ultimately leading to right-sided heart failure. There are similarities in the blood pattern and clinical findings in anaphylactic and septic shock and AFE. Circulating amniotic fluid may also cause DIC.

*Possible predisposing factors or cause*

No clear risk factors for AFE are discernible from previous cases,[12] although a weak link between intrapartum placental abruption and AFE has been identified.

*Evidence does suggest that earlier diagnosis may lead to better outcomes.*

*Signs and symptoms*

- A sudden change in the woman's behaviour or mood may be an early feature of the onset of hypoxia.
- Maternal anxiety and feelings of doom.
- Dyspnoea, tachypnoea, cyanosis.
- Pink frothy sputum.
- Hypotension.
- Convulsions may occur (can precede respiratory symptoms).
- Bleeding per vaginam/haemorrhage.
- Shock/collapse.

*Subsequent picture and complications*

- Hypoxia may cause permanent neurological damage.
- Massive haemorrhage may occur as a result of DIC (➔ see Disseminated intravascular coagulation, p. 500).
- Acute renal failure as a result of hypotension.
- Anoxia and neurological damage to fetus.
- Death of both mother and fetus.

*Management*

- The woman's life may depend on early detection and immediate action by the midwife.[13]
- Call for the emergency resuscitation team, including the obstetrician and anaesthetist. Inform the haematologist and the chest physician on call.
- Assess airway and breathing—give 100% oxygen via a face mask initially. Use a pulse oximeter.
- Assess the BP and pulse. For the maintenance of circulation and to combat hypotension, site/help site an IV infusion. Diuretics and drugs which support the cardiac muscles to contract effectively (dopamine and digoxin) may be given to the woman.
- Take bloods and dispatch for FBC, cross-match 4 units, coagulation screen, U/E, blood glucose, blood culture, blood gases.
- Organize an ECG and portable chest X-ray.
- The anaesthetist may insert a pulmonary artery catheter to aid fluid replacement and monitor for fluid overload.
- After initial IV infusion has been given to improve the BP, the midwife may be asked to restrict fluids to prevent pulmonary oedema and respiratory distress.
- A urinary catheter is sited and strict fluid balance maintained. Output should be 25–30mL/h.
- Treat DIC—FFP and platelets should be administered immediately, or whole blood if available.
- It may be necessary for the anaesthetic team to intubate the woman to maintain adequate oxygenation.
- The team may need to deliver the baby by an emergency Caesarean section within 15min to minimize anoxia and prevent neurological damage to the baby and to facilitate maternal resuscitation.
- Cardiopulmonary arrest may occur which has a low rate of survival, but if the woman survives, her condition will be monitored in intensive care.

Any suspected or proven case of AFE should be reported to the UK register.

### References

12 UK Obstetric Surveillance System (2015). *Amniotic fluid embolism.* Available at: 🔗 www.npeu. ox.ac.uk/ukoss/current-surveillance/amf.

13 Arulkumaran S, Symonds IM, Fowlie A (2004). *Oxford Handbook of Obstetrics and Gynaecology.* Oxford: Oxford University Press.

# Acute uterine inversion

### Definition
This is a rare complication of labour. The uterus turns inside out and pro-lapses into the vagina. It happens suddenly during the third stage of labour. It can be a cause of maternal death because of shock and haemorrhage.

### Factors associated with acute uterine inversion
- Adherent placenta.
- Fundal placenta.
- Short umbilical cord.
- More common in primiparae.
- Macrosomic fetus.
- Atonic uterus (sometimes with sudden cough or sneeze).
- Distended uterus suddenly emptied.

### Types of acute inversion
- Incomplete inversion when the body of the uterus does not extend beyond the cervical rim.
- Complete inversion when the body of the uterus extends as far as the introitus.
- Prolapse of the uterus through the introitus.

### Prevention
The reason why inversion happens is not fully understood. However, acute inversion may sometimes be aggravated by mismanagement of the third stage of labour.[14]

The midwife should *never*:
- Use fundal pressure to expel the placenta (Crede's manoeuvre)
- Use excessive controlled cord traction (CCT)
- Attempt to deliver the placenta without signs of separation
- Use CCT when the uterus is relaxed
- Use CCT, omitting to guard the uterus with the left hand above the symphysis pubis.

### Signs and symptoms
- The placenta may/may not be separated.
- Haemorrhage is usually present whether or not the placenta is separated.
- Shock due to:
  - Blood loss
  - Pain.
- On abdominal palpation, the fundus of the uterus cannot be located, or if inversion is incomplete a concave shape may be felt.
- A bluish, bleeding mass may be present in the vagina or at the introitus. It is the interior of the fundus of the uterus.
- Incomplete inversion is more difficult to identify. Extreme shock and pain (possibly caused by tension on the peritoneum, ovaries, and nerves of the broad ligament) may be out of proportion to the amount of haemorrhage and may be a clue to diagnosis.

## Management
- Call for the obstetric and anaesthetic team.
- The best opportunity for replacing the uterus is as soon as the inversion occurs. This is especially important in the community situation. This will avoid blood loss and shock.
- The woman should be laid flat. The foot of the bed should be raised.
- The woman should be given an explanation to gain her consent and cooperation and have adequate analgesia.

## Johnson's manoeuvre
- It may be possible to speedily reduce an inversion if the midwife recognizes the condition immediately and applies gentle pressure to the uterus, starting at the point nearest to the cervix and working towards the fundus. Thus the inverted uterus is pushed back, following the angle of the vagina, through the cervix, then directing the push upwards towards the umbilicus to restore the normal position.
- If the placenta is not delivered and not bleeding, it should be left *in situ* to avoid haemorrhage. The inverted uterus cannot contract.
- If the woman's condition is stable, there is some bleeding because of apparent separation, and she has adequate analgesia, the placenta can be removed if this facilitates repositioning.
- IV ergometrine 0.25mg or 5 units of oxytocin slowly administered will secure a good contraction once the uterus is established in place.

## Shock
- If there is severe bleeding and hypotension, the woman must be treated immediately and urgently for shock.
- Two IV infusions are sited using a large-bore cannula, and IV fluid commenced to help fast replacement of fluid and allow administration of drugs.
- Respirations, pulse and BP, and oxygen saturation are monitored.
- Bloods are obtained for FBC and platelets, G&S and cross-match, and coagulation.
- Analgesia should be given urgently.
- Catheterize the bladder and monitor output.
- Transfer to theatre at the earliest opportunity.

## Other methods to help replacement
- Manual replacement of the uterus may be complicated by the development of a retraction ring between upper and lower segments or a tight cervix. The anaesthetist may give IV drugs to relax the uterus such as terbutaline 0.25mg or ritodrine 6mg before the obstetrician attempts replacement. However, this relaxation of the uterus may also be achieved by giving the woman a general anaesthetic.
- Under general anaesthetic, hydrostatic repositioning may be effective. The obstetrician replaces the inverted uterus in the vagina and 'seals off' the external labia with one hand. Several litres of warm saline are infused into the posterior vaginal fornix via an IV giving set. The fluid exerts pressure evenly over the uterus and pushes it back into position. The manual and hydrostatic methods may be used together.

- Operative procedures are successful as a last resort. Laparotomy may be necessary under general anaesthetic. Forceps are placed on the round ligaments. The obstetrician pulls gently on the ligaments whilst a second operator pushes the uterus upwards from the vagina.
- The hand is kept inside the uterus until oxytocin (e.g. 5 units IV) has produced a firm effective contraction.
- Oxytocin (e.g. IV 20 units in 500mL of normal saline via a pump over 4h) should then be administered to keep the uterus contracted and to prevent recurrence. IV oxytocin should be used with caution in hypovolaemia.

### Post-partum
- The woman should be observed in a high-dependency area until stable.
- Broad-spectrum antibiotics should be given for 5 days minimum.

### Reference
14 Arulkumaran S, Symonds IM, Fowlie A (2004). *Oxford Handbook of Obstetrics and Gynaecology*. Oxford: Oxford University Press.

# Uterine rupture

## Definition

## Types

## Risk factors associated with a risk of rupture during labour

## Prevention

# Uterine rupture

### Definition

This is a dangerous complication of pregnancy and labour when there is a laceration of the uterine wall. Tears may extend to uterine vessels and haemorrhage ensue. Rupture of the gravid uterus is a devastating complication of pregnancy with high maternal and fetal mortality and morbidity:

- 6.2% of uterine ruptures are associated with perinatal death
- 14–33% of women with uterine rupture require an emergency hysterectomy
- In a systematic review of VBAC, the uterine rupture rate was 3 per 1000 VBACs. Maternal mortality rate for trial of labour was 3.8 per 100 000 and 13.4 per 100 000 for elective repeat Caesarean.[15]

### Types

*Incomplete*

- The depth of the myometrium may be torn, but the perimetrium remains intact.
- The external myometrium may be torn, but the laceration does not extend into the body of the uterus. This may lead to intraperitoneal haemorrhage.

*Complete*

All layers of the uterus are involved. There is direct communication between the uterine and abdominal cavities and the fetus may be expelled from the uterus into the abdominal cavity.

### Risk factors associated with risk of rupture during labour

- Scar rupture following a Caesarean section (both lower and upper segment incision), hysterotomy, myomectomy, previous rupture repair. Scar dehiscence is the most common cause of rupture.
- Spontaneous rupture resulting from strong uterine contractions. It is sometimes associated with use of oxytocin, especially in multiparous women or with obstructed labour.
- Traumatic rupture from instruments, e.g. a high rotational forceps delivery or from manipulation (e.g. internal podalic version and breech extraction of second twin) when there is previous scarring.
- Trauma may occur as a result of accident.

### Prevention

*For women with a uterine scar*

- On admission to the labour ward, the midwife should ensure that a birth plan discussion is documented in the notes by a senior obstetrician and that the woman is satisfied with the plan.
- If VBAC is anticipated, good progress in labour should be observed and any fetal heart abnormalities reported to the obstetrician by the midwife.
- If augmentation of labour is indicated, IV oxytocin must be prescribed by the registrar and administered with care.

- Induction should be overseen by a consultant obstetrician and proceedings documented carefully in the case notes. Amniotomy is the preferred method. However, one or two doses of dinoprostone gel 1mg PV (prostaglandin) may be given, but repeat doses should preferably be avoided and further management discussed. Propess® pessary may be used with caution—remove after 12h.[16]

*Spontaneous rupture*
- If oxytocin is used to induce or augment labour, the midwife should be vigilant that contractions occur no more than four in 10min and last approximately 60s. The amount of oxytocin given should be carefully monitored in multiparous women.
- The midwife should consider disproportion or abnormal presentation when labour is delayed.

## Silent rupture
- Associated with previous Caesarean section and partial scar separation—perhaps some blood loss PV but no haemorrhage at the site of scar dehiscence.
- Mildly raised maternal pulse (>100bpm), pale.
- Some abdominal pain, scar tenderness. Epidural may sometimes mask the pain.
- Contractions may continue but no progress in labour.
- Irregularities of fetal heart, but, if diagnosed, fetus born alive.

*Typical signs*
- Develops over an hour or two.
- Low abdominal pain, unlike contraction pain, continuous.
- Tenderness on abdominal palpation.
- Vomiting.
- Faintness, pale.
- Blood loss PV, variable amount.
- Rising pulse.
- Cessation of previously efficient uterine contractions.
- Signs of fetal compromise, variable decelerations, bradycardia.
- If undiagnosed—hypotension and shock, absent FHR.

## Violent rupture
- Strong uterine contraction. The woman reports 'something giving way' and sharp pain in lower abdomen.
- Chest or shoulder tip pain and sudden shortness of breath.
- Contractions cease and the abdominal pain is continuous.
- The woman has a sense of foreboding that something serious has happened. She becomes anxious.
- Blood loss PV/gross haematuria.
- On abdominal palpation, the fetus is felt close to the fingers and the presenting part can be moved easily and may not be in the pelvis. Abdominal palpation may reveal obvious fetal parts as the fetus passes either partially or totally out of the uterus and into the abdominal cavity, with a high risk of intrapartum death.
- Maternal tachycardia, shock, and collapse soon occur.
- The FHR is profoundly bradycardic or absent.

## Management

- Briefly explain to the woman and partner.
- Alert the senior obstetric and anaesthetic team.
- The consultant should be called.
- Ensure IV access with large-bore (16 gauge) cannula and commence IV infusion; infuse quickly.
- Give the woman oxygen via a face mask.
- Alert theatre staff to prepare urgently for laparotomy.
- Follow the protocol for major obstetric haemorrhage. Cross-match 6 units (➔ see Major obstetric haemorrhage, p. 490).
- Transfer the woman to theatre immediately in the hope of delivering a live baby if the FHR is still recordable.

➔ See Emergency lower segment Caesarean section, p. 465.

*Postnatally*

- Admit the woman to the HDU.
- Close monitoring of maternal condition, especially fluid balance and oxygen saturation.
- Prescribe broad-spectrum antibiotics for 5 days.

## References

15 Guise JM, Eden K, Emeis C, et al. (2010). Vaginal birth after cesarean: new insights. *Evid Rep Technol Assess (Full Rep)* 191: 1–397.

16 Turgut A, Ozler A, Siddik Evsen M, et al. (2013). Uterine rupture revisited: predisposing factors, clinical features, management and outcomes from a tertiary care center in Turkey. *Pak J Med Sci* 29: 753–7.

## Further reading

Fox NS, Gerber RS, Mourad M, et al. (2014). Pregnancy outcomes in patients with prior uterine rupture or dehiscence. *Obstet Gynecol* 123: 785.

Ronel D, Wiznitzer A, Sergienko R, Zlotnik A, Sheiner E (2012). Trends, risk factors and pregnancy outcome in women with uterine rupture. *Arch Gynecol Obstet* 285: 317–21.

Walsh CA, Baxi LV (2007). Rupture of the primigravid uterus: a review of the literature. *Obstet Gynecol Surv* 62: 327–34.

# Shock

Acute shock results in collapse; the body is unable to receive oxygen and nutrition and to excrete waste. Shock must be reversed quickly to avoid chronic conditions and death.

## Causes specific to childbearing

- PPH.
- Uterine rupture or inversion.
- Undiagnosed intra-abdominal or genital tract haematoma.
- AFE.
- Eclampsia.

## Causes that may complicate childbearing

- Thromboembolism.
- PE, pulmonary oedema, Mendelson's syndrome.
- Sepsis (endotoxic/bacteraemic shock).
- Allergy (anaphylactic shock).
- Metabolic or endocrine (e.g. diabetic collapse).
- Haemorrhage from organ rupture or aneurysm.
- Epilepsy, cerebrovascular accident, subarachnoid haemorrhage.
- Heart failure, arrhythmias, myocardial infarction (➔ see also Cardiac conditions, p. 186).
- Substance misuse or overdose.

## Signs and symptoms

- Pale, cold, clammy, fingernails blue grey.
- Dry mouth, thirsty.
- Initially BP is maintained, then it falls.
- Increasing pulse rate—thready and weak.
- Increased respiratory rate—fast and shallow.
- Oliguria, anuria if low BP (systolic <80mmHg) continues.
- Dizzy, restless, lethargic, sometimes in acute pain.
- Mood change, altering consciousness.

## Management

The first priority is resuscitation, but, at the same time, it is necessary to think about the cause, so that treatment can be given.

- Call for emergency equipment and help from the obstetric and anaesthetic team.
- Explain briefly to the woman's partner, and acknowledge anxiety. Give information as available.
- Position the woman flat or in recovery position if semi-conscious.
- Assess breathing and give oxygen via a face mask.
- Assess vital signs, BP, pulse, oxygen saturation.
- Site, or help site, large-bore (14 gauge) IV cannulae, enough to replace fluids.
- Take blood as indicated and requested by the obstetrician for FBC, G&S or cross-match, U/E, LFTs, coagulation screen, blood cultures, and blood glucose.

- Support the anaesthetist to take and dispatch any arterial bloods for blood gases, to site a CVP line, and to monitor readings.
- Catheterize the woman and measure urine output hourly. Anuria, oliguria, and blood staining of the urine indicate low renal blood flow.
- Help the team to facilitate a speedy delivery of the baby if necessary.
- Assist the obstetrician to perform a full clinical, including neurological, examination.

## Addressing the cause of shock

Be ready with the following information at the onset of collapse, to help with diagnosis of the cause:

Has the woman:
- Delivered baby and placenta?
- Had excessive blood loss?
- Been in pain, if so what area of the body?
- Had a fit?
- Any medical history of, for example, PIH, diabetes, epilepsy, heart condition?
- Been given any medication?
- Had pyrexia?

### Haemorrhage

For the diagnosis of haemorrhage, → see Major obstetric haemorrhage, p. 490).

### Septic shock

For the diagnosis of septic shock, → see Sepsis, p. 180.

Very rarely, you may see the following.

### Anaphylactic shock

Anaphylaxis is a severe and potentially fatal systemic hypersensitivity reaction which occurs because the woman has been exposed to an antigen against which she has been previously sensitized. Typically this may occur following the administration of medicines such as anaesthetic agents or antibiotics.[17] It is characterized by a combination of life-threatening airway, breathing, or circulatory problems with skin or mucosal changes. The body releases histamine when challenged with the antigen, which dilates arteries and makes capillaries more permeable. There is always a rapid onset and progression of symptoms—the BP falls and signs of shock are present.

- Record the time of onset of the reaction and the circumstances immediately before the onset of symptoms to help to identify the possible trigger.
- Document the acute clinical features of the suspected anaphylactic reaction (rapidly developing, life-threatening problems involving the airway [pharyngeal or laryngeal oedema] and/or breathing [bronchospasm with tachypnoea] and/or circulation [hypotension and/or tachycardia] and, in most cases, associated skin and mucosal changes).
- Adrenaline, ephedrine, antihistamines, or corticosteroids may be given by the anaesthetist.

- Take timed blood samples for mast cell tryptase testing as follows:
  - A sample as soon as possible after emergency treatment has started
  - A second sample ideally within 1–2h (but no later than 4h) from the onset of symptoms.
- After emergency treatment for suspected anaphylaxis, offer a referral to a specialist allergy service (age-appropriate where possible) consisting of health-care professionals with the skills and competencies necessary to accurately investigate, diagnose, monitor, and provide ongoing management of, and patient education about, suspected anaphylaxis.

*Cardiorespiratory collapse*
- A fall in cardiac output occurs as a result of heart failure. Venous return is reduced. The lungs become congested with blood.
- Arrange chest X-ray, arterial gases, ECG, FBC, U/E.

*Neurological conditions*
- Indicated by an alteration in consciousness when cardiorespiratory signs are not present.
- An MRI scan of the brain may be needed.

*Diabetic collapse*
- The woman will typically be an insulin-dependent diabetic.
- The woman may become uncooperative, distant, and confused.
- She will feel faint, sweating but clammy.
- Give a drink with sugar if possible—unconsciousness will not then occur. If it does, it is quickly reversed by a glucagon injection or IV glucose fluids.

*Drug toxicity/overdose collapse*
Drug toxicity/overdose should be considered in all cases of collapse, and illicit drug use/overdose should be remembered as a potential cause of collapse outside of hospital.

## Reference

17 Mulla ZD, Ebrahim MS, Gonzalez JL (2010). Anaphylaxis in the obstetric patient: analysis of a statewide hospital discharge database. *Ann Allergy Asthma Immunol* 104: 55–9.

# Maternal resuscitation

Cardiopulmonary arrest is estimated to occur once in every 30 000 late pregnancies and somewhere between 0.14 and 6/1000 (14 and 600/100 000) births.[18] As it is such a rare event, with potentially devastating consequences, it is essential that caregivers are skilled in initial effective resuscitation techniques and are able to investigate and diagnose the cause of the collapse to allow appropriate, directed continuing management. Basic resuscitation skills are an essential requirement of all midwives, who should be familiar with resuscitation guidelines and the location and use of resuscitation equipment provided.

Although the incidence of arrest is low, there are emergency situations that may result in cardiopulmonary arrest necessitating resuscitation:[18,19]

- Acidosis
- Anaphylaxis
- Anaesthetic complications
- Cardiac disease: myocardial ischaemia/infarction, aortic dissection, cardiomyopathy
- Cerebral aneurysm
- Embolism: pulmonary, coronary, AFE
- Epilepsy
- Haemorrhage/DIC
- Hypertension, pre-eclampsia, eclampsia
- Hypoglycaemia
- Hypo-/hyperthermia
- Hypoxia, hyper-/hypokalaemia
- Placental abruption/praevia
- Ruptured liver/spleen
- Septic shock
- Tamponade
- Tension pneumothorax
- Thromboembolism
- Total spinal block
- Toxins
- Trauma
- Uterine atony
- Uterine inversion
- Uterine rupture.

## Responsibility of the midwife

- Provide effective basic life support to ensure adequate circulation and perfusion of vital organs.
- Participate in, and often initiate, advanced life support.

## In pregnancy

- Oxygen consumption is increased; therefore, oxygen supply to the brain will diminish more rapidly than in a non-pregnant person.
- To optimize fetal outcome, support should be given to the mother.
- Basic life support should be initiated immediately.

## Resuscitation in a hospital setting

If a woman collapses or is found collapsed:

- Pull the emergency buzzer/shout for help
- Assess responsiveness. Gently shake her shoulders and shout
- If she *responds*:
  - Send for medical assistance
  - Position in left lateral
  - Maintain airway
  - Give oxygen via a non-rebreathe mask 14L/min
  - Monitor vital signs
  - Consider venous cannulation
  - Stay with her until medical review and investigations.
- If there is no response, check breathing and circulation. This can be done simultaneously. Take no more than 10s.

*Airway*

With your hand on the woman's forehead, gently tilt her head back; remove any visible obstruction from the mouth; place your fingertips on the point of her chin, and lift the chin to open the airway. If trauma to the head or neck is suspected, avoid this head tilt manoeuvre. Instead a jaw thrust should be performed.

*Breathing*

- *Look* for chest movements.
- *Listen* for breath sounds.
- *Feel* for air on your cheek.

*Circulation*

- Feel for a carotid pulse.
- If she is not breathing, a 'maternal cardiac arrest emergency' should be declared and activated immediately. Ensure that the cardiac arrest team has been called, and the defibrillator and emergency equipment have been sent for, as well as an obstetrician capable of performing a Caesarean delivery. The neonatal team should be called early if delivery is likely.
- If >20 weeks pregnant, ensure that aorto-caval compression is prevented to optimize the cardiac output produced from chest compressions. Place the woman in a supine position on a firm, flat surface (e.g. use a backboard) with left manual uterine displacement. Manual uterine displacement should be performed using two hands from the left side of the patient; the designated provider must pull leftward and upward (if downward force is inadvertently applied, inferior vena caval compression may worsen). Left lateral tilt of the patient to a full 30° (i.e. raise the right side of the pelvis with a pillow or wedge) can also be used, but this position may make the provision of adequate chest compressions more challenging as the force transmitted to the chest wall is reduced.
- Commence cardiopulmonary resuscitation (CPR).
- CPR should be commenced with 30 chest compressions; observe chest movements. Start high-quality chest compressions at a rate of 100/min immediately to optimize maternal and fetal outcomes.

*To perform chest compressions*

- Place the heel of one hand over the lower half of the sternum; place the heel of the other hand on top of the first hand, and extend or interlock the fingers. Do not apply pressure over the ribs, upper abdomen, or tip of the sternum. For women in the third trimester of pregnancy, it is recommended during resuscitation to place the hand 2–3cm higher on the sternum than in non-pregnant individuals. From above the woman, with arms straight, press down to depress the sternum 4–5cm. Release the pressure and repeat at a rate of about 100/min. Take equal time with compression and release to allow the chest to recoil.
- After 30 compressions, check the airway position and give two more breaths. Continue this ratio of two breaths to 30 compressions until advanced life support is in place. In the ideal situation, it would be advisable to deliver cardiac compressions continuously without pauses as this increases the chances of survival. This is only possible once an endotracheal tube or an advanced airway has been placed.
- The resuscitation team should rotate its team members every 2min because compressions are physically rigorous and provider fatigue develops rapidly.
- If other staff are present whilst waiting for the arrest team to arrive, they should:
  - Apply ECG monitor/defibrillator pads
  - Monitor pulse oximetry
  - Monitor BP
  - Cannulate using ×2 large-bore (16 gauge, grey) Venflon®
  - Obtain bloods for urgent cross-match, FBC, coagulation screen, U/E, blood glucose, LFTs, and arterial blood gas
  - Make notes of times, actions, and any fluid/drug treatment.

## Considerations in pregnancy

*Airway*

It may be difficult to maintain an airway, and intubation may be difficult due to:
- Neck obesity
- Enlarged breasts
- Glottic oedema.

A bag–valve–mask is preferred, with two staff working together, one holding the mask and maintaining the airway and the other giving inflation breaths and chest compressions. If a pocket mask is nearby, use this until more help and equipment arrive and connect to oxygen as soon as possible. If the woman is unconscious, a Guedel airway can be used to help maintain the airway.

*Breathing*

Due to delayed gastric emptying, reduced tone of stomach muscle sphincter, and increased pressure on the stomach from the gravid uterus, there is an *increased risk of regurgitation and pulmonary aspiration*. Early intubation using cricoid pressure is preferable.[20]

Until the airway is protected by the insertion of a cuffed tracheal tube, aspiration can occur. Give each ventilation slowly over 2s, with volumes just sufficient to produce a visible chest rise (400–600mL). Allow the chest to deflate following each breath.

*Circulation*
There is an increased circulatory demand in pregnancy.
• Pressure on the major vessels (aorto-caval compression) should be relieved by left lateral displacement of the uterus. This will improve venous return and cardiac output. Placing a Cardiff wedge or pillow under the right side will achieve this by tilting the woman by approximately 30°. Alternatively, raising her right hip, or manual displacement of the uterus to the left and upwards, will suffice until suitable equipment arrives.
• Chest compression may be more difficult in this position.

## Advanced life support
Treat arrhythmias according to standard protocols.
• Avoid lidocaine when epidural anaesthesia has been used, as high levels of local anaesthetic may be present in the blood. Amiodarone is an alternative antiarrhythmic drug.
• If 5min of in-hospital resuscitation is unsuccessful, an emergency Caesarean section is indicated to save the fetus (in the third trimester) and improve the prognosis for the mother. Advanced life support should continue during and after the procedure.[20]

## Resuscitation out of the hospital setting
Follow basic life support guidelines; assess responsiveness and breathing. If no response and no breathing, start high-quality chest compressions at a rate of 100/min immediately to optimize maternal and fetal outcomes. If you are alone, you may need to use your knee to tilt the woman onto her left side; a cushion or clothing might have to be used whilst you call for assistance.

Send for medical assistance. An emergency ambulance should be sent for; clear instructions are important, stating 'I have an unconscious, pregnant woman who is not breathing, we are at [address]', as this should influence the type of assistance that is sent. In the home setting, a partner, friend, or neighbour could be given clear instructions and asked to call an ambulance.

If alone and without the use of a phone, you will have to decide whether to start resuscitation or go for help. This might be influenced by the condition/cause of collapse and available equipment; however, if there is no breathing and/or pulse, it is advisable to call for medical assistance before attempting resuscitation, to ensure that advanced life support and defibrillation are available as soon as possible. If the likely cause of unconsciousness is a breathing problem, i.e. drugs/alcohol, 1min of CPR should be performed before going for help.

On arrival of the ambulance, basic life support should continue. Advanced life support may be initiated, depending on the skills of the team that arrives, and the woman should be transferred to hospital as soon as possible. The hospital should be notified of her pending arrival so that preparations can be made.

## Cross-infection

All community midwives should carry equipment that will protect them when performing basic life support. Key fobs are available containing a single-use mask which, when placed over the victim's mouth to perform mouth-to-mouth resuscitation, will give some protection against cross-infection. Pocket masks are also available with one-way valves, which will prevent transmission of bacteria.

In the hospital, the midwife should wait for equipment to arrive before attempting ventilations. Chest compressions can be performed whilst waiting. Gloves and eye protection must be worn, and considerable care taken with needles and sharp instruments.

## Jaw thrust manoeuvre

Used to open the upper airway with minimal movement of the cervical spine. Using both hands, place the forefingers behind the angle of the jaw. Keeping the head and neck still, push the jaw forward and upwards; this will push the tongue forwards and away from the pharynx.

## References

18 Royal College of Obstetricians and Gynaecologists (2011). *Maternal collapse in pregnancy and the puerperium. Green-top guideline No. 56.* Available at: ℛ www.rcog.org.uk/globalassets/documents/guidelines/gtg56.pdf.

19 Institute of Obstetricians and Gynaecologists, Royal College of Physicians of Ireland, Health Service Executive (2014). *Clinical practice guideline: resuscitation for the pregnant woman.* Available at: ℛ www.hse.ie/eng/about/Who/clinical/natclinprog/obsandgynaeprogramme/resuscitationpregnantwoman.pdf.

20 Resuscitation Council (UK) (2015). *Resuscitation guidelines 2015.* Available at: ℛ www.resus.org.uk/pages/guide.htm.

## Guidelines for admission to critical care

# Guidelines for admission to critical care

Maternal critical care, high-dependency care, and high-risk maternity care are not interchangeable terms. The RCOG/Royal College of Anaesthetists (RCoA) Maternal Critical Care Group[21] reiterates that the terms 'high dependency' and 'intensive care' be replaced by the term 'critical care'. This also supports earlier proposals that the care required by an individual be independent of location, coining the phrase 'critical care without walls'.

Within the term, care is subdivided into four levels, dependent on organ support and the level of monitoring required independent of diagnosis:
• Level 0—care for women whose needs can be met on a normal ward
• Level 1—care is provided for women at high risk of their condition deteriorating, needing more frequent monitoring
• Level 2—care is for women who need invasive monitoring or support for a single organ system
• Level 3—care is for women needing advanced respiratory support alone or basic respiratory support along with support for an additional organ.

Policy for admission may vary between units, depending on facilities and available personnel. Admission to level 2 care should be considered in the following situations:
• Ante- or postnatal hypertensive women whose condition is deteriorating, e.g. when the BP is difficult to control, LFTs are abnormal, and signs of fulminating pre-eclampsia or cerebral agitation are present
• Women who experience major haemorrhage which is causing maternal compromise
• Women who experience blood loss of 1000mL or more
• Women suspected of having PE or having signs of respiratory distress, hypoxia, or tachycardia
• Following LSCS, when the woman has insulin-dependent diabetes mellitus and a sliding scale with insulin and glucose is in progress
• Any woman having had general anaesthesia
• Women who receive diamorphine via an epidural catheter
• Women showing signs of shock, septicaemia, and anaphylaxis
• Status epilepticus
• Women diagnosed with pulmonary oedema or suspected AFE
• Any woman requiring continuous oxygen therapy
• Women suffering from HELLP syndrome or DIC (➔ see Disseminated intravascular coagulation, p. 500)
• Any woman with an underlying medical or surgical condition which is compromising maternal condition, e.g. known symptomatic heart condition
• Cardiac arrhythmia requiring continuous ECG monitoring
• Women requiring a CVP or arterial line
• Woman transferred back from a general ICU.

## Guidelines for transfer out of level 2 to level 3 care

The woman requiring level 3 care is unstable and requires multiple organ monitoring/support. The level of dependency is an important factor in determining appropriateness of level 3 care. A woman needs urgent attention in the following situations (if there is no improvement in 2h, seek consultant review for transfer to level 3):

- Women with chronic impairment of one or more organ systems, sufficient to restrict daily activities, and who require support for an acute reversible failure of another organ system
- A woman not responding to commands.
- The woman with deteriorating respiratory rate not responding to treatment:
  - Inability to maintain own airway
  - Requiring advanced respiratory support (mechanical ventilation).
  - Oxygen saturation of <90% despite 60% inspired oxygen.
- Pulse of <40bpm or >130bpm.
- Oliguria: urine output of <30mL/h for 3 consecutive hours.

## Reference

21 Maternal Critical Care Working Group (2011). *Providing equity of critical and maternity care for the critically ill pregnant or recently pregnant woman.* Available at: ℜ www.rcog.org.uk/globalassets/documents/guidelines/prov_eq_matandcritcare.pdf.

# Maternal mortality

The Confidential Enquiry into Maternal and Child Health report (2011) has been replaced by the MBRRACE report (2014). The purpose of its enquiry remains to assist in identifying factors that may be detrimental to maternal health and to assist in improving the care that mothers receive in pregnancy and when they are newly delivered. The report includes topic-specific reviews of deaths and morbidity due to sepsis, and deaths from haemorrhage, AFE, and anaesthetic-related, neurological, and other indirect causes.

The MBRRACE report (2014) found that in 2009–2012, 357 women died during or within 6 weeks of the end of their pregnancy in the UK. This represents a statistically significant decrease in the maternal mortality rate, which is now 10.12 per 100 000 maternities.

Direct maternal deaths have halved; this decrease is predominantly due to a reduction in deaths due to direct (obstetric) causes; the mortality rate from hypertensive disorders of pregnancy is now the lowest since the inception of the Confidential Enquiry in 1952. However, there has been no significant change in the rate of indirect maternal death over the last 10 years and the rate of indirect maternal deaths (6.87 per 100 000 maternities) is now twice that of direct deaths (3.25 per 100 000 maternities).

- Two-thirds of these women died from medical and mental health problems in pregnancy and only one-third from direct complications of pregnancy such as bleeding.
- Three-quarters of women who died had medical or mental health problems *before* they became pregnant.
- The most common cause of indirect death, and the largest cause of maternal deaths overall, was psychiatric illness. It is clear that maternal deaths from indirect (medical and psychiatric) causes are still not being addressed effectively.

The MBRRACE report[22] aimed to evaluate all the factors playing a part in women's deaths, and further analysis reinforces the need to ensure that maternity services are designed to meet the needs of all women and, in particular, those who are vulnerable or disadvantaged in any way.

Risk factors for maternal deaths are identified as follows

- Social disadvantage: women were up to 20 times more likely to die if they lived in families where both partners were unemployed, compared to those from more advantaged groups. Single mothers were three times more likely to die than those in stable relationships.
- Poor communities: in the most deprived areas of England, women had a 45% higher death rate compared with women from more affluent areas.
- Minority ethnic groups: women from groups other than white were three times more likely to die. Black African women, including asylum seekers and newly arrived refugees, had a seven times higher mortality rate than white women and had problems accessing the service.
- Late booking or poor attendance: 20% of the women who died booked for care after 22 weeks or had missed over four routine antenatal visits.
- Obesity: 35% of all the women who died were obese.
- Domestic violence: 14% of all the women who died disclosed that they were subject to violence in the home.
- Substance abuse: 8% of women who died were substance misusers.

The MBRRACE report[22] has provided an overview of the findings and recommendations specifically related to midwives and their practice. This is intended to stimulate debate on what lessons can be learnt from the management of the women who died. There are detailed recommendations on antenatal care and specific guidance for developing ways to meet the needs of women in the above-named groups.

## Reference

22 Knight M, Kenyon S, Brocklehurst P, Neilson J, Shakespeare J, Kurinczuk JJ (eds.) on behalf of MBRRACE-UK (2014). *Saving Lives, Improving Mothers' Care—Lessons learned to inform future maternity care from the UK and Ireland Confidential Enquiries into Maternal Deaths and Morbidity 2009–12*. Oxford: National Perinatal Epidemiology Unit, University of Oxford. Available at: ℘ www.npeu.ox.ac.uk/downloads/files/mbrrace-uk/reports/Saving%20Lives%20Improving%20 Mothers%20Care%20report%202014%20Full.pdf.

# Fetal emergencies during pregnancy, labour, and postnatally

## *In utero* transfer

The midwife may be asked to transfer a woman in preterm labour to a unit with a vacant cot at specialist neonatal facilities. The ambulance service will provide transport. The decision to transfer lies with the senior obstetrician, but the midwife involved should feel confident about the transfer.

She or he should have the time and opportunity to assess the woman's progress in labour and should discuss alternative arrangements if, for example:
• The woman is experiencing, or has recently experienced, fresh bleeding
• The woman is experiencing frequent strong contractions regularly and is distressed
• The woman is severely pre-eclamptic.

The midwife dealing with the transfer must:
• Ensure that the obstetric team which will be receiving the woman is identified and agree to the transfer
• Liaise with the ward or unit that will accommodate the woman
• Establish IV access
• Ensure that all medications have been given as prescribed
• Ensure that all information, including the receiving consultant's name, is recorded in the notes
• Ensure that a photocopy of the woman's hospital notes and summary is available for the receiving hospital
• Ensure that facilities are available to monitor and care for the woman during transit
• Arrange an ambulance and arrange for support by trained paramedical staff during the transfer
• Ensure that the woman and the woman's partner and family understand the rationale for transfer and that the family are able to visit
• Arrange transport for the midwife's return to base since the ambulance service will not routinely do this.

The midwife should travel with the woman and give care and support as appropriate on the journey, ensuring that the woman is comfortable at her destination before returning home.

# Hypoxia and asphyxia

The fetus has increased oxygen-carrying capacity because it has a high fetal Hb and a relatively high cardiac output. However, fetal oxygen supply can be reduced as a result of changes in:
- Maternal oxygenation and blood flow (cardiac or respiratory disease or maternal hypotension as a result of supine position, epidural, haemorrhage, or shock)
- Uterine blood flow (during labour, each strong uterine contraction temporarily restricts the blood/oxygen supply to the placenta; this may be more severe if oxytocin is used and contractions are hypertonic)
- Placental sufficiency (PIH)
- Fetal circulation (cord compression, abnormal fetal cardiac function).

## Fetal responses to hypoxia

In hypoxia, oxygen supply is insufficient for tissue energy requirements.
- Heart rate increases to increase cardiac output.
- Blood flow is directed to main organs (heart, brain).
- Reduced fetal activity/movement and, in chronic situations, IUGR.
- Eventually glucose and liver glycogen are metabolized (anaerobic metabolism—without oxygen) to provide energy to maintain organ function. This results in the production/accumulation of lactic acid, and metabolic acidosis occurs with a fall in blood pH and a rise in base deficit.
- As the fetus becomes acidotic with depleted glycogen reserves, bradycardia develops.
- The fetus may pass meconium into the liquor.

Glycogen stores are used up quickly and the length of time the fetus can withstand hypoxia depends on reserves. Asphyxia will occur if hypoxia continues. Finally, energy balance cannot be maintained and tissue damage, then organ failure, will ensue. A growth-retarded fetus (IUGR) with low glycogen stores will be particularly susceptible to asphyxia.

## Detecting hypoxia in labour

- The normal fetus is well able to withstand normal labour stress, but if the fetus has already been compromised during pregnancy, it may be even more vulnerable during labour. Fetal surveillance during labour therefore depends on an assessment of risk (➔ see The partogram, p. 280) and, if indicated, institute continuous monitoring (CTG).
- Abnormal FHR patterns may indicate fetal hypoxia and asphyxia. The most frequently noted abnormalities include loss of baseline variability, baseline tachycardia, and decelerations.
- A deceleration is a transient fall (>15 beats) in the baseline rate for >15s, classified as:
  - *Early*: deceleration occurs at the beginning and returns to the baseline at the end of the contraction, and is usually a repeating pattern of similar decelerations
  - *Variable*: decelerations that do not necessarily occur with the contraction. They may occur in isolation and vary in depth and shape
  - *Late*: deceleration may occur partway through the contraction or following it, with the lowest point >20s after the height of the contraction
  - *Isolated prolonged*: a deceleration that lasts 60–90s.

- NICE guidelines[1] suggest analysis of the CTG to facilitate early detection of fetal compromise. They suggest that abnormal patterns are non-reassuring if one of the following features is present, but otherwise the trace is reassuring:
  - Abnormal baseline rate
  - Reduced baseline variability
  - Decelerations present.

Abnormal patterns may be regarded as *pathological* if two or more non-reassuring features are found or one or more abnormal features are present (Table 23.1).

Table 23.1 Classification of fetal heart reading

| Classification | Baseline (bpm) | Variability | Decelerations |
|---|---|---|---|
| Normal (reassuring) | 110–160 | +5 | None or early |
| Non-reassuring | 100–109 161–180 | <5 for 30b 90min | *Variable decelerations:*<br>• Dropping from baseline by 60bpm or less and taking 60s or less to recover<br>• Present for over 90min<br>• Occurring with over 50% of contractions<br>OR<br>*Variable decelerations:*<br>• Dropping from baseline by >60bpm or taking over 60s to recover<br>• Present for up to 30min<br>• Occurring with over 50% of contractions<br>OR<br>*Late decelerations:*<br>• Present for up to 30min<br>• Occurring with over 50% of contractions |
| Abnormal (pathological) | <100 >180 | <5 for +90min | *Non-reassuring variable decelerations* (see row above):<br>• Still observed 30min after starting conservative measures<br>• Occurring with over 50% of contractions<br>OR<br>*Late decelerations:*<br>• Present for over 30min<br>• Do not improve with conservative measures<br>• Occurring with over 50% of contractions<br>OR<br>*Bradycardia* or a single prolonged deceleration lasting 3min or more |

- A CTG recording with loss of baseline variability and accompanied by shallow late decelerations is particularly pathological and should be reported.
- A rare occurrence in labour is a sinusoidal trace—a regular, smooth, sine wave-like baseline with loss of variability, but with normal baseline. It is associated with hypoxia as a result of severe fetal anaemia, FMH, diabetes, prolonged pregnancy, or cord compression.

### A non-reassuring fetal heart

It is important to recognize that management of care should be holistic and not simply related to CTG patterns. Factors other than hypoxia may make the fetal heart appear abnormal. You should ask:

- Is the pattern precipitated by care procedures, maternal position, or temperature/pulse?
- Is this client high-risk?
- What is the rate of progress in labour?
- What is the current cervical dilatation?
- Is the liquor meconium stained?

### Initial intervention

NICE[1] suggests the following guidance for intervention (Table 23.2).

### Fetal blood sampling

A sample of blood is obtained from the fetal scalp and tested for a lowering of blood pH, which is indicative of metabolic acidosis. Indications include:

- An FHR pattern which is assessed to be suspicious or pathological
- Meconium-stained liquor noted during labour if the fetus is 34–37 weeks' gestation.

*FBS is avoided if:*

- There is HIV, hepatitis B or C, herpes simplex, or other viral blood-borne infection in the mother
- Gestation <34 weeks
- Clotting disorders in the fetus are suspected.

Under these circumstances, inform the consultant obstetrician; delivery may be the best option.

*Procedure*

Be sensitive to the needs of the parents. Explain the procedure and obtain verbal consent. Preserve the woman's dignity and provide support and adequate pain relief.

- Encourage the woman into the left lateral position or the lithotomy position with a wedge support to prevent supine hypotension.
- The obstetrician uses an amnioscope to view the fetal scalp.
- The area in view is cleaned and ethyl chloride is sprayed on to the scalp to stimulate hyperaemia.
- Sterile grease is smeared on the scalp to facilitate collection of the fetal blood sample into a pre-heparinized capillary tube.
- A small incision is made and 0.4mL of blood is collected.
- The obstetrician ensures wound haemostasis.

Table 23.2 Categories of intervention

| Category | Definition | Interpretation | Management |
|---|---|---|---|
| CTG is normal/ reassuring | All three features are normal/ reassuring | Normal CTG, no non-reassuring or abnormal features, healthy fetus | • Continue CTG and normal care<br>• If CTG was started because of concerns arising from intermittent auscultation, remove CTG after 20min if there are no non-reassuring or abnormal features and no ongoing risk factors |
| CTG is non-reassuring and suggests need for conservative measures | One non-reassuring feature AND Two normal/ reassuring features | Combination of features that may be associated with increased risk of fetal acidosis; if accelerations are present, acidosis is unlikely | • Think about possible underlying causes<br>• If the baseline FHR is over 160bpm, check the woman's temperature and pulse. If either are raised, offer fluids and paracetamol<br>• Start one or more conservative measures:<br>  • Encourage the woman to mobilize or adopt a left lateral position, and in particular to avoid being supine<br>  • Offer oral or IV fluids<br>  • Reduce contraction frequency by stopping oxytocin if being used and/or offering tocolysis<br>• Inform coordinating midwife and obstetrician |
| CTG is abnormal and indicates need for conservative measures AND further testing | One abnormal feature OR Two non-reassuring features | Combination of features that is more likely to be associated with fetal acidosis | • Think about possible underlying causes<br>• If the baseline FHR is over 180bpm, check the woman's temperature and pulse. If either are raised, offer fluids and paracetamol<br>• Start one or more conservative measures (➊ see row 'CTG is non-reassuring ...' above for details)<br>• Inform coordinating midwife and obstetrician<br>• Offer to take an FBS (for lactate or pH) after implementing conservative measures, or expedite birth if an FBS cannot be obtained and no accelerations are seen as a result of scalp stimulation<br>• Take action sooner than 30min if late decelerations are accompanied by tachycardia and/or reduced baseline variability<br>• Inform the consultant obstetrician if any FBS result is abnormal<br>• Discuss with the consultant obstetrician if an FBS cannot be obtained or a third FBS is thought to be needed |

- Sometimes obtaining an adequate sample is problematic. Repeated attempts should be avoided.
- Discuss the plan of management with the obstetric consultant.
- The pH measurement is done straightaway using a pH meter:
  - pH >7.25 is regarded as normal
  - pH <7.20 is regarded as indicative of fetal acidosis. Urgent delivery is necessary
  - pH between these readings suggests the fetus may be on the verge of acidosis and the sample should always be repeated in 30min to obtain an improved reading.
- Cord blood samples should be obtained at delivery.

### Cord blood samples: fetal pH at delivery

Oxygen from the maternal blood diffuses to the fetus via the placenta and cord vein. Deoxygenated blood returns via the cord arteries to the placenta and carbon dioxide diffuses to the maternal blood.[2]

- Thus cord arterial blood should give an indication of the fetal acid–base balance.
- Venous blood should reflect the maternal acid–base status and placental function.
- Cord blood samples should be considered if:
  - An emergency Caesarean section is performed
  - A forceps delivery is performed
  - FBS is taken during labour
  - The Apgar score at 5min after delivery is 7 or less.

#### Double clamping

When there has been active management of the third stage, it may be recommended that the cord be double-clamped at delivery:

- Clamp the cord as usual near the baby's umbilicus
- Clamp a second time to allow for cutting of the cord
- Leave 10–15cm between the second and a third clamp, which preserves blood in a segment of the cord.

#### Obtaining the samples

- Arterial and venous samples are obtained from the cord in a pre-heparinized syringe.
- The result should remain accurate for up to 10min at room temperature.
- Ensure that there is no air in the syringes, that they are capped, and that the heparin is mixed with the sample by rolling the syringe between the fingers.

#### Measurements

The following measurements are obtained (Tables 23.3 and 23.4):

- pH: measure of acidity or alkalinity
- $pO_2$: oxygen tension in the blood (unit in kilopascal, kPa)
- $pCO_2$: carbon dioxide measure (unit in kilopascal, kPa).

Table 23.3 Normal arterial blood gas values

|  | Artery | Vein |
|---|---|---|
| pH | 7.26 (7.05–7.38) | 7.35 (7.17–7.48) |
| pCO$_2$ (kPa) | 7.3 (4.9–10.7) | 5.3 (3.5–7.9) |
| Base deficit | 2.4 (2.5–9.7) | 3.0 (–1.0–8.9) |

From reference 2.

Table 23.4 Criteria for diagnosis of acidosis—analysis of blood gases results

|  | Respiratory | Metabolic | Mixed |
|---|---|---|---|
| pCO$_2$ | High | Normal | High |
| pO$_2$ | Normal | Low | Low |
| HCO$_3$⁻ (bicarbonate) | Normal | Low | Low |
| Base deficit | Normal | High | High |

- Base deficit: an indirect measure of anaerobic metabolism. It allows distinction between a low pH caused by a build-up of carbon dioxide (respiratory acidosis) and that caused by a build-up of metabolic acids as a result of anaerobic metabolism (metabolic acidosis). The former is resolved quickly at birth when the lungs are inflated; the latter indicates that a significant period of hypoxia has occurred which may affect the baby in the neonatal period
- Cord blood results are influenced by the mode of delivery, gestational age, and analgesia during labour.

What should you expect to find in a baby who has intrapartum asphyxia?
- Metabolic acidosis in the cord sample.
- Need for resuscitation at birth.
- Evidence of organ dysfunction in the neonatal period: convulsions due to CNS malfunction.
- Hypotension, poor cardiac function, hypoxia.
- Blood and oxygen redistributed from peripheral organs results in respiratory distress, renal failure, and hepatic damage.
- Neonatal hypoglycaemia resulting from depletion of liver glycogen.

### References

1 National Institute for Health and Care Excellence (2014). *Intrapartum care for healthy women and babies.* NICE guidelines CG190. Available at: ℘ www.nice.org.uk/guidance/cg190/resources/cg190-intrapartum-care-interpretation-of-cardiotocograph-traces-table2.
2 The Practice Development Team (2010). *Jessop Wing Labour Ward guidelines 2010.* Sheffield Teaching Hospitals NHS Trust (quoted from Plymouth Perinatal Research Group, 1994).

# Cord presentation and cord prolapse

Cord presentation and cord prolapse occur in any situation where the presenting part is poorly applied to the lower segment of the uterus or is high in the pelvic cavity, making it possible for a loop of cord to slip down in front of the presenting part. When vaginal birth is not imminent, a Caesarean section is the recommended mode of delivery in cases of cord presentation or prolapse, in order to prevent hypoxic acidosis.[3]

## Definitions

- *Cord presentation*: the umbilical cord lies in front of the presenting part with the membranes intact (Fig. 23.1).
- *Cord prolapse*: the umbilical cord lies in front of the presenting part and the membranes have ruptured (Fig. 23.2).
- *Occult cord prolapse*: the cord lies alongside, but not in front of, the presenting part.

## Predisposing conditions

- High or ill-fitting presenting part.
- High parity: due to a weakened lower uterine segment or loss of abdominal muscle tone, there is an increased incidence of non-engagement of the presenting part until labour is well established.
- Prematurity: the size of the fetus in relation to the uterus constitutes a high risk of cord prolapse, hence there is a high mortality rate associated with prematurity.
- Multiple pregnancy: especially malpresentation of the second twin.
- Malpresentation: breech presentation is particularly vulnerable, especially complete or footling breech. The close proximity of the umbilicus to the buttocks is an added risk. Other malpresentations, such as shoulder presentation or transverse lie, carry a high risk of cord prolapse.
- Polyhydramnios: the cord may be swept down with a gush of liquor if the membranes rupture spontaneously.
- Obstetric practices and interventions may possibly make a difference to the incidence of cord prolapse, dependent on the intrapartum practices of individual hospitals, such as ARM in early labour, displacement of the presenting part during a vaginal examination.
- Long umbilical cord: usually associated with one of the above.

## Cord prolapse

Where there are factors that predispose to cord prolapse, a vaginal examination should be undertaken following SROM. Cord prolapse should be suspected when there is an abnormal FHR pattern, especially if such changes commence soon after membrane rupture, either spontaneous or artificial. The risks to the fetus are hypoxia or death.

## Diagnosis

- The cord is felt below or beside the presenting part on vaginal examination.
- A loop of the cord may be felt in the vagina or the cord may be visible at the vulva.
- There may be bradycardia.

Fig. 23.1 Cord presentation.

Fig. 23.2 Cord prolapse.

## Management

- Call for medical aid and preparations should be made for immediate birth in theatre.
- Explain the situation to the mother.
- Carry out a vaginal examination.
- If an oxytocic infusion is running, this should be stopped immediately.
- Relieve pressure on the umbilical cord by keeping your fingers in the vagina to push the presenting part away from the umbilical cord.
- Assist the woman to move into the knee–chest position, which helps to relieve compression of the umbilical cord (Fig. 23.3). Alternatively, the exaggerated Sim's position (Fig. 23.4) may be adopted, by lying her on her side with a wedge or pillow to raise her hips. The foot of the bed can be elevated.
- Monitor the FHR.
- Urgent delivery.
- In some units, alternative management may involve displacing the presenting part by filling the bladder with 500mL of normal saline. The catheter is then clamped and the fingers may then be withdrawn from the vagina. The clamp is released when the incision for LSCS is being made and therefore delivery is imminent.
- Tocolysis can be considered whilst preparing for a Caesarean section if there are persistent FHR abnormalities after attempts to prevent compression mechanically, particularly when birth is likely to be delayed.[3]

## Cord presentation

- Will usually have been diagnosed on vaginal examination.
- May be associated with deceleration of the FHR.
- Do *not* rupture the membranes.
- Discontinue the vaginal examination.
- Call for medical assistance.
- Monitor the FHR.
- Encourage the woman to adopt a position as above that will reduce the occurrence of cord compression.
- Expedite delivery as soon as possible—LSCS is the most likely outcome.

Although the measures described above are potentially useful during preparation for birth, they must not result in unnecessary delay.[3] Cord presentation and cord prolapse constitute a serious threat to fetal well-being. In order to reduce mortality and morbidity, it is important that urgent delivery is initiated. This will usually be by a Caesarean section if the fetus is alive and delivery is not imminent. In some instances, with a multiparous woman, a second-stage vaginal delivery may be possible. In the community, where the fetus is alive, arrange urgent transfer to hospital.

Fig. 23.3 Knee–chest position (relieves compression on the prolapsed cord).

Fig. 23.4 Sim's position.

### Reference

3 Royal College of Obstetricians and Gynaecologists (2014). *Umbilical cord prolapse. Green-top guideline No. 50.* Available at: ℬ www.rcog.org.uk/globalassets/documents/guidelines/gtg-50-umbilicalcordprolapse-2014.pdf.

# Vasa praevia

- This is a rare occurrence when a *fetal* blood vessel is situated over the cervical os and therefore is in front of the presenting part.
- There may be a velamentous insertion of the cord (or possibly a succenturiate lobe), resulting in a fetal vessel running through the membranes.

## Diagnosis

- The presence of the vessel might be suspected during vaginal examination whilst the membranes are still intact.
- If a careful speculum examination is performed with a good light, it might be possible to see the vessel.

## Rupture of the vessel

- This may occur if the membranes rupture.
- The fetus may die unless quickly delivered.

## Signs and symptoms

- Minimal fresh red loss occurring typically at the rupture of the membranes.
- On monitoring the fetal heart, there are signs of fetal compromise which are disproportionate to the amount of blood loss.
- There may be a sinusoidal fetal heart pattern sometimes seen when the fetus is severely anaemic. This is characterized by increased variability of >15 beats and resembles a sine wave with 2–6 cycles/min.

## Immediate care

The midwife should:
- Recognize the risk of fetal asphyxia (➔ see Hypoxia and asphyxia, p. 530)
- Call for help speedily from the obstetric registrar and team
- Continue to record a CTG
- If fetal compromise is apparent, prepare the woman for a very urgent Caesarean section (➔ see Emergency lower segment Caesarean section, p. 465) if this is the first stage of labour
- If delivery is imminent or the woman is multiparous in the second stage of labour, encourage pushing or/and if requested prepare for forceps/ ventouse delivery
- Call the paediatrician to the delivery
- Double-clamp the cord and obtain blood for blood gases and also for Hb estimation in the baby.

The paediatric team will transfer the baby to the SCBU for observation and treatment. S/he may require a blood transfusion.

# Undiagnosed breech presentation

### Definition

In a breech, the fetal buttocks, knees, or feet present at the cervix as opposed to the fetal head. The feet may be alongside the buttocks (complete breech presentation 5–10%); the legs may be extended against the trunk and the feet lying against the face (frank breech presentation 50–70%); or one or both feet or knees may be prolapsed into the maternal vagina (incomplete breech presentation 10–30%) (➔ see Recognition and management of breech presentation, p. 224).

### Incidence and management options

The unexpected diagnosis of breech presentation upon admission in labour affects approximately one in 100 women at term[4] and presents an ethical dilemma for health professionals involved, particularly when this occurs in the context of midwifery-led care. Perinatal mortality is increased 2- to 4-fold with breech presentation, regardless of the mode of delivery, although most of these deaths are associated with malformations, prematurity, and intrauterine fetal demise.[4]

Delivery by a Caesarean section for breech presentation had increased markedly in the last 20 years following the publication of the Term Breech Trial.[5] However, there are benefits and risks associated with both a Caesarean delivery and a vaginal breech birth and it is recognized that there is currently no conclusive evidence of the benefit of a Caesarean section performed in active labour (>3cm).[4,6] Management should therefore be discussed between the woman, midwife, and obstetrician, to facilitate an informed choice.

Diagnosis of breech for the first time during labour is not a contraindication for vaginal breech birth, providing the following criteria are met:[6]

• No contraindication to vaginal birth (e.g. placenta praevia, compromised fetus)
• The pelvis is clinically adequate. NB. Clinical judgement is adequate. There is no role for routine pelvimetry
• Frank or complete breech presentation (not footling or kneeling)
• Baby expected to weigh >2500g and <3800g
• The fetal neck is not hyper-extended in labour (by ultrasound). Cervical spine injury is predominantly observed when the fetus has a hyper-extended head prior to delivery
• No previous Caesarean section
• Emergency Caesarean facilities are available
• Appropriately prepared and experienced clinicians are available for the birth (midwife, obstetrician, paediatrician, anaesthetist).

Current data indicate that 50% of breech presentations may be considered suitable candidates for vaginal delivery and that 60–82% of elective vaginal breech births are successful.[7]

The midwife has a responsibility to provide women with appropriate evidence in a supportive and enabling way, rather than one which is conflicted or coercive. If birth is not imminent, the woman must provide verbal informed consent to proceed with a vaginal breech birth.

## Management of vaginal breech birth

There are three types of vaginal breech delivery.

### Spontaneous breech delivery

No traction or manipulation of the infant is used. This occurs predominantly in very preterm, often pre-viable, deliveries.

### Assisted breech delivery

This is the most common type of vaginal breech delivery. The infant is allowed to spontaneously deliver up to the umbilicus, and then manoeuvres are initiated to assist in the delivery of the remainder of the body, arms, and head if required.

### Total breech extraction

The fetal feet are grasped, and the entire fetus is extracted. Total breech extraction should be used only for a non-cephalic second twin; it should not be used for a singleton fetus because the cervix may not be adequately dilated to allow the passage of the fetal head. As long as the FHR is stable in this situation, it is permissible to manage expectantly to allow the cervix to completely dilate around the breech. Total breech extraction for the single ton breech is associated with a birth injury rate of 25% and a mortality rate of approximately 10%.

(➔ For detailed management and care, see Breech delivery, p.468.)

### References

4  Walker S (2013). Undiagnosed breech: towards a woman-centred approach. *Br J Midwifery* 21: 316–22.
5  Royal College of Obstetricians and Gynaecologists (2006). *Breech presentation, management. Green-top guideline No. 20b.* (This guideline is currently being revised, with publication anticipated late 2016.) Available at: ℜ www.rcog.org.uk/en/guidelines-research-services/guidelines/gtg20b/.
6  Alarab M, Regan C, O'Connell MP, Keane DP, O'Herlihy C, Foley ME (2004). Singleton vaginal breech delivery at term: still a safe option. *Obstet Gynecol* 103: 407–12.
7  Hannah ME, Hannah WJ, Hewson SA, *et al.* (2000). Planned caesarean section versus planned vaginal birth for breech presentation at term: a randomised multicentre trial. *Lancet* 356: 1375–83.

# Shoulder dystocia

### Definition

Shoulder dystocia (SD) is defined as a vaginal cephalic delivery that requires additional obstetric manoeuvres to deliver the fetus after the head has delivered and gentle traction has failed.[8] It generally involves impaction of the anterior shoulder behind the symphysis pubis, or the posterior shoulder on the sacrum, which impedes the spontaneous delivery of the baby.

### Incidence

There is a wide variation in the reported incidence of SD. Studies involving the largest number of vaginal deliveries report incidences of between 0.58% and 0.70% of such deliveries.[8]

- Maternal morbidity is increased, particularly the incidence of PPH (11%) as well as third- and fourth-degree perineal tears (3.8%). Incidences remain unchanged by the number or type of manoeuvres required to effect delivery.[8]
- Perinatal mortality can be between 2.6% and 29%, with surviving babies at risk of long-term morbidity. Brachial plexus injury (BPI) is one of the most important fetal complications of SD, complicating 0.43/1000 live births in the UK.[8]

SD is one of the most frightening emergencies experienced, as it is difficult to predict and the midwife facilitating the birth may be working alone. All midwives should be aware of the methods for both predicting and diagnosing SD and the techniques required to facilitate delivery.

### Predisposing factors

Risk assessments for the prediction of SD are insufficiently predictive to allow prevention of the large majority of cases.[8] Conventional risk factors predicted only 16% of SD that resulted in infant morbidity.

A number of antenatal and intrapartum characteristics have been reported to be associated with SD, but statistical modelling has shown that these risk factors have a low positive predictive value, both singly and in combination:

- *Fetal size and SD*: there is a relationship, but it is not a good predictor—partly because fetal size is difficult to determine accurately, but also because the large majority of infants with a birthweight of ≥4500g do not develop SD. Equally important, 48% of births complicated by SD occur in infants who weigh <4000g
- *Infants of diabetic mothers* have a 2- to 4-fold increased risk of SD compared with infants of the same birthweight born to non-diabetic mothers
- Maternal obesity: maternal BMI >30kg/m$^2$
- Post-dates >41 weeks' gestation
- Previous SD
- Prolonged first and/or second stage of labour
- Operative delivery, especially mid-cavity instrumental delivery for delay.

Timely management of SD requires prompt recognition. The attendant midwife should routinely observe for:

- Difficulty with delivery of the face and chin
- The head remaining tightly applied to the vulva: the baby's head is pressing so tightly against the perineum that it is impossible to insert a finger into the vagina, and the baby's face becomes suffused and discoloured
- The head retracting (turtle neck sign): failure of the baby's chin to escape the perineum
- Failure of restitution of the fetal head
- Failure of the shoulders to descend.

Routine traction in an *axial* direction can be used to diagnose SD, but any other traction should be avoided. Axial traction is traction in line with the fetal spine, i.e. without lateral deviation.

## Management

NOTE THE TIME OF THE DELIVERY OF THE HEAD.

*Maternal pushing should be discouraged, as this may exacerbate impaction of the shoulders.* The following mnemonic HELPERR is recommended by the RCOG:[8]

### H = HELP

Call for help: obstetrician, anaesthetist, midwives, paediatric team, and support workers.

### E = EVALUATE for EPISIOTOMY

An episiotomy is not always necessary. Episiotomy scissors open, symphysiotomy tray available.

### L = LEGS

Lie the bed flat; remove pillows, and elevate the woman's knees to her shoulders (McRobert's position; Fig. 23.5).

### P = PRESSURE: SUPRAPUBIC

Apply constant pressure for 30s, from the side of the fetal back in a downward and lateral direction just above the maternal symphysis pubis and then rocking pressure for 30s (Fig. 23.6). *Fundal pressure should NOT be used* during the management of SD. It is associated with a high neonatal complication rate and may result in uterine rupture.

### E = ENTER THE PELVIS

- Episiotomy if required (to gain access to the vagina).

*Consider INTERNAL MANOEUVRES.*

*Rubin's 2*

- Pressure on the posterior aspect of the baby's anterior shoulder; try to get the baby's shoulders into an oblique diameter (Fig. 23.7).
- Continue pressure and rotate the baby by 180° (the baby's anterior shoulder should now be posterior).

**Fig. 23.5** McRobert's manoeuvre.

**Fig. 23.6** Suprapubic pressure: reduce the bisacromial diameter and rotate the baby's anterior shoulder forwards (towards the fetal chest).

**Fig. 23.7** Rubin's 2 manoeuvre: rotate the anterior shoulder forwards.

### Wood's screw

In combination with Rubin's 2, add pressure on the anterior aspect of the posterior shoulder (Fig. 23.8).

### Reverse Wood's

Pressure on the posterior aspect of the baby's posterior shoulder; try to get the baby's shoulders into an oblique diameter (Fig. 23.9).

• Continue pressure and rotate the baby by 180° (the baby's posterior shoulder becomes anterior).

### OR, IF EASIER:

### R = REMOVE THE POSTERIOR ARM

The midwife's hand enters posteriorly along the arm, flexes the arm, and grasps the hand, sweeping the baby's arm across his chest and face to deliver.

**Fig. 23.8** Wood's screw manoeuvre: rotate the anterior shoulder forwards and the posterior shoulder backwards in conjunction.

**Fig. 23.9** Reverse Wood's manoeuvre: rotate the posterior shoulder forwards.

*R = ROLL ONTO ALL FOURS/REPEAT MANOEUVRES*

*Gaskin manoeuvre*

Place the mother in an all-fours position—change of position may dislodge the anterior shoulder and may facilitate access for repeat of internal manoeuvres.

*Consider other options*

*The last three options would need to be performed by an obstetrician.* They are last resort measures:

- Fracture the fetal clavicle
- Perform a symphysiotomy (division of the symphysis)
- Attempt the Zavanelli manoeuvre (cephalic replacement and delivery by a Caesarean).

*Document all actions* on the SD proforma, including the head-to-body delivery interval, the order of manoeuvres, and the cord pH.

*Debrief*—full and clear explanations should be given to the parents. The professionals involved should be offered the chance to discuss the case in a supportive environment.

It is difficult to recommend an absolute time limit for the management of SD as there are no conclusive data available, but there appears to be a very low rate of hypoxic–ischaemic injury if delivery is expedited within up to 5min.[8]

## Reference

8 Royal College of Obstetricians and Gynaecologists (2012). *Shoulder dystocia. Green-top guideline No. 42,* 2nd edn. Available at: ℘ www.rcog.org.uk/globalassets/documents/guidelines/gtg_42.pdf.

# Guidelines for admission to neonatal intensive care unit

A *premature* baby as defined by the WHO is any baby born alive before 37 completed weeks of gestation.[9] There are sub-categories of preterm birth, based on gestational age:

- Extremely preterm (<28 weeks)
- Very preterm (28 to <32 weeks)
- Moderate to late preterm (32 to <37 weeks).

A *small-for-dates baby* is a baby whose weight falls below the 10th percentile for its gestational age.

These definitions indicate that a baby can be both premature and small-for-dates, or term and small-for-dates.

## Incidence

### Worldwide

Every year, an estimated 15 million babies are born preterm (before 37 completed weeks of gestation), and this number is rising.[9,10]

- Preterm birth complications are the leading cause of death among children under 5 years of age, responsible for nearly 1 million deaths in 2013.
- Three-quarters of them could be saved with current cost-effective interventions.
- Across 184 countries, the rate of preterm birth ranges from 5% to 18% of babies born.

### In England and Wales

- In 2012, 7.3% of live births were preterm (under 37 weeks' gestation). The majority (95%) occur after 28 weeks.[11]
- Nearly 85% of all babies born prematurely will have a very low birthweight (under 1000g), compared to 94% of babies born under 24 weeks.
- Preterm birth rates have remained steady (7.3% in 2009, 7.1% in 2010, 7.2% in 2011, and 7.3% in 2012).
- In 2012, the infant mortality rate for babies born preterm (between 24 and 36 weeks) was 23.6 deaths per 1000 live births, 15.5% lower than the rate for preterm babies born in 2008 (27.6 deaths per 1000 live births).
- 10% of preterm births were to mothers aged 40 and over, compared to 6.8% in mothers aged 20–24. For babies born in 2012, only 6% of singleton births were preterm, compared with more than half (56%) of multiple births.
- In 2012, the infant mortality rate for babies born preterm was higher for single births than for multiple births (24.8 and 19.9 deaths per 1000 live births respectively).

### In Scotland

- The percentage of preterm (born before 37 completed weeks) singleton babies rose from 5.2% in 1975/76 to a peak of 6.7% in 2003/04 and fell to 5.9% in 2011/12.[12]

*Northern Ireland*
- Does not currently compile figures on premature births.

## Survival rates

In England, survival rates of very premature babies increased from 40% in 1995 to 53% in 2006. Survival increases by 9.5% for each week if the baby is born at 23 weeks, and 16% per week if the baby is born at 25 weeks. Survival rates for the rest of the UK countries are not available.

## Current structure of neonatal care in the UK

*Transitional care units (TCUs)*

These are usually based on a maternity ward away from the intensive and high-dependency care contexts, thus keeping the baby with or near to its mother and cared for by midwives or neonatal nurses. Babies needing this level of care usually require treatment for jaundice or infections, or they may be small but are otherwise well.

*Special care units (SCUs)*

These provide special care for their own local population. They are based in all maternity hospitals, for the care of small babies from 32 weeks' gestation. They also provide, by agreement with their neonatal network, some high-dependency services; they usually have two or three intensive cots and may keep the baby if it can be managed within that context. They can also provide emergency treatment and stabilization for the smaller, sicker babies, until transfer to the regional unit can be arranged.

*Local neonatal units (LNUs)*

These provide special care and high-dependency care and a restricted volume of intensive care (as agreed locally) and would expect to transfer babies who require complex or longer-term intensive care to a NICU. They provide full expert intensive care, the only difference being that they do not provide surgery and will transfer any baby requiring surgery to the nearest surgical unit.

*Neonatal intensive care unit (NICU)*

These are larger ICUs that provide the whole range of medical (and sometimes surgical) neonatal care for their local population and additional care for babies and their families referred from the neonatal network in which they are based, and also from other networks when necessary to deal with peaks of demand or requests for specialist care not available elsewhere. Many will be sited within perinatal centres that are able to offer similarly complex obstetric care. These units will also require close working arrangements with all of the relevant paediatric sub-specialties. It is preferable to transfer the baby *in utero* as, once born, its survival depends on provision of a stable thermal environment and effective management of oxygenation. Transferring a small, sick baby in the back of an ambulance can prove to be very hazardous. The baby returns to the referring unit once he or she is well enough.

## Criteria for admission to the NICU

In 1990, the Human Fertilization and Embryology Act stated that a baby is capable of surviving from 24 weeks of pregnancy. Viable gestational age is considered by law to be 24 weeks, whatever the baby's weight.[13]

- Clinical condition requiring constant monitoring, <34 weeks' gestation or birthweight <1800 g (follow local guidelines for gestation and birthweight limits).
- Any baby who has severe congenital abnormalities requiring emergency management and/or surgery.
- Term babies who have birth asphyxia, meconium aspiration, or respiratory difficulties requiring extensive resuscitation at birth:
  - Unwell baby
  - Respiratory distress or cyanosis
  - Apnoeic or cyanotic attacks
  - Signs of encephalopathy
  - Jaundice needing intensive phototherapy or exchange transfusion
  - Major congenital abnormality likely to threaten immediate survival
  - Seizures
  - Inability to tolerate enteral feeds with vomiting and/or abdominal distension and/or hypoglycaemia (blood glucose <2.6mmol/L)
  - Suspicion of sepsis
  - Symptomatic hypoglycaemia or hypoglycaemia not responding to treatment
  - Neonatal abstinence syndrome requiring treatment
  - Mother admitted to the ICU.
- Social reasons for admission, e.g. adoption.

Babies with congenital abnormalities who are not seriously ill, e.g. babies with Down's syndrome who are otherwise well, stay with their mothers on the maternity ward or in the TCU (➔ see Guidelines for admission to transitional care, p. 554).

## References

9 World Health Organization (2015). *Preterm birth*. Fact sheet No. 363. Geneva: World Health Organization. Available at: ℘ www.who.int/mediacentre/factsheets/fs363/en/.

10 Blencowe H, Cousens S, Oestergaard M, *et al.* (2012). National, regional and worldwide estimates of preterm birth. *Lancet* 379: 2162–72.

11 Office for National Statistics (2013). *Gestation-specific infant mortality in England and Wales, 2011*. Available at: ℘ webarchive.nationalarchives.gov.uk/20160105160709/http://www.ons.gov.uk/ons/dcp171778_329137.pdf.

12 Information Services Division (2013). *Births in Scottish hospitals: year ending 31st March 2012*. Edinburgh: Information Services Division Scotland. Available at: ℘ www.isdscotland.org/Health-Topics/Maternity-and-Births/Publications/2013-08-27/2013-08-27-Births-Report.pdf?34511965514.

13 British Association of Perinatal Medicine (2010). *Service standards for hospitals providing neonatal care*, 3rd edn. Available at: ℘ www.bapm.org/publications/documents/guidelines/BAPM_Standards_Final_Aug2010.pdf.

## Further reading

National Institute for Health and Care Excellence (2013). *Preterm labour and birth*. Available at: ℘ www.nice.org.uk/guidance/indevelopment/gid-cgwave0660/documents.

# Guidelines for admission to transitional care

The TCU provides care for those babies who require more than normal postnatal care but do not require admission to the neonatal unit. It is an environment where infants requiring specific nursing and medical management can be cared for without being separated from their mothers. Transitional care is instrumental in the development of attachment between the mother and infant, as it allows 24h parenting. Moderately compromised babies gain weight more quickly and are discharged earlier with less chance of readmission than if they were cared for in a standard neonatal unit. The typical length of stay varies between 2 and 3 days and 3 weeks.

The criteria for admission to the TCU are more difficult to define than those to the NICU; generally, the mother must not need inpatient midwifery or obstetric care, but the baby needs more care than can be provided on the postnatal ward. In a busy obstetric unit, over a 6-month period, approximately 150 babies weighing >1.5kg will be admitted to the neonatal unit, for an average of 3.7 special care days each. It is likely that most of these infants could be cared for on a transitional care ward, reserving neonatal care facilities for sicker infants.

## Admission criteria

- Babies between 34+0 and 34+6 weeks' gestation at birth who are otherwise well; they may be admitted directly from the delivery suite, depending on the mother's condition.
- Babies with a birthweight of >1.5kg, unless requiring admission to the neonatal unit.
- Babies who require regular tube feeding but are otherwise well.
- Babies requiring treatment for neonatal abstinence syndrome due to maternal substance use (➔ see Neonatal abstinence syndrome, p. 756).
- Babies of insulin-dependent diabetic mothers requiring increased monitoring or management of low blood sugars.
- Babies on low-flow oxygen establishing feeding prior to discharge.
- Babies requiring double phototherapy.
- Hypothermic babies.
- Dehydrated babies.
- Babies requiring increased observation, e.g. traumatic delivery.
- Babies with congenital abnormalities such as cleft lip and palate.
- Unaccompanied babies, e.g. for adoption, babies whose mothers are in level 3 critical care.[14]
- Babies with a birth plan that identifies the need for additional support or observation of parenting capacity (this will be for a maximum of 7 days).[14]

It may be possible to extend the admission criteria, if the ward is well established and adequately staffed, to include babies requiring palliative care.

## Not for admission to transitional care

- Sick babies requiring the care of a neonatal unit, e.g.:
  - Any baby requiring extensive resuscitation and/or ventilatory support
  - Any baby requiring oxygen therapy
  - Any baby requiring IV fluids.
- Babies who can be cared for on a normal postnatal ward, e.g.:
  - Babies who only require IV cannulation and antibiotics
  - Babies who are slow to feed with no excessive clinical symptoms of hypoglycaemia/dehydration
  - Multiple-birth babies who are clinically well.
- Sick babies for foster care or adoption are treated in a neonatal unit whether or not they meet admission criteria for a transitional care ward.

## The following (otherwise well) babies should be managed on the postnatal ward

- Gestation of 35 completed weeks or more; birthweight >2kg and not fulfilling criteria above.
- Babies only requiring phototherapy.
- Babies requiring a hot cot or incubator to maintain temperature only.
- Mothers and babies requiring breastfeeding support or babies requiring cup feeds.
- Well babies on IV antibiotics.
- Babies only requiring blood sugar monitoring, other than infants of insulin-dependent diabetic mothers.
- Babies requiring physiological observations only (e.g. as per meconium aspiration policy, risk of GBS policy, etc.).

## Reference

14 Roland D, Madar J, Connolly G (2010). The Newborn Early Warning (NEW) system: development of an at-risk infant intervention system. *Infant* 6: 116–29.

## Further reading

National Institute for Health and Care Excellence (2006). *Postnatal care up to 8 weeks after birth.* NICE guidelines CG37. Available at: ℞ www.nice.org.uk/guidance/cg37.

Roberton J (2005). *Roberton's Textbook of Neonatology*, 4th edn. London: Churchill Livingstone.

# Neonatal resuscitation

## Stimuli resulting in the initiation of respiration
- At birth, gas exchange changes from placental to alveolar.
- As the fetus is propelled down the birth canal, a negative intrathoracic pressure is exerted, so that on delivery air is sucked into the lungs.
- Clamping and cutting the cord. For uncompromised babies, a delay in cord clamping of at least 1min from the complete delivery of the infant is now recommended.[15] As yet there is insufficient evidence to recommend an appropriate time for clamping the cord in babies who are severely compromised at birth and babies requiring resuscitation; resuscitative intervention remains the priority.
- Physical stimuli: tactile, cold, and gravity.[16]

## Changes from fetal to normal circulation
- The first breath increases $PaO_2$ and closes the ductus arteriosus between the aorta and pulmonary artery, allowing more blood to flow to the lungs.
- There is a decrease in the pulmonary vascular resistance and an increase in blood flow from the lungs.
- The increased left atrial pressure and decreased right atrial pressure closes the foramen ovale.[16]

## Prevent hypothermia
- The intrauterine environment is 1.5°C higher than the maternal temperature.
- The temperature of a newborn is approximately 37.8°C. The core temperature of a wet, asphyxiated infant will decrease by 5°C in as many minutes.
- Surfactant production is decreased if the body temperature goes <35°C.
- The baby will increase oxygen intake by breathing rapidly, using up glycogen stores to produce body heat, leading to hypoglycaemia.[16]

## Preparation for delivery
Ensure that:
- Personnel capable of initiating resuscitation are always available
- A person capable of complete resuscitation is in attendance for all high-risk deliveries
- Resuscitaire® and overhead heater and dry and warmed towels are prepared. For preterm infants, delivery room temperatures should be at least 26°C
- Set oxygen at 21% (equivalent of air). For term infants, air should be used for resuscitation at birth. If, despite effective ventilation, oxygenation (ideally guided by pulse oximetry) remains unacceptable, use of a higher concentration of oxygen should be considered.[16]
- Set inflation pressure 30cmH₂O
- Face masks (varying sizes) are available
- Suction and suction tubes (varying sizes) are available

- Food-grade plastic wrap or bag: preterm babies of <28 weeks' gestation should be completely covered in plastic wrap or a bag up to their necks without drying, immediately after birth. They should remain wrapped until their temperature has been checked after admission
- Laryngoscopes, endotracheal tubes, and connections are at hand
- Medications are readily available.[16]

### Initial assessment at birth

- Start the clock.
- Dry and warm the baby.
- Assess:
  - Colour
  - Breathing
  - Heart rate by listening with a stethoscope or palpate the base of the cord
  - Tone
  - Response to stimuli.

These observations form the basis of assessment and re-assessment throughout the resuscitation.

Provided the airway is clear, most babies who are apnoeic at birth will resuscitate themselves.[16]

### ABC of resuscitation

Call for help.

- *Airway*. To secure a clear airway:
  - Hold the head in a neutral position
  - Do not flex or overextend the neck
  - Jaw thrust will be needed if the baby is very floppy; with one or two fingers under each side of the angle of the jaw, push forwards and outwards.[16] These manoeuvres may be all that is required to initiate breathing.
- *Breathing*. If not breathing:
  - Administer five inflation breaths
  - Inflation pressure sustained at 30cmH$_2$O for 2–3s
  - This will sufficiently aerate the lungs
  - As the first few inflations will be replacing lung fluid with air, chest movement will not be detected until the fourth or fifth inflation.
- *Circulation*. If the heart rate is <60bpm and not increasing despite adequate lung inflations:
  - Start chest compressions and ventilation breaths at a ratio of 3:1 for 30s
  - After 30s, check the heart rate
  - If the heart rate is >60bpm but <100bpm, continue with ventilation breaths only at a rate of 30–40/min
  - After 30s, check the heart rate
  - If there is still no response despite adequate inflation, ventilation, and chest compressions, emergency drugs may be needed.[16]

### Chest compression

There are two methods:
- The two-thumb method
- The two-finger method.

The main principles for both are the same, using the lower third of the sternum, one finger's breadth below the nipple line:
- Rate: 90/min
- Ratio: three compressions to one ventilation/inhalation
- Depth: one-third of the depth of the baby's chest (1–2cm)
- Action: well controlled, not jerky or erratic.

Allow for expansion after each compression to facilitate venous return.[16]

Emergency drugs are given if adequate ventilation and effective chest compressions have failed to increase the heart rate above 60bpm. They are given to increase cardiac output and improve cardiac and cerebral perfusion. They are usually administered through an umbilical venous catheter.
- *Adrenaline:* improves cerebral and cardiac perfusion:
  - Dose 10–30 micrograms/kg; 0.1mL of 1:10 000 solution can be given via an endotracheal tube but is less effective.
- *Sodium bicarbonate:* reverses acidosis, 'kick-starts' the heart:
  - Dose 1–2mmol/kg; 2–4mL of 4.2% solution.

If there is no response to adrenaline and sodium bicarbonate, use:
- *Glucose:* 2.5mL/kg of 10% solution.

Occasionally volume expansion may help. Use:
- Plasma, whole blood, or normal saline: 10mL/kg.

In addition:
- Naloxone 100 micrograms/Kg can be administered at intervals of 1 minute, up to a maximum dose of 2mg to reverse the effects of pethidine given during labour. Do not use this if the mother has been taking opiate drugs during pregnancy
- Calcium 2mL/kg of 10% solution. Give when the heart rate remains below 80bpm, despite a minimum of 30s of adequate ventilation with 100% oxygen, chest compressions, and the administration of adrenaline or if the heart rate is 0 and there is no response to ventilation despite the administration of adrenaline and cardiac compressions.

### Tracheal intubation

Is indicated where there is:
- Ineffective face mask ventilation
- The need for tracheal suction at the level of or below the vocal cords due to thick meconium
- Extreme prematurity and surfactant administration (➔ see Respiratory distress syndrome in the newborn, p. 748)
- Prolonged ventilation
- During transfer from the labour ward/theatre to the neonatal unit
- Some congenital abnormalities where the baby has abnormalities of the face and neck, e.g. a cystic hygroma which is large enough to obstruct the airway
- Lung pathology due to diaphragmatic hernia, pneumothorax, hypoplastic lungs, and hydrops.

## Meconium-stained liquor

- Meconium aspiration syndrome (MAS) is a problem associated with term babies.
- If peristalsis is stimulated by hypoxia *in utero,* the anal sphincter relaxes and the fetus will pass meconium into the amniotic fluid.
- The asphyxia also causes the fetus to make gasping movements, taking the meconium into the lungs.
- Aspiration can occur at any time, but the risk is greatest with intrauterine asphyxia.[16]

### Management of meconium-stained liquor

In the presence of any degree of meconium:[15]

- Do not suction the baby's upper airways (nasopharynx and oropharynx) before birth of the shoulders and trunk
- Do not routinely suction the baby's upper airways (nasopharynx and oropharynx) if the baby has normal respiration, heart rate, and tone
- Do not routinely intubate if the baby has normal respiration, heart rate, and tone.

### Thin meconium

May be an 'innocent' finding due to fetal maturation processes. It is often associated with post-term deliveries.

- A small amount of meconium with light staining and no particulate material presents minimal risk of aspiration.
- The baby will be lively and have cried and breathed spontaneously.
- Assess and treat as any other birth.

If there has been non-significant meconium, observe the baby at 1 and 2h of age in all birth settings.

### Thick particulate meconium

- Is a marker of fetal hypoxia
- Increases the risk of aspiration.
- The infant will be depressed and not making any respiratory effort.
- Attempt to remove the meconium before initiating normal respiration.
- Do not stimulate or ventilate.
- Place the infant under a radiant heater on the Resuscitaire®.
- If there has been significant meconium and the baby does not have normal respiration, heart rate, and tone, follow nationally accredited guidelines on neonatal resuscitation:[15]
  - Examine the upper airway for residual meconium
  - Suck out under direct vision using a large-sized catheter or a Yankauer® sucker
  - The trachea should be intubated and meconium suctioned from the lower airways. This may require several attempts.[16]
- Dry the baby and keep warm.

If there has been significant meconium and the baby is healthy, closely observe the baby within a unit with immediate access to a neonatologist. Perform these observations at 1 and 2h of age and then 2-hourly until 12h of age.[15]

If any of the following are observed after any degree of meconium, ask a neonatologist to assess the baby (transfer both the woman and baby if they are at home or in a free-standing midwifery unit, following the general principles for transfer of care):[15]

- Respiratory rate above 60/min
- The presence of grunting
- Heart rate below 100 or above 160bpm
- Capillary refill time above 3s
- Body temperature of 38°C or above, or 37.5°C on two occasions 30min apart
- Oxygen saturation below 95% (measuring oxygen saturation is optional after non-significant meconium)
- Presence of central cyanosis, confirmed by pulse oximetry if available.

Explain the findings to the woman, and inform her about what to look out for and who to talk to if she has any concerns.

## Management of babies born to women with pre-labour rupture of membranes at term

Closely observe any baby born to a woman with pre-labour rupture of the membranes (>24h before the onset of established labour) at term for the first 12h of life (at 1h, 2h, 6h, and 12h) in all settings. Include assessment of:

- Temperature
- Heart rate
- Respiratory rate
- Presence of respiratory grunting
- Significant subcostal recession
- Presence of nasal flare
- Presence of central cyanosis, confirmed by pulse oximetry if available
- Lack of tone (floppiness), general well-being, and feeding
- Skin perfusion assessed by capillary refill.

If any of these are observed, ask a neonatologist to assess the baby (transfer both the woman and baby if they are at home or in a free-standing midwifery unit), following the general principles for transfer of care:

- If there are no signs of infection in the woman, do not give antibiotics to either the woman or the baby, even if the membranes have been ruptured for over 24h
- If there is evidence of infection in the woman, prescribe a full course of broad-spectrum IV antibiotics
- Blood, CSF, and/or surface culture tests are not required in an asymptomatic baby.

Advise women with pre-labour rupture of the membranes to inform their health-care professionals immediately of any concerns they have about their baby's well-being in the first 5 days after birth, particularly in the first 12h when the risk of infection is greatest.

## Post-resuscitation care

- Babies who receive minimal or no resuscitation can normally be handed straight to the parents. Routine observations will be made.
- Babies who receive prolonged resuscitation will need to be transferred to the NICU. This will involve:
  - Stabilization
  - Safe transfer
  - Identification and treatment of problems.
- Babies with MAS will require antibiotics, physiotherapy, and suction to remove the meconium from the lungs. They are also at risk of a pneumothorax due to the meconium blocking the airways.[16]
- Newly born infants born at term or near term with evolving moderate to severe hypoxic–ischaemic encephalopathy should, where possible, be treated with therapeutic hypothermia.[16]

### Communication and record keeping

- An accurate written record detailing the resuscitation events is vital, as it can help to protect practitioners if defence of their actions is required.
- All documentation should be legible, signed, dated, and timed.
- Parents need a clear, detailed account of the baby's problems and further treatments, should the baby require specialized care and transfer to the NICU.[16]

### When to stop

Hospitals will have their own policies in place regarding when to stop resuscitation, usually based on the following factors:

- No cardiac output after 15min
- No respiratory effort after 30min, despite effective ventilation and chest compressions.

When all reversible factors have been eliminated, the decision to stop is made by the most senior clinician available.[16]

## References

15 Resuscitation Council (UK) (2015). *Newborn life support guidelines*. London: Resuscitation Council. Available at: ℜ www.resus.org.uk/resuscitation-guidelines/.
16 National Institute for Health and Care Excellence (2014). *Intrapartum care for healthy women and babies*. NICE guidelines CG190. Available at: ℜ www.nice.org.uk/guidance/cg190.

# Perinatal mortality

Perinatal mortality is defined as the sum of all stillbirths and neonatal deaths in the first week of life. The rate is expressed as numbers of deaths per thousand births.

In June 2015, MBRRACE[17] produced a report on stillbirth, neonatal, and post-neonatal mortality during 2013. This is the first UK perinatal surveillance report produced under the auspices of the Maternal, Newborn and Infant Clinical Outcome Review Programme (MNI-CORP).

MBRRACE-UK has introduced two important changes to the data collection compared to previous surveillance reports:
- The introduction of a new system for classifying deaths: the Cause of Death and Associated Conditions (CODAC) classification system will provide: (a) a greater understanding of the factors associated with antepartum stillbirths; and (b) sufficient detail about the cause of death to allow the effect of serious congenital anomalies to be adequately identified and, where appropriate, excluded from the analyses.
- The widening of inclusion criteria to include all late fetal losses as well as neonatal deaths at 22+0 to 23+6 weeks' gestational age. Such losses, which have been collected at times in the past, are not part of the statutory 'death certification' process.

Despite the fact that the birth rate has risen by 12% between 2003 and 2013, the rate and the number of stillbirths and neonatal deaths fell in the UK. The fall equates to >1000 fewer deaths. In 2013, the extended perinatal mortality rate in the UK was 6.0 per 1000 total births, comprising 4.2 stillbirths per 1000 total births and 1.8 neonatal deaths per 1000 live births.

Significant variations in the rates of extended perinatal mortality across the UK persist. Stabilized and adjusted perinatal mortality rates varied from 5.4 to 7.1 per 1000 total births. Pregnancies to women living in areas with the highest levels of social deprivation in the UK are over 50% more likely to end in stillbirth or neonatal death. Babies of black or black British and Asian or Asian British ethnicity had the highest risk of extended perinatal mortality with rates of 9.8 and 8.8 per 1000 total births, respectively. Both these findings show that inequalities in perinatal outcomes persist in the UK.

For those where a diagnosis had been made, the leading cause of stillbirth during 2013 (excluding terminations of pregnancy and births <24+0 weeks' gestational age) were:
- Placental (19.1%)
- Intrapartum event (8.8%)
- Congenital anomaly (5.9%)
- Umbilical cord (3.9%)
- Maternal (3.4%)
- Fetal (3.0%)
- Infection (2.6%).

For those where a diagnosis had been made, the leading cause of neonatal death during 2013 (excluding terminations of pregnancy and births <24+0 weeks' gestational age) were:

- Congenital anomaly (22.4%)
- Neurological (14.1%)
- Extreme prematurity (13.2%)
- Cardiorespiratory (11.0%)
- Intrapartum event (6.5%)
- Gastrointestinal (4.7%)
- Infection (4.2%)
- Multi-organ failure (2.0%).

Just under 9% of stillbirths and 7% of neonatal deaths were attributed to an intrapartum cause highlighting one particular group of deaths where perinatal care provision should be targeted for improvement.

Whilst the CODAC classification system gives far wider insight into where different management of the mother, or baby, may have led to a different outcome, fewer than half of the stillbirths and only a quarter of the neonatal deaths were consented for full post-mortem. Whilst a post-mortem following stillbirth may not provide a definitive diagnosis of the cause of death, the process can exclude some of the potential causes and provide valuable information for the counselling of parents for future pregnancies. Similarly, for neonatal deaths, a post-mortem may identify conditions or congenital anomalies that would contribute important information for parental counselling. Units should therefore ensure that a post-mortem examination is offered in all cases of stillbirth and neonatal death in order to improve future pregnancy counselling of parents.

### Reference

17 Manktelow BM, Smith LK, Evans TA, et al., on behalf of the MBRRACE-UK collaboration (2015). *Perinatal Mortality Surveillance Report UK Perinatal Deaths for Births from January to December 2013*. Leicester: The Infant Mortality and Morbidity Group, Department of Health Sciences, University of Leicester. Available at: ℬ www.npeu.ox.ac.uk/mbrrace-uk/reports.

# Intrauterine death and stillbirth

## Definition
Intrauterine fetal death (IUFD) refers to death of the fetus at any stage in the pregnancy after the first trimester and before the onset of labour. The fetus may be retained in the uterus for weeks or be born a few days following intrauterine death.

A stillbirth is a baby born after 24 weeks' gestation which shows no signs of life. A baby born before 24 weeks is defined (from a medical viewpoint) as a spontaneous abortion.

## Factors associated with intrauterine death
Parents should be advised that no specific cause is found in 25–60% of IUFDs.[18]

*Maternal*
- Social factors, e.g. low socio-economic status.
- Maternal age (teenagers and >35 years).
- Less formal education.
- Lack of antenatal care.
- Smoking, alcohol, and drug misuse.
- Obesity/excessive weight gain in pregnancy.
- Viruses/infection: rubella, CMV, toxoplasmosis, listeriosis.
- Exposure to environmental hazards:
  - Lead, cadmium, mercury
  - Air pollution.
- Direct trauma to the abdomen.
- Placental dysfunction: abruption, placenta praevia.
- PIH, cholestasis of pregnancy.
- Poor previous obstetric history: abortions, preterm labour, stillbirth.
- Maternal illness: diabetes, renal disease, severe anaemia, epilepsy, antiphospholipid syndrome.

*Fetal*
- Fetal malformation (e.g. associated with diabetes).
- Fetal anoxia.
- Severe IUGR.
- Rh incompatibility.
- Multiple pregnancy (especially monozygotic twins).
- Cord accidents, compression, entanglement, true knot.

## Complications of intrauterine death
- DIC may occur if the fetus is retained >3–4 weeks.
- Induction of labour may be prolonged or difficult.
- The woman and her partner are at risk of psychological trauma.

## Signs
Signs will depend on the time lapse since intrauterine death:
- No fetal movements will be felt by the woman
- No fetal heart heard with the abdominal transducer

- The uterus may be smaller than expected for dates
- The woman may experience full breasts and may produce milk
- Any hypertension may settle
- There may be a brownish discharge PV.

## Diagnosis

- Ultrasound scan will confirm no heartbeat.
- Spalding's sign: overlap and misalignment of fetal skull bones.
- Robert's sign: gas in the great vessels and heart of the fetus (1–2 days).
- Fetal curl: there is arching of the fetal spine.

## Management of care

- The woman who presents with anxieties about reduced or no fetal movements should be seen urgently.
- Be sensitive to her anxiety. You may be able to reassure the woman quickly by hearing the fetal heart using the CTG or Sonicaid®. When doing this, it is important to differentiate the fetal and maternal pulses. Caution must be used, as auscultation of the fetal heart with a Pinard stethoscope or Doppler ultrasound is insufficiently accurate and should not be used to diagnose a suspected IUFD.[19] Auscultation can give false reassurance; maternal pelvic blood flow can result in an apparently 'normal' FHR pattern with an external Doppler.
- Ideally, real-time ultrasonography should be available at all times; this is essential for the accurate diagnosis of IUFD. If the fetal heart is not heard (or the pregnancy is <20 weeks and the FHR is not easily audible), explain the findings and contact an experienced ultrasonographer and a registrar to assess by ultrasound whether or not the FHR is present.
- The diagnosis of intrauterine death should be confirmed by two experts.
- Women booked under midwifery-led care should be transferred to consultant-led care. However, continuity of midwifery care should still be given high priority in order to facilitate adequate support and coordination of information throughout the episode. A midwife specializing in bereavement care may be available.

*When giving bad news note that:*
- Support for the woman should be sought from her partner/family/ friends.
- Health-care professionals should offer support to help the women and their partners and/or family cope with the emotional and physical consequences of the death. This should include offering information about specialist support.[20]
- Information should be clear and honest, given in a way sensitive to individual needs and feelings. Parents will always remember the way the news is delivered and the attitudes of staff.
- The parents may react with shock or 'numbness' or disbelief. Some may experience physical symptoms. Mothers should be prepared for the possibility of passive fetal movement after the scan to diagnose IUFD; a repeat scan should be offered.[19]
- Parents need time to receive the information.

- Any information given may need to be repeated, and distressed clients may need the information to be written down so that they can review it later.
- Support for staff is also important.
- The SoM, community midwife, health visitor liaison, and GP should be informed of the intrauterine death as soon as possible after diagnosis.

**Induction of labour**

- An obstetric consultant should discuss a plan for care and delivery with the parents.
- Once the diagnosis is made, in the event of an IUFD, if the woman appears to be physically well, her membranes are intact, and there is no evidence of infection or bleeding, she should be offered a choice of immediate induction of labour or expectant management.[20] Some women will want to wait a day or two; others will request induction of labour as soon as practical.
- Immediate induction of labour is the preferred management option if the death of the fetus is thought to be related to maternal complications such as placental abruption, PIH, or infection, or there is evidence of ruptured membranes or bleeding.[20]
- A full explanation should be given of the procedures, a possible time scale, and how the baby may look at delivery. Obtain consent for treatment. Those close to the couple should be encouraged to stay and give support.
- Ensure that the room for induction of labour is comfortable, and remove any inappropriate items (e.g. fetal monitor).
- Take IV samples of blood to test for FBC/platelets and G&S. Obtain a clotting screen if the intrauterine death occurred >3 weeks previously. Other samples may be requested, depending on the clinical picture.

*Induction regimen*

- Mifepristone 200mg is given orally and the woman may go home and return in 36–48h.
- On readmission: the choice of vaginal PGE2 or vaginal misoprostol 800 micrograms given PV should be offered. The choice and dose of vaginal prostaglandin should take into account the clinical circumstances, the availability of preparations, and the local protocol; for women who have had a previous Caesarean section, the risk of uterine rupture is increased. The dose of vaginal prostaglandin should be reduced accordingly, particularly in the third trimester.[20]
- Misoprostol 400 micrograms is given PV 3h later.
- This is repeated 3h with up to five doses. The regimen should be continued even when the cervix dilates, to maintain uterine activity.
- If delivery does not occur, the senior obstetrician should be informed. After 24h, it is safe to repeat the five doses of misoprostol.
- ARM should be avoided until delivery is imminent because:
  - There is a risk of infection
  - The fetal skull is cushioned by the waters.
- Choice in analgesia is important. Opiates may be given or an epidural if there is no coagulopathy.
- Syntometrine® is indicated at delivery. Be aware that PPH may occur.

INTRAUTERINE DEATH AND STILLBIRTH 567

## Care immediately after birth

- Support the parents, and, if they are willing, encourage them to look at and hold the baby. They should be left alone with the baby for a period of time if they so wish.
- Acknowledge the parents' feelings of loss. A few kind words, a clasped hand or a hug, or a small posy of flowers from staff can enrich the few memories the couple take away.
- The obstetric registrar or consultant should see the baby and complete a stillbirth certificate. It is important that this is obtained early in the proceedings because the parents will need it to make arrangements for registration and burial.
- Weigh the baby and measure his or her length. The parents may want to help with bathing and dressing the baby. They will wish to give the baby a name. Photographs, a lock of hair, handprints, and footprints are taken and transferred to a card as a keepsake.
- Carefully label the baby with the mother's identification details.
- Enquire whether the parents would like to see the hospital chaplain or other persons who may provide spiritual support.

## Administration

It is good practice to complete a bereavement checklist and to have a communication book to ensure that all administration is recorded efficiently (Table 23.5).

## Investigations into the cause of fetal loss

- To complete the process of grieving for their baby, the parents often need to know the cause of death.
- Certain blood, tissue samples, and swabs may be requested from the mother, fetus, and placenta, and are important for obtaining accurate information for counselling the parents at a later date (Table 23.6).
- The placenta may be sent to histology for examination.
- A post mortem may be indicated. A senior obstetrician or midwife should obtain consent after a full, but sensitive, explanation of the procedure. The parents should be given written information about the examination and have an opportunity to read it before consent.
- Photographs of the baby may be required and can be requested from medical photography.
- An appointment with the consultant should be arranged 4–6 weeks after the stillbirth to discuss any findings.

## Transfer to the community

- If the woman is physically well after the delivery, the parents may want to go home and return, as they wish, to see the baby and discuss further arrangements. The baby will be kept in the hospital until decisions have been made about a post-mortem and funeral.
- If the fetal death occurred unexpectedly in labour, it is especially important that the parents be given plenty of time to talk through the incident with staff involved at the earliest opportunity.
- The parents need to know what might have been the cause; otherwise some in their grief may irrationally blame themselves or others. A mutually convenient appointment should be arranged.

Table 23.5 Example of bereavement checklist for labour ward

| | Signature | Date |
|---|---|---|
| Name of doctor examining baby after delivery | | |
| Mother informed of death by | | |
| Father informed of death by | | |
| New page in bereavement diary | | |
| Notes marked with SANDS logo | | |
| Cancellation card Bounty advertising | | |
| Community midwife informed ASAP<br>Name:        Phone:<br>Is a visit wanted at home? | | |
| GP informed.<br>Name:        Phone:<br>Is a visit wanted at home? | | |
| Cancel antenatal clinic appointment | | |
| Health visitor (HV) referral form:<br>HV notified by phone | | |
| Inform chaplaincy | | |
| Parents given time to handle baby | | |
| Four Polaroid photographs taken | | |
| Medical illustration card completed | | |
| Hand- and footprints/hair taken | | |
| Computer details completed | | |
| Congenital anomalies registered | | |
| Mortuary identification labels attached ×2 | | |
| SANDS booklet and other literature given | | |

- Anti-D may be given prophylactically to Rh-negative women.
- If the woman's pregnancy was >20 weeks' gestation and she has no history of PIH, she may be given a prescription for cabergoline 1mg, to be taken on the first post-partum day. This will help to suppress lactation.
- Give the woman and her partner literature that puts them in touch with other parents who have been bereaved, e.g. the Stillbirth and Neonatal Death Society (SANDS). The Child Bereavement Trust provides support for parents and siblings.
- Mark the hospital notes with the SANDS teardrop logo, indicating a perinatal bereavement.
- Where possible, postal advertising for pregnancy is cancelled.
- Some units keep a remembrance book and hold yearly memorial services for parents and families who have experienced the loss of a baby.

Table 23.6 Example of checklist for maternal, placenta, and fetal investigations

| Maternal investigations | Bloods | Signature | Date | Required |
|---|---|---|---|---|
| Viral studies: toxoplasmosis, CMV, herpes, rubella | Virology | | | (Yes/no) |
| Blood group, antibodies, Kleihauer | BTS | | | Regardless of blood group |
| Haemoglobin | Haematology | | | |
| Listeriosis | Microbiology | | | |
| Fetal and placental | Bloods | Signature | Date | Required |
| Viral PCR studies: toxoplasmosis, CMV, herpes, rubella | Virology | | | |
| Blood group and Coombs' test | BTS | | | |
| Haemoglobin | Paediatric vial, haematology | | | |
| Chromosome analysis | Paediatric vial, cytogenetics; plus sample of membrane, placenta, and cord. Send in culture solution to cytogenetics (consent required) | | | |
| Placental swabs | From maternal surface and fetal surface; bacteriology | | | |
| Placenta to histology | Send as soon as possible regardless of whether a post-mortem is required | | | |

CMV, cytomegalovirus; BTS Blood Transfusion Service; PCR, polymerase chain reaction.

Adapted from Bereavement guidelines (2004). Jessop Wing Sheffield Teaching Hospitals Trust.

## Registration and funeral arrangements

- If the gestation is <24 weeks, no registration is required.
- All stillborn babies after 24 weeks' gestation require a stillbirth certificate.
- This certificate is taken by the parents to the registrar of births and deaths at the registry so that the registration of the stillbirth can take place.
- The registration should be completed within 42 days.
- Unless legally married, the woman and her partner should attend together if the father's name is to be registered on the certificate.
- The parents should ask for a copy of the certificate for themselves.
- The registrar will issue a certificate of disposal following a stillbirth.
- This, when given to the funeral directors, allows them to proceed with arrangements for the funeral.
- The hospital may arrange the funeral, or parents may arrange a private cremation or burial if they wish.

For further information, ➜ see Bereavement care, p. 624.

## References

18 Silver RM, Varner MW, Reddy U, et al. (2007). Work-up of stillbirth: a review of the evidence. *Am J Obstet Gynecol* **5**: 433–44.

19 Royal College of Obstetricians and Gynaecologists (2010). *Late intrauterine fetal death and stillbirth. Green-top guideline No. 55.* Available at: ℳ www.rcog.org.uk/globalassets/documents/guidelines/gtg_55.pdf.

20 National Institute for Health and Care Excellence (2008). Induction of labour in specific circumstances. In: National Institute for Health and Care Excellence. *Inducing labour.* NICE guidelines CG70. Available at: ℳ www.nice.org.uk/guidance/cg70/chapter/guidance#induction-of- labour-in-specific-circumstances.

# Part 4

# Postnatal care

# Postnatal care

# Principles of postnatal care

The principles of postnatal care are mother- and family-centred to meet her physical, psychological, and emotional needs in recovering from the birth experience and caring for her baby. In providing effective postnatal care, the midwife must ensure:

- The mother and her family are treated with kindness, respect, and dignity
- Excellent communication that respects the views, values, and beliefs of the woman, partner, and her family
- A documented, individualized care plan developed in partnership with the mother and reviewed at each contact
- Timely and relevant information to enable her to promote her own and her baby's health and well-being and recognize and respond to any problems arising
- The mother is encouraged to make informed decisions about her care and any treatment needed
- The mother's emotional well-being is monitored and what family and social support she has in the postnatal period. Encourage the mother and her partner and family to tell the midwife about any changes in mood, emotional state, and behaviour that are outside of her normal pattern
- Contact details of all health-care professionals involved in her care
- The mother knows the signs and symptoms of potentially life-threatening conditions and how to summon help from the midwife or doctor or emergency services, if required
- Contemporaneous and accurate records about maternal and neonatal health and well-being, information and advice given, agreed in partnership with the mother, and readily available to all health-care professionals involved in her care.

The midwife must ensure that postnatal care complies with the following:
- Department of Health (2007). *Maternity Matters*. London: Department of Health
- National Institute for Health and Care Excellence (2006), reviewed 2014, *Routine Postnatal Care of Women and their Babies*. Clinical guideline 37. London: NICE.
- National Institute for Health and Care Excellence (2014). *Antenatal and Postnatal Mental Health*. Clinical guideline 192. London: NICE.

# Physiological aspects of postnatal care

## Aim

- To ensure optimal physical health and to detect deviations from normal.
- A methodical top-to-toe examination, accompanied by a discussion about her health.
- Exact interpretation of the findings will depend on:
  - Whether the woman had a normal pregnancy and a spontaneous vaginal birth
  - Pre-existing health or obstetric problems
  - Problems occurring in labour.

## Physiological changes

- Involution of the uterus and other parts of the genital tract.
- Initiation of lactation.
- Physiological changes in other body systems.

## Vital signs

- Temperature: normal range 36–37°C. Once returned to the normal range after birth, it is unnecessary to check it routinely, unless the mother complains of, or shows, signs that suggest infection: feeling unwell, flu-like symptoms, or actual signs of infection.
- Pulse: normal range 65–80bpm. A rapid pulse rate may also indicate infection.
- Respiratory rate: normal range 12–16/min at rest.
- BP: should return to normal within 24h of birth. Unless the BP was raised pre-pregnancy, during pregnancy, and/or labour, there is no need to monitor routinely postnatally.

# Involution of the uterus

## Definition
The return of the uterus to its pre-pregnant size, tone, and position.

## Process
- Ischaemia: the uterine muscle contracts and retracts, restricting the blood flow within the uterus.
- Phagocytosis: redundant fibrous and elastic tissue is broken down.
- Autolysis: muscle fibres are digested by proteolytic enzymes (lysozymes).
- All the waste products pass into the bloodstream and are eliminated via the kidneys.
- The decidual lining of the uterus is shed in the vaginal blood loss, and the new endometrium begins to develop from about 10 days after birth and is completed by 6 weeks.
- Uterine size decreases from 15cm × 11cm × 7.5cm to 7.5cm × 5cm × 2.5cm by 6 weeks.
- Uterine weight decreases from 1000g immediately after birth to 60g by 6 weeks. At the end of the first week, it weighs about 500g.
- Rate of involution: there is a steady decrease by 1cm/day. On the first day, it is 12cm above the symphysis pubis and by the seventh day it is approximately 5cm above the symphysis pubis. By day 10, it is barely palpable, if at all.
- Involution will be slower after a Caesarean section.
- Involution will be delayed if there is retention of placental tissue or blood clot, particularly if associated with infection.

## Assessment of postnatal uterine involution
- Discuss the need for uterine assessment with the mother.
- Obtain verbal consent.
- Ask her to empty her bladder if she has not done so in the last half hour.
- Ensure privacy.
- Ask her to lie on her back, with her head well supported.
- Cover her legs and abdomen.
- Wash your hands thoroughly.
- Ask the mother to expose her abdomen.
- Talk to the mother throughout the examination; explain what you are doing and why, and answer her questions.
- Face the mother and place the lower edge of the examining hand on the abdomen at the level of the umbilicus.
- Palpate gently inwards towards the spine and gently move downwards until the uterine fundus is located.
- Note the level of the uterine fundus and the degree of uterine contraction and retraction.
- Note any pain, tenderness, or uterine bulkiness.
- Ask her about her vaginal loss: odour, amount, abnormal colour, or any concerns at all about her loss.

- Discuss the findings with the mother.
- Document the findings in the mother's records.
- Report any abnormalities to the doctor without delay.

## Practice points

▶ It is important that:

- Wherever possible, the same midwife carries out the regular postnatal examination, to monitor normal involution and detect early deviations from normal
- The uterus remains contracted and retracted and centrally positioned in the lower abdomen
- Daily uterine palpation is unnecessary after the first 3 days, unless there is any reason for concern or deviations from normal are apparent. The midwife should use her discretion.

# Vaginal blood loss

- Blood is the major component of vaginal loss in the first few days.
- As uterine involution progresses, the vaginal loss changes to stale blood products, lanugo, vernix, and other debris from the products of conception, leucocytes, and organisms.
- Towards the end of the second week, the discharge is yellowish white, consisting of cervical mucus, leucocytes, and organisms.
- This process may take as long as 3 weeks, and research has shown that there is a wide variation in the amount, colour, and duration of vaginal loss in the first 12 weeks post-partum.

**Practice point**

▶ It is important that the midwife asks focused questions about the nature of the vaginal loss, to determine whether it is normal or not.

# The perineum

- Even if the perineum remains intact at the time of birth, women experience bruising of the vaginal and perineal tissues for the first few days.
- Women may be embarrassed about exposing the perineum after birth, so, unless there is a clinical indication, i.e. pain or evidence of infection, routine daily observation by the midwife is unnecessary and may actually serve to introduce infection, when strict handwashing before and after the procedure and the wearing of disposable gloves is not carried out.
- Ask her specific questions about perineal pain and soreness.
- Dependent on the suturing technique used and on the suture material, sutures may have to be removed approximately 1 week after birth. However, absorbable, non-irritant suture material is now increasingly used.

**Practice points**

- The first few days after birth can be difficult physically, emotionally, and psychologically for a woman with perineal trauma, restricting her mobility, her rest and sleep, the enjoyment of her baby, and the ability to find a comfortable position for feeding, particularly if breastfeeding.
- Long-term physical and psychological trauma may be the result, and the midwife must be sensitive and supportive of the mother at this time.

# Perineal pain

- If the mother has sustained perineal trauma, the midwife may wish to inspect the perineum daily for the first few days, to ascertain the comfort of any sutures, wound healing, and cleanliness.
- If she has interrupted sutures, removal of a particularly tight suture may be all that is required to ease perineal pain and tension.
- Advice should be given, as appropriate, about cleansing and changing the sanitary pad regularly, to avoid infection.
- Vaginal blood loss can also be assessed, as can the presence of haemorrhoids.

Pain relief may be achieved in a number of ways:
- Try the simple remedies first such as a bath, bidet, or cool water poured over the perineum.
- Bath additives, such as salt or Savlon®, have been shown in research to be of no added value, neither have treatments such as ultrasound, infrared heat, or pulsed electromagnetic energy in promoting healing or reducing pain.
- Keeping the area clean and dry, with pain relief, as above, allows healing.
- Oral analgesia, such as paracetamol, may be administered 4- to 6-hourly.
- Lavender oil or tea tree essential oils—five drops added to bath water or applied as a topical compress. Both can be applied directly to the skin.
- Homeopathic remedies, such as arnica, calendula, and Bellis perennis, may be applied topically or taken orally, but the mother must be referred to a registered homeopathy practitioner should she wish to use homeopathic remedies.

## Practice points

- If administering any of the above treatments, ensure personal knowledge and competence with regard to the current research evidence and the use of complementary therapies, or refer the mother to an appropriately trained complementary therapist.
- Document all examination, findings, and treatments clearly in the mother's and/or your notes.

# Circulation

- The increased blood volume of pregnancy is gradually reabsorbed and excreted in the diuresis of the first few days after birth.
- Oedema of the feet and ankles may be experienced, even if not experienced in pregnancy.
- Check that the woman's BP is not abnormally raised, and advise her to mobilize, avoid long periods of standing, and elevate the feet and legs when sitting.
- The swelling should be bilateral and without pain. Swelling in one leg accompanied by pain in the calf or femoral area may indicate a DVT (➔ see Deep vein thrombosis, p. 196 and ➔ Principles of thromboprophylaxis, p. 200, for further details).

## Legs

- ▶ It is important to observe for swelling, oedema, inflammation, colour, and pain, particularly in a woman confined to bed or mobilizing in a limited way, essential after an operative delivery.
- ▶▶ Any abnormality may be due to a DVT and medical aid should be sought immediately.

## Haemoglobin level

- It should not be necessary to routinely check in fit, healthy women where blood loss at birth has had no detrimental effect.
- In a mother who has had a traumatic birth and/or sustained a heavy blood loss, an FBC may be undertaken on the third postnatal day.
- Generally it is not now done unless clinically indicated.

# General health

## General observations

- Overall body temperature.
- Abnormal body odour that may suggest an infection.
- Overall colour and complexion, e.g. flushed or pale.

## Skin

- Skin texture and tone will return to normal soon after birth.
- Any skin irritation caused by obstetric cholestasis or skin stretching will soon resolve. A moisturizing lotion is all that is normally required to ease irritation and any dry feeling.

## Nutrition

- Encourage the mother to maintain a balanced diet as much as possible and to include as much fresh food as possible.
- Adequate water intake is important, at least 2L a day.
- Adequate fluid and nutrition are essential for lactation, to encourage normal gastrointestinal activity and resume normal bowel action as soon as possible.

## Bowel action

- This should return to normal in 2–3 days after birth.
- Fresh fruit, vegetables, and a good fluid intake will encourage this.
- After a Caesarean section, it may take a day or so longer, particularly if diet and fluids have been restricted in the first few hours after operation.

## Practice point

The mother may be afraid of rupturing any perineal sutures, so supporting the perineum with a pad may help during the first bowel action.

# Urinary output

- A marked diuresis will occur in the first 2–3 days after birth, but there should be no dysuria (pain on micturition).
- There may be some soreness from perineal trauma.
- Ask the mother whether she is passing urine normally and whether there is any discomfort or any stress incontinence.
- The bladder neck and urethra may have been damaged during labour and birth, which could result in a lack of sensation to pass urine in the first couple of days. This can lead to retention with overflow, causing intense pain and discomfort, urinary tract infection, and sub-involution of the uterus, a cause of primary or secondary PPH.

## Practice points

- ▶ Passing very small amounts of urine is often a sign of retention with overflow. Palpate the bladder after she has been to the toilet. If a portable ultrasound bladder scanner is available, the midwife may scan the bladder to estimate the amount of urine retained.
- If the mother has difficulty in passing urine, try the simple remedies first, such as running water, asking her to sit on the bidet or in a bath of warm water, in an attempt to stimulate micturition.
- Oral fluids should not be restricted, but encouraged.
- If a mother has difficulty with micturition, burning sensation, or pain with micturition, obtain a midstream specimen of urine in a sterile container and send for laboratory culture.
- Initial inspection of the urine for colour, clarity, and odour will yield useful information if an infection is suspected.

# Psychological and emotional aspects of postnatal care

- Psychological and emotional well-being and positive mental health are as important as the physical aspects of care.
- Postnatal emotional and psychological changes following childbirth are commonly experienced by women.
- Midwives have an important role in the early detection of psychological problems and have a responsibility as part of the multi-professional team, to ensure that women are referred appropriately and receive support and care.
- Psychological conditions in the postnatal period cover a spectrum of conditions that vary from mild to severe.
- At each postnatal contact, the mother should be asked about her emotional well-being, what family and social support she has, and her usual coping strategies with day-to-day matters.[1]
- Good communication, listening to what the mother is telling you, and responding appropriately will do much to alleviate situations causing the mother anxiety, most commonly concerning baby care and feeding.
- The mother and her partner should be offered the opportunity to talk about their birth experiences and ask questions about the care they received and the events of labour. (For further information, ➔ see Postnatal afterthoughts for parents, p. 617.)
- The mother and her partner/family should be encouraged to tell the midwife about any changes in mood, emotional state, and behaviour that are outside the woman's normal pattern.[1,2]
- The midwife must always be able to recognize the risks, signs, and symptoms of domestic abuse and know whom to contact for advice and management.[2,3]

## Temporary mood alteration (post-partum 'blues')

This is a transient, self-limiting condition, often referred to as 'baby blues'. It occurs between the third and tenth days, although it occurs most often around the fourth day. It is considered a normal reaction to childbirth and between 50% and 80% will experience the condition.[1]

### Symptoms

These include:
- Tearfulness
- Mood swings
- Irritability.

The condition usually resolves spontaneously within a day or two, although women with postnatal depression have been shown to have higher occurrences of the baby blues. Provide emotional support and reassurance that it is a temporary condition that will resolve.

# References

1 National Institute for Health and Care Excellence (2006). *Routine postnatal care of women and their babies*. NICE guidelines CG37, reviewed 2014. London: National Institute for Health and Care Excellence.
2 National Institute for Health and Care Excellence (2014). *Antenatal and postnatal mental health: clinical management and service guidance*. NICE guidelines CG192. London: National Institute for Health and Care Excellence.
3 Department of Health (2013). *Guidelines for health professionals on domestic violence*. Available at: ℛ www.gov.uk/government/publications/guidance-for-health-professionals-on-domestic-violence.

# Transfer home from hospital

- The exact timing of transfer home is normally negotiated between the mother and the midwife, and is dependent on her circumstances and needs.
- Care is transferred back to the community midwife, if the model of care operating locally has not involved the named community midwife in her care in hospital.
- Examine the mother to ensure that she is physically fit to go home, and ensure that the baby has been fully examined by a paediatrician or a midwife appropriately trained and competent to undertake this first complete examination of the newborn. Community midwives now also undertake this examination in the UK for mothers who have had a home birth, or they may carry out the examination on the first visit after transfer home.
- Explain to the mother about the continued support by her community midwife; give her her personal notes, duly completed to date, and letters for her family doctor and community midwife, containing the relevant details about the birth and progress of the mother and baby to date.
- This is accompanied by a range of leaflets and details of how to get advice and support night and day, e.g. the telephone number of the community midwife, postnatal ward, community midwifery office, and infant feeding adviser.
- The mother makes her own arrangements for transport home.
- The importance of car safety for the mother and baby should be stressed, although it is the mother's/parents' responsibility to ensure that the baby is transported in a car seat, appropriately secured in the car.
- On no account must the midwife have any involvement in the process of putting the baby in the car seat or securing the seat in the car.
- It is important that the transfer home between the hospital and community midwife is seamless, in that there is continuity of care and no conflicting advice, and records clearly show the progress and problems to date and advice given.

# Parent education

## Aims

- To promote health improvement.
- To give appropriate information and support.
- To develop confidence in parenting skills.
- To facilitate parental involvement in decision-making.
- To provide emotional and psychological support for the new parents.
- To encourage peer support.

## Practice points

- The social, emotional, and psychological needs of parents are as important as the physical skills of caring for the baby.
- Every mother/parent has differing needs.
- Certain groups have special needs, e.g. the young, single, women with disability, ethnic minorities, women whose first language is not English, women with learning difficulties, asylum seekers, refugees.
- Do not forget the men!
- Preparation for parenthood begins in childhood, in the home, in school, and the social environment, e.g. television, books, magazines.
- Continuity of care and carer, as far as possible, will enable the mother to express her concerns, fears, and anxieties more freely, and will enable the midwife to be more effective in educational activities.
- Every meeting with new parents is an opportunity for health education, health promotion, parent education, or referral to other health or social care professionals or agencies that can more effectively address or meet their needs.
- Use each care setting as an educational opportunity.
- Small groups aid discussion and can encourage women/parents to air their problems, learn from each other, and aid peer support for new parents. With the development of local children's centres in the UK, the opportunity for networking and developing social networks of support for the mother also offers the midwife and other health and social care professionals the ideal opportunity for health education and promotion.
- When offering group sessions, consider the target group and its needs carefully. You may need to offer a choice of groups and times.
- Be realistic about what can be achieved in a series of meetings.

## Main educational activities

*The mother*

- Adequate rest and sleep.
- Well-balanced diet.
- Personal hygiene, particularly of the vulval and perineal area.
- Prevention of infection.
- Healthy lifestyle, e.g. smoking cessation.
- Postnatal exercises and encouragement to continue with them for at least 6 weeks.
- Resuming normal exercise regimens, e.g. returning to the gym.
- Continuing contact with health-care professionals for personal support and infant care, e.g. immunizations and child development.
- Emotional and psychological well-being.

*The baby*

- Provide a safe, child-friendly environment.
- Teach infant care skills.
- Cord care.
- Hygiene.
- Room temperature—keep the baby warm but not overheated.
- Prevention of infection.
- Breastfeeding (→ see Chapter 28 for further information):
  - Establishing and maintaining lactation
  - Correct fixing technique
  - Hand expression technique
  - Safe storage of expressed breast milk.
- Formula feeding:
  - Sterilization of feeding and other equipment
  - Making up feeds safely
  - Choosing the correct formula
  - Storage of made-up feeds
  - The dos and don'ts of formula feeding.
- Responding to and interpreting baby's cry.
- Getting to know the baby.
- Sleep patterns.
- General behaviour.
- Car seats and safety.
- Prevention of sudden infant death.
- Risks of co-sleeping with parents.

*Emotional*

- Effect of the new baby in the home.
- Changing roles and responsibilities.
- Relationship with the partner and family.
- Sibling jealousy.
- Psychological adaptation to parenthood.

*Father/partner*

- Increasing involvement in the care of the immediate family.
- Important adjustments.
- Aid his/her partner in adjusting to motherhood.
- Jealousy of the baby.
- Sharing his/her partner.
- Supporting his/her partner.
- Sharing baby care.
- Helping with other children and care of the home.
- Encourage him/her to be as involved as possible.
- Paternity leave entitlement.

*Sexual*

- Resumption of sexual relationships.
- Dyspareunia.
- Contraception.
- Sexual health.
- Cervical screening.

# Post-operative care

- The most common reason for post-operative care is a Caesarean section, but reasons may include manual removal of the placenta or dealing with persistent post-birth bleeding from the genital tract.
- Immediate post-operative care is normally undertaken in the theatre recovery room by theatre staff, but in many cases the midwife will find herself undertaking this care.
- Clear and accurate documentation of all aspects of care is vital.
- Post-operative observations of the mother will consist of observation and management of:
  - Vital signs and level of consciousness, if she has had a general anaesthetic
  - Epidural site and degree of anaesthesia
  - Pain
  - Vaginal blood loss
  - Wound drain
  - IV fluids and the cannula area
  - Bladder drainage (if a urinary catheter is *in situ*).
- As soon as possible after the birth, the mother should have skin-to-skin contact with her baby, as would happen in a normal birth. If her condition/level of consciousness do not immediately allow this, then the father could undertake the initial skin-to-skin contact, until the mother is able to (➔ see Breast crawl and skin-to-skin, p. 378).
- Once the mother's condition is stable and she is fully conscious, she is transferred to the postnatal ward with her baby.
- A Caesarean section is a major abdominal surgery, and if it was undertaken following a complicated or traumatic labour, the mother has to recover from the physical and mental stress of labour, as well as from the anaesthetic and the operation.

## Immediate care

*Position*

- General anaesthetic: nurse her in the left lateral or 'recovery' position until fully conscious.
- Epidural or spinal anaesthesia: as directed by the anaesthetist, particularly noting her respiratory rate, because of the narcotic analgesia given.
- Gradually sit her up as soon as possible, provided her BP is stable.

*Observations*

The frequency of the observations carried out will be according to local policy and practice guidelines, but generally will follow this pattern for the first 12h:

- BP and pulse rate: half-hourly for the first 2h, hourly for 2h, then 4-hourly
- Wound and wound drain inspection, as above
- Vaginal blood loss, as above
- Temperature: 2-hourly for the first 4h, then 4-hourly.

*Analgesia*

Post-operative pain relief can be given in a number of ways:

- Epidural opioid (observe respiratory rate)
- IV opioid: patient-controlled device
- Subcutaneous opioid or other similar analgesia
- IM opioid; never use in conjunction with an epidural opioid
- Rectal, e.g. diclofenac
- Oral drugs, e.g. dihydrocodeine or paracetamol
- An antiemetic, such as cyclizine, may be prescribed and given IM or subcutaneously, to counteract nausea or vomiting caused by opioid drugs.

## Care on the postnatal ward

Unless the baby has been transferred to the neonatal unit, the mother and baby should be transferred together and stay together. Attachment should be encouraged and a clip-on cot, which fits on to the mother's bed, will make it easier for the mother to touch and handle her baby.

The midwife should employ a model of care that ensures a holistic and integrated approach to meeting the individual woman's needs and encouraging increasing self-care, but limiting over-exertion.

*Observations*

Continue the regimen begun in the theatre recovery room for the first 12h:

- BP and pulse rate: half-hourly for the first 2h, hourly for 2h, then 4-hourly
- Wound and wound drain inspection, as above
- Vaginal blood loss, as above
- Temperature: 2-hourly for the first 4h, then 4-hourly
- The IV infusion is usually removed 8–12h after the operation, once the mother's BP is stable and she is tolerating oral fluids.

## Wound care

- Prophylactic antibiotics may be prescribed to reduce the incidence of wound infection; the regimen and route of administration are dependent on local policy and practice, e.g. IV, IM, or oral.
- The principle of wound care is to keep it dry and clean. The dressing is usually removed after 24h, if one has been applied initially.
- If the woman is obese and lower abdominal skinfolds are present, allowing the wound to become warm and moist, the dressing may be left on.
- Offer advice about drying the wound thoroughly after a shower.
- Observe the wound for the following, reporting any occurrence to the doctor:
    - *Infection*: hot, tender, inflamed area, pyrexia; obtain a swab for laboratory culture
    - *Haematoma*: pain, hard to touch, tender.
- Broad-spectrum antibiotics will usually be started at this point, if they are not being taken prophylactically. They may be given IV or subcutaneously or taken orally, depending on local policy.

## Thromboprophylaxis

(→ See Principles of thromboprophylaxis, p. 200.)

- PE and thromboembolic disease are the main causes of direct maternal death in the UK.[4]
- Encourage the mother to move her legs, with leg stretching and ankle rotation exercises, at least every hour.
- Administer LMWH tinzaparin subcutaneously, daily for 48–72h.
- Measure the woman for thromboembolic prevention stockings prior to the operation and ensure they are put on prior to the operation and worn until full mobility is regained.
- Encourage mobilization as soon as possible.

## Urine output

- An indwelling catheter is usually *in situ* for the first 24–48h post-operatively, after which it is removed.
- Observe and record the urine output carefully and empty the catheter bag; measure and record the amount 6- to 8-hourly. Never let the drainage bag get too full, as this can be very uncomfortable, cumbersome, and embarrassing for the mother, as she begins to mobilize.
- The mother should be encouraged to use the bidet when she is able to get up, to keep the vulva and catheter area clean.
- It is good practice to obtain and send a catheter specimen of urine to the lab at the time of removal of the catheter, or any time before that if the mother is complaining of pain, which could be associated with a urinary tract infection.
- After catheter removal, it is important to ask the mother about her ability to pass urine and the amount passed.
- Observe and palpate the abdomen for evidence of retention of urine at least twice a day for the first day.
- At first, the bladder may not be completely emptied and a bladder scan after passing urine will estimate the residual urine in the bladder. This should be <30mL as bladder tone gradually returns.
- Report any haematuria to the doctor.

## Fluid and nutrition

- The mother is encouraged to drink plenty and to gradually introduce a light diet. Plain water is the fluid of choice if there are any problems with nausea or vomiting following general anaesthesia, until this has passed.
- If there has been trauma to any part of the pelvic structures or handling of the bowel, the surgeon will usually request water only by mouth until bowel sounds return, 24–48h after surgery, to avoid the risk of paralytic ileus.
- Appetite will vary from woman to woman, and those who have had a general anaesthetic will be less keen to eat initially.

## Mood and feelings

- After a general anaesthetic, some women feel very tired and have a sense of detachment for several days.
- She may not relate well to the baby immediately.
- She may feel guilty, disappointed, or a failure at not achieving a normal birth.
- Pain and the analgesia given may make her sleepy.
- She will need help with caring for and feeding her baby.

## Reference

4 Knight M, Kenyon S, Brocklehurst P, Neilson J, Shakespeare J, Kurinczuk JJ (eds.) on behalf of MBRRACE-UK (2014). *Saving Lives, Improving Mothers' Care: Lessons learned to inform future maternity care from the UK and Ireland Confidential Enquiries into Maternal Deaths and Morbidity 2009–12.* Oxford: National Perinatal Epidemiology Unit, University of Oxford. Available at: ℘ www.npeu.ox.ac.uk/mbrrace-uk/reports.

# Postnatal care of the breasts

The advice that is given to the mother on the care of the breasts postnatally will depend upon her choice of infant feeding method.

## Postnatal care for breastfeeding mothers

- Mothers are no longer advised to wash their breasts before each feed, as the use of soap may remove the natural oils that keep the nipples and areola supple.
- Advise mothers that adequate personal hygiene is sufficient.
- A supportive well-fitting maternity bra may add to the mother's comfort, but care should be taken that it does not dig into the breast tissue.
- There is no evidence to support the use of creams, ointments, sprays, or tinctures to prevent nipple soreness and in some cases these have been shown to increase the incidence of soreness.
- Provide help and assistance to ensure correct positioning and attachment of the baby at the breast.
- The duration and frequency of feeds should not be restricted.
- For mothers with specific problems, ⮕ see Breastfeeding problems, p. 800.

## Breast care for mothers who are bottle-feeding

The mother should be informed that although she is not breastfeeding the milk will still 'come in' between 2 and 4 days postnatally. Advise the mother:

- To handle her breasts as little as possible
- To wear a good supporting bra
- Not to express the milk as this will encourage further milk production
- To use heat and cold, either via a shower or soaking in the bath, to help relieve discomfort
- To take mild analgesics, e.g. paracetamol, to help relieve the discomfort.

Reassure the mother that this is a transient condition that will resolve within 24–48h.

Occasionally, pharmacological preparations (bromocriptine and cabergoline) may be used for the suppression of lactation. Bromocriptine has adverse side effects and therefore cabergoline is usually the drug of choice.

# Care of the mother with pre-existing medical conditions

Two-thirds of mothers who die during pregnancy and up to 1 year after birth have pre-existing medical and mental health problems.[5]

## Diabetes

Most diabetic women can return to normal management of their diabetes after the birth, as soon as the first meal is taken. In GDM, there is a rapid return to normal and usually no further insulin is required.

If the mother is insulin-dependent:

- The dosage of insulin should reflect the blood glucose measurement
- Energy requirements vary considerably in the postnatal period, especially if the mother breastfeeds
- Most women need extra carbohydrates if breastfeeding, 40–90g/day.
- The mother may experience more hypoglycaemic episodes and may need a snack when feeding her baby at night.
- Many breastfeeding diabetics find that their insulin requirements are lower because of the energy expenditure of lactation. This remains so whilst fully breastfeeding and needs adjustment when the baby starts weaning.

## Epilepsy

Women are often concerned about how they will manage once their baby is born, and there may be safety issues for some women with epilepsy. Precautions aim to minimize any risk to the baby and mother but maximize opportunities for bonding. The mother should be advised to avoid extreme tiredness (this makes seizures more likely), which can be difficult with the demands of a new baby! The woman's partner helping to settle the baby after feeds at night or helping with formula feeds helps protect against exhaustion. Where the mother has sudden, frequent, or unpredictable seizures, the following safety measures are recommended:

- The mother can feed her baby whilst sitting on the floor, supported by cushions
- Changing the baby's nappy can take place at floor level on a changing mat
- Bathing the baby should take place when the mother is least likely to experience a seizure or when there is someone there to assist if necessary. Alternatively, washing the baby on a towel instead of immersion in water might be preferable.

🚫 AEDs are excreted in breast milk, but breastfeeding is safe, and it should be recommended if this is the mother's preferred choice, as it may even help wean the baby from the higher levels of AEDs to which he or she was exposed *in utero*. Mothers should watch for drowsiness in their infants.

A postnatal epilepsy review should take place at 6 weeks and the mother should be seen by a specialist at 12 weeks.[5,6] If the dose of AEDs was increased during pregnancy, this may need to be gradually reduced under supervision.

Effective contraception must be discussed with a woman taking AEDs and the contraceptive pill should be avoided if possible, because drug interactions reduce its effectiveness.

## References

5 Knight M, Kenyon S, Brocklehurst P, Neilson J, Shakespeare J, Kurinczuk JJ (eds.) on behalf of MBRRACE-UK (2014). *Saving Lives, Improving Mothers' Care: Lessons learned to inform future maternity care from the UK and Ireland Confidential Enquiries into Maternal Deaths and Morbidity 2009–12*. Oxford: National Perinatal Epidemiology Unit, University of Oxford. Available at: ℘ www.npeu.ox.ac.uk/mbrrace-uk/reports.
6 National Institute for Health and Care Excellence (2012). *Epilepsies: diagnosis and management*. NICE guidelines CG137. Available at: ℘ www.nice.org.uk/guidance/CG137.

# Disorders of the postnatal period

# The uterus

- The uterus that is deviated to one side, usually to the right, is usually the result of a full bladder. If the mother cannot empty her bladder, or the bladder still palpates as full after voiding urine, catheterization of the bladder is required to remove the urine, allow the uterus to involute normally, and prevent urinary tract infection.
- As a precaution, an MSU should be sent to the laboratory for bacterial culture.
- Constipation may also inhibit the rate of uterine involution.

## Sub-involution of the uterus

- The uterus fails to involute at the expected rate and feels wide and 'boggy' on palpation.
- The vaginal blood loss is markedly brighter red and heavier than normal.
- The mother may be passing clots of blood and/or her loss may smell offensive. This may indicate a genital tract infection or retained products of conception.
- The mother may also feel unwell and have a raised temperature and pulse rate.
- Seek urgent medical aid to investigate and treat the cause.
- The usual treatment is a course of antibiotics and, if retained products are suspected, an evacuation of the uterus under general anaesthesia, to prevent infection and PPH.
- Thereafter, undertake twice-daily monitoring of vital signs, palpation of the uterus and monitor vaginal blood loss, until the situation returns to normal.

## Practice point

▶ It is so important that, at the birth, you check the placenta for completeness and note any apparent missing pieces of cotyledon or membrane in the birth records. This information must be passed to the midwife giving postnatal care.

# Ruptured postpartum haemorrhage

## Definition

## Signs and symptoms

## More serious

## Immediate action

# Primary post-partum haemorrhage

### Definition
Profuse bleeding from the genital tract from after completion of the third stage of labour until 24h after birth.

### Signs and symptoms
- Sudden or excessive vaginal blood loss.
- The uterus may feel enlarged, soft, and 'boggy' on palpation.
- Pallor.
- Rising pulse rate. Tachycardia common, but bradycardia may develop.
- Falling BP: a late sign of deteriorating maternal condition.

### More serious
- Maternal collapse.
- Altered level of consciousness: drowsy, restless.
- Heavy blood loss.

### Immediate action
- Summon medical aid.
- Summon other colleagues if able to.
- Stop the bleeding. If the uterus feels soft and relaxed:
    - Rub up a contraction by massaging the uterine fundus gently in a circular motion
    - When contracted, stop the massage.
- Administer a uterotonic drug:
    - Oxytocin 5–10 units IM (effective in 2–2.5min)
    - Oxytocin/ergometrine 1mL IM (effective in 2–2.5min)
    - Ergometrine 0.25–0.5mg IV (effective in 45s).
- Consider further resuscitative measures according to maternal response.
- Put the baby to the breast.
- Empty the bladder by catheter.
- Empty the uterus: gentle pressure on the contracted uterus, in an attempt to expel any retained placental tissue, membranes, or blood clots.
- If the bleeding continues and the uterus is well contracted, consider other causes of bleeding:
    - Cervical tear
    - Deep vaginal wall tear
    - Perineal trauma
    - Uterine rupture (rare).
- Attempt to locate the source of the bleeding. Direct pressure can be applied to a lower vaginal or perineal tear.
- A vaginal pack can be inserted to attempt to arrest bleeding from higher up the genital tract, as a first-aid measure.
- Keep all pads and linen to assess blood loss.

- If possible, and if trained to do so, ask a colleague to cannulate a suitable vein in the arm or hand, with a cannula suitably large enough to administer blood, and commence IV fluids—sodium chloride 0.9% or Hartmann's solution 1L.
- Record vital signs every 5–15min, according to the mother's condition.

This emergency may occur in the home, when the mother may be alone, and the community midwife may be the first person to arrive.

- Tell the mother to leave the access door unlocked and lie down flat until you arrive.
- If severe or uncontrolled blood loss, summon urgent aid, as determined by local policy—either the emergency obstetric unit or a paramedic ambulance.
- Reassure the mother and others present; warn her of the possible need for theatre for exploration and treating the cause of the bleeding under general anaesthesia.
- Accompany the mother to hospital with her baby.

## Afterwards

- Continue IV therapy according to prescription.
- Monitor the BP, pulse rate, temperature, and respirations, as described above.
- Monitor vaginal blood loss.
- Administer antibiotics as prescribed, usually IV at first.
- Monitor the mother for signs of infection.
- Give psychological support and reassurance to the mother, partner, and others concerned, and explain what happened and the ongoing care.

# Secondary post-partum haemorrhage

### Definition
- Profuse bleeding from the genital tract, occurring after the first 24h until 6 weeks after birth.
- It most commonly occurs between 7 and 14 days after birth.

### Signs and symptoms
- Often preceded by a heavy red loss, which may be offensive and accompanied by sub-involution of the uterus. Some clots or pieces of membrane may be seen.
- Tachycardia and low-grade pyrexia will indicate the presence of infection.

### Management
- Massage the uterus, if palpable, to encourage uterine contraction.
- Summon medical aid, according to local policy.
- Ensure the bladder is empty; catheterize if necessary.
- To control bleeding:
  - If bleeding is severe, give 250–500 micrograms of ergometrine maleate IV, or IM if you are unable/not trained and competent to administer IV drugs.
- Insert an IV cannula if competent to do so, and start an IV infusion of sodium chloride 0.9%. Otherwise, get the equipment ready for an IV-competent midwife, doctor, or paramedic to carry out this procedure.

### Practice point
▶▶ This emergency normally occurs in the home 7–14 days after birth. Transfer the mother to hospital as quickly as possible via a paramedic ambulance and accompany her, continuing to carry out emergency procedures, as required.

# Maternal collapse within 24h without bleeding

## Possible causes
- Inversion of the uterus.
- AFE.
- PE.
- Cerebrovascular accident.
- Fitting: eclamptic fit, even with no previous signs of hypertension or pre-eclampsia.

## Midwifery management
- Ensure a safe environment.
- Summon emergency medical aid and help from other midwives in the vicinity.
- Lay her down flat.
- Commence basic emergency care:
    - Airway—ensure it is patent
    - Breathing—ensure she is breathing. Monitor the respiratory rate and depth of respirations
    - Circulation—check the pulse rate.
- If trained and able, ask a colleague to insert an IV cannula and commence IV fluids, e.g. Hartmann's solution 1L. This is best done as soon as possible, before her veins collapse as her BP falls.
- If collapse is total and she has stopped breathing, and her pulse is weak or absent, initiate the emergency resuscitation procedure drill until help arrives.

# Hypertensive disorders

- All women who have pre-existing hypertension and hypertensive disorders of pregnancy can develop eclampsia in the hours and days following birth.
- Although postnatal eclampsia is rare, it is not unknown for a woman with a history of a normal BP to develop postnatal pre-eclampsia or eclampsia.
- Continue monitoring the BP twice daily for at least 3 days after birth, until you are sure it is back within the normal range and there are no other signs of pre-eclampsia.
- Keep accurate records of the recordings in the mother's records.
- If necessary, the doctor may prescribe antihypertensive treatment, in which case regular BP recording must be continued until the BP has been back within normal range and stable for at least 24h.

## Essential hypertension

- This woman was hypertensive prior to pregnancy and has probably required an increase in her medication in pregnancy.
- Continue monitoring the BP daily for 48h, then daily whilst the antihypertensive medication is satisfactorily readjusted and the BP is stable within normal limits.
- If the mother is breastfeeding, check that the medication is not harmful to the baby. If the medication is contraindicated in breastfeeding, discuss it with the doctor to find one that is suitable.

## Practice point

- ▶ It is essential that the BP is controlled within the normal range to prevent eclampsia, cerebrovascular accident, and renal damage.
- Monitor the urine output, as well as monitoring the BP in the early postnatal period.

# Circulatory disorders

## Varicose veins

- Generally, these start in pregnancy and are due to hormonal relaxation of the veins, increased venous pressure, and increasing weight as pregnancy progresses.
- Most common in the legs but may present as vulval or femoral varicosities.
- Generally they regress after birth.
- Some women have pre-existing varicose veins and for some women they become worse with successive pregnancies and increasing age.

### Signs and symptoms

- They may become inflamed and painful, particularly in the early postnatal period.
- Vulval varicose veins may rupture during the second stage of labour, from pressure of the fetal head or from perineal tearing, and can be a cause of significant haemorrhage.
- May predispose to an increased risk of DVT.

### Treatment

- Early ambulation and walking out each day is encouraged.
- Rest with legs raised, whenever possible.
- Local anti-inflammatory treatment and oral analgesia.
- ▶ Support stockings should *not* be worn, as they restrict blood flow in the legs. Support tights are better.
- In subsequent years, some women will require surgical treatment for varicose veins.

## Superficial thrombophlebitis

### Signs and symptoms

Localized inflammation and tenderness around the affected varicose vein and perhaps a mild pyrexia.

### Treatment

- Support, anti-embolic stockings.
- Early ambulation. Support when sitting, with the leg raised on a footstool or preferably on the bed in the acute stage.
- Anti-inflammatory drugs (care if breastfeeding).

## Deep vein thrombosis

### Signs and symptoms

- Unilateral oedema in the affected leg.
- Calf pain and stiffness.
- Difficulty in walking.
- Positive Homan's sign.

### Treatment

- Urgent referral to the doctor is required.
- If necessary, transfer the woman back to hospital medical services by ambulance.
- Anticoagulant therapy must be started as soon as possible—IV heparin initially for 24–48h, followed by daily subcutaneous tinzaparin injection of 3500 or 4500mg.

- Observe and monitor the woman for signs and symptoms of PE.
- Document all observations and treatment in her notes.

## Pulmonary embolism

- PE remains a major cause of maternal death worldwide and is the most common cause in the UK.[1]
- Early ambulation for all women is the most effective form of prevention.
- Women most at risk are those with:
  - Previous history of DVT or PE
  - Pre-existing or pregnancy-induced medical or obstetric complications resulting in prolonged immobility
  - Epidural anaesthesia
  - Operative birth
  - Prolonged labour
  - Anaemia.

### Signs and symptoms

- Severe chest pain.
- Breathlessness.
- Gasping for breath.
- Fear.
- Tachycardia.
- Shallow, gasping respirations.
- Sweating, pallor.
- Cyanosis, particularly at the peripheries and around the mouth.

### Treatment

- Ensure a safe environment.
- Summon emergency medical aid and help from other midwives in the vicinity.
- Ask for an emergency trolley and a defibrillator.
- Lay her down flat.
- Commence basic emergency care:
  - Airway—ensure it is patent
  - Breathing—ensure she is breathing. Monitor the respiratory rate and depth of respirations
  - Circulation—check the pulse rate.
- If trained and able, ask a colleague to insert an IV cannula and commence IV fluids, e.g. Hartmann's solution 1L. This is best done as soon as possible, before her veins collapse as her BP falls.
- If collapse is total and she has stopped breathing, and her pulse is weak or absent, initiate the emergency resuscitation procedure drill until help arrives.

### Practice points

- ► PE is the biggest major cause of direct maternal deaths in the UK.[1]
- ► It is essential that all midwives know and practise the emergency drills regularly, in order that, should an emergency occur, the emergency procedure works well and all know what to do.

## Reference

1 Knight M, Kenyon S, Brocklehurst P, Neilson J, Shakespeare J, Kurinczuk JJ (eds.) on behalf of MBRRACE-UK (2014). *Saving Lives, Improving Mothers' Care: Lessons learned to inform future maternity care from the UK and Ireland Confidential Enquiries into Maternal Deaths and Morbidity 2009–12.* Oxford: National Perinatal Epidemiology Unit, University of Oxford. Available at: ℘ www.npeu. ox.ac.uk/mbrrace-uk/reports.

# Postnatal pain

- *'After pains'*: the most common cause of postnatal pain is experienced as the uterine involution and pelvic musculature return to normal. All women experience them to some degree, from mild discomfort to pain equivalent to moderate labour pains. It is caused by the release of oxytocin to cause uterine contraction and retraction and is exacerbated in a breastfeeding mother, in response to suckling and the 'let down' response. An appropriate analgesic, taken prior to breastfeeding, will usually help. The pain is intermittent in nature.
- *Abdominal or pelvic pain* may also be associated with a full bladder, constipation, flatus, intrauterine infection, or, in rare cases, a pelvic vein thrombosis.
- *Pain in the uterus*, which is constant or present on abdominal palpation, is most likely due to infection. Other signs, such as a raised temperature and pulse rate, and heavy, offensive vaginal blood loss, may be present.
- *Symphysis pubis pain* occurs 8–60h after birth and may inhibit mobility. Whenever possible, the midwife should seek the support of the obstetric physiotherapist. Bed rest with the hips adducted and analgesia may be supplemented by a pelvic binder, an elasticated support bandage, or a trochanteric belt. Lying on her side in bed helps reduce symphysis pubis separation. Elbow crutches or a walking frame may be needed to support weight-bearing for several weeks. She will also need considerable help with the baby's care.

# Headache

## General headache

As with the general population, there are many causes of postnatal headache. The duration, severity, and frequency are important in the postnatal period.

- Tiredness, lack of sleep, the hot and dry environment of the postnatal ward, dehydration, worrying about her baby, her ability as a mother, and infant feeding, particularly establishing breastfeeding, may all cause tension and anxiety, leading to headache.
- Simple analgesia, such as paracetamol or ibuprofen, should be effective in these situations.
- Ensure that she drinks sufficient fluid, particularly water.
- ▶ A walk in the fresh air, in the cooler part of the day, will also often help, as will support and encouragement with baby care.

## Epidural anaesthesia

- Headache arising from a dural tap once the mother is mobile again, and is worse when she is standing. The headache may be accompanied by neck stiffness, vomiting, and visual disturbances.
- The anaesthetist must be informed to manage the leakage of CSF.
- She may already have returned home and will require readmission to hospital with her baby.

## High blood pressure

- It is most important to monitor the BP if there has been a pre-existing raised BP.
- ▶ An untreated raised BP will cause increasing headache and may lead to fits or a cerebrovascular accident.

## Psychological stress

- It is important that issues pertinent to birth are explored sensitively in privacy, and also other issues that may be worrying her.
- Take time to explore her feelings and ascertain whether there are problems at home, e.g. domestic abuse.
- Deal sensitively and confidentially with any issues that arise, with the mother's permission; this may mean referral to other members of the multidisciplinary team.

# Urinary tract disorders

The physiological changes that occurred in pregnancy and labour may take up to 6 weeks to resolve after birth, hence the potential for urinary problems and infection is considerable.

Problems are relatively common in the immediate postnatal period and usually resolve as the pelvic floor regains its muscle tone and the pelvic structures return to the pre-pregnant state. However, for a small number of women, the problem persists for weeks or months.

## Common disorders

- Difficulty in voiding urine.
- Frequency of micturition.
- Acute retention of urine.
- Cystitis.
- Urinary tract infection.

Most at risk are those with:

- Antenatal asymptomatic bacteriuria
- Antenatal urinary tract infection or pyelonephritis
- Catheterization in labour
- Epidural or spinal anaesthetic
- Long second stage with slow progress
- Vaginal delivery of a large baby
- Instrumental delivery, particularly forceps, causing trauma to the bladder and urethra
- Perineal trauma, particularly vulval grazes and tears
- Lax abdominal wall.

*Management*
- Determine the cause.
- Catheterize if retention of urine is present.
- Reassure the mother.
- Give analgesia if required.
- Exclude a urinary tract infection through laboratory culture of an MSU.
- Postnatal pelvic floor exercises.

## Acute retention of urine

- Usually caused by trauma to the bladder and urethra during labour.
- The bladder feels hard and distended abdominally.
- Lower abdominal severe discomfort and pain, if sensation is present.
- After an epidural or spinal anaesthetic, the sensation to pass urine may be lost for a number of hours.
- The uterus is higher in the abdomen than it should be and is displaced to one side.

*Management*
- Catheterize to remove the urine, and withdraw the catheter.
- Advise the mother to drink plenty of fluid, and keep an accurate fluid balance chart until you are sure the crisis period is over.
- An indwelling catheter must not be left in at this stage.

- Encourage her to void urine at regular intervals, to regain bladder tone.
- If retention reoccurs, an indwelling catheter may be inserted for 24–48h, to help the bladder regain its tone.

## Urinary tract infection

*Signs and symptoms*

- Frequency of urine.
- Dysuria.
- Urine may be cloudy in appearance and have an offensive odour.
- Dip test the urine for increased protein, leucocytes, nitrites, and blood.
- Rise in temperature.
- Feeling unwell.

*Treatment*

- Obtain an MSU and send to the laboratory for microscopy.
- Report to the doctor.
- Commence broad-spectrum antibiotics, usually trimethoprim or nitrofurantoin as first line, and change, if necessary, once the results of laboratory microscopy are known.
- Ask the mother to drink at least 3L of fluid a day.
- Maintain an accurate fluid balance chart.
- Repeat the MSU once the antibiotic course is completed to ensure the infection is successfully treated.

## Pyelonephritis

*Signs and symptoms*

- As above, but more severe.
- The woman looks and feels very unwell and has flu-like symptoms.
- Pain radiating from the loin to the groin, usually unilaterally.
- Pyrexia.
- Rigors.
- Vomiting.
- Lack of any appetite.
- Urine smells offensive, has an acid reaction, and is 'cloudy' in appearance.
- On laboratory microscopy, pus cells are seen in the urine.

*Treatment*

- Notify the doctor.
- Give antipyretic drugs.
- Commence a broad-spectrum antibiotic immediately and change, if necessary, according to the result of the microscopy.
- IV fluids for the duration of the period of vomiting.
- She should drink at least 3L of fluid a day.
- Maintain an accurate fluid balance chart.
- Repeat an MSU after the antibiotic treatment is completed.
- Help with baby care.

## Stress incontinence

The precise role of pregnancy and birth in the immediate and long-term problem is unclear, but stress incontinence is usually linked to pelvic floor stretching and nerve damage during childbirth. Approximately one in five women complain of stress incontinence at 3 months post-partum, and many of these women are still symptomatic several years later.

Most at risk are:
- The older mother
- Long second stage of labour
- Vaginal birth of a large baby.

*Management*
- Encourage postnatal pelvic floor exercises, as these have longer-term benefits.
- Refer the woman to a specialist physiotherapist.
- Encourage regular exercise.

## Vesico-vaginal fistula

A rare complication when a fistula (hole) develops between the bladder or the urethra and the vagina, through the anterior vaginal wall. There are two main causes:
- Damage during labour, caused by prolonged pressure of the fetal head against the symphysis pubis:
  - The damaged tissue takes 1–2 weeks to break down, after which the mother becomes incontinent of urine
  - Surgical repair and antibiotics are required
  - This should never be seen where there are professionally skilled attendants present during labour and birth. Prolonged labour and/or obstructed labour should be quickly diagnosed and immediate delivery by a Caesarean section carried out. It is more common in situations where this skilled help is not available.
- Direct trauma to the bladder during difficult instrumental delivery, notably with forceps:
  - Incontinence occurs almost immediately
  - Initial treatment is with antibiotics and continuous bladder drainage for 2–3 weeks, to encourage spontaneous healing
  - If this fails, surgical repair is required.

# Bowel disorders

- Difficulties in regaining normal bowel function are common in the first few postnatal days and are a common problem for the midwife to deal with.
- Most women are embarrassed to talk about bowel problems, but it is important to ascertain her normal pre-pregnancy bowel habits, to determine what is normal for her.
- Bowel problems are common in the latter stage of the pregnancy, due to the relaxing effects of progesterone on the smooth muscle of the bowel, diminishing peristaltic movement. The relative dehydration and lack of dietary intake in labour exacerbate this, along with pelvic pressure and pushing in the second stage of labour.
- Inform the mother about the importance of drinking plenty of water and eating a diet high in fibre, fruit, and vegetables, to regain normal bowel action.

## Haemorrhoids

- These are swollen varicose veins of the lower rectum and anal margin.
- They may be present in pregnancy and exacerbated by pelvic pressure and pushing in the second stage of labour.
- Perineal trauma may exacerbate the pain and discomfort of haemorrhoids.
- They may occur for the first time in the early postnatal period.
- Instrumental delivery, particularly forceps, is twice as likely to cause haemorrhoids.

*Management*
- Dietary advice: high fibre, plenty of fruit, vegetables, and fluids.
- Avoidance of constipation.
- Proprietary treatments in the form of creams or suppositories may be bought or prescribed by the independent midwife prescriber or doctor.
- Compress of cypress and lavender essential oils in a 1% dilution of grapeseed or vegetable oil. This may also be added to bath water (lavender oil used alone: three drops on a pad may be applied directly to the perineal skin).
- Oral analgesia such as paracetamol. Codeine should be avoided, as it can cause constipation.

## Constipation

- A common problem of the early postnatal period.
- It is usually 2–3 days after birth when the mother has a bowel movement, especially if perineal sutures are painful or after operative birth.
- A mild aperient may be offered 24–48h after birth, but research has shown that laxatives are generally unnecessary.
- Irritant laxatives, such as senna and bisacodyl, or other herbal remedies may cause maternal discomfort and diarrhoea in breastfed infants.
- A balanced diet, with plenty of fruit and vegetables, and plenty of fluids is all that is required.

# Postnatal afterthoughts for parents

This is often referred to as debriefing, but the use of this term is contentious.

- Postnatal afterthoughts discussion is the responsibility of every midwife.
- ▶ Offer every mother and others present at the birth, such as partner, friend, or grandparents, the opportunity to discuss the events.
- Appropriate and effective communication is vital to this process and should be handled with empathy and understanding.
- Honesty is essential and euphemisms should be avoided.
- Even if you consider the birth to have been normal, with no complications, there still needs to be an opportunity for the parents to ask any questions and for you to ensure that explanations have been understood.
- As the midwife present at the birth, you should set aside time for discussion with the parents before you leave the labour ward or home, and definitely within 24h of the birth.
- It is particularly important to offer a clear explanation of events and the reasons for a particular course of action to those who have experienced traumatic events or complications in labour, as soon as possible. Appropriate documentation is essential to this process.
- The effects of intense pain, use of technological or operative intervention, and insensitive and/or disrespectful care from one or more carers in labour can cause intense distress.
- One discussion may be insufficient; more questions may arise as the parents contemplate on events and possible/actual long-term consequences. Providing an opportunity to discuss these, together with good support from the midwife and, where appropriate, the doctor involved, will, in the majority of cases, prevent further long-term consequences such as postnatal depression or post-traumatic stress disorder.
- Women (and their partners) will react differently. Experiences that some will understand as necessary and normal and will eventually overcome will be intensely distressing to others and may become ingrained in their psyche, adversely affecting their relationship with their partner and baby.
- In some cases, parents may need more specialist help such as professional counselling and psychological or psychiatric care.
- Women who experience nightmares and flashbacks need specialized help. The sensitive support of a midwife will be essential, should they ever embark on a future pregnancy.
- ▶ In an increasingly litigious world, provision of a postnatal afterthoughts service could prove cost-effective in reducing complaints and legal action. The majority of complaints and threats of legal action arise from the fact that parents want someone to listen to them, to give them a clear explanation, and to say 'sorry', where appropriate.
- Many maternity units are identifying and training specialist midwives to lead this service, provide specialist discussion and counselling for the parents, and advise midwifery managers on professional development and risk management issues that may arise.

# Postnatal afterthoughts for midwives

- Midwives also need the opportunity to reflect and discuss events after caring for a woman who has experienced traumatic complications during childbirth.
- Reflection with senior midwifery colleagues or an SoM can put the events in perspective and help the midwife learn from the experience.
- It is also important to reflect on the midwife's actions and records and, where appropriate, praise their actions and assure them that they have done nothing wrong.
- All those present at the birth must be given the opportunity to work through their feelings and obtain support.
- In the UK, the SoM should provide the confidential support required, identify any professional development required for the midwife, and draw up an action plan to meet any identified need.

# Psychological and mental health disorders

- Mental health disorders in the antenatal and postnatal period can have serious consequences for the mother, her baby, and other family members. They may be pre-existing or occur for the first time in pregnancy or the postnatal period.[2]
- There should be clearly specified care pathways in each NHS trust to enable the midwife to make an appropriate referral.[2]
- Women who require inpatient care for a mental disorder within 12 months of childbirth should be admitted to a specialist mother and baby unit, wherever possible.[2]

## Postnatal psychosis

This condition is at the other end of the spectrum to baby blues and is the most severe form of psychiatric morbidity. It is the least common of the postnatal psychological conditions, but different studies report varying levels of incidence from 1:500 to 1:1500. It is usually sudden and dramatic in onset and usually occurs very early, within the first week, the majority presenting before the 16th day postnatally.

### Symptoms

These may be variable but can include:
- Changes in mood state
- Irrational behaviour
- Restlessness and agitation
- Fear
- Perplexity, as the woman loses touch with reality
- Suspicion
- Insomnia
- Episodes of mania where the mother becomes hyperactive
- Neglect of basic needs
- Hallucinations and morbid delusional thoughts
- Profound depression.

Twenty-five per cent of women admitted for postnatal psychosis within 3 months of birth will have been consulted for psychological symptoms in pregnancy; 50% will have had symptoms of anxiety or depression in pregnancy; and 50% will have non-puerperal episodes of psychosis and/or a family history of mental illness.

▶▶ There should be immediate referral to the mental health team, as the condition will usually warrant admission to hospital. Prognosis is good, but there is a high risk of recurrence in subsequent pregnancy.

The psychotropic drugs often used in the treatment of postnatal psychosis and for other long-term mental health conditions make it imperative that the woman understands the need for effective contraception and the risks of severe damage to the fetus in a subsequent unplanned pregnancy. The midwife should encourage her to attend the contraception and sexual health clinic for effective contraceptive management.

## Reference

2 National Institute for Health and Care Excellence (2014). *Antenatal and postnatal mental health: clinical management and service guidance*. NICE guidelines CG192. London: National Institute for Health and Care Excellence.

# Postnatal depression

Postnatal depression refers to depression with its onset during the first postnatal year. It is a non-psychotic depressive disorder that varies in severity and is not fundamentally different from depression occurring at other points in a woman's life. The incidence varies according to different reports but it is thought that around 10–15% of women suffer from postnatal depression following childbirth. However, this may only be the tip of the iceberg, as many incidences go unreported and untreated.

## Symptoms

There is a wide range of symptoms that the mother may exhibit, including:
- Anxiety
- Panic attacks
- Tension and irritability
- Feelings of despair and emptiness
- Exhaustion
- Lack of concentration
- Rejection of the partner or baby
- Inappropriate or obsessional thoughts
- Loss of libido
- Physical symptoms
- Desire for sleep
- Feels better in the morning
- Guilt and anxiety about the baby
- Preoccupied with the baby's health.

## Aetiology

There has been wide research into the causes of postnatal depression, but no one single cause is apparent. It has been linked with both physiological and psychosocial factors.

*Physiological factors*
- Genetic background.
- Hormonal changes.
- Oestrogen is seen as being more significant than progesterone.
- Thyroid dysfunction.

*Psychosocial factors*
- Events surrounding the birth.
- Difficult to care for the baby.
- Previous history of depression.
- Age of the mother.
- Prior experience with babies.
- Stressful life events.
- Marital stress.
- Inadequate postnatal sexual relations.
- Mother's own childhood experiences.
- Social condition.
- Personality.
- Linked with parenthood rather than pregnancy or birth experiences.

## Effects of postnatal depression on the family

A review of research revealed that postnatal depression had profound and long-lasting effects on both the children and the families of women. It can have adverse effects on the children's emotional and intellectual development, and boys appear to be affected more than girls.

## Detection

Early diagnosis and treatment is important not only for the woman, but also her family. The midwife has an important role in recognizing women at high risk of postnatal depression and the early signs of postnatal depression.

- Assess the mother's emotional state as part of the routine postnatal care.
- The Edinburgh Postnatal Depression Scale, or other validated assessment tool, is useful in assisting the diagnosis of the condition.
- If you suspect that the mother may be affected, be sensitive and reassuring and refer to appropriate resources.

## Treatment

A wide range of treatments has been suggested for postnatal depression. The treatment required will depend upon the severity of the illness and the support available for the woman. For some women, the condition will resolve spontaneously, but for many, the condition will become chronic and may last for the first year or longer following the birth. The report into maternal death[3] has shown suicide to be the leading cause of maternal death in the first year after birth.

Treatments may include:
- Social and emotional support
- Self-help groups
- Prophylactic progesterone
- Oestrogen treatment
- Placentophagy
- Psychotropic drugs
- Electroconvulsive therapy.

## Reference

3 Knight M, Kenyon S, Brocklehurst P, Neilson J, Shakespeare J, Kurinczuk JJ (eds.) on behalf of MBRRACE-UK (2014). *Saving Lives, Improving Mothers' Care: Lessons learned to inform future maternity care from the UK and Ireland Confidential Enquiries into Maternal Deaths and Morbidity 2009–12.* Oxford: National Perinatal Epidemiology Unit, University of Oxford. Available at: ℜ www.npeu. ox.ac.uk/mbrrace-uk/reports.

# Bereavement care

- This section refers to loss of a non-viable fetus, stillbirth, or neonatal death.
- Legal definitions and requirements stated are those currently required in the UK.
- Please check your own local policies and procedures.
- ▶ The disposal of a baby's body is of immense importance and therapeutic value to the parents. It can be the means towards the healing of the inner hurt sustained in the death of their child. Poorly managed, it can be the foundation of severe psychological damage.
- ▶ Respect and facilitate religious customs and rituals. Time spent in getting everything right will save many years of heartache.

### Aims for the midwife

- To achieve optimal communication with families when their baby dies before, during, or soon after birth.
- To ensure parents are fully aware of, and understand, all the choices open to them.
- To help parents to face the reality of the situation as they grieve for their baby.
- To act as an advocate for the family, demonstrating sensitivity whilst maintaining professional boundaries.
- To ensure that the family's cultural and religious traditions are respected.
- To provide families with a choice of appropriate follow-up support and counselling arrangements.

### Post-mortem examination

- This may be legally required in certain circumstances, particularly for a neonatal death. It may also be requested by the parents.
- Explain sensitively the reason for the post-mortem examination.
- One of the parents will be required to sign the consent form.
- If the parents refuse consent, their wishes must be respected, unless the death has been reported to the coroner (in Scotland the Procurator Fiscal), in which case the coroner will order the post-mortem. Try to avoid this, if at all possible, as it will cause unnecessary distress.

*Practice point*

❶ If the baby is to have a post-mortem, the body must be kept dry and not bathed after birth.

### The non-viable fetus

- *Definition*: a fetus born dead before the legal age of viability, i.e. before 24 weeks' gestation.
- After 16 weeks', but before 24 weeks', gestation, the parents may be given the opportunity to have their baby buried, either by the hospital making the arrangements or by the parents making their own funeral arrangements.

- The law requires that the funeral director undertaking such a burial is given a letter signed by the qualified health-care professional present at the birth.
- It is also possible to arrange for the hospital chaplain or a minister of the parents' own choice to officiate. This applies to all religious faiths.

## Stillbirth

- *Definition*: a baby who neither breathes nor shows any other sign of life after being completely expelled from its mother after 24 completed weeks' gestation.
- The Certificate of Stillbirth must be completed by the midwife present at the birth. This is given to the parents to register the stillbirth with the local Registrar of Births and Deaths, which must be done within 42 days and before the baby can be buried or cremated.
- Encourage the parents to give the baby a name, as forenames cannot be added to the certificate retrospectively.
- Inform your SoM and lead midwife of the stillbirth.

## Neonatal death

- *Definition*: a baby born alive, but who dies within 28 days of birth.
- You will have completed the notification of birth in the normal way and the doctor certifying the baby's death will issue the death certificate.
- Both the birth and the death must be registered by the parents within 5 days. This often occurs simultaneously.
- Encourage the parents to give the baby a name, as forenames cannot be added to the certificate retrospectively.

## Baby's body

- Handle the baby sensitively and respectfully at all times.
- Wash or bathe the baby to remove traces of blood, unless a post-mortem examination is to be carried out. Wear gloves for this procedure.
- The mother or father can bathe the baby if they wish. Allow sufficient time for this to be done properly.
- Dress the baby in its own clothes, disposable nappy, and bonnet, if possible.
- Apply small waterproof dressings to any wounds.

## Photographs

- Take at least two photographs of the baby after consent gained and give one to the parents.
- If they do not wish to keep the photo, seal it in an envelope and save in the mother's notes. She may ask for it at a later date.
- Encourage the parents and family to take as many photos as they wish. Have a camera and film ready for their use, if required.
- Offer a professional photograph taken by the hospital photographer.

**Mementos**
- Footprints and handprints, a lock of hair, cot card, and name bracelets need to be collected for the memento folder.
- Parental permission *must* be obtained before obtaining a lock of hair.
- Small toys or other mementos may be kept with the baby.

**Religious customs and ceremonies**
- Ask the parents, at the outset, about any religious customs or ceremonies they wish to be observed. They may wish to make their own arrangements or the hospital chaplain will facilitate this for them.
- The parents may appreciate a simple blessing and naming ceremony.

**Parent information booklet**
- It is important that all information for parents, including helpful leaflets, booklets, support group and website addresses, and telephone numbers, should be made available in each maternity unit.
- Go through this page by page to help the parents understand the help and support available.

**The environment**
- This is so important and should be as homely and non-clinical as possible.
- Each maternity unit should have a 'quiet room' to ensure the family is not disturbed.
- A door notice asking others to respect their privacy should be available for them to use at their discretion when they feel the need for privacy.
- Encourage the parents to see and cuddle the baby.
- Allow the family to be alone with the baby for as long as they wish.
- Have a Moses basket or a cot available to put the baby in when they are ready.
- Have a telephone in the room for the parents to use. The hospital switchboard may need to be informed, so that they can connect calls sensitively.
- After the baby has been taken to the mortuary, the parents may ask for it to be brought back to the ward, whilst the mother is in hospital, or to visit it in the mortuary viewing room.

**Transport of the baby's body**
- Inform the mortuary technician when the baby is to be collected and whether or not a post-mortem is required.
- Inform the porter when the baby is ready to be collected.
- Refer to local guidelines as the arrangements may differ slightly, depending on the location.

**Arranging the funeral**
- In the cases of both stillbirth and neonatal deaths, the Registrar of Births and Deaths will issue the Certificate for Burial or Cremation once the death has been officially registered.

- The parents may wish the burial or cremation arrangements to be made by the hospital, or they may make their own arrangements. The hospital chaplain or a minister/religious leader of their own choice may officiate.
- Occasionally, parents may ask to take the baby home. This can be arranged and the undertaker will collect the baby from home for the funeral. This usually requires additional paperwork and the police may need to be informed.

## Memorial book

- This may be kept in the hospital chapel and should be on view at all times.
- Invite the parents to place the baby's name and date of birth in the book. There should also be a space for a short verse.
- If the parents cannot do this themselves, the hospital chaplain may do it for them.

## Memorial service

- A memorial service, which may be multi-faith, may be held annually, to which all families and staff are invited, to remember newborn babies who have died.
- Parents and families will decide for themselves how many years they wish to attend. They should never be excluded by time limit or other obstacles.

## Counselling

- Encourage parents to talk to staff about how they feel. Set aside time to do this.
- It is helpful if the maternity unit has one or two midwives, trained in counselling skills and experienced in dealing with families in this situation, to lead this work.
- Home visits can be arranged, if the parents do not wish to return to the maternity unit for counselling.
- Some parents may need longer counselling and psychological support than you are able to offer, in which case establish appropriate referral mechanisms.

## Further reading

Child Bereavement UK. Available at: ℜ www.childbereavementuk.org.
The Stillbirth and Neonatal Death Society. Available at: ℜ www.uk-sands.org/support.

# Part 5

# Contraception

# Contraception

# Contraception

Important points for the midwife to remember:
- Any discussion about contraception is both sensitive and highly personal to individual women and their partners
- You need to be knowledgeable both about the range of contraceptive methods available and the local services available to best meet the woman's needs
- Ensure that you have up-to-date information on the full range of contraceptive methods available in the locality, access to relevant appropriate websites, NICE guidelines, and useful books that might help (➔ see Contraceptive methods, p. 633).
- Allow enough time for discussion, and ensure an appropriate environment to maintain confidentiality and allow a relaxed discussion, ideally in the woman's home.
- Encourage discussion.
- Offer any leaflets and suitable websites available to support information given.
- Remember that to be effective, the chosen contraception must be used properly, and therefore acceptable to the woman and ideally to her partner.
- As with any other form of treatment, informed decision-making and consent are required.
- Brand names of contraceptives apply to the UK, but these will vary throughout the world.

## Contraception following abortion/miscarriage
- First trimester: hormonal contraception can be commenced or recommended immediately.
- Second trimester: hormonal contraception should not be commenced or recommended until at least 21 days after abortion or miscarriage until uterine changes have reverted to the pre-pregnant state.
- However, there will be exceptions to consider in individual cases, when effective contraception is paramount.

## Contraception after giving birth
- Normally, hormonal contraceptive methods are not commenced until at least 21 days after birth.
- However, should the need for contraception be the paramount concern, it may be started sooner.

## Important points to remember
- *Never recommend the combined oral contraceptive pill to a breastfeeding woman.* Oestrogen will inhibit the release of prolactin and suppress her lactation within 24h.
- Giving progesterone whilst the postnatal vaginal loss is still present may cause an increase in the amount of blood loss and prolong the bleeding time.
- Progesterone-only methods, if started too soon in a breastfeeding mother, may also cause suppression of lactation.

# Contraceptive methods

The topics in Table 26.1 will be discussed in this chapter:

**Table 26.1** Contraceptive methods

| Hormonal | |
|---|---|
| Combined oestrogen and progesterone | Combined pill |
| | Skin patch |
| | Vaginal ring |
| Progesterone only | Oral progesterone-only pill |
| | Injectables |
| | Implant |
| | Intrauterine system |
| Emergency contraception | *Oral pills* |
| *Non-hormonal* | *Intrauterine device* |
| Barrier | Male condom |
| | Female condom |
| | Diaphragm and cervical cap |
| Natural | Breastfeeding |
| Sterilization | Fertility awareness |
| | Male sterilization |
| | Female sterilization |

# Further reading

British Association for Sexual Health and HIV. Available at: ℜ www.bashh.org.uk.
Everett S (2014). *Handbook of Contraception and Reproductive Sexual Health*, 3rd edn. London: Routledge.
Faculty of Sexual and Reproductive Healthcare. Available at: ℜ www.fsrh.org/home/.
Faculty of Sexual and Reproductive Healthcare (2016). *UK medical eligibility criteria for contraceptive use (UKMEC, 2016)*. London: Faculty of Sexual and Reproductive Healthcare. Available at: ℜ ukmec.pagelizard.com/2016.
Guillebaud J, MacGregor A (2012). *Contraception: Your Questions Answered*, 6th edn. Edinburgh: Churchill Livingstone.
International Planned Parenthood Federation. Available at: ℜ www.ippf.org.
*Journal of Family Planning and Reproductive Health Care*. Available at: jfprhc.bmj.com/.
National Institute for Health and Care Excellence (2006). *Routine Postnatal Care of Women and their Babies*. NICE guidelines CG37, reviewed 2014. London: National Institute for Health and Care Excellence.
National Institute for Health and Care Excellence (2007). *Long-acting Reversible Contraception*. NICE guidelines CG30. London: National Institute for Health and Care Excellence.
The Family Planning Association. Available at: ℜ www.fpa.org.uk.
World Health Organization. *Family planning*. Available at: ℜ www.who.int/topics/family_planning/en/.

# Lactational amenorrhoea method

### How does it work?

The lactational amenorrhoea method (LAM) will inhibit ovulation if the following criteria are all met:

- *Amenorrhoea* since the postnatal vaginal blood loss ceased
- *Full lactation*: the mother is fully supplying the baby's nutritional needs day and night
- *The baby is <6 months old*.

In these circumstances, the operating prolactin levels inhibit gonadotrophin release from the anterior pituitary gland, thus inhibiting ovulation, and the risk of pregnancy occurring is only approximately 2% (i.e. 98% effective as contraception) (Fig. 26.1).

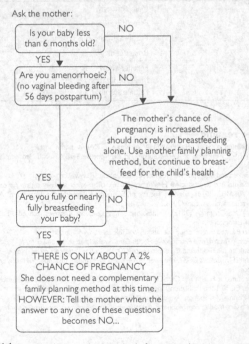

**Fig. 26.1** Lactational amenorrhoea method of contraception.
Reproduced with permission from Institute of Reproductive Health, Georgetown University.

## Efficacy

- A WHO multicentre study[1] supports this, with a reported pregnancy rate in the first 6 months after childbirth of 0.9–1.2%.
- Prolactin levels are highest during the night, and to ensure that LAM works, it is essential to continue night-time feeding as long as possible.
- The failure rate will increase if the mother is not fully breastfeeding, and in the Western world women are encouraged and motivated to stop night feeding as soon as possible and the baby is encouraged to sleep the night through by giving supplementary solids in the evening.
- Before modern times, LAM was the only contraceptive method available and is still the only method available to women in many parts of the world.

## Additional contraception

- Many women choose to rely on an additional method such as the condom or the progesterone-only pill (POP).
- If the mother is using the POP whilst fully breastfeeding, it is unnecessary to give emergency contraception if a pill is missed.
- If a breastfeeding mother chooses a POP, the amount passed to the baby in the breast milk is the equivalent of one POP in 2 years, considerably less progesterone than in formula milk.[2]
- As soon as the baby begins to be weaned or the mother has a period, it is important that, if she wants effective oral hormonal contraception, she is switched to the desogestrel progesterone only or the combined contraceptive pill. All methods available are fully discussed.

## Return of ovulation

- The time taken for return of ovulation depends on the frequency, intensity, and duration of feeding, maintenance of night feeds, and introduction of supplementary feeding.
- Midwives should be confident in recommending this method to mothers, *provided the criteria are met in full*.

## References

1 [No authors listed] (1999). The World Health Organization multinational study of breast-feeding and lactational amenorrhea method. III. Pregnancy during breast-feeding. World Health Organization Task Force on Methods for the Natural Regulation of Fertility. *Fertil Steril* 72: 431–40.
2 Guillebaud J (2012). *Contraception Today*, 7th edn. London: Informing Healthcare.

## Further reading

Fertility UK. Fertility Awareness. Available at: ℡ www.fertilityuk.org.

# Combined oral contraceptive: 'the pill'

## Contents

Each tablet contains a combination of oestrogen and progesterone. Most brands contain 30 micrograms of ethinylestradiol and a progestogen.

In the UK, the combined oral contraceptive pill is the most commonly used form of contraception. It:

- Is highly effective
- Is convenient
- Is not related to intercourse
- Is reversible
- Reduces the incidence of ectopic pregnancy
- Causes lighter and less painful periods
- Possibly helps to reduce premenstrual symptoms
- Protects against ovarian and endometrial cancer.

## When is it taken?

- Ideally, the woman should start the first pack on the first full day of menstrual bleeding and definitely within the first 5 days of the cycle. If this is done, then FSH inhibition will be complete for that cycle, and no additional contraception will be necessary.
- If the pill is started later than the fifth day of the cycle, she should use a condom every time sexual intercourse occurs in the next 7 days. After that, the hormonal control will be established.
- It is not started in the latter half of the menstrual cycle, because of the risk of pregnancy.
- Tell the woman to take one pill daily, at approximately the same time every day, choosing a time of day that is most convenient and best remembered. She should follow the arrows on the pack until all 21 pills have been taken. Then she will have a 7-day break, during which a withdrawal bleed—the 'period'—will occur. The next pack should be commenced 7 days later. The golden rule to remember is that the day she takes the first pill in the first pack is the day she always starts a new pack.

## Follow-up

- Normally, the first prescription is for 3 months, with an appointment to return to clinic in 8–10 weeks for review.
- Unless there are any menstrual irregularities or other side effects are evident, follow-up and repeat prescription is then 6–12 months, depending on local policy.

## Points to remember

- A useful tip for an effective pill-taking regime is to ask the woman to make a note of the day she started the pill for the first time, i.e. the day she will always start a new pack.
- She should make a note of the new pack start date. Again, a paper diary, an electronic diary, or a mobile phone calendar and alarm can be used.
- A reliable downloadable smartphone app is available at ℬ www. knowyourcontraceptives.co.uk.
- Missed pill: there is a 'window' of 12h, during which a pill may be taken later than normal and still be within the normal regime. If >12h late, then advise her to follow the regime given in ➡ When the pill may not be effective (p. 638).
- If the woman smokes, she must be warned of the increased risk of coronary heart disease and VTE.
- After giving birth:
  - Ideally the combined pill should not be started until at least 21 days after birth, to allow the body to recover physiologically from birth and to avoid increasing the thromboembolic risk
  - However, there are some women for whom the risk of further pregnancy is high and who need highly effective contraception. In this case, refer the woman to the contraception and sexual health clinic for appropriate management
  - The combined pill should never be given to a breastfeeding mother, as the oestrogen component will suppress her lactation within 24–48h
  - If a breastfeeding mother requires hormonal contraception, then advise a progesterone-only method
  - If the combined pill is started whilst the mother still has a vaginal blood loss, the progesterone component will cause bleeding to become heavier and more prolonged. Be aware of this and also warn the mother
  - The combined pill should be avoided, wherever possible, in a mother who has reduced mobility following birth, e.g. after a Caesarean section, because of the increased thromboembolic risk.
- BP and personal and family medical history are checked annually for any significant changes that may signal caution or discontinuation of this method of contraception, notably cardiovascular issues such as hypertension, heart attacks, and stroke or thromboembolic disorders.

# When the pill may not be effective

### Missed pill(s)

- If the pill for that day is taken >12h late, advise the woman to take the missed pill as soon as it is remembered and to take the next scheduled pill at its normal time. In practice, what often happens is that two pills are taken together.
- Up to two pills can be missed anywhere in the pack (only one if taking a 20-microgram pill). No additional contraception is needed.
- If three or more pills are missed (two if taking a 20-microgram pill), take the last pill missed as soon as it is remembered. Leave any earlier missed pills in the pack. Use an extra method of contraception for the next 7 days (the male condom is the easiest).
- If three or more pills have been missed and the woman has had unprotected sex in the last few days, advise her to consider emergency contraception, as she may be at risk of pregnancy.
- If seven or more pills are left from now until the end of this cycle, she should continue taking the pill in the normal way to the end of the pack and have the normal 7-day break. The normal withdrawal bleed should occur.
- If fewer than seven pills are left from now until the end of this cycle, she should continue to the end of the pack, but not have the 7-day break. Tell her to start the new pack immediately and follow the normal daily regime to complete the pack in the normal way. In this case, there will be no withdrawal bleed between the two packs, but there should be a normal withdrawal bleed at the end of the second pack.

*Points to remember*

- She should only take one missed pill. If >1 pill has been missed, advise her to leave the other missed pills in the pack. If this happens, it is important that a condom is used for every act of sexual intercourse for the next 7 days.
- When a pill has been missed for >12h in a cycle, the risk of pregnancy is increased. Any disturbance in the menstrual cycle as a result should be followed up with a pregnancy test.

### Antibiotic therapy

During any period of broad-spectrum antibiotic therapy, she should continue to take her pill as normal, and no additional contraception is required. However, to be extra safe, for all acts of sexual intercourse during the antibiotic course and for the next 7 days, additional condom protection should be used.

### Antiretroviral therapy

Drug interactions between the antiretroviral drugs and the combined hormonal contraceptive may alter the effectiveness of the combined hormonal contraceptive and consistent additional use of the condom should be recommended during therapy.

## Nausea and vomiting

If the woman vomits within 3h of taking the pill, she may not have absorbed sufficient of the oestrogen component to suppress ovulation effectively, so missed pill rules should be followed. In this case, a condom should also be used for every act of sexual intercourse for the duration of the episode of illness involving vomiting and for the next 7 days, to allow the contraceptive effect to return.

## Drug interactions

Certain drugs may inhibit the absorption/reduce the effectiveness of the pill, so it is imperative that you check whether or not the woman is taking any other medication when discussing the possible use of the pill.

The main interacting drugs are:

- Enzyme-inducing anticonvulsants used in the treatment of epilepsy, tuberculosis, and HIV
- Antibiotics/anti-infectives and antifungals
- St John's Wort (a herbal complementary medicine often taken by women).

Refer her to the contraception and sexual health clinic or GP for review of the drug regime.

Advise her that St John's Wort *must not* be taken when using combined hormonal contraception.

## Further reading

Faculty of Sexual and Reproductive Healthcare (2016). *UK medical eligibility criteria for contraceptive use (UKMEC, 2016)*. London: Faculty of Sexual and Reproductive Healthcare. Available at: ℅ ukmec.pagelizard.com/2016.

# Contraceptive patch

The 'pill in a patch' first became available in the UK in 2003. It is a combination oestrogen and progesterone drug and can be given to any woman who is suitable for the combined pill. Each pack contains 3 months' supply.

## Using the patch

She should:

- Start using the patch on the first day of the next period or no sooner than day 21 after giving birth or having a second-trimester abortion. After a first-trimester abortion, she can start immediately. Ask her to note the start day. This is most easily done using the calendar wheel on the underside of the box lid provided to store the patches
- Place the patch on any part of the body, *except the breasts*, where it is unseen and where clothes are unlikely to rub excessively. The adhesive will allow normal activity, bathing, sport, and swimming
- Leave the patch in position for 7 days and then change the patch weekly for the next 3 weeks. After the 3 completed weeks, tell her to then have a 7-day break, during which withdrawal bleeding will occur.

## Points to remember

- Remind her not to place the patch on the breasts.
- Remind her to check daily that the patch is firmly in place.
- If the patch comes off, she must replace it with a new one within 24h for continuous contraception. If left off for over 24h, the 7-day rule applies and should intercourse occur in the following 7 days, condoms should be used. Lack of condom use warrants the use of emergency contraception if the patch was off for >24h.
- She should restart the next cycle with a new patch.
- She should report any side effects to the doctor or contraception and sexual health clinic supplying the patch.
- This method is expensive.
- Contraindications to its use are as for the combined pill.
- ❶ Care should be taken when prescribing this form of contraceptive for any woman who has a sensitive skin or allergy. Monitor her for evidence of skin irritation or allergy, even though the patch is hypoallergenic, and ask her to return immediately if skin irritation should occur, but to continue to wear the patch until an alternative method of contraception is organized.
- Additional support is available from the company making the patch in the form of:
  - A 24h telephone helpline
  - Online support
  - Text message reminder on patch change day.

# Contraceptive vaginal ring

- The 'pill in a ring' is designed as an alternative to taking a pill daily. Known as NuvaRing® in the UK.
- It is a combination oestrogen and progesterone drug and can be given to any woman who is suitable for the combined pill.
- Each ring lasts for 3 weeks, i.e. one ring per menstrual cycle, with a ring-free week in the fourth week, during which a withdrawal bleed 'period' will occur.
- The daily release of hormone is 15 micrograms ethinylestradiol and 120 micrograms etonogestrel. Hormone release occurs continuously and the body does not store the drug. It is designed to inhibit ovulation.

## Using the ring

She should:

- Insert the vaginal ring on the first day of the next period or no sooner than day 21 after giving birth or having a second-trimester abortion. After a first-trimester abortion, she can start immediately. Ask her to note the start day. This is the day that she will always insert a new ring.
- Place the ring as high in the vagina as she can, a similar technique to inserting a tampon.
- Leave the ring in position for 21 days. After the three completed weeks, tell her to then have a 7-day break, during which withdrawal bleeding will occur.
- Remove the ring 3 weeks after insertion on the same day of the week at about the same time of the day that it was inserted. Hook the index finger under the forward rim or hold the rim between the index and middle fingers and pull it out.

## Points to remember

- Remind her to check regularly that the ring is firmly in place.
- If the ring is accidentally expelled and is left outside of the vagina for <3h, contraceptive efficacy is not reduced. Replace the ring in the vagina.
- If the ring is out of the vagina for >3 continuous hours during weeks 1 and 2, contraceptive efficacy may be reduced. She should reinsert the ring as soon as she can. Additional contraception, normally in the form of the male condom, should be used for the next 7 days.
- If the ring is out of the vagina for >3 continuous hours in week 3, she should discard that ring. She can at that point either:
  - Insert a new ring immediately for another 3 weeks, or
  - Have a withdrawal bleed and insert a new ring no later than 7 days from the time the previous ring was removed or expelled. Additional contraception, normally in the form of the male condom, should be used for the next 7 days.
- She should report any side effects to the doctor or contraception and sexual health clinic supplying the ring.
- This method is expensive.
- Contraindications to its use are as for the combined pill.
- ❶ Care should be taken when prescribing this form of contraceptive for any woman who has lax pelvic floor tone.

## Storage

- The NuvaRing® can be stored for up to 4 months at 25°C.
- Avoid storing in direct sunlight or at temperatures above 30°C.

# Progesterone-only pill

## Contents

Tablets containing progesterone only. Dispensed in packs containing either 28 or 35 days' pills, dependent on the brand.

Designed to prevent implantation of the fertilized ovum, which, depending on personal beliefs about when life begins, may not be acceptable to all women. However, in long-term users of the POP, ovulation does become inhibited.

The desogestrel pill has a different mode of action to standard POPs and is the first-choice POP in women under 40 who need highly effective contraception. It is designed to inhibit ovulation; in clinical trials, ovulation was inhibited in 99% of cycles at 7 and 12 months after initiation and has been shown to be as effective as the combined pill.

## Indications

There are a number of indications for the POP:

- The woman's choice
- Breastfeeding: all POPs secrete a very small amount of progestogen to the infant, the equivalent of one POP in 2 years, which is much less than the progesterone level found in dried cow's milk.[3] POPs do not interfere with lactation
- Hypertension
- Migraine (particularly focal migraine/migraine with aura)
- Diabetes
- Obesity
- Older women, particularly smokers over 35 years of age
- Side effects of the combined pill
- SCD.

## When is it taken?

- Advise the woman to choose a time of day that is most convenient and best remembered. A useful tip to help her remember is to set an alarm/use a reliable downloadable app on her mobile phone. Her partner or other close relative could be of help in reminding her, if she is liable to forget.
- Ideally, the woman should start the first pack on the first full day of menstrual bleeding. If this is done, there is no need for additional contraception in the first cycle.
- However, if the pill is started later than the second day of the cycle, it is advisable to use condoms every time sexual intercourse occurs in the next 7 days. After that, the hormonal control will be established. This advice also applies when started postnatally in a non-breastfeeding woman who has not yet had her first period following birth.
- It is not started in the latter half of the menstrual cycle, because of the risk of pregnancy, even if full sexual intercourse has not occurred.

### Missed pill

- When a pill has been missed for >3h window (12h with desogestrel POP), advise the woman to take the missed pill as soon as she remembers it and to continue with her normal pill-taking routine.
- Only the *last* missed pill should be taken, if she has missed >1.
- Additional barrier protection should be used if any sexual contact occurs in the next 48h, e.g. male condom.
- Additional emergency contraception may be used, particularly if >1 pill has been missed (➔ see Emergency contraception, p. 678).

### Follow-up

- Normally, the first prescription is for 3 months, with an appointment to return to clinic in 8–10 weeks for review.
- Unless any menstrual irregularities or other side effects are evident, follow-up and repeat prescription are then 6–12 months, dependent on local policy.
- Check the BP and personal and family medical history annually, to check for any significant changes that may signal caution or discontinuation of this method of contraception, which is rare.

### Points to remember

- ▶ There is only a 3h 'window' during which a pill may be taken late, but still be 'safe'. If >3h late, this must be classed as a missed pill. The exception to this rule is the desogestrel POP, which has a 12h window.
- If a breastfeeding mother requires hormonal contraception, the POP is ideal.
- The POP is highly effective if taken regularly each day, without any missed pills or breaks.
- In women over 30, it is almost as effective as the combined pill.
- A useful tip for an effective pill-taking regime is to ask the woman to make a note of the day she started the pill for the first time, i.e. the day she will always start a new pack.
- ▶ There are no pill-free days. The next pack must be started immediately.
- She should make a note of the new pack start date. A reliable downloadable app from ➔ www.knowyourcontraceptives.co.uk can be recommended.

### Following birth

- Ideally the POP should not be started until at least 21 days after birth, to allow the body to recover physiologically from birth. However, there are some women for whom the risk of further pregnancy is high and who need highly effective contraception. In this case, refer the woman to the contraception and sexual health clinic for appropriate management.
- If the POP is started whilst the mother still has a vaginal blood loss, it will cause bleeding to become heavier and more prolonged. Be aware of this and also warn the mother.
- The POP is a better choice than a combined oral contraceptive in a mother who has reduced mobility following birth, e.g. after a Caesarean section, because of the increased thromboembolic risk.

### Antibiotic therapy

Any period of antibiotic therapy will not affect the uptake of this pill and the woman should continue to take it as normal. No additional barrier protection is required.

### Antiretroviral therapy

HIV-positive women on antiretroviral therapy should be advised to use consistent additional barrier contraception.

### Nausea and vomiting

If the woman vomits within 3h of taking the pill, she may not have absorbed a sufficient amount of the pill for it to be effective. In this case, a condom should also be used for every act of sexual intercourse for the duration of the episode of illness involving vomiting and for the next 7 days, to allow the contraceptive effect to return. If she does not follow this advice, additional emergency contraception may be required (➔ see Emergency contraception, p. 678).

### Drug interactions and the pill

Certain drugs *may* inhibit absorption or reduce the effectiveness of the POP, so it is imperative to check whether or not the woman is taking any other medication when discussing possible use of the pill. However, it is very unusual to find a drug that will inhibit the POP uptake and effectiveness.

### Reference

3 Guillebaud J (2012). *Contraception Today*, 7th edn. London: Informing Healthcare.

# Implant

# Implant

Known as Nexplanon® in the UK, but likely to have other brand names elsewhere. The contraceptive implant offers 3 years' contraception, being most effective in the first 2 years.

## Content

The implant is a single rate-limiting polymer capsule, 4cm long and 2mm in diameter, containing 68mg etonogestrel, which is released at over 30 micrograms/day to inhibit ovulation.

## Benefits

- Long-term effective contraception. Zero failure rate in initial clinical trials.
- One insertion.
- No daily pill-taking regime.
- Non-intercourse-related.

## Mode of action

- The subdermal implant is inserted into the underside of the upper arm by a doctor, midwife, or nurse trained and competent in the technique.
- The hormone is released directly into the surrounding interstitial tissue and absorbed by capillaries into the bloodstream.
- Ovulation is suppressed at the level of the hypothalamus; therefore, the luteal phase of the menstrual cycle is deficient, preventing implantation, should ovulation and fertilization occur.

## Insertion

- Insertion is a minor surgical procedure under local anaesthetic (Fig. 26.2).
- The preloaded single-capsule system is contained within a sterile, disposable applicator and is an easy and rapid subdermal injection technique.
- The implant should be inserted at the beginning of the menstrual cycle, ideally on day 1. If inserted on day 1, the serum etonogestrel levels will be sufficient for ovulation inhibition within the first day and no further contraception will be required in that cycle.
- If inserted on the second day or later, then it is important to recommend 7 days of extra barrier contraception, if sexual intercourse occurs within this period.

## Points to remember

- Following first-trimester abortion, the implant can be inserted immediately.
- Following second-trimester abortion, it is wise to wait 21 days before insertion, because of the side effect of prolonged or heavy bleeding.
- After giving birth, again it is wise to wait 21 days for the above reason.
- At any time, it is important to remember that for some women the risk of repeated pregnancy is greater than the risk of early insertion.
- When changing from another form of hormonal contraception, it is important that there is planned change. Remind the woman to use condoms as additional protection for the first 7 days following insertion.

**Fig. 26.2** Nexplanon® capsule showing the position in the arm.
Reproduced with permission from the Family Planning Association, 2014.

## Follow-up
- Apart from a check of the insertion site to ensure there is no infection, it is not necessary to give any routine follow-up appointments.
- Give the woman the card that comes in the implant packaging which tells her the date of insertion and the date for removal.
- It is only necessary for her to return if there are any problems.

## Suitable for
- Most women across the age range.
- Women who cannot take oestrogen or who have oestrogen-related side effects.
- Diabetics, although possible adjustment of insulin dose may be required.
- Women weighing >70kg, but it may have reduced efficacy, particularly in the third year. In this case, the implant may be changed sooner than 3 years.
- Breastfeeding women, although a tiny amount of hormone may get into breast milk.
- Hypertensive women, as there is no adverse effect on BP.
- Older women and smokers who are at risk of cardiovascular incidents with oestrogen.
- Blood levels of hormone are steady, rather than fluctuating, as with injectable or oral POP. Absence of high-dose progesterone effects, as occur with Depo-Provera®.

**Side effects**
- Disturbance of menstrual bleeding pattern:
    - 25% of women experience some change, with irregular cycles, intermenstrual bleeding, spotting, or prolonged bleeding in the first 6 months
    - 80% of problems settle without further management
    - 35% have normal cycles and no problems in the first 6 months
    - 20% become amenorrhoeic
    - Bleeding problems are normally successfully managed with short- or long-term additional combined oral contraceptive or POP
    - Do a full STI screen for all women with nuisance bleeding
    - Bleeding problems are the most common reason for early removal.
- Other possible effects:
    - Acne
    - Headaches
    - Abdominal pain
    - Weight gain
    - Breast pain
    - Dizziness
    - Mood swings
    - Hair loss.
- Functional ovarian cysts:
    - These are usually asymptomatic and managed conservatively
    - They will resolve on removal of the implant.
- Ectopic pregnancy: rare in implant users.

**Return of fertility**
- Plasma levels of etonogestrel are too low to measure 48h after removal and normal ovulatory cycles return within the first month after removal.
- The subsequent conception rate is comparable with that of women not using contraception, and you can therefore reassure women that the implant alone will not adversely affect their future fertility.

**Drug interactions**
- Antibiotics, except rifampicin and griseofulvin, do not affect effectiveness.
- Anti-epileptic treatment with enzyme-inducing drugs may reduce efficacy slightly. Advise additional consistent condom use.

**Metabolic effects**
- Minimal effects on carbohydrate metabolism, LFTs, blood coagulation, immunoglobulins, and serum cortisol levels have been reported.
- Lipoprotein levels: there should be a small fall in total triglycerides and cholesterol. The high-density lipoprotein (HDL)/cholesterol ratio is unchanged or improved.
- These minimal metabolic effects make this a very suitable form of contraception for almost all women.

# Injectables

### Content

- The most common injectable contraceptive in use is Depo-Provera® (depot medroxyprogesterone acetate) 150mg, given every 12 weeks, but the interval may be extended up to 14 weeks.[1]
- Depo may be given at 11 or 10 weeks for women who have some bleeding near the end of the 12-week depo cycle.
- Sayana Press® is a new subcutaneous version, given every 13 weeks.
- Noristerat® (norethisterone enantate) 200mg, given by IM injection every 8 weeks. Noristerat® is oily and must be warmed to near body temperature prior to administration. Normally, only used for those women who have persistent vaginal bleeding problems with Depo-Provera® and who wish to continue to use an injectable method.

### Method of administration

- For both drugs, the first dose should be given in the first 5 days of the menstrual cycle.
- For maximum effect, injection should be on day 1.
- If given later than day 2, it is important to advise the woman to use extra barrier precautions for the next 7 days, if sexual intercourse occurs.
- Depo-Provera® is given by deep IM injection into the gluteus muscle of the buttock, in the upper outer quadrant. It is important that the injection site is not rubbed afterwards, as this will accelerate breakdown of the drug and make it less effective.
- Sayana Press® is given subcutaneously in the upper thigh or lower abdomen and suitable for self-administration at home after teaching the technique in clinic and provision of a small sharps bin for used injection equipment.

### After giving birth

- Normally given no sooner than 21 days after childbirth to avoid prolonged or heavy bleeding, but can be given within 5 days of birth if not breastfeeding.
- Ideally wait 6 weeks before injection in a breastfeeding mother, if she chooses additional hormonal contraception. By this time, the infant's enzyme system will be more fully developed and able to effectively metabolize any of the drug transmitted in the breast milk.

### After abortion

- First trimester: can be given immediately.
- Second trimester: ideally wait 2 weeks.

### Return of fertility

- ▶ After the last dose, return of fertility is commonly delayed (median 9 months) and the woman should be told this clearly.
- There is no evidence that injectable contraceptives cause permanent infertility.
- Over 80% of women are expected to conceive within 15 months of their last injection.

## Benefits

The injectable progesterone-only method offers effective short- or long-term contraception.

- 0–1 failure per 100 woman years.
- Non-intercourse-related.
- May be used in spite of a previous history of thrombosis.
- Ideal for women awaiting surgery, including sterilization.
- Suitable for women whose partners are awaiting a vasectomy and post-operative confirmation of clear sperm count. *It is important to stress the need to continue with effective contraception until the sperm count is clear or for 6 months after a vasectomy.*
- Studies show no adverse effect on BP.
- Positively beneficial in women with endometriosis, epilepsy, sickle-cell anaemia, and PID.
- Suitable for women being immunized against rubella. One dose will be effective.
- Minimal metabolic effects.

## Effects

- Suppression of ovulation.
- Amenorrhoea usual within 6 months.
- Not reversible for the duration of the injection.
- Injectables are safer than combined oral contraceptives.
- Delay in return of fertility (median 9 months).

## Side effects

*Irregular bleeding*
- This is the most common side effect, usually in the first 3-month cycle.
- It usually resolves with a second injection, which may be given early (not less than 4 weeks after the previous dose). For further management, refer to the contraception and sexual health clinic.

*Amenorrhoea*
- At least 90% of users have ceased having periods by 6 months.
- Prolonged amenorrhoea may cause hypo-oestrogenism, adverse lipid effects, and osteoporosis.
- When this form of contraception is administered over a long period of time, the woman should be reviewed at least once every 2 years by a doctor specializing in contraception or a specialist nurse prescriber. A bone mineral density scan may be undertaken.

*Weight gain*
- This may be slow and insidious or rapid and marked. Most women gain 0.5–2.0kg in the first year, and 10–12kg after 4–6 years of use.
- Progesterone use may increase the appetite, a similar effect to that of high progesterone levels in pregnancy. Weigh the woman regularly if weight gain is apparent or suspected.
- The evidence is that this weight gain is as a result of increased fat and not secondary to an anabolic effect or fluid retention.

*Mood*
- Some women on Depo-Provera® complain of premenstrual-type depression.
- Others have reported marked mood swings, which were not there before they started to use Depo-Provera®.
- For postnatal mothers, these progestogenic side effects may exacerbate postnatal depression.
- Women with a history of endogenous depression should not be given Depo-Provera® if there is a suitable alternative.
- Hormone replacement therapy (HRT) on reaching menopause is advisable for women with a history of prolonged use of Depo-Provera®.

*Bone mineral density changes*
- Large, well-controlled studies show there is a risk of reduction in mineral density with prolonged use.
- The evidence is that structure and bone mass return to normal once the drug is no longer taken.
- Care with women over 45 to ensure they do not enter the menopause with a reduced bone mineral density as it is irreversible after the menopause.
- A bone scan should be undertaken every 5 years during prolonged use to detect any reduction in bone mineral density.

### Reference
4 World Health Organization (2004). *Selected Practice Recommendations for Contraceptive Use*, 2nd edn. Geneva: World Health Organization.

# The intrauterine system

## Content

- The IUS, known as Mirena®, is a long-acting reversible contraceptive inserted into the uterus, mounted on a Nova T IUD frame.
- It contains a silastic capsule along its shaft, which secretes levonorgestrel 20 micrograms daily.
- It is licensed for 5 years' duration. If left longer than this, the contraceptive effect of the IUD will continue, but the progestogenic effects will cease.
- A smaller version, Jaydess®, is now available for nulliparous and women with a short-length uterus, containing a smaller amount of levonorgestrel, licensed for 3 years' duration and which will maintain light monthly periods.

## Indications for use

There are two main uses:

- Contraception, particularly in women who have heavy menstrual periods. After pregnancy, a woman may experience a notable and debilitating increase in menstrual flow and the IUS is ideal in these cases
- Menorrhagia: the use of an IUS may prevent the need for a hysterectomy.

Other conditions: endometriosis, chronic pelvic pain, dysmenorrhoea, and anaemia associated with heavy menstrual bleeding where there is no pathological cause.

It is NOT used for post-coital emergency contraception.

## How does the intrauterine system work?

In addition to the foreign body effect of the IUD, there is the additional progestogenic effect:

- Frequency of ovulation is reduced
- Cervical mucus thickens to inhibit the passage of sperm through the cervix
- The foreign body reaction within the uterus causes the release of leucocytes and prostaglandins from the endometrium, making the environment hostile to the blastocyst
- The endometrium is thinned
- Menstrual bleeding becomes much lighter. This is in direct contrast to the copper IUD, which may cause heavier menstrual bleeding
- Irregular spotting or bleeding may occur in the first few months after insertion but diminishes after the first 3 months.

### The intrauterine system and breastfeeding

The IUS and other progesterone-only contraceptives are not shown to affect milk supply or infant growth.

The risk of intrauterine perforation is increased in a lactating mother and fitting should ideally be delayed until at least 12 weeks post-birth.

### Fitting

For infection screen, when it is fitted, and insertion notes and other information, ➲ see Intrauterine devices, p. 656. As with other IUDs, it MUST be fitted by a doctor or nurse trained and competent in the technique, assessing suitability and dealing with possible immediate complications.

The Mirena® is not normally fitted in a nullipara; Jaydess® is normally fitted in these women.

# Intrauterine devices

- These are small polyethylene and copper devices, which come in a variety of shapes and sizes and are inserted into the uterus (Fig. 26.3).
- IUDs provide excellent contraception, have the benefit of no 'user failures', and are the most popular form of contraception in some parts of the world, e.g. China.
- It is a myth that a nulliparous woman cannot be fitted with an IUD. Developments in IUDs now make this possible —shorter and narrower, ideal for nulliparae and young women.
- In some parts of the world, the IUD had received a negative press but is now increasing in popularity again, as the newer IUDs are able to offer up to 10 years' contraceptive protection, and longer in the older woman whose fertility is declining towards menopause.
- It is unsuitable for a woman who has a true copper allergy and for certain other women with uterine abnormalities, previous or current PID or bacterial endocarditis, or those whose lifestyle puts them at high risk of pelvic infection. Other contraindications include past ectopic pregnancy, established immunosuppression, menorrhagia, unexplained vaginal or uterine bleeding, and heart valve replacement.
- It is important that the midwife knows the woman's medical, obstetric, gynaecological, and sexual history before advising her about an IUD.

## How does the intrauterine device work?

- The mode of action is not exactly known, but it is thought that the main mechanism of the copper is in preventing fertilization, by altering the composition of tubal and uterine fluids. In this way, the IUD does not cause abortion. Within the uterus, the IUD causes a foreign body reaction within the endometrium, with increased numbers of leucocytes.
- If fertilization does occur, then the IUD will stop implantation in the uterus, but this would normally occur only if the woman keeps the device *in situ* longer than the recommended number of years for the copper content of the individual device to be effective. For the different IUDs, this period ranges from 5 to 10 years, with the majority being licensed for 10 years.
- ▶ The IUD provides excellent post-coital emergency contraception for the above reason and may be removed after the next normal period or left *in situ* for long-term contraception.
- As the woman gets older, her fertility declines, so the IUD is more effective in women over 30. If an IUD is fitted in a woman over 40, it need not be changed and is removed at the time of the menopause.

(A)

Nova T380

(B)

Multiload Cu375

(C)

Gyne T380

**Fig. 26.3** Intrauterine devices.
Reproduced with permission from Andrews, G. (ed.), *Women's Sexual Health*, Elsevier 2005.

### When is it inserted?

- *After first-trimester abortion*: it can be inserted immediately.
- *After second-trimester abortion*: wait 2–4 weeks to allow uterine involution and avoid the risk of expulsion.
- *After a vaginal birth*: wait at least 6 weeks to allow full uterine involution. If breastfeeding, the mother may be at increased risk of uterine perforation, and, if fully breastfeeding day and night, she could wait up to 12 weeks to have her IUD inserted, because breastfeeding will prevent ovulation.
- *After a Caesarean section*: wait at least 8 weeks to allow uterine muscle healing. If breastfeeding, the above applies.
- The IUD will be inserted by a doctor or nurse trained in the technique.
- Ideally insertion takes place at the end of a period, when the cervix is more receptive to facilitate insertion.

### ▶ Pre-insertion infection screen

- Prior to insertion, it is good practice to check for any current evidence of infection that could be extended into the uterine cavity with insertion. Explain this to the woman.
- The vagina and cervix are inspected and endocervical or low vaginal swabs taken for chlamydia and gonorrhoea and a high vaginal swab for other infections such as bacterial vaginosis, if required. Ideally this is done and results are known, so that any infection can be treated before the IUD is inserted.
- In the case of emergency post-coital contraception, the swabs are taken at the time of insertion and infection subsequently treated, if necessary. Swabs should be repeated 2 weeks later, if required.

### Insertion

- This is an aseptic procedure throughout.
- It is normal practice to insert lidocaine 2% gel around the cervix prior to the procedure. This not only reduces any discomfort felt, but also helps to relax the cervix during uterine sounding and IUD insertion.
- It also helps to advise the woman to take some simple analgesia, such as paracetamol or ibuprofen, about 1h prior to her appointment.
- It also helps to advise her to have a proper meal and be well hydrated 2h prior to the procedure, as low blood sugar may contribute to her feeling faint during or following the procedure.
- ▶ The woman's colour, pulse rate, and any evidence of reduced consciousness are monitored to detect any evidence of shock.
- Once inserted, the monofilament threads are trimmed to approximately 3cm outside the cervix.
- At follow-up, 4–6 weeks later, the threads may be further trimmed to 2cm outside the cervix, leaving enough to facilitate later removal.
- Teach the woman to feel for the threads after every period, to ensure that the device remains *in situ*. If she cannot feel them, she should return to the clinic where the IUD was inserted.

## Advantages
- Provides long-term, highly effective, reversible contraception.
- It is immediately effective.
- It is not related to intercourse.
- There are no tablets to remember.
- Very low morbidity.
- Once removed, the woman's fertility immediately returns to normal.

## Disadvantages
- Periods may be longer, heavier, and more painful, particularly the first couple of days.
- The woman may experience intermenstrual bleeding or spotting, particularly in the first 3 months.
- Infection: a small percentage of women may develop a pelvic infection, particularly in the first few weeks after insertion, which should be treated promptly with appropriate antibiotics. Pelvic infection is more likely in younger and nulliparous women and in those who are at risk of STIs.

## Follow-up
- Normally the first appointment is at least 1 week after the next expected period, or up to 3 months, depending on local policy.
- This is to ensure that the IUD is comfortable, with no pain or discomfort, that there is no evidence of infection, and that no part of the IUD can be felt or seen in the cervical canal, and to trim the threads once the IUD is settled in position.
- It is important to advise the woman to keep her follow-up appointment, even though she may not be experiencing any problems with her IUD.

## Removal
The IUD is usually removed during a period. If removed later in the menstrual cycle, advise the woman to use an additional contraceptive method for 7 days prior to removal or avoid any sexual intercourse to avoid a possible pregnancy.

## Problems with the intrauterine device
Most problems occurring after IUD insertion can be attributed to a faulty insertion technique:
- Failure to check the position and length of the uterine body and obstructions in the uterus such as submucous fibroids or a septate or bicornuate uterus
- The actual insertion technique was faulty.

## Infection
Symptoms of infection may include pain during or after intercourse, unusual vaginal discharge, irregular bleeding, and lower abdominal or back pain.

Actinomyces-like organisms may be found in the genital tract of women with an IUD inserted. These potentially threaten future fertility and may be life-threatening if untreated.

❶ If any signs or symptoms of infection, such as abnormal vaginal discharge, pain, dyspareunia, and tenderness, the woman must be immediately referred to a doctor for investigation and treatment. Ideally, this should be at a contraception and sexual health clinic. The IUD may have to be removed.

## Bleeding

- Intermittent bleeding and spotting may occur for the first two or three cycles after insertion, after which it normally settles down.
- Warn the woman that this might occur.
- Periods may be heavier with an IUD fitted.

## Ectopic pregnancy

It is a myth that an IUD will cause ectopic pregnancy. The main cause is infection of the Fallopian tubes, with one or both tubes being affected. The IUD is highly effective at preventing uterine pregnancy and very few sperm actually penetrate the copper-containing uterine fluid to reach the egg in the Fallopian tube to be able to cause fertilization.[5]

## Points to remember

- A modern copper-bearing IUD is a highly effective form of short- or long-term contraception, with an efficacy rate of over 99%. IUDs now on the market can have a copper efficiency of up to 10 years.
- Know her history for contraindications before advising a woman about an IUD.
- It does not cause abortion.
- Advise her about insertion after abortion or birth, particularly if breastfeeding.
- It is more effective than the oral form of emergency contraception, particularly between 3 and 5 days after intercourse in the fertile period of the woman's menstrual cycle.
- More effective in women over 30.
- An infection screen is good practice, wherever possible, prior to IUD insertion.
- Advise her to take a simple analgesic about 1–2h before a planned insertion, which will help with discomfort during insertion and any lower abdominal cramps in the hours after insertion.
- Advise her to have a normal meal and drink about 2h prior to her appointment to help any feelings of faintness or dizziness during or after insertion.
- Advise the woman of the importance of checking for her threads after every period. If she cannot feel them, the doctor or specialist nurse will check and an ultrasound scan will be advised to locate the IUD, if necessary.
- Advise her of the importance of attending follow-up appointments.
- Advise her to report any signs and symptoms of infection promptly, to prevent any possible long-term damage to her reproductive tract.

## Reference

5 Guillebaud J (2008). *Contraception Today*, 7th edn. London: Taylor and Francis.

# Female condom

- The female condom is a well-lubricated, loose-fitting polyurethane sheath, with an outer rim, designed to keep the condom outside the vagina in use, and a loose inner ring, with a retaining action similar to the diaphragm, designed to fit behind the suprapubic bone and over the cervix.
- It is easy to obtain over the counter, as well as at contraception and sexual health clinics, and does not need medical supervision. It is made in one size only and full instructions are contained in the packet. Each condom is individually packaged; they come in packs of three and each condom is single use only.

## How is it used?

- For effective use, it must be used before there is any genital contact. Remind the woman that, before opening the packet, she should push the condom well away from the edge of the packet that is to be torn to release the condom.
- The condom is inserted into the vagina, using the inner ring as a guide, as far as possible along the posterior vaginal wall towards the posterior cervical fornix. The outer ring lies flat against the body, outside the vulva, which helps prevent the condom from being drawn up into the vagina during intercourse. It can be inserted any time before sexual intercourse and when correctly in place it will feel loose and comfortable. The man needs to be careful that the penis is not inserted between the condom and the vaginal wall. After use, it should be carefully disposed of and *not* flushed down the toilet (Fig. 26.4).
- Additional spermicides or lubricants of any kind can be used, although this should not be necessary, as the condom is very well lubricated.

## Advantages

- The condom, when used carefully and consistently, is extremely effective in preventing pregnancy.
- Similarly, it is effective in preventing STIs and HIV.
- It is easy to obtain and use and requires no medical supervision.
- It does not require additional spermicide.
- It can be used with oil-based products.
- Polyurethane is stronger than latex. It is much less likely to split or break in use than the male condom.
- It does not require male erection before use.
- It may protect the woman against cancer of the cervix by preventing the transmission of HPV.
- The woman can take responsibility for contraception and STI prevention.

1

Gently insert the inner ring into the vagina. Feel the inner ring go up and move into place.

2

Place the index finger on the inside and push the inner ring up as far as it will go. Ensure the sheath is not twisted. The outer ring on the outside of the vagina.

3

The female condom is now in place and ready for use with your partner.

4

When you are ready, gently guide your partner's penis into sheath's opening with care to make sure that it enters properly—be careful the penis is not entering on the side, between the sheath and the vagina wall.

5

To remove the condom, twist the outer ring and gently pull condom out.

6

Wrap the condom in the package or tissue and throw it in the rubbish bin. Do not put it into the toilet.

**Fig. 26.4** Female condom.

Reproduced with permission from Andrews, G. (ed.), Women's Sexual Health, Elsevier 2005.

**Disadvantages**

- It needs forward planning each time.
- It needs to be used carefully to be effective.
- It can interrupt sex.
- It can get pushed into the vagina during intercourse.
- It needs to be carefully disposed of.
- For women unable to touch their genital area with comfort, it is not a good method to recommend.

**Points to remember**

- In the first few weeks after birth, intercourse may be uncomfortable or sore. Advise her to use an additional lubricant, if necessary.
- Advise the woman about the availability of emergency contraception, in case of failure to use or failure in use.
- If a mother is not breastfeeding or is post-abortion, her risk of pregnancy, even in the first menstrual cycle, is real. We have all seen the woman who comes for her postnatal examination and is pregnant again!
- For the mother who is fully breastfeeding day and night, the risk of pregnancy is minimal. If this woman chooses to use a female condom, although it is very well lubricated, she may need additional lubrication because of the very low oestrogen levels whilst breastfeeding.
- If one or more partners are sensitive or allergic to latex, this is a useful alternative.
- She may use additional spermicides to increase efficacy of the condom.
- Emphasize that the condom is a 'once-only' use and should never be reused.
- In the UK, all contraception is free of charge and the midwife can offer the woman a supply of female condoms. Make sure you know where the local contraception and sexual health clinics are located to be able to advise her on further supplies.
- Remind her to check that the condom she is purchasing has the nationally agreed quality mark, e.g. the British Kite mark or the European Community CE mark.

# Diaphragms and cervical caps

Diaphragms and cervical caps fit into the vagina and cover the cervix, providing a barrier to sperm, thus preventing fertilization.

Fitting and teaching of the method must be done by a doctor, nurse, or midwife trained and competent to do so. Accurate fitting is essential to their success in use.

## How are they used?

- Diaphragms, in particular, are simple to use, once taught by a doctor or nurse experienced in fitting and teaching the use of this method (Fig. 26.5).
- The diaphragm comes in sizes from 55mm to 100mm, and careful measuring and fitting are important.
- It can be inserted well ahead of intercourse and need not affect spontaneity.
- If >3h have elapsed since spermicide was applied, it must be reapplied before intercourse, normally in the form of a spermicidal pessary.
- The spermicide should be reapplied before repeated acts of intercourse.
- ▶ It must be left in place for at least 6h after intercourse.

## Efficacy

- When used carefully and consistently, with spermicide, they have a 92–96% success rate.
- Typically the efficacy rate is 82–90%, with a spermicide.
- The failure rate depends on how effectively the woman uses the diaphragm or cervical cap.
- Age is relevant, as the woman aged 25 is generally more fertile than a woman aged 40+.

## Disadvantages

- Requires motivation and needs to be used carefully and consistently.
- Needs to be used with a spermicide cream or gel for maximum effectiveness. Some women find the additional spermicide messy and unacceptable.
- No protection against HIV.
- May increase the incidence of cystitis and urinary tract infection (particularly if the diaphragm is too big).
- The woman must be comfortable with handling and exploring her body.
- Psychosexual problems may become apparent during discussion and teaching diaphragm or cervical cap fitting.

## Advantages

- There is little reduction in sexual sensitivity.
- It may give some protection against cervical cancer and sexually transmitted diseases if the cervix is covered.
- No hormones to take.
- It is under the control of the woman.

**Fig. 26.5** Diaphragm fitted correctly.
Reproduced with permission from Andrews, G. (ed.), Women's Sexual Health, Elsevier 2005.

## Contraindications
- Poor vaginal muscle tone, bladder or uterine prolapse.
- Allergy to spermicide or latex.
- Undiagnosed genital tract bleeding.
- Congenital abnormality such as two cervices or septal wall defects in the vagina.
- Current vaginal, cervical, or pelvic infection.
- Recurrent urinary tract infections.
- Past history of toxic shock syndrome.
- Women unable to touch their genital area.

## Side effects
- Urinary tract infection.
- Vaginal irritation.
- Toxic shock syndrome if left in longer than 30h.

## Points to remember
- ► After any pregnancy, the diaphragm or cap should be refitted. This is particularly important after a full-term pregnancy.
- Fitting should be delayed until at least 6 weeks after birth to allow for return of pelvic tone.
- Advise the woman to have a diaphragm or cap properly fitted by a competent nurse, doctor, or midwife.
- If her weight varies by >7lb (3kg), the fitting should be professionally re-assessed.
- The diaphragm must be checked regularly for deterioration or holes.
- A new diaphragm should be fitted following any episode of treated vaginal infection.
- Only water-based lubricants should be used, as any other preparations damage the latex rubber.

# Fertility awareness (natural family planning)

- Fertility awareness methods are natural, requiring no medical intervention, but do require competent education in their use (Fig. 26.6).
- Natural methods of family planning are widely and successfully used, particularly in certain religious groups.
- Natural fertility awareness methods involve observation of female body changes within the woman's menstrual cycle, in order to detect ovulation, either to use as contraception or to achieve pregnancy in the fertile period.
- There are four main methods of natural family planning and fertility awareness:
  - Temperature method
  - Calendar method
  - Cervical mucus method (Billing's method)
  - A combination of the above, known as the symptothermal method, which is the most effective and preferable method.

## After pregnancy

▶ Because of the hormonal changes in pregnancy, it is important to remind the woman that this method should not be relied on until she has had at least three normal periods after abortion or birth. This is to ensure that her natural hormonal levels are back to normal.

## Changing from a hormonal method of contraception

▶ As above, she should wait until at least three normal periods after discontinuing the hormonal method. She can learn the method but not rely on it until the hormonal contraceptive effects are no longer active.

## Breastfeeding

- ▶ This method cannot be used whilst a mother is breastfeeding, because of altered hormone levels (➲ see Lactational amenorrhoea method, p. 634) for further details).
- She should wait until she has ceased breastfeeding and had at least three normal periods.
- She may need additional contraception in the intervening period.

## Efficacy

- This depends on consistency and conscientiousness of method use.
- The efficacy rate varies from 80% to 90%.

## Disadvantages

- Cannot be used immediately after pregnancy.
- Requires motivation and conscientiousness in use.
- Requires observation and recording of daily body changes.
- Requires specialist teaching.
- Takes time to learn (typically 3–6 months).
- Basal body temperature is affected by illness, alcohol, disturbed sleep, anxiety, and stress.

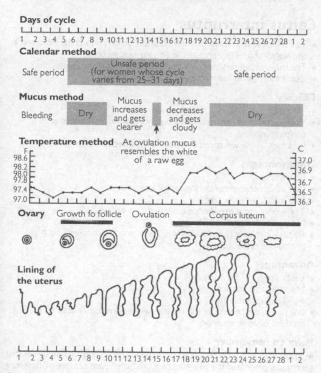

**Days of cycle**

1 2 3 4 5 6 7 8 9 10 11 12 13 14 15 16 17 18 19 20 21 22 23 24 25 26 27 28 1 2

**Calendar method**

| Safe period | Unsafe period (for women whose cycle varies from 25–31 days) | Safe period |

**Mucus method**

| Bleeding | Dry | Mucus increases and gets clearer | Mucus decreases and gets cloudy | Dry |

**Temperature method**   At ovulation mucus resembles the white of a raw egg

F: 98.6 98.2 98.0 97.8 97.4 97.0
C: 37.0 36.9 36.7 36.5 36.3

**Ovary**   Growth fo follicle   Ovulation   Corpus luteum

**Lining of the uterus**

1 2 3 4 5 6 7 8 9 10 11 12 13 14 15 16 17 18 19 20 21 22 23 24 25 26 27 28 1 2

Fig. 26.6 Summary of fertility awareness methods.

- Some cold and flu remedies can inhibit cervical mucus production.
- A vaginal infection will make it difficult to detect changes in the cervical mucus.

## Advantages

- It is under the control of the couple, once learnt.
- No side effects.
- Can be used to avoid or achieve pregnancy.
- Detects the beginning and end of the fertile period.
- Helps couples learn about their fertility and recognize body changes.
- Competent teaching will help her interpret those factors that may affect her temperature or cervical mucus secretion.
- Acceptable to a number of religious beliefs and cultures.

## Further reading

Fertility UK. Fertility Awareness. Available at: ℘ www.fertilityuk.org.

# Coitus interruptus

- The oldest known form of contraception, referred to in the Bible and in the Koran and widely acceptable on religious grounds.
- The male withdraws his penis from the woman prior to ejaculation.
- Commonly called 'withdrawal' or 'being careful'.

## Efficacy

- Variable.
- With careful and consistent use, it may be up to 96% effective as contraception.
- Less careful use will result in it being 80% effective, at best.

## Disadvantages

- Low efficacy.
- May inhibit enjoyment during sexual intercourse.
- May lead to erectile problems.
- The woman may experience anxiety that it will work.
- No protection against STIs or HIV.
- Efficacy is markedly reduced in men with erectile problems such as premature ejaculation.

## Advantages

- Easily used.
- No clinic appointments.
- Religious acceptability.
- It is under the control of the couple, when consciously used as a method of contraception.

## Point to remember

▶ In discussing this method, it is important to remember to emphasize that sperm are present in the pre-ejaculate, and therefore capable of fertilizing the female, even when full intercourse with ejaculation has not occurred.

# Male condom

- This is the easiest form of contraception to obtain and use, and second only in popularity of use to the oral contraceptive pill in the under-30 age group, and to sterilization in the over 30s, in the UK.
- For a large proportion of the population, it is a completely acceptable method.
- For those who have become used to alternative methods not related to intercourse, it may be completely unacceptable, even on a temporary basis.
- Male condoms come in various sizes, shapes, colours, and flavours, and are now produced from hypoallergenic latex.
- A non-latex polyurethane condom Avanti® is available if either partner is allergic to latex.
- The main reason that men do not like to use them is the lack of sensitivity during sexual activity, but manufacturers are continually making attempts to overcome this problem.

## How is it used?

- ▶ For effective use, it must be used before there is any genital contact.
- Remind the woman that before opening the packet she should ensure that the condom is well away from the edge that is to be torn to release the condom.
- The closed end of the condom—the 'teat'—is squeezed to expel any air and to leave about 1cm to receive the ejaculated semen.
- It is then gently rolled down the full length of the erect penis.
- After ejaculation, hold the condom firmly at the rim, to avoid any semen being spilt as the penis is withdrawn.
- It is then carefully and hygienically disposed of, *but not down the toilet.*

## Advantages

- The condom, when used carefully and consistently, is extremely effective in preventing pregnancy.
- Similarly, it is effective in preventing STIs and HIV.
- It is easy to obtain and use, and requires no medical supervision.
- It may protect the woman against cancer of the cervix by preventing transmission of HPV.
- The man can take responsibility for contraception and sexually shared infection prevention.

## Disadvantages

- It needs forward planning each time.
- It needs to be used carefully to be effective.
- It may interrupt sex, although putting it on can be part of the enjoyment of foreplay.
- There may be possible loss of sensitivity during intercourse or loss of erection.
- It can slip off or split.
- It needs to be disposed of carefully.

**Points to remember**

- In the first few weeks after birth, intercourse may be uncomfortable or sore. Advise the woman to use a water-based lubricant, if necessary.
- ▶ Oil-based lubricants will interact with the latex and encourage the condom to split and should not be used. Baby oil will destroy up to 95% of the strength of condoms within 15min. Avoid ad hoc use of products from the kitchen or bathroom cupboards!
- Advise the woman about the availability of emergency contraception, in case of failure to use or failure in use.
- If a mother is not breastfeeding or is post-abortion, her risk of pregnancy, even in the first menstrual cycle, is real. We have all seen the woman who comes for her postnatal examination and is pregnant again!
- For the mother who is fully breastfeeding day and night, the risk of pregnancy is minimal. If this woman chooses to use a condom, she may need additional water-based lubrication, because of the very low oestrogen levels whilst breastfeeding.
- If one or more partners is sensitive or allergic to latex, a hypoallergenic non latex condom Avanti® is available.
- Because of allergic reactions, most manufacturers do not now coat the condom with nonoxynol-9 spermicide. For added protection, a spermicidal pessary or cream may be used.
- Emphasize that the condom is a 'once-only' use and should never be reused.
- In the UK, all contraception is free of charge and the midwife can offer the woman a supply of condoms.
- Make sure you know where the local contraception and sexual health clinics are located to be able to advise her on further supplies.
- Remind the woman to check that any condom supplied or purchased has a recognized quality mark, e.g. the British Kite mark or the European Community CE mark.
- Condom use is the only method proven to be effective against the transmission of HIV.

# Male sterilization

## Vasectomy

- Vasectomy has become a popular method of permanent contraception in the UK.
- It is simpler to carry out than female sterilization and is commonly done under local anaesthetic as an outpatient, in the contraception and sexual health clinic, or in the doctor's surgery.
- Vasectomy is a minor surgical procedure, involving incision, location, and excision of the vas deferens, preventing sperm from the epididymis from reaching the seminal vesicles. Sperm cannot then be ejaculated and the man becomes infertile, once the vas deferens has been cleared of sperm, which takes approximately 3 months (Fig. 26.7).

## Efficacy

- Highly effective.
- The immediate failure rate is 1:1000, with a later failure rate of 1:3000 to 1:7000.

## Disadvantages

- Not easily reversible and must be regarded as permanent.
- Requires a surgical procedure.
- Requires a local or general anaesthetic.
- ❶ Because vasectomy is not immediately effective, alternative contraception is required until two consecutive clear sperm counts are obtained.
- ❶ If a man does not produce the required two sperm specimens after surgery, the couple must be warned to wait at least 3 months before discontinuing the additional contraception.

## Advantages

- Permanent.
- Highly effective.
- Safe and simple procedure.
- Anxiety of unplanned pregnancy removed.

## Contraindications

- Urological problems.
- Relationship problems.
- Indecision by either partner, if a partner is involved.

## Side effects

- Possibility of infection.
- Haematoma.
- Sperm granulation.

**Fig. 26.7** Male sterilization.

Reproduced with permission from Andrews, G. (ed.), Women's Sexual Health, Elsevier 2005.

## Counselling prior to vasectomy

- This is extremely important, because of the permanency of the method.
- Consider issues of regret and grief for loss of fertility.
- Ensure that the couple considers all the possible different scenarios that may affect their decision, particularly in respect of current children or future relationship breakdown.
- A particular worry of a lot of men is about their ability to maintain erections and have sexual intercourse following vasectomy. Vasectomy does not affect libido or erections, and they will ejaculate normally, but the ejaculate will not contain sperm.
- Contraception is required for at least 3 months following vasectomy.
- There is no proven link between vasectomy and the incidence of testicular or prostatic cancer.
- Ensure that the decision that is made is without the influence or coercion from health-care professionals.

# Female sterilization

- This is the only permanent form of female contraception.
- Normally a day-care procedure under regional or general anaesthesia (Fig. 26.8).
- Involves incising and dissecting or blocking the Fallopian tubes, preventing fertilization.
- It is performed either by laparoscopy, mini-laparotomy, or vaginally.

## Efficacy

Highly effective, with an efficacy rate of 99.4–99.8 per 100 woman years.

## Disadvantages

- Involves a surgical procedure and an anaesthetic.
- Not easily reversed and must be regarded as permanent.
- If it fails, there is a greater risk of ectopic pregnancy.

## Advantages

- Permanent.
- Effective immediately.
- The anxiety of unplanned pregnancy is removed.
- The ultimate decision is the woman's.

## Contraindications

- Indecision by either partner (if a partner is involved).
- Relationship problems.
- Psychiatric illness.
- A health problem or disability that may increase the risk of the surgical procedure.

## Relative contraindications

- Obesity may be a contraindication for laparoscopy.
- Request for sterilization for a young woman under 25 years old.

## Counselling prior to sterilization

- This is extremely important, because of the permanency of the method.
- ► Post-operative regret and grief for lost fertility happens in at least 10% of sterilized women and this must be discussed and the procedure considered thoroughly.
- Whenever possible, discussion should be undertaken with the couple together, to get each partner's perspective.

## Practice points

- When discussing sterilization, it is important to emphasize that sterilization is not normally carried out at the time of termination of pregnancy, vaginal birth, or Caesarean section, due to the increased vascularity of the tissue involved. This will increase the failure rate.
- In the UK, sterilization reversal is not carried out on the NHS, except in very exceptional circumstances.

**Fig. 26.8** Female sterilization techniques.
Reproduced with permission from Andrews, G. (ed.), Women's Sexual Health, Elsevier 2005.

- Termination of pregnancy or birth is an emotive time and a decision for sterilization made at this time is fraught with potential future psychological and psychosexual problems.
- It is normal to wait at least 6 weeks following termination of pregnancy or birth.
- Unless the mother is fully breastfeeding, effective contraception in the interim period is essential to prevent pregnancy.

# Emergency contraception

There are three forms of emergency post-coital contraception:
• The levonorgestrel-only oral preparation, commonly known as the 'morning-after pill', although this terminology should be discouraged, as it is misleading
• The ulipristal acetate oral preparation, known in the UK as ellaOne®, with increased effectiveness from 72h and up to 5 days post-coitally over levonorgestrel
• A copper IUD.

NB. The 'Mirena®' IUS should not be used for this purpose.

## How do they work?

• These methods inhibit implantation, should unwanted conception have occurred.
• The primary action of ulipristal is to delay or inhibit ovulation and alter the endometrium, which may also contribute to efficacy.
• This must be explained carefully, as personal beliefs about whether life begins at conception or at implantation may affect a woman's decision about whether to take the emergency contraception pill or to have an IUD inserted.

## Oral pill

• The Levonorgestrel tablet is taken within 72h of unprotected sexual intercourse or contraceptive failure to give maximum protection, but it can be taken up to 5 days after intercourse. If taken within 24h, the efficacy rate is 99.6%, and 98.9% at 72h.
• The ulipristal[6] tablet is taken orally as soon as possible, but no later than 120h after, unprotected sexual intercourse or contraceptive failure.
• In explaining the mode of action and efficacy of the emergency contraceptive pill, it is vital to ensure that the woman clearly understands that this relates only to the immediately preceding 72h, even if there are multiple episodes of intercourse within this period.
• ❶ Any episodes in the current cycle occurring prior to this 72h period may have already resulted in pregnancy and render emergency contraception totally ineffective.
• Treatment with levonorgestrel may be repeated in any menstrual cycle, if necessary. However, ulipristal is not currently recommended to be used more than once per cycle, as the efficacy of repeated exposure has not been assessed.
• Ulipristal has been shown to be more effective compared to levonorgestrel in women who are categorized as overweight or obese and in women aged under 35 and in mid cycle.
• There is no evidence of any effect on the fetus, if taken in early pregnancy.
• If there is any doubt about whether pregnancy is possible, carry out a reliable pregnancy test prior to administration. The trophoblast embeds in the uterus in 5–7 days after conception and a reliable dipstick test, which takes a maximum of 5min, should give the answer.

- It is professionally responsible for the midwife to discuss ongoing reliable methods of contraception with the woman and to give her information or refer her to a contraception and sexual health clinic, or a doctor or nurse trained and currently up-to-date with contraceptive methods, if hormonal methods are required, or to a midwife or nurse competent in the non-hormonal methods.

*Side effects*
- Virtually none.
- The period may be heavier than normal but should occur at the expected time.

*Contraindications*
- Current or suspected pregnancy.
- No other absolute contraindications.

*Follow-up*
- Normally 1 week after the next expected period, i.e. approximately 3 weeks.
- If a normal period has not occurred, carry out a pregnancy test.

## Intrauterine device
- It can be inserted up to 5 days following unprotected intercourse or up to 5 days after the earliest calculation of the day of ovulation. This latter point clearly relies on the woman knowing her own menstrual cycle pattern, in order for the doctor or nurse/midwife to calculate and fit the IUD, *in good faith*, e.g. up to day 20 in a 28-day cycle.
- Advise a copper IUD, normally one of the cheaper varieties, with the minimum 5-year lifespan on the copper component. This can then be removed at the end of the next period.
- Discussion with the woman may reveal that she would like to keep the IUD as a long-term method of contraception, longer than 5 years, in which case an IUD with an 8- to 10-year copper licence will be fitted.

*Pre-insertion infection screen*
- Not possible in this circumstance. Take swabs at the time of fitting, along with visual inspection for evidence of an existing infection. Antibiotics are prescribed, if necessary.
- For remaining details about IUD insertion, ➔ see Intrauterine devices, p. 656.

*Follow-up*
- Normally 1 week after the next expected period.
- If a normal period has occurred, the IUD can be removed.
- If the period has not occurred, a pregnancy test should be carried out.
- It is good practice to offer an infection screen at this point or to refer the woman to the appropriate clinic.

## Reference
6 Faculty of Sexual and Reproductive Healthcare, Clinical Effectiveness Unit (2009). *New product review (October 2009) Ulipristal acetate (ellaOne®)*. Available at: ℰ www.fsrh.org/documents/cec-ceu-newproductreview-ellaone-oct-2009/.

# Care of the newborn

# Care of the newborn

# Examination of the newborn: monitoring progress

The purpose of the examination of the newborn is to monitor the normal progress of the baby and for early detection of deviations from normal.

During the examination, advice can be given to the parents about minor disorders (→ see Minor disorders of the newborn, p. 694) and safe baby care practice, such as the correct amount and type of clothing and bedding needed and the correct sleeping position, to reduce the risk of sudden infant death syndrome (SIDS). Information can also be gained about the baby's overall feeding and sleeping pattern.

The midwife will monitor and record the following information.

- With the mother's permission, the baby should be undressed and examined in a draught-free environment. Care is taken not to expose the baby longer than necessary and he/she should be re-dressed as quickly as possible to maintain body temperature.
- Colour: the baby should not be pale, cyanosed, or jaundiced. The skin is inspected for rashes and spots.
- Temperature: the chest and back should feel warm. If the hands and feet are cool, mittens and bootees can be put on.
- Respirations: should be regular, up to 40/min with no dyspnoea or expiratory grunt.
- Muscle tone should be neither floppy nor stiff.
- The eyes, nose, and mouth should be inspected for discharge or other signs of infection.
- The umbilicus is inspected for signs of cord separation and advice given about washing the umbilicus as part of the daily bath. The cord may need to be cleaned during the nappy change and warm tap water is sufficient for this purpose. The cord usually separates during the first 10 days of life.
- The nappy area is inspected for signs of rashes and the mother can be asked whether the baby is passing urine and stools regularly.
- The baby should pass urine during the first 24h after birth and then urine output is governed by the baby's intake of food and fluid. Wet nappies signify a good fluid intake.
- The first stools will be meconium, a soft black sticky substance which accumulates in the gut in fetal life. Passage of meconium confirms the patency of the lower gut.
- After a few days of feeding, the stools change colour to green/brown as the milk starts to be digested. Passage of a changing stool confirms the patency of the upper digestive tract.
- Yellow stools confirm that milk is being fully digested. A breastfeeding baby may pass stools several times per day or only once every few days, depending on its intake. Formula-fed babies should pass stools each day.

- Weight should be recorded on the tenth day to ensure the baby has regained its birthweight. Weight recording between birth and the tenth day would be performed if there were any other concerns about the baby's progress. Evidence-based local midwifery guidelines on weighing should be followed.
- If the mother expresses any concerns that the baby is not progressing as expected, advice should be given and the baby re-examined later the same day. A baby showing signs of illness, such as lethargy, poor tone, and breathing or feeding difficulties, needs to be referred to a paediatrician *as a matter of priority*.

# Reflexes in the newborn

Reflexes are incorporated into the neurological examination performed by the paediatrician or a suitably trained midwife following birth. Reflexes are involuntary reactions to external stimuli such as touch, sound, and light. Certain stimuli evoke specific reactions that give reassurance regarding a normal neuromuscular development. Inborn reflexes are movement patterns that develop during fetal life and are crucial for survival of the newborn. All reflexes have their own time span—an infant exhibiting reflexes after this time indicates neurological impairment.

## Common reflexes observed in the newborn infant

- *Rooting reflex*: a very common reflex observed by midwives. When the cheek is brushed lightly with the finger, a soft object, or the nipple, the baby's head will turn to the side being stimulated and he or she will open their mouth wide. A mother wishing to breastfeed will be advised to use this reflex to encourage the baby to open the mouth to receive the nipple and ensure successful attachment to the breast.
- *Grasping reflex*: stroking or applying pressure to the palm of the hand will result in the baby making a clenched fist. This reflex is very strong in the newborn baby. A weak reflex may indicate neurological disturbance.
- *Sucking reflex*: when the root of the baby's mouth is touched with a clean finger or a teat, the baby spontaneously starts to suck. This response begins at about 32 weeks' gestation but is not fully developed until 36 weeks' gestation. Therefore, premature babies may well have a weak sucking reflex.
- *Moro reflex*: also known as the 'startle' reflex. This reflex is initiated by startling the baby, usually by supporting the baby supine on the hand and forearm. When the baby is relaxed, the head is suddenly dropped back a few centimetres. The baby then flings his or her arms open, with the hands open and fingers curled in slightly. This is followed by drawing the arms back towards the chest in an embrace-like position. This may be accompanied by the baby grimacing or crying. This reflex may also be stimulated by sudden noise.
- *Walking or stepping reflex*: the significance of this reflex is not fully understood. When the baby is held under the arms in an upright position over a flat surface, the baby will make stepping movements forwards.
- *Tonic neck reflex*: with the baby lying on his or her back, when the head is turned to one side, one arm and leg are extended in the direction that the baby's head is facing. The opposite arm and leg are in a flexed position.
- *Babinski reflex*: stroking the sole of the foot from heel to toe will result in the baby's toes fanning out and the foot turns inwards. This reflex is present until the age of 2 years.

# Screening tests

Screening tests aim to identify the likelihood of potential abnormality within a normal population. During the early neonatal period, various tests and examinations may be undertaken to detect specific abnormalities that could undermine the infant's health. Screening procedures are only appropriate when diagnostic tests are available that are inexpensive, simple, and specific to the condition. Effective treatment or intervention should also be readily available before the onset of symptoms or pathology is apparent. Early diagnosis of some conditions can result in curtailing disease processes that have devastating effects on the individual. An excellent example is the screening test for phenylketonuria (PKU)—early diagnosis of this inborn error of metabolism prevents severe mental impairment by prescribing a specialized diet.

## Hearing

Approximately 1–2 babies in 1000 are born with hearing loss in one or both ears. Recent technological advances have led to major improvements in screening methods for detecting hearing loss in the neonate.

Early detection of hearing loss in infancy ensures that full investigation into the cause and possible therapy or treatment can be commenced that will be important for the baby's speech development.

### Oto-acoustic emissions (OAE) test

- This test is done as early as possible; many maternity units perform this test within the first 24h of birth.
- A trained hearing test screener or health visitor undertakes the test, which only takes a few moments to perform.
- The test is non-invasive, using a small soft-tipped earpiece placed in the outer ear, which transmits clicking sounds to the inner ear. A computer detects how the ears respond to sound emissions.
- A strong response to the test indicates the unlikehood of hearing impairment. The result of the test is given immediately to the parents by the screener.
- If there is no clear response to the test, then a second test is arranged. Various reasons may make it difficult to test a baby's hearing: the baby was unsettled; an accumulation of fluid in the ear after birth; and background noise at the time of the test.
- Parents may also be given checklists to monitor their baby's hearing at key stages of development.

### Automated auditory brainstem response (AABR)

- This is a similar test to the OAE using computer technology; it takes slightly longer.
- Three small sensors are placed on the baby's head; headphones are placed over the ears, and a series of clicking sounds is transmitted. The computer measures how well the baby's ears respond to sound.
  If the second test shows a poor response, then referral to the audiology department is necessary for further tests and follow-up.

## Further reading

Public Health England (2013, updated 2015). *NHS newborn hearing screening: programme overview.* Available at: 🖰 www.gov.uk/guidance/newborn-hearing-screening-programme-overview.

# Growth

Due to physical and psychological limitations, the baby is reliant on its mother to provide dedicated care to enable its ongoing survival, growth, and development. Providing the baby has been born with no physical or neurological abnormalities, it will require the following in order to grow and develop normally:

- Nutritional needs met
- Safe environment
- Adequate exercise, rest, and sleep
- Psychological/emotional stimulation.

To some extent, the physical growth and development of the baby depends on the nutritional status of the mother before, during, and after pregnancy (especially if breastfeeding), as well as the adequacy of the infant's diet if bottle-feeding.

- Nutrition—establishing infant nutrition in the early days is an essential part of midwifery care of the newborn, whether the baby is breastfeeding or bottle-feeding. Observation of the baby's feeding technique is important to ensure correct attachment to the breast or the baby's sucking and swallowing behaviour if bottle-feeding.
- Environment:
  - *Safety*: ensuring that the environment is free from potential hazards/ dangers that may impair adequate growth such as tight clothing. Over-swaddling the baby may restrict movement. Avoid a smoky environment. There is some debate about the practice of bed sharing; parents should be encouraged to carefully weigh up the risks and benefits
  - *Thermoregulation*: in mature infants, heat loss may pose a problem to the baby's survival and health status due to the immaturity of the heat regulatory system. Because of the baby's immobility and lack of ability to shiver, there is still a risk of hypothermia if the environment is not adequately warm. If the baby is cold, the nape of the neck may still feel warm; therefore, it is best to check the skin of the abdomen for a more reliable assessment of the temperature. Observing the baby's behaviour is crucial; initially babies may generate more heat by crying and creating activity. However, in the later stages of hypothermia, the baby may become lethargic, with a poor response to stimuli, even though their pallor may be deceivingly healthy
  - *Prevention of infection*: during the first 6 months of life, babies are at increased risk of infection due to immaturity of the immune system. Care should be taken to ensure sound hygiene standards when caring for or handling newborn babies. Infection can seriously undermine a baby's health and growth, leading to morbidity and sometimes mortality.
- Psychological development—although the baby sleeps for long periods during the first 6–8 weeks, it is important to communicate and provide sensory stimulation during the wakeful times and at feed time. It is well known that emotional deprivation results in poor growth and delayed development.

Indicators of sound nourishment and adequate growth are:
- Steady increase in weight and length
- Regular sleeping patterns
- Regular daily elimination
- Active, alert, and responsive during wakeful times
- Firm muscles and moderate amount of subcutaneous fat.

Some predisposing/inhibiting factors may need to be considered when assessing growth:
- Cultural and hereditary factors—small/large stature, diet.
- Prematurity—it may take some time for the premature baby to catch up with the normal parameters. The baby may still be on a strict feeding regime on discharge from hospital; consequently parents may require extra support and reassurance from the midwife. The baby's stomach capacity is much smaller and the sucking reflex may still be weak. In some instances, the baby may still be receiving partial nutrition via a nasogastric route, which may require the support of a neonatal nurse.
- SGA—depends on the reason for the lack of adequate growth *in utero*. If the baby is nutritionally deficient, this may have far-reaching effects, which may not necessarily be rectified post-delivery. Lack of essential minerals *in utero* and early neonatal life has been linked with suboptimal brain development and impaired physical growth. These babies are increasingly discharged home much earlier; therefore, the parents may need extra support from the midwife/neonatal nurse until they are confident in their abilities to maintain the healthy growth and development for their baby.
- Babies of diabetic mothers—due to high glucose levels *in utero*, there may be a period of readjustment before normal feeding patterns are established.
- Congenital abnormalities—some abnormalities may deter the ability to feed properly, therefore potentially causing difficulty:
  - Cleft lip and cleft palate—special teats may need to be used
  - Oesophageal atresia
  - Pyloric stenosis—projectile vomiting occurs between the third and fifth week of life and affects males more than females.
- Twins—there may be inherited differences in feeding and growth patterns; it is therefore important to monitor both babies to ensure that they both progress along normal parameters. The mother will require extra support and input from the midwife to ensure she retains the healthy growth and development of both infants.

In order to monitor a baby's growth and development, various checks may be carried out:
- Weight—in most units, the routine weighing of healthy term infants is not carried out, as most babies may lose up to 10% of their birthweight within the first week of life. Thereafter, most babies will have regained their birthweight by 10 days. It is usual for babies to gain approximately 200g per week, although individual differences need to be taken into account, as outlined above.

- Length—the measurement at birth gives a baseline for the baby's further growth. Debate about measuring length accurately is crucial if using it to monitor adequate growth patterns. A correct supine stadiometer should be used and two people are required for the procedure.
- Head circumference—measurements for the head circumference at birth and up to 24h may be inaccurate due to moulding. Some units delay this measurement until 24–48h post-birth. The head circumference provides a good baseline for later comparisons. An unusually large or small head circumference indicates abnormality.
- Percentile charts are the most common means of assessing growth; usually these consist of graphs plotting the upper, lower, and midpoint levels of average growth patterns—the baby's weight, length, and head circumference readings can be plotted and compared with normal expectations. Babies below the ninth centile will have reduced glycogen stores and are therefore more prone to hypothermia and hypoglycaemia.
- Feed charts may be employed where strict feeding regimens are important to ensure that exact calorific requirement are provided.

# Minor disorders of the newborn

# Minor disorders of the newborn

### Skin rashes

Babies commonly present with non-infective skin rashes within the first few weeks of life, which usually resolve spontaneously without treatment.

- *Erythema toxicum*: also known as urticaria neonatorum, is a blotchy red rash with pinhead papules, which usually occurs within the first week of life and normally disappears within a day or two.
- *Heat rashes*: appear as reddened areas, often in the skinfolds and have hard pinpoint centres. The rash resolves quickly when the baby cools down.
- *Milia*: also known as a sweat rash, is seen in babies who become overheated and is due to blocked sweat glands. Less clothing and fewer cot blankets should be used and more fresh air may help.

Other skin rashes that may occur but require remedial action include:

- *Chafing or intertrigo*: this is due to inadequate drying of the skin, particularly in the groin or axilla area, after washing or bathing. The skin should be dried using a dabbing movement with the towel and then a slight dusting of antiseptic power applied
- *Sore buttocks*: presents as soreness and excoriation around the anus and buttocks and is usually a result of frequent loose stools. It is more common in formula-fed babies than breastfed babies. Other causes may include infrequent nappy changes, poor hygiene, incorrect laundering of nappies, diet, and infections such as candidiasis (thrush). It is usually very painful. Treatment includes identifying the cause, good hygiene, and exposure of the buttocks to the air. If candidiasis infection is thought to be present, the mouth should also be examined and treatment with local and oral nystatin is required. If sore buttocks persist for more than a day or two, medical advice should be sought.

*Any rash* that presents as watery filled pustules or appears infected should be seen by the paediatrician or family doctor without delay.

### Nappy rash (ammoniacal dermatitis)

The skin beneath the nappy area becomes red and excoriated. This usually results from infrequent changing of the nappies (either cloth or disposable), hot weather, and the use of plastic pants. Increased contact of urine with the skin leads to production of ammonia and chemical burns. The condition is preventable by avoiding the precipitants and the use of commercial barrier creams. However, care should be taken with their application as they can cause the one-way process design of disposable nappies to become ineffective by blocking the perforations within the nappy linings. This will result in the urine not being able to soak through into the inner lining of the nappy, which may exacerbate the condition.

Treatment involves the protection of the damaged skin and exposure of the skin in a warm, dry atmosphere to promote healing of the excoriated skin. Care needs to be taken to prevent secondary infection. If this occurs, refer for a medical opinion.

## Breast engorgement

Breast engorgement may occur in both male and female babies on or about the third day of life. The drop in serum oestrogen levels following the separation of the mother and baby at birth stimulates the breasts to secrete milk. No treatment is required as the condition will resolve spontaneously. Mothers must be advised not to squeeze the breasts as this may result in infection.

## Pseudo-menstruation

A bloodstained vaginal discharge may occur in baby girls. This is due to oestrogen withdrawal following separation of the mother and baby. The mother should be reassured that it is a normal physiological process, which will resolve without treatment.

## Constipation

Constipation is defined as the difficult passage of infrequent dry, i.e. hard, stools. A baby's constipated stool resembles rabbit droppings or gravel in its size and consistency. Not all hard stools are constipated. The stools of a formula-fed baby will be bulkier, firmer, and often drier than that of a breastfed baby. Babies will often appear to strain, even when passing normal soft stools.

Constipation is unusual in breastfed babies although they may not pass a stool for 2–3 days once feeding is established, but this is quite normal, provided that the stool is of a normal soft consistency. Constipation most commonly occurs in formula-fed babies. If a formula-fed baby is constipated, the following should be considered:

• Are the feeds being made up correctly, i.e. is the formula being added to the water and not vice versa?
• Is anything being added to the feed, e.g. baby rice, baby rusks?

All of these will result in a reduced fluid:solids ratio, which will result in the baby receiving inadequate fluids. If either is occurring, advise the mother appropriately. If neither of the above are occurring, advise the mother to offer the baby small amounts of extra boiled, cooled water between feeds and, if constipation still persists, to seek medical attention.

## Regurgitation

Regurgitation is the effortless posseting of small amounts of milk following a feed. It usually occurs after a large feed and is usually of no importance. A newborn baby may have swallowed liquor amnii, blood, or mucus shortly before or during the process of being born. If following birth, he or she vomits watery fluid or mucus, possibly streaked with blood, reassure the mother that it is usually of no significance.

Vomiting other than this may well be abnormal and should be referred to the paediatrician. Possible causes may be:

• Feeding errors
• Infection
• Intracranial injury
• Congenital malformation
• Haemorrhagic disease of the newborn
• Metabolic disorders.

The colour, quantity, frequency, and timing in relation to feeding should be observed and recorded, and whether or not it is projectile.

# Neonatal temperature control

Temperature is controlled from the heat-losing centre and the heat-promoting centre of the hypothalamus, an area of the brain near to the pituitary gland. The mechanisms controlled by these centres are immature in the newborn, especially if premature.[1,2]

- The newborn temperature should be maintained between 36.5°C and 37°C.
- Hypothermia in the newborn is defined as a temperature below 35°C.[1,2]

## Non-shivering thermogenesis

Newborns have a limited ability to sweat and shiver. Non-shivering thermogenesis (NST) is used by newborns to keep warm and is initiated by:

- Oxygenation
- Separation from the placenta: cutting the cord maximizes NST
- Cutaneous cooling: cold receptors in the skin stimulate noradrenaline and thyroxine release, which stimulate brown fat.

### Brown fat

- It is found around the neck and between the scapulae, across the clavicle line and the sternum.
- It also surrounds the major thoracic vessels and pads the kidneys.
- The cells contain a nucleus, glycogen, mitochondria (which release energy), and multiple fat vacuoles in the cytoplasm (a source of energy).
- The presence of the mitochondrial enzyme thermogenin means that, when the fat is oxidized, it releases heat rather than other forms of energy.
- It has a high concentration of stored triglycerides and a rich capillary network, and is densely innervated.
- It increases in amount during gestation.[2]

## Heat loss

Heat is lost during birth, resuscitation, and transportation.
Mechanisms of heat loss are:

- *Conduction* from cold surfaces
- *Radiation* from surrounding objects
- *Convection* from the air
- *Evaporation*: insensible water loss from the skin, especially in the preterm infant.

Thermoneutrality is the environmental temperature at which minimal rates of oxygen consumption and energy expenditure occur.[2]

## Effects of hypothermia (cold stress)

- Increases pulmonary vascular resistance, reducing oxygenation.
- Decreases surfactant production and efficiency, giving rise to atelectasis which worsens hypoxia.
- Poor perfusion causes an increase in anaerobic metabolism, worsening acidosis.
- Acidosis increases the pulmonary artery pressure, decreasing the amount of flow of blood through the lungs, leading to hypoxia.

- Increased acidosis also leads to displacement of unconjugated bilirubin from binding sites, risking hyperbilirubinaemia.
- Increased use of glucose, due to the increase in metabolism, leads to hypoglycaemia and reduces the energy available for growth.
- Poor cardiac output and reduced blood flow to the gastrointestinal tract causes ischaemia, which can lead to necrotizing enterocolitis (NEC).
- Pulmonary haemorrhage can also occur due to left ventricular failure and damage to the pulmonary capillaries, leading to leakage of fluid and cells from the alveoli.[2]

## Hyperthermia

Hyperthermia is unusual in the newborn and is normally the result of environmental factors or pyrexia due to sepsis.

Usually in sepsis, there is a vast difference between core and peripheral temperatures. Low core temperatures indicate thermal stress. A difference between core and peripheral temperatures of >2–3°C indicates thermal stress that can be due to:
- Sepsis
- Patent ductus arteriosus
- Hypervolaemia
- Catecholamine infusions.

The factors that lead to hyperthermia are:
- Large surface area
- Limited insulation
- Limited ability to sweat.

Sweating, seen on the forehead and temples, can occur in term babies in response to overheating. This can lead to:
- Hypotension secondary to vasodilation
- Dehydration, following insensible water loss.[2]

## Maintaining the neonatal temperature

### Assessment

The different methods of assessing the baby's temperature are:
- Electronic axilla: most commonly used
- Rectal: occasionally used with caution as it can cause damage, but it can give a more accurate estimation of the core temperature in the newborn
- Skin probes: may also be used during resuscitation or incubation
- Infrared tympanic: can be used but is not very accurate in the newborn as the ears are still full of fluid from the delivery.[3]

### Care at birth

- The temperature of the fetus is at least 1°C higher than that of the mother, due to heat exchange via the placenta.
- The drop in ambient temperature at delivery is more marked when the wet infant is delivered into a cool environment.
- A healthy term baby will respond by increasing heat production.
- Drying and wrapping the baby in warm towels will enable it to maintain its temperature.

- 'Kangaroo care' helps to keep the baby warm. Putting the baby in skin-to-skin contact on the mother's chest stimulates the mother to alter her temperature to the needs of the baby.[2,3]

*Premature babies*
- Delivery rooms can be cool and draughty, which increases convective heat loss.
- The body temperature of a 1kg infant can decrease by 1°C every 5min.
- Set the radiant warmer to maximum and have warm towels ready.
- Remember, the head is a large surface area for heat loss, so place a hat on the baby if he or she requires extensive resuscitation and transfer to the NICU.
- During resuscitation and transportation to the NICU, use plastic bags to contain the infant's body. The plastic next to the skin helps to cut down the transepidermal fluid loss through the immature skin of premature babies.
- Once the baby is in the incubator environment, the 87% humidity will also help the baby to warm up.[2,3]

## Equipment used to maintain temperature in the newborn

*Radiant heaters*
- Provide dry heat directly on to the skin.
- Are used mainly at delivery or during interventions.
- Increase insensible, evaporative, and convective heat loss.

The infant will increase its metabolic rate as it tries to produce neutral thermal conditions. Radiant heaters are not used for long with very premature or ill babies.

*Incubators*
- Provide an enclosed protected space.
- As a result of their double-glazed design, they reduce radiation heat loss, surrounding the infant with a 'curtain' of heat, even when the doors are open.
- Enable the administration of humidity (87%) to help cut down evaporation (insensible) heat and fluid loss.
- Enable the administration of oxygen.
- Reduce noise, because the portholes and doors are cushioned.

*Controlling temperature*
Incubators control temperature in three ways:
- Servo control: if the infant's temperature decreases, the incubator will increase its heat automatically to compensate. This is not used for premature infants as the decrease in temperature needs to be observed as an early and subtle sign that the infant is becoming unwell, perhaps with an infection.
- Air temperature: this can be altered according to the changes in the infant's condition and is the method used for premature and ill babies as it allows for an observation to be recorded and recognized as a sign that the baby is unwell.
- Air temperature probe: this hangs near to the infant and maintains a consistent set temperature, leading to less fluctuation.

*Radiant hood warmer*

This can be used independently of the incubator's main source. It is preferred for very premature infants as it:

- Cuts down on handling
- The hood warmer reduces oxygen consumption, which can be 8.8% higher under a standard radiant warmer
- Provides a better thermal environment for controlling transepidermal water loss.[2,3]

## If a baby in an incubator becomes cold

- Turn up the incubator temperature by 0.5°C.
- Put a hat on the baby.
- Check the baby's colour, heart rate, respiration rate, blood sugar, activity, feeding, and aspirate.

If still cold after 1h:

- Turn up the incubator temperature by another 0.5°C.
- Inform the medical staff, especially if the baby remains unwell. This could be an early indication of infection and may lead to an examination and full infection screening.[2,3]

*General points*

- Most incubators will be double-glazed to keep warm whilst the doors are open. Do not keep the doors open for longer than necessary.
- Check the baby's temperature before commencing cares or procedures. Let the baby warm up in between episodes of handling.
- Warm the air and oxygen.
- Overhead heaters provide dry heat only.
- Humidity may be required.[2,3]

## Cot-nursed babies who become cold

- Use a hat.
- Add extra clothes and covers.
- Use an overhead radiant heater.
- Observe the baby closely for signs of infection.
- Inform the medical staff if the baby does not respond or if he or she appears unwell.[2,3]

## References

1 Fleming PJ, Blair PS, Bacon C, et al. (1996). Environment of infants during sleep and risk for SIDS: results of 1993–1995 case centred study for confidential enquiry into stillbirths and deaths in infancy. *BMJ* 313: 191–5.

2 Fellows P (2010). Management of thermal stability. In: Boxwell G, ed. *Neonatal Intensive Care Nursing*, 3rd edn. London: Routledge, pp. 87–111.

3 Bailey J (2000). Temperature measurement in the preterm infant: a literature review. *J Neonatal Nurs* 6: 28–32.

# Hypoglycaemia

Healthy term newborns who are breastfeeding on demand *need not* be screened for hypoglycaemia and need no supplementary foods or fluids. They do not develop 'symptomatic' hypoglycaemia as a result of simple underfeeding.

Babies at high risk of hypoglycaemia can be identified as follows:
• Preterm baby <37 weeks
• Weight <2.5kg
• Apgar <5 at 1min and/or <7 at 5min
• Fetal blood sample pH <7.2
• Umbilical venous/arterial pH <7.1.

If a baby meets one or more of the above criteria, the following protocol is instigated.
1. Breastfeed and give skin-to-skin contact as soon as possible after birth.
2. Two hours post-delivery, blood glucose analysis is required.
3. Then 3h feeds and pre-feed blood glucose analysis for 12h.
4. Discontinue blood glucose analysis after 12h if pre-feed results are at/or >2.6mmol/L.
5. Continue 3h feeds and assessment of vital signs for 24h.
6. Document results and actions taken.
• If the baby fails to feed at 3h intervals assist the mother to express her milk.
• Offer expressed breast milk (EBM) obtained via a cup/pipette.
• Leave the baby to rest.
• After 24h if baby is well, extend feeds to 3–4h, then introduce demand feeding as tolerated.
• Assess the baby's vital signs and feeding at each shift until transfer to community.
• Infants of diabetic mothers (insulin-dependent or gestational diabetic) require active management.
• Thirty minutes post-delivery, blood glucose analysis is required, then offer the baby a breastfeed, irrespective of the result.
• If the baby fails to feed well, offer any EBM obtained, with additional formula milk if required.
• The baby must receive as much milk as possible, but at least 5mL/kg birthweight should be given. The total volume taken should be controlled by the baby's appetite.
• Then 3h feeds, pre-feed blood glucose analysis, and assessment of vital signs for 24h.
• Discontinue blood glucose analysis after 24h if pre-feed results are at/or >2.6mmol/L.
• Document results and actions taken.
• If pre-feed blood glucose analysis is <2.6mmol/L, inform the paediatrician.
• Offer the baby a breastfeed. If the baby fails to feed well, offer any EBM obtained, with additional formula milk if required.

- The baby must receive as much milk as possible, but at least 5mL/kg birthweight should be given. The total volume taken should be controlled by the baby's appetite.
- Repeat blood glucose analysis 1h post-feed. If blood glucose is <2.6mmol/L, the baby requires paediatric assessment.
- If blood glucose analysis is at/or >2.6mmol/L, follow the protocol as before.

# Advice to parents: reducing the risk of sudden infant death syndrome

Cot death, or SIDS, is the sudden unexpected death of an apparently well baby aged from birth to 2 years. Over 300 babies still die of cot death a year in the UK. The UK rate was 0.33/1000 live births in 2013.[4]

Although there is no guaranteed method of preventing cot deaths, the risk can be reduced by following the Department of Health and The Lullaby Trust guidelines.[5] This leaflet should be given to, and discussed with, all new mothers prior to taking a baby home from hospital. Since parents and carers have been following the risk reduction advice, the number of babies dying has fallen by over 70%. Health professionals can explore the research behind the recommendations by downloading a fact file from the The Lullaby Trust website.[6]

▶ The recommendations that should be given to parents are as follows.
• Place your baby on their back to sleep in a cot in a room with you.
• Do not smoke in pregnancy or let anyone smoke in the same room as the baby.
• Do not share a bed with your baby if you have been drinking alcohol, if you take drugs, or if you are smoker.
• Never sleep with your baby on a sofa or armchair.
• Do not let your baby get too hot. Keep your baby's head uncovered. Their blanket should be tucked no higher than their shoulders.
• Place your baby in the feet-to-foot position (with their feet at the end of the cot or pram).

Other factors that can help reduce the risk are:[5]
• Breastfeeding
• Keeping the baby in the same room as the parents for the first 6 months
• Using sheets and lightweight blankets. Do not use duvets, quilts, pillows, or similar thick bedding
• Keeping the bedroom at a comfortable, but not hot, temperature (18°C)
• The baby should never sleep with a hot water bottle or next to a radiator, heater, or fire, or in direct sunlight
• Using a dummy, but if breastfeeding do not give the baby a dummy until they are 1 month old.

## References

4  The Lullaby Trust (2015). *Statistics on SIDS*. Available at: ℗ www.lullabytrust.org.uk/statistics.
5  NHS Choices (2015). *Sudden infant death syndrome (SIDS)*. Available at: ℗ www.nhs.uk/ Conditions/Sudden-infant-death-syndrome/Pages/Introduction.aspx.
6  The Lullaby Trust (2014). *The Lullaby Trust: evidence base*. Available at: ℗ www.lullabytrust.org. uk/file/Evidence-Base-updated-Oct-14.pdf.

# Bed sharing

Bed sharing is a controversial issue and has been linked to cot deaths. Many mothers will take their babies into bed to feed and provide comfort without intending to fall sleep. Bed sharing has been shown to promote breastfeeding; therefore, it is important that midwives give the mothers the correct information to enable mothers to continue breastfeeding, whilst at the same time reducing the risk of cot death.[7]

## Recommendations whilst in hospital

▶ Mothers should be constantly supervised if bed sharing and co-sleeping if they are:

- Under the effects of a general anaesthetic
- Immobile due to a spinal anaesthetic
- Taking drugs that may cause drowsiness
- Seriously ill, e.g. high temperature, large blood loss, severe hypertension
- Excessively tired
- Have a condition that affects mobility or sensory or spatial awareness, e.g. multiple sclerosis, blindness
- Very obese
- Likely to have a temporary loss of consciousness, e.g. if she is diabetic or epileptic.

Bed sharing and co-sleeping are contraindicated if:

- A mother is a smoker
- The baby is preterm or ill.

## Advice to mothers at home

Mothers should always be given the UNICEF leaflet 'Sharing a bed with your baby' prior to transfer home.[8] It is recommended that babies share their mother's room for at least the first 6 months, as this assists breastfeeding and protects against cot death.

### When mothers should not sleep with their babies

If they or their partners:

- Are smokers
- Have drunk alcohol
- Have taken any drug (legal or illegal) which makes them drowsy
- Have a condition that affects their awareness of their baby
- Are overtired to the point that they could not readily respond to their baby.

### Reducing the risk of accidents and overheating

- Parents should *never* sleep with their baby on a sofa or armchair.
- The bed must be firm and flat.
- Ensure the baby cannot fall out of bed or get stuck between the mattress and wall.
- Make sure the room is not too hot (16–18°C is ideal).
- The baby should not be overdressed.
- Bedclothes must not overheat the baby or cover the baby's head.
- Never leave the baby alone in or on the bed.

- The partner should be informed if the baby is in bed.
- If an older child is also bed sharing, there should be an adult (you or your partner) between the child and the baby.
- Never share your bed with pets and your baby.

Mothers who are bottle-feeding should be advised to put their babies back into their cot after feeding, as mothers who bottle-feed can sometimes turn their backs on their babies when they have fallen asleep.

## References

7 UNICEF UK Baby Friendly Initiative (2004). *Babies sharing their mothers' bed while in hospital: a sample policy*. London: UNICEF UK Baby Friendly Initiative. Available at: ℘ www.babyfriendly.org.uk.
8 UNICEF UK Baby Friendly Initiative (2014). *Statement on co-sleeping following publication of new NICE postnatal guidance*. Available at: ℘ www.unicef.org.uk/Documents/Baby_Friendly/Infosheets/statement_NICE_guidance_co-sleeping_2014.12.pdf.

## Neonatal infection

The incidence of infection in the newborn has declined over the past 10 years due to the increased use of antenatal antibiotics and more effective management of premature rupture of the membranes.[9]

### Definitions
- Very early onset: <24h.
- Early onset: 1–7 days.
- Late onset: >7 days.
- Nosocomial infection: hospital-acquired.
- Bacteraemia: the presence of viable bacteria in the blood.
- Septicaemia: systemic disease caused by the multiplication of organisms in the blood.
- Sepsis: the presence of pus-forming and other pathogenic organisms in the blood.[9]

### Infections acquired in the antenatal period

Amniotic fluid has bactericidal properties and the membranes provide a physical barrier. If these defences are breached, the fetus will be infected by direct aspiration into the lungs, causing pneumonia and bacteraemia.
- GBS is the most common cause of early-onset septicaemia and meningitis.
- Mycoplasmas found in the maternal genital tract can cause premature labour.
- GBS and mycoplasmas have also been found where the membranes remain intact.

Other organisms that ascend the genital tract and contaminate the amniotic fluid are:
- *Bacteroides* spp.
- *Escherichia coli*
- *Clostridium* spp.
- *Peptococcus* spp.

#### Infections acquired via the placenta
- *Listeria monocytogenes* causes placentitis.
- Viruses, such as CMV, herpes, and that causing rubella, and the parasitic protozoan *Toxoplasma* sp. also affect placental function, resulting in growth retardation and congenital abnormalities.
- Intrauterine infection with parvovirus B19 is associated with fetal anaemia.
- Vertical transmission of HIV from the mother to the fetus through the placenta is thought to be related to the maternal viral burden, disease stage, and immune response.

### Intrapartum infection

Factors that increase the likelihood of intrapartum infection are:
- Premature labour
- Maternal pyrexia
- Prolonged rupture of the membranes.

Causative organisms include:
• GBS: the most common
• Herpes simplex: acquired through contact with genital secretions
• Hepatitis B: acquired through contact with vaginal secretions
• HIV: attributed to contact with infected secretions.

*Sexually transmitted diseases* are on the increase in the UK and are transmitted during vaginal delivery. These include:
• Chlamydiosis
• Syphilis
• Gonorrhoea—in the newborn, this can cause conjunctivitis, which can develop into pneumonia.[9,10]

▶▶ All health-care workers are strongly advised to use universal precautions routinely when in contact with maternal and fetal blood and other body fluids.[11]

## Late-onset and nosocomial infections

Occur due to:
• Maternal contact
• Contact with hospital personnel (cross-infection)
• Contact with inanimate objects.

The most common causative organisms are:
• *Klebsiella* spp.
• *Escherichia coli*
• Coagulase-negative *Staphylococcus*
• *Staphylococcus aureus*
• *Pseudomonas aeruginosa*.[11]

*Risk factors for nosocomial infections*
• Low birthweight with a depressed immunological function.
• Underlying disease.
• Raised gastric pH and poor nutritional status requiring total parenteral nutrition.
• Excessive use of antibiotics.
• Multiple IV site access, the presence of an endotracheal tube and central lines.
• Long hospital stay.
• Poor compliance of staff with infection control and poor handwashing.
• Shared equipment, overcrowding, and inadequate staffing.
• The presence of opportunistic organisms.[9,10]

## Defences

*Physical defences*
• The skin.
• Mucous membranes.
• Gastric secretions.
• Tears.
• Urine pH.
• Ciliated epithelium.

All are affected by immaturity, poor skin keratinization, and invasive procedures.

*Non-specific defences*
- Phagocytes (neutrophils and monocytes).
- Natural killer cells.
- Inflammatory responses.
- Antimicrobial proteins.
- Complement activation.
- Serum opsonins.
- Polymorphonuclear neutrophils.

All of these are immature as there is little or no transmission via the placenta. Their ability to release complement is reduced until 6–18 months. This deficiency in phagocytosis and opsonization is pertinent in the case of GBS and is further compounded by prematurity.

*T and B cells*
- Generated from the bone marrow.
- T cells are responsible for cell-mediated immunity.
- B cells confer humoral immunity from which antibodies are produced.

*Humoral immunoglobulins*
There is some evidence of transfer, which gives the newborn some protection:
- *Maternal IgG* is transferred from 22 weeks and increases by 30 weeks, giving the fetus passive immunity
- *IgM* does not cross the placenta, so immunity to acute maternal infection at the time of delivery is not provided
- *IgA* is secretory, present in saliva, sweat, tears, intestinal secretions, and colostrum
- *IgD* is present on the surface of lymphocytes to control activation and suppression of B cells
- *IgE* is present in low quantities in the serum but in higher quantities in the respiratory and gastrointestinal tracts.[9,10]

## Signs of neonatal infection

▶ Early detection is crucial (Table 27.1) or the infection will overwhelm the baby, leading to:
- Septicaemia
- Meningitis
- Death.

Indicators may be apparent in the maternal history such as:
- Maternal pyrexia
- Prolonged rupture of membranes
- Length of gestation of the fetus.

The midwife or nurse caring for the baby will often 'feel' that the baby is 'not as well as it was'. Neonatologists in practice will act on this observation, especially if it comes from an experienced neonatal nurse, and it often leads to examination and an infection screening.[9,10]

**Table 27.1** Signs of neonatal infection

| Common signs | Uncommon signs |
| --- | --- |
| Pallor | Purpura |
| Poor feeding | Omphalitis |
| Tachycardia/arrhythmia | Vasomotor instability |
| Decreased peripheral perfusion | Bleeding |
| Unstable BP | Pustules |
| Abdominal distension | Bulging fontanelle |
| Apnoea | Splenomegaly |
| Lethargy | Rash |
| Hyperbilirubinaemia | Diarrhoea |
| Recession/grunting/cyanosis | Seizures |
| Tachypnoea | |
| Unstable temperature | |

## Investigations

- *Surface swabs* taken from multiple sites are useful when late infection is suspected or on admission to the NICU. The optimal site is a deep ear swab or a swab of obvious lesions in later-onset infection.
- *Blood cultures* are mandatory before starting antibiotics.
- *Total neutrophil count* is more reliable than a total white cell count. The immature-to-total ratio is a good indicator of infection.
- *CRP*: a level of >6mg/L is a sign of infection. This is used to measure the course of infection and response to treatment. Levels should return to normal 96h after starting treatment.
- *Platelet count*: due to increased destruction, aggregation and adhesion occur, but this is usually a late finding in about 50% of cases.
- *CSF*: lumbar punctures are carried out to rule out bacterial meningitis.
  - The sample should be clear.
  - *CSF white cell level* <30mm$^3$ with >66% neutrophils.
  - *CSF protein levels* of >1g/L in a term baby or 2g/L in a premature baby are suspicious of meningitis.
  - *CSF glucose level* should be approximately 70–80% of the plasma glucose level.
- *Urine*: usually collected as a bag sample or suprapubic tap. The long-term effects of urinary infection can be renal scaring and atrophy.[9,10]

## Management of the infected infant

- *Supportive therapy and broad-spectrum antibiotics*: begin as soon as the infection screening is complete.
- *Ventilation* may be needed and is mandatory in cases of GBS, due to associated pulmonary vasoconstriction and the development of pulmonary hypotension.

- *Cardiovascular support*: the infant will be shocked. Management of the BP and perfusion are necessary. A decrease in circulating blood volume can cause prerenal failure.
- *Peripheral perfusion and capillary refill time* must be kept within normal limits.
- *Volume replacement* with plasma or blood helps to provide immunoglobulins and clotting factors.
- *Dopamine and dobutamine and plasma*: are used to treat hypotension.
- *Acid–base balance*: maintained with ventilation, fluid replacement, and inotropes.
- *Sodium bicarbonate*: use with caution to help correct acidosis where all other treatments have failed. It can improve acidaemia, myocardial contractility, and surfactant production, and lower pulmonary vascular resistance.
- *Fluid and electrolyte balance*: record carefully. This can be complicated by the inappropriate secretion of antidiuretic hormone due to severe hypoxia or meningitis.
- *Hyponatraemia* can result from inappropriate antidiuretic hormone secretion.
- *Sodium and potassium losses* increase when the baby has NEC or in the diuretic phase of acute tubular necrosis following low renal perfusion rates.
- *Hypoglycaemia* can occur due to increased metabolic demands.
- *Haematological management*: keep a record of all bloods taken and treatment with top-up transfusions, especially in small premature babies.
- *Bruising, oozing, and petechiae* due to consumptive coagulopathy: treat with platelet transfusions, plasma, and vitamin K.
- *Exchange transfusion*: in extreme cases, this can wash out coagulation inhibitors and supply missing coagulation factors and opsonins, and increase the oxygen-carrying capacity of the blood.[9,10]

## Antibiotic therapies and sensitivities

(See Table 27.2.)
- *Gentamicin levels*: check after five half-lives at steady state or after 3–5 doses have been given, to avoid the occurrence of troughs in blood levels.
- *Metronidazole* is used to treat Gram-negative anaerobic bacilli, such as *Bacteroides*, and is useful for the treatment of NEC.
- Despite the increase in meticillin-resistant *Staphylococcus aureus* (MRSA), some penicillins are useful to treat *Staphylococcus aureus* and *Staphylococcus epidermidis*.
- *Vancomycin* is active against staphylococci, enterococci, and other Gram-positive bacteria; it is also used for treating MRSA.
- Meticillin has been replaced by *nafcillin*.
- *Ticarcillin* is a semi-synthetic penicillin used for treating *Pseudomonas* spp.[10]

**Table 27.2** Antibiotic therapies and sensitivities

| Penicillins | Aminoglycosides | Cephalosporins | Vancomycin |
|---|---|---|---|
| Streptococci | Gram-negative organisms | Gram-negative bacilli | Staphylococci |
| Pneumococci | Have a synergistic effect when used with penicillin to treat GBS | Meningococci | Enterococci |
| Meningococci | | Gonococci | Gram-positive bacteria |
| Gonococci | | *Haemophilus influenzae* | Used to treat MRSA |
| *Treponema pallidum* | | *Pseudomonas* spp. | |

## References

9 Boxwell G (2010). Neonatal infection. In: Boxwell G, ed. *Neonatal Intensive Care Nursing*, 2nd edn. London: Routledge, pp. 302–24.
10 Bedford Russell A, Isaacs D (2012). Infection in the newborn. In: Rennie JM, ed. *Textbook of Neonatology*, 5th edn. London: Churchill Livingstone, pp. 1013–64.
11 Department of Health (1990). *Guidance for clinical health-care workers: protection against infection with HIV and hepatitis viruses: recommendations of Expert Advisory Group on AIDS*. London: HMSO.

## Neonatal jaundice

Jaundice is one of the most common problems in the newborn period as all infants undergo changes in bilirubin metabolism at birth.[12]

- *Physiological jaundice* is a normal process seen in about 60% of term and up to 80% of premature infants within the first week of life. It is a transitional change, leading to an excessive build-up of bilirubin in the blood, which gives the baby a jaundiced (yellow) colour.[13]
- *Pathological jaundice* refers to jaundice that arises from pathological factors that alter the usual processes involved in bilirubin metabolism such as blood group incompatibility, excessive bruising, and sepsis.[14]

### Newborn physiological jaundice

- Newborns have high Hb levels (180–200g/L).
- The short life of the baby's RBCs produces a high rate of Hb breakdown (haemolysis) compared to adults.
- Each gram of Hb produces 34–35mg of indirect (unconjugated) bilirubin.
- β-glucuronidase from fetal life may still be active in the gut.
- This changes conjugated bilirubin into unconjugated bilirubin.
- *In utero*, this would have been excreted via the placenta and the maternal circulation. This is known as the enterohepatic circulation.
- After birth, this unconjugated bilirubin can be reabsorbed into the enterohepatic circulation, causing a further build-up in the baby's blood.

### Indirect unconjugated bilirubin

- Has not been unconjugated by the liver.
- Is fat-soluble and cannot be excreted in the bile or urine.
- It builds up in the blood and can be deposited in the fatty tissue of the skin, leading to jaundice.
- If levels rise very high, it is deposited in the fatty tissue in the brain, which can lead to kernicterus and brain damage.
- The body metabolizes unconjugated (indirect) bilirubin in the liver, changing it into conjugated (direct) bilirubin.

### Direct conjugated bilirubin

- Is water-soluble.
- Can be excreted by the biliary system into the intestines and stools.
- A small amount can be reabsorbed in the colon and excreted in the urine.

Newborns are also deficient in:

- Albumin for binding, which will carry the unconjugated bilirubin to the liver
- Ligandins (Y and Z carrier proteins)—these are needed to transport the unconjugated bilirubin across the space of Diss, which surrounds the hepatocytes in the liver. The bilirubin is then able to cross the hepatocyte cell membrane
- Glucuronyl transferase, an enzyme in the hepatocyte, which helps to conjugate the bilirubin
- Glucose substrate which is needed to provide energy for the enzyme reactions to take place.[14]

## Patterns of jaundice

Jaundice developing within the first 24h may be due to:
• Rh disease
• ABO incompatibility
• Congenital infection
• Glucose-6-phosphate dehydrogenase (G6PD) deficiency.

Those jaundiced at 48h may have:
• Physiological jaundice
• Acquired infection
• Undetected haemolytic disease.

Jaundice lasting beyond 10 days may indicate:
• Breastfeeding jaundice
• Chronic or late infection
• Hepatitis
• Obstruction, e.g. biliary atresia
• Inborn errors of metabolism, e.g. PKU, cystic fibrosis
• Hypothyroidism.

### ABO incompatibility
• The incidence is one in five births. A mother who is group O and whose baby is group A or B has naturally occurring anti-A or anti-B lysins (antibodies), which destroy the fetal RBCs, leading to newborn jaundice.

### Glucose-6-phosphate dehydrogenase deficiency
This is an X-linked recessive condition. G6PD maintains the integrity of the RBC membrane, so a lack of this enzyme leads to excessive haemolysis. This condition can be triggered by infection or sulfonamides.[15]

### Breastfeeding jaundice
• Breastfeeding jaundice is early in onset, seen by 2–4 days.
• The majority of infants with raised serum bilirubin where no other cause can be found are usually breastfed.
• There is an increase in enterohepatic shunting. This process normally exists in the fetus where β-glucuronidase in the gut unconjugates the conjugated bilirubin in order to return unconjugated bilirubin via the placenta to the maternal circulation for excretion by the mother. The fetus is not able to excrete it through its bowel until after birth. Breastfed babies excrete less bilirubin in their stools, keeping conjugated bilirubin in the intestines for longer, thus increasing the chance that the β-glucuronidase will unconjugate it before it is excreted.
• Decreased fluid intake leads to altered liver conjugation and clearance.
• Inadequate calorific intake causes an increase in fat metabolism to meet energy needs, which interferes with bilirubin uptake by the liver.
• Human milk also contains β-glucuronidase, which increases enterohepatic shunting and indirect bilirubin levels in the blood.
• Supplementation of breastfeeding infants with water is counterproductive as it decreases milk intake, and therefore lowers production due to a lack of stimulation of the breast.[13]

## Assessment of infants with jaundice

All infants are at risk of jaundice. Factors that increase this risk must be identified.

*Factors that increase the risk*
- Fetomaternal blood group incompatibility (haemolysis).
- Birth trauma (RBC destruction and increased bilirubin production).
- Congenital abnormalities of the gastrointestinal tract.
- Delayed cord clamping.
- Delayed passage of meconium/delayed feeding (increases enterohepatic shunting).
- Sepsis (leads to RBC destruction and altered hepatic clearance).

*Other risk factors*
- Low birthweight.
- Prematurity.
- Premature rupture of membranes.
- Increased weight loss, delayed feeding, and dehydration.
- Swallowed/sequestered blood from trauma, cephalic haematoma, and surgery.

*Problems that interfere with bilirubin metabolism*
- Hypoxia.
- Asphyxia.
- Hypoglycaemia.
- Hypothermia.

## Preventative strategies

- Give Rh D Ig to Rh D-negative mothers within 72h of delivery of each baby.
- Avoid trauma in labour.
- Prevention of hypothermia.
- Prevent hypoxia and hypoglycaemia.
- Early feeding/increased frequency of breastfeeding.

## Examination

Assess:
- Skin and sclera
- Activity.

Note:
- Birth trauma
- Length of gestation.

NICE[13] now recommends that all babies who are more likely to develop jaundice in the first 72h should be assessed at every opportunity, in order to identify those needing intervention.
- Measure and record bilirubin level within 2h of all babies with suspected jaundice, especially in the first 24h of life.[13]
- Continue to measure the bilirubin level every 6h for all babies with suspected or obvious jaundice.[13]

- Use a transcutaneous bilirubinometer (TBM), which is a small hand-held device placed against the baby's chest as this is more accurate than visual inspection alone. If a TBM is not available or it indicates a level >250mmol/L, check the result by measuring the serum bilirubin.[13]
- Serum bilirubin is used to determine bilirubin levels in the first 24h and for babies <35 weeks' gestation. It is also a guide to treatment.[13]

## Investigations

Laboratory estimation of serum bilirubin levels is required for all ill term and premature infants. The levels are reported as total bilirubin and the direct (conjugated) component.
- Hb/haematocrit.
- Reticulocyte count.
- Maternal and infant blood groups.

Investigate cases of prolonged jaundice for liver function and thyroid problems. To detect spherocytes and a diagnosis of congenital spherocytosis, carry out an RBC smear.

### Total bilirubin
- This is an accurate reflection of indirect (unconjugated) bilirubin because the direct (conjugated) component is usually very low.
- Exceptions can occur where there is significant Rh incompatibility or in infants with elevated bilirubin levels after 2 weeks. The bilirubin in these cases will be mainly direct (conjugated).

### Blood group testing
#### Direct Coombs' test
This is a measure of antibody-coated blood cells. It is a direct measure of the amount of maternal antibody coating the infant's RBCs.
- If antibody is present, it will be a *positive direct result*.
- Infants with Rh incompatibility will have a positive direct response.
- Infants with ABO incompatibility will have a negative or weakly positive result.

#### Indirect Coombs' test
This measures the effects of a sample of the infant's serum, thought to contain antibodies, on the RBCs of an unrelated adult. If antibody is present, the components will interact and coat these adult RBCs, giving a *positive indirect result*.

#### Kleihauer's test
This detects the presence of fetal blood cells in the maternal circulation. This normally occurs during separation of the placenta from the uterus following delivery of the baby. The presence of fetal cells in the maternal circulation indicates a risk of antibodies being formed if the mother is Rh-negative and the fetal blood cells are Rh-positive.[16]

## Management
- Phototherapy.
- Exchange transfusion will be used in cases where the rise in bilirubin levels cannot be controlled by the use of phototherapy.

**Phototherapy**

The light used in phototherapy reduces bilirubin levels by:

• Photoisomerization, which converts indirect bilirubin to water-soluble photoisomers. The light energy rearranges the molecules in the chemical group to produce photobilirubin and rearranges the atoms to produce lumirubin. These can be excreted into the bile without conjugation. This isomerization is thought to be the most important in terms of bilirubin elimination.

• Photosensitized oxidation is a minor pathway, by which the bilirubin molecule absorbs light energy which is then transferred to oxygen, forming a reactive oxygen molecule. Bilirubin is then oxidized, forming a water-soluble product which is excreted in the urine with no need for conjugation.

*Strength of light*

A blue-green light of a wavelength in the range of 425–475nm is used. Blue, green, and turquoise light (the blue-green spectrum) are considered the most effective. The recommended irradiance is approximately 10cm if fluorescent tubes are used.[17]

*Light sources*

• *Overhead strip lights* incorporated into a unit which is designed to fit closely over the incubator hood to give maximum efficiency, maintaining the effectiveness of the treatment.

• *Fibreoptic paddles* used underneath the baby, often used in conjunction with overhead lights.

• *Fibreoptic blankets* ('*Biliblankets*®') can be used if the baby is well enough to be held. The light source, a tungsten halogen lamp, is linked to a woven fibreoptic pad via a fibreoptic cable.

• *Bilibed*, a bed with lights incorporated into the base. The baby lies on the bed and is covered with a sleeping bag attached to the base.[18]

*Recording the levels*

• The bilirubin levels are plotted on a chart to indicate when treatment is needed.

• The charts differ for gestational age and for the degree of illness.

• The more premature, ill baby will be treated at lower levels than a term, well infant who may not need any treatment.

• Incorporated into the charts are also levels at which an exchange transfusion may be required if phototherapy is not enough to control the rising levels of bilirubin.[17]

*In practice*

• Commence phototherapy as soon as bilirubin levels start to rise, using the charts as a guide.

• Give the parents a full explanation of the cause and treatment.

• Turn the incubator temperature down to accommodate extra heat from the lights and record the infant's temperature frequently.

• The baby should be naked, but cover the gonads.

• Turn the baby regularly to get maximum exposure.

• Protect the baby's eyes with goggles.

- Change nappies frequently, because of diarrhoea.
- Calculate extra fluid into the daily requirements of premature babies, to allow for insensible water losses.
- Do not use creams on the skin, because of burning.
- Observe for skin rashes and irritation.
- Treatment is continuous until levels start to fall, usually by 3–4 days from starting treatment.
- Physiological jaundice should have resolved by 10 days. If the jaundice persists beyond this time, investigate other causes.[13]

*Advantages*
- Cheap.
- Effective.
- Non-invasive.

*Disadvantages*
- Makes observation difficult.
- Can upset the baby's water and electrolyte balance.

## References

12 Ives NK (2015). Management of neonatal jaundice. *Paediatrics and Child Health* 25: 276–81.
13 National Institute for Health and Care Excellence (2010). *Jaundice in newborn babies under 28 days*. NICE guidelines CG98. Available at: ℐ www.nice.org.uk/guidance/cg98.
14 Coad J (2012) *Anatomy and Physiology for Midwives*. London: Churchill Livingstone Elsevier.
15 Rimon D, Pyeritz R, Korf B (2013). *Emery & Rimoin's Principles and Practice of Medical Genetics*. London: Elsevier.
16 Polin R, Yoder M (2014). *Workbook in Practical Neonatology*. Philadelphia: Elsevier Saunders.
17 Lissauer T, Fanaroff A (2011). *Neonatology at a Glance*. Oxford: Wiley-Blackwell.
18 Day C (1995). Phototherapy for neonates: a step by step guide. *J Neonatal Nurs* 3: 4.

# Vomiting in the newborn

- Vomiting small amounts of milk after feeding is a common event in healthy babies during the first 2 weeks of life. It is physiological and universal.
- The normal baby swallows a variable amount of air during a feed which can be expelled easily by sitting the baby upright and gently rubbing his or her back.
- A teaspoon or two of milk is often regurgitated within the first 10min after feeding. This is known as posseting and is considered to be a normal response.[19,20]
- Vomiting has many possible causes, most of which are simple and benign. Should the vomiting become persistent, then more serious causes will be considered.[19]

## Causes

The causes of vomiting can be non-organic or organic.

- Non-organic:
  - Overfeeding
  - Incorrect preparation of feeds
  - Overstimulation and excessive handling
  - Crying
  - Air swallowing.
- Organic:
  - Infection
  - Gastroenteritis
  - Meningitis
  - Otitis media
  - Gastro-oesophageal reflux
  - Gastritis from swallowed meconium or blood
  - Bowel obstruction
  - Pyloric stenosis
  - Hiatus hernia
  - Feeding intolerance/allergy
  - Metabolic disorders.

Bile-stained vomiting may indicate malrotation of the bowel.[20,21] Bile-stained or projectile vomiting may indicate intussusception of the bowel.

The cause can be determined by a taking a history of:

- Feeding technique
- Description of the vomiting
- Preparation of the feed
- Other symptoms.

## Investigations

If the history and physical examination of the baby prove inconclusive, the following investigations are carried out:

- U/E.
- Abdominal X-ray for bowel obstruction.
- Oesophageal pH monitoring.

- Barium swallow and follow-through for:
  - Oesophageal anomalies
  - Hiatus hernia
  - Gut malrotation.
- Abdominal ultrasound examination for:
  - Malrotation
  - Gastric outlet obstruction.
- Infection screen, including:
  - Blood cultures
  - Urine microscopy
  - CSF culture.
- Arterial blood gases for:
  - Alkalosis with pyloric stenosis
  - Persistent acidosis with inborn errors of metabolism
  - Serum electrolytes
  - Hypokalaemia in paralytic ileus
  - Hypochloraemic alkalosis in pyloric stenosis.[20]
- Metabolic screen for:
  - Urine amino and organic acids
  - Plasma amino acids
  - Lactate.[20,21]

## Management

Management involves identifying and treating the cause and maintaining the baby's fluid balance.

▶ Throughout the period of investigation and management, the midwife must remember the need for accurate and detailed documentation, and the need for advice, support, and clear explanations to the parents.

The above list of investigations is not necessary for every vomiting baby. Vomiting can often be transient and attention to the frequency and volume of feeds is enough to improve the situation.[20,21]

### Abdominal distension

Feeding should be stopped where there is vomiting accompanied by mild to moderate abdominal distension. Carry out an abdominal X-ray. If this is satisfactory but the baby continues to vomit when feeds are reintroduced, stop feeding for 3 days to rest the gut and provide fluids and electrolytes via an IV line, then gradually reintroduce enteral feeding again.

### Feeding intolerance

This is not common in the newborn but should be considered where simple remedies have failed to improve the baby's condition or if there is a family history of feeding intolerance. It may then be necessary to introduce the baby to a soya-based formula.

### Irritation due to swallowed fluids

During birth, amniotic fluid, meconium, and mucus can be swallowed, which can irritate the stomach, causing gastritis and the rejection of early feeds. A small stomach washout via a nasogastric tube can usually cure the problem.[19]

*Vomited blood*

Vomited blood in the first few days is usually swallowed maternal blood. This can be distinguished easily from the baby's own blood as it will not contain any fetal Hb.

*Vomited bile*

▶ Vomited bile is more serious and can indicate intestinal obstruction, which can occur at different levels in the gut. An abdominal scan will confirm or exclude this as the problem. Bile-stained vomiting may also occur with a cerebral disorder such as intracranial bleeding or meningitis.[19]

*Gastro-oesophageal reflux*

This is characterized by repeated small vomits occurring shortly after feeds. It is caused by an incompetent lower gastro-oesophageal sphincter and is common in:

● Preterm babies
● Babies who have neurological abnormalities causing hypo- or hypertonia
● Following surgery for repair of a diaphragmatic hernia or oesophageal atresia.

The baby may fail to thrive due to loss of calories in the vomit and there is a risk of aspiration into the lungs. The problem can be treated in several ways:

● Thickening feeds with:
  • Nestargel®
  • Carobel®
  • Thixo-D®.
● Nursing the baby in a prone position with the cot tilted up 30–40°.
● Drugs such as:
  • Gaviscon® 1–2g with each feed, but this can cause constipation
  • Antacids, such as cimetidine, can help to relieve gastritis.

Where medical treatment fails, fundoplication will be tried.

The natural history is for a gradual improvement as the baby grows and the condition is usually better by the end of the first year of life.[19,21]

*Projectile vomiting*

Projectile vomiting usually indicates pyloric stenosis. This is more common after the first month of life and rarely occurs in the first week. There is usually a family history and it is more common in boys.

Diagnosis can be made by observing visible peristalsis and a palpable 'tumour' in the area of the pyloric sphincter (the muscle that regulates the flow of milk from the oesophagus into the stomach).

Because this muscle is too tight, the milk stays in the oesophagus for longer. The amount of milk in the oesophagus increases as the baby feeds and it is forcibly ejected. Treatment usually involves surgery to split the muscle (Ramstedt's operation).[21]

## References

19 Johnston PGB, Flood K (2002). *The Newborn Child*, 9th edn. London: Churchill Livingstone.
20 Mupanemunda RH, Watkinson M (2004). *Key Topics in Neonatology*, 2nd edn. Oxford: Bios Scientific.
21 Sinha S, Miall L (2012). *Essentials Neonatal Medicine (Essentials)*, 5th edn. London: Wiley.

# Metabolic disorders and the neonatal blood spot test

Although these conditions can present in the neonatal period, diagnosis is difficult or delayed because the clinical signs may not be specific to an individual disorder or to an inborn error of metabolism. Routine screening is designed to detect the affected infants before symptoms develop, allowing treatment to be initiated as soon as possible.[22]

## Genetic inheritance

These conditions are usually inherited as autosomal recessive conditions, which have the following pattern:[22]

- Both parents are normal and do not have the condition
- Both parents are carriers of a faulty gene
- Both carrier genes from both parents must be inherited to produce a child with the condition
- This gives a 1:4 risk of having an affected child with the condition with each pregnancy
- 2:4 will be normal, but carriers of the faulty gene
- 1:4 will be normal, non-carrier.

## Clinical presentation

- There may be a family history of neonatal death or siblings with a known inborn error of metabolism.
- A period of 'well-being' followed by illness and collapse.
- Infection may be suspected and a full infection screening done, but the baby will not respond to treatment.
- Parental consanguinity.[22]

## General signs and symptoms

- Unexplained metabolic acidosis.
- Reducing substances in the urine.
- Feeding difficulties/vomiting/diarrhoea.
- Hepatomegaly.
- Convulsions/cerebral oedema.
- Ketosis/hypoglycaemia/hyperglycaemia.
- Respiratory distress.
- Bradycardia/apnoea.
- Hypothermia.
- Abnormal tone (hypertonia or opisthotonus).
- Axial hypotonia.
- Smelly urine.
- Do not forget that antibiotics also make the urine smell of yeast.[22]

## Initial investigations

- *Non-specific* blood and urine tests, with the test results available within a few hours, can place the error within a diagnostic category, allowing appropriate emergency treatment to be instigated. These are available in all units providing neonatal care:
  - FBC
  - U/E
  - Blood gas
  - Blood ammonia
  - Urine-reducing substances
  - Urine ketones.
- A *presumptive diagnosis* from the urine and blood can be available within a few days. Second-line investigations available in each region include:
  - Urine amino acids
  - Urine organic acids
  - Plasma amino acids
  - Blood and CSF lactate
  - Beutler test for galactosaemia
  - Plasma carnitine.
- A *definitive diagnosis* requires specific enzyme or genetic analysis and can take weeks or months. Specialized investigations available at a supra-regional level are:
  - Specific enzyme assays on blood or skin fibroblasts, e.g. lysosomal enzyme studies
  - DNA mutation analysis
  - Special metabolite studies, e.g. long-chain fatty acids, bile acid analysis.[22]

## Screening

Routine neonatal screening is offered for five disorders:
- PKU
- Congenital hypothyroidism
- Cystic fibrosis
- Medium-chain acyl CoA dehydrogenase deficiency (MCADD)
- Sickle-cell disorders and thalassaemia major.[22]

### Collecting the sample

Parents will receive an information leaflet and have the reasons for the test explained to them in the third trimester of the pregnancy. The reasons should also be discussed with them again just before the procedure is carried out.

The health professional responsible for the baby will usually take the sample on day 6 of milk feeding and will also record the event in the maternity notes.

### Gathering equipment

- Parent information leaflet.
- Blood spot card and envelope.
- Gloves.
- Automated lancet device.
- Cotton wool.
- Spot plaster.
- Maternity record.[23]

*The procedure*

- With the consent of the parents, offer the baby a pacifier with sucrose on it, to lessen pain responses.
- Wash the heel with sterile water and an alcohol swab, then leave to dry for 30s.
- Lance the heel on the plantar surface beyond the lateral and medial limits of the calcaneus. Avoid the posterior curvature of the heel.
- Allow the blood to fill the circle by natural flow.
- Apply the drop to one side of the card.
- Fill all the circles completely. Avoid layering the blood and ensure that the blood permeates through to the back of the card.
- Wipe the foot and apply gentle pressure and a plaster if required.
- Comfort the baby.
- Complete the records and inform the parents how and when they will receive the results.
- Send the card within 12h of the sample being taken.[23]

## Phenylketonuria

- The incidence in Britain is 1:10 000 births.
- ❶ If it is not treated, it leads to permanent brain damage.
- It is treated with a diet restricting phenylalanine.
- The baby is born with a normal blood phenylalanine level.
- There is a block in the normal metabolic pathway, preventing conversion of unused phenylalanine into tyrosine.
- The baby quickly shows a marked rise in blood phenylalanine when given feeds containing protein.

*Screening*

▶ It takes a few days for levels of blood phenylalanine to accumulate; therefore, the screening test is usually done after 6 days of milk feeding or at least 48h of IV feed containing protein.

*Guthrie's test*

Introduced by Dr Robert Guthrie, this test was originally based on inhibition of bacterial growth. It is now carried out using a fluorometric assay to test for PKU. A 6.25mm diameter disc is punched out of a dried blood spot on a blood-screening card. Water is added and the sample is then left to dry. Reagents are added to cause the phenylalanine to fluoresce and the fluorescence is measured. Any rise in serum phenylalanine above a given standard stands out on the chart. This will be followed up with further tests on the original sample before confirmation of the diagnosis with the parents.[24,25]

## Congenital hypothyroidism

- The incidence in Britain is 1:3500 births.
- It is due to an absent or a small thyroid gland and reduced/absent thyroxine production.
- Thyroid-stimulating hormone (TSH) levels will be increased.
- ❶ If it is not treated, the individual will have a decreased IQ.
- Treatment is a regular daily dose of thyroxine to replace the missing hormone.[25,26]

- The baby may:
  - Have prolonged jaundice beyond 10 days
  - Be lethargic
  - Be feeding poorly
  - Be constipated
  - Have an odd appearance with a large tongue
  - Have a hoarse cry.

*Screening*

The test involves punching a small hole out of the blood-screening card. A radioactive marker is added to the blood spot; the sample is left overnight and the TSH is measured the next day.

## Cystic fibrosis

- Affects about one baby in 2500.
- It affects the digestion and causes chronic lung disease.
- There is no cure for cystic fibrosis, but early detection improves the quality of life.

*Screening*

- The initial screening test measures immune reactive trypsinogen (IRT) in the blood, which will be increased if the baby has cystic fibrosis.
- The IRT can be raised in normal babies due to other factors.
- If levels are raised, a DNA test is carried out.
- It is estimated that one in 25 people in the UK carries the cystic fibrosis delta F508 gene mutation.
- If the delta F508 gene is found on both alleles in the child, then he or she definitely has cystic fibrosis.
- If the delta F508 gene is found on one allele, the child will be a carrier.
- If the IRT is still raised at this time, it confirms the diagnosis of cystic fibrosis.[25,27]

## Sickle-cell disorders and thalassaemia major

- In *sickle-cell disorders*, the RBCs become sickle-shaped, causing anaemia and making the baby more prone to serious infections.
- These cells can also block the small blood vessels, causing pain.
- A baby with sickle cells needs treatment with antibiotics to prevent serious infections.
- In *thalassaemia major*, the baby does not make enough Hb and becomes severely anaemic, needing regular blood transfusions to remain well.

All parents in these situations will be carriers and are usually offered genetic counselling. Children Living with Inherited Metabolic Diseases (CLIMB) is a support group for parents and health professionals.[25]

## Medium-chain acyl CoA dehydrogenase deficiency

- Incidence: 1:10 000–20 000 births.
- About 1:80 people are carriers and do not have any symptoms.
- It is due to a lack of an enzyme needed to metabolize fat into energy.

- It becomes apparent if the child has long periods between meals:
  - Children with MCADD cannot break down the fat quickly enough to provide energy
  - This leads to a hold-up in the breakdown of medium-chain fats, due to the lack of the correct enzyme
  - The banked-up medium-chain fats form toxic substances, which lead to life-threatening symptoms or death.
- MCADD has no apparent symptoms at birth.
- The most acute presentations occur within the first 2 years of life.
- It is not possible to predict which children will develop symptoms.
- Symptoms occur if the child is not feeding well or is ill with an infection.
- The child becomes:
  - Drowsy and may vomit
  - Hypoglycaemic
  - Comatose, due to low blood sugar and also the build-up of the toxins.
- Most children with this condition will be well as long as they eat regularly. The main problem occurs when the child has additional viral illnesses with a sore throat, vomiting, and diarrhoea, which makes them reluctant to eat or drink.
- The body also requires increased energy to cope with the infection, so children with MCADD need to eat more often during such infections.

*Management of MCADD*

- The main focus for treatment is to prevent a 'metabolic crisis'.
- Closely monitor the child to determine 'safe' time periods between meals.
- Follow a strict feeding schedule.
- If the child becomes unwell and drowsy or vomits, give glucose supplements and refer to a doctor.
- There is no cure for MCADD, but with early detection and monitoring, the child can lead a normal life, and the 'safe' time between meals increases with age.[25,28]

## References

22 Jones S, Wraith JE (2012). Inborn errors of metabolism in the neonate. In: Rennie JM, ed. *Textbook of Neonatology*, 5th edn. London: Churchill Livingstone, pp. 906–19.
23 UK Newborn Screening Programme Centre (2012). *Health professional handbook. A guide to newborn blood spot screening for healthcare professionals.* Available at: ℅ www.gov.uk/government/uploads/system/uploads/attachment_data/file/390977/Health_Professional_Handbook_2012_v1.0_December_2012.pdf.
24 National Society for Phenylketonuria. Available at: ℅ www.nspku.org.uk.
25 NHS Choices (2015). *Newborn blood spot test.* Available at: ℅ www.nhs.uk/conditions/pregnancy-and-baby/pages/newborn-blood-spot-test.aspx.
26 Great Ormond Street Hospital for Children NHS Foundation Trust (2015). *Congenital hypothyroidism.* Available at: ℅ www.gosh.nhs.uk/medical-information/search-medical-conditions/congenital-hypothyroidism.
27 Smyth AR, Bell SC, Bojcin S, et al. (2014). European Cystic Fibrosis Society Standards of Care: Best Practice guidelines. *J Cyst Fibros* **13**(Suppl 1): S23–42.
28 Climb National Information Centre for Metabolic Diseases (2013). *Medium chain acyl-CoA dehydrogenase deficiency.* Available at: ℅ www.climb.org.uk/IMD/Mike/MediumChainAcylCoA DehydrogenaseDeficiency.pdf.

# Developmental dysplasia of the hip

In its severest form, developmental dysplasia of the hip (DDH) is one of the most common congenital malformations.[29] Neonatal screening programmes, based on clinical screening examinations, have been established for >40 years, but their effectiveness remains controversial. The longer-term outcomes of DDH with its contribution to premature degenerative hip disorders in adult life, and the benefits and harms of newborn screening, are not clearly understood. High-quality studies of the adult outcomes of DDH and the childhood origins of early degenerative hip disease are needed, as are randomized trials to assess the effectiveness and safety of neonatal screening and early treatment.[30]

It is becoming more common for midwives with appropriate training to be responsible for screening the hips as part of the holistic assessment of the newborn. Approximately 1.5 per 1000 babies is born with a dislocatable or subluxable hip. This used to be called congenital dislocation of the hips, but the terminology has changed to reflect its potentially progressive nature.

If the condition remains untreated, the hip will function well initially but ultimately lead to problems with walking and premature degenerative disease of the hip.

## Risk factors
- Breech presentation.
- Family history of hip dysplasia.
- Increased birthweight.
- Females more at risk than males.
- First baby more at risk than subsequent babies.

## Diagnosis
The diagnosis is made in the first instance by physical examination and then confirmed by ultrasound scan. Two methods are used.
- Ortolani's manoeuvre detects a dislocatable but reducible hip
- Barlow's manoeuvre is a provocation test for an unstable hip.

## Carrying out the examination
- Consent is obtained from the parents before the test is carried out and then performed in their presence.
- Ortolani's—the baby must be relaxed and on a firm surface.
  - The hip is flexed to 90° and then gently abducted (an outward movement away from the body).
  - The examiner's finger on the outer part of the hip can detect the 'clunk' as the head of the femur slides into the hip socket.
  - This differs from the benign click of soft tissues snapping over bony prominences during the manoeuvre.
- Barlow's—the hip is flexed to 90°, and then the leg is adducted (an inward movement towards the body) and gently pushed backwards.
  - The hip will 'clunk' as the head of the femur dislocates.
- ▶ These tests are not forceful and should not cause any discomfort.

Should either test be positive, the result should be sensitively explained to the parents and arrangements made to confirm the diagnosis by ultrasound scan. Following diagnosis, the most common treatment is for the baby to wear a Pavlik's harness or hip spica cast which gently keeps the hips in abduction until the hip capsule tightens and the hips are kept in place by the normal action of the ligaments.

## References

29 Dezateux C, Rosendhal K (2007). Developmental dysplasia of the hip. *Lancet* 369: 1541–52.
30 Sewell MD, Rosendhal K, Eastwood DM (2009). Developmental dysplasia of the hip. *BMJ* 339: b4454.

## Further reading

Stricker SJ, Barone SR (2001). Tips about hips in children. *International Pediatrics* 16: 196–206.

# Birth injuries

Birth injuries are most commonly caused by trauma or mechanical difficulty at delivery. Head injuries are most common, followed by injury to the limbs, internal organs, and the skin.

## Head injury

- *Cephalhaematoma and caput succedaneum* are common birth injuries (➔ see Examination of the newborn: monitoring progress, p. 684).
- *Hypoxia* is the most common cause of cerebral injury following birth. This may result in intracranial haemorrhage or oedema. Occasionally cerebral trauma may result in cerebral palsy; this is often linked to pregnancy complications such as pre-eclampsia.
- *Tentorial tears*: these are due to the fetal skull being exposed to excessive, rapid, or abnormal moulding, which exerts pressure and stress on the cranium. If this pressure is stretched to its limit, the underlying soft tissues of the brain are vulnerable to tearing (the tentorium cerebelli and the falx cerebri). The source of the bleeding is usually from rupture of the great cerebral vein.
- *Fractured skull*: serious fracture to the skull is extremely rare. Where a woman may have a severely immobilized sacrococcygeal joint and coccyx, this can cause abnormal compression to the fetal head, which may result in a small depressed fracture of one of the frontal bones. Unusual or excessive moulding may produce a fine linear fracture of the cranial bone. Neither of these injuries requires treatment.
- *Facial paralysis*: this injury is usually caused by trauma at delivery. Damage to a branch of cranial nerve VII occurs when pressure is applied on the facial nerve as the head emerges at delivery. The affected side shows no movement when the baby cries; the eye is permanently open, and the mouth droops. This may affect the baby's feeding ability if severe. Invariably, full recovery occurs within hours or up to several days. Care of the affected eye is important to prevent corneal damage.

## Other injuries

- *Dislocations and fractures*: the humerus or clavicle may be fractured in a difficult shoulder dystocia. Occasionally, the femur may be fractured, and in a mismanaged breech delivery the newborn's hip may be dislocated.
- *Sternomastoid haematoma*: this may occur following traction to expedite delivery of the head or shoulders. Swelling occurs to the sternomastoid muscle due to blood oozing from a torn blood vessel. Shortening of the muscle results in the head twisting to one side; this is commonly known as torticollis or wry neck. This condition takes several weeks to subside and rarely causes permanent damage.
- *Klumpke's palsy*: this is caused by traction on the arm when delivering the shoulders, resulting in damage to the lower brachial plexus. Paralysis to the hand and a wrist drop occur and sometimes a fracture is also apparent. Physiotherapy is the main treatment and recovery is usually slow.

- *Erb's palsy*: this is caused by excessive traction on the neck during a breech or cephalic presentation, resulting in damage to the upper brachial plexus. The arm hangs loosely from the shoulder with the palm of the hand turned backwards in the 'waiter's tip' position. Physiotherapy is the main treatment; again this may be slow, but the condition does usually resolve completely.
- *Injury to abdominal organs*: this usually occurs after inappropriate handling of the baby during a breech delivery, causing rupture of the liver or spleen.
- *Skin injuries*: bruising and/or abrasions are sometimes a result of application of forceps. More extensive bruising accompanied by soft tissue swelling may result from a ventouse delivery; this usually resolves within a few days. Abrasions may also be noted due to application of a scalp electrode in labour. Small superficial haemorrhages of the head, face, and neck may resemble cyanosis but are due to congestion of blood vessels in the head. This may occur due to trauma or a precipitate delivery—no treatment is required.

## Practice points

- ▶ Birth injuries still cause a significant number of unnecessary perinatal deaths.
- ▶ Good antenatal surveillance and skilful labour care may go some way to prevent such injuries.
- ▶ Careful observation of the newborn in the postnatal period, particularly after a traumatic or difficult birth, is essential to enable abnormal signs and symptoms to be detected promptly.

# Congenital abnormalities

The incidence of congenital abnormalities varies between 2% and 7% of live births. They are classified into two groups: malformations and deformations. Malformations result from disturbed early embryonic growth, e.g. congenital heart disease. Deformations result from late changes to normal structures by pathological processes or intrauterine forces.[31]

## Causes

- Teratogens: substances like chemicals, drugs, viruses, or radiation.
- Excessive alcohol intake: fetal alcohol syndrome.
- Infections, e.g. rubella.
- Chemicals, e.g. mercury.
- Maternal disease, e.g. diabetes, maternal PKU.

## Examination

The most obvious defects will be detected shortly after birth during the neonatal examination.[32]

### The face

- There is a wide range of recognizable features called dysmorphic features which may suggest congenital abnormality.
- The position of the eyes in relation to the nasal bridge should be noted. If they are too far apart, this is called hypertelorism, and if they are too close together this is called hypotelorism.
- Low-set ears are seen in a variety of conditions, including Potter's syndrome.
- Cleft lip and/or palate occurs in 14.6 per 10 000 births.
- A large or protruding tongue may suggest hypothyroidism or Down's syndrome.
- An underdeveloped jaw, called micrognathia, is seen in Pierre Robin syndrome.

### The chest

- It should be symmetrical and move equally on respiration.
- A small chest may occur with hypoplastic lungs and in a variety of rare syndromes.

### The abdomen

- Distension suggests intestinal obstruction.
- A scaphoid abdomen suggests a diaphragmatic hernia.
- An umbilical hernia may be present.
- The anus should be patent.

### The genitalia

- Testes should be present in the scrotum in 98% of full-term boys.
- Hypospadias occurs if the opening of the urethra is on the underside of the penis.
- Epispadias occurs if the urethral opening is on the upper side of the penis.
- A hydrocele (fluid-filled cyst) may be present in the scrotum. No treatment is required as they usually spontaneously resolve.

- The size of the outer labia in girls is governed by gestational age. By term, they should completely cover the inner labia.
- The clitoris is variable in size. If large, consider adrenogenital syndrome, especially if the labia are also fused.

*The extremities*

- Mild postural deformities may be present in the feet. The ankle joint should be able to be passively moved through its range of normal movements. Abnormalities include talipes.
- The hips are examined to detect a dislocatable or dislocated hip.
- There should be a range of normal movements in the arms.
- Examination of the hands may reveal a single palmar crease in Down's syndrome.

## References

31 Sinha S, Miall L (2012). *Essentials Neonatal Medicine*, 5th edn. Oxford: Wiley.
32 Baston H, Durward H (2010). *Examination of the Newborn. A Practical Guide*, 2nd edn. London: Routledge, pp. 65–91.

## Further reading

Davies L, McDonald S (2008). *Examination of the Newborn and Neonatal Health: A Multidimensional Approach*. Edinburgh: Churchill Livingstone.

# Heart murmurs in the newborn

Murmurs are caused by the sound of turbulent blood flow into the chambers and vessels of the heart. This will usually be detected during the neonatal examination undertaken prior to the baby being discharged home from hospital after the birth.

Increasingly this holistic examination is being performed by suitably trained midwives as part of the continuing care given to all mothers and babies. Community midwives undertaking the assessment in the mother's home have clear referral guidelines to follow if a problem is detected. It is common for babies to have a heart murmur in the first 24h following birth. This is the time during which two structures of the fetal circulation complete their closure in response to the onset of respirations and the establishment of a normal pulmonary circulation.

The two structures are:
- The foramen ovale—an opening in the atrial septum
- The ductus arteriosus—a vessel connecting the pulmonary artery to the aorta. This normally closes within 24h.

Another examination is carried out at the age of 6 weeks on all babies, during which the heart is examined again.

## Significance of heart murmurs

In one study, murmurs were detected in 0.6% of babies, of whom around half had a cardiac malformation.[33] Some babies who were later diagnosed with cardiac malformations had a normal neonatal examination.[34] The study concluded that the neonatal examination only detects 44% of cardiac malformations, but if a murmur is heard there is a 54% chance of it being due to a cardiac malformation. Occasionally heart murmurs are not diagnosed for several months.

## Management

▶ Babies presenting with a murmur during examination should be referred to a consultant paediatrician. This needs to be sensitively explained to parents who are waiting to go home with their baby after this examination takes place.

If the consultant suspects an abnormal murmur, an echocardiogram is arranged. If a problem is suspected, the baby will be referred to a cardiologist for more detailed investigations.

Other signs that may become apparent in the baby in the first few days of life if there is a cardiac malformation are:
- Tachypnoea
- Feeding difficulties
- Cyanosis around the lips
- Failure to gain weight.

Provided the baby is otherwise well and there are no feeding problems, parents may take the baby home in the interim period whilst awaiting appointments and tests.

The two most common cardiac defects in children are:
- Ventricular septal defect
- Atrial septal defect.

## References

33 Ainsworth SB, Wylie JP, Wren C (1999). Prevalence and clinical significance of cardiac murmurs in neonates. *Arch Dis Child Fetal Neonatal Ed* **80**: F43–5.
34 Azhar AS, Habib HS (2007). Accuracy of the initial evaluation of heart murmurs in neonates: do we need an echocardiogram? *Pediatr Cardiol* **27**: 234–7.

# Management of the small-for-gestational-age baby

## Definition

A small-for-gestational-age baby is any baby whose weight falls below the tenth percentile for its gestational age.[35]

A baby can be premature and small-for-dates, or term and small-for-dates, e.g.:

- A baby born at 28 weeks who weighs 500g
- A term baby who weighs 2500g.

## Determination

- Gestational age is calculated using ultrasound scanning where measurement and comparison of the fetal skull and femur enable determination of the age in days, size, and weight.
- Whether the baby is the correct size for its gestational age or if it is growth restricted can also be determined.[36]

## Causes

The SGA baby will have been starved *in utero* due to poor placental supply of nutrients. Some of the causes relate to poor maternal health; others relate to socio-economic factors, and some are fetal, e.g.:

- PIH
- APH
- Congenital infection
- Multiple pregnancy
- Some congenital abnormalities
- Poor diet
- Smoking
- Alcohol
- Drug abuse
- Poor housing
- Unemployment.[37]

There may be genetic and racial inheritance reasons for why babies appear small when weighed and measured using standard percentile charts designed for the average European Caucasian population. This is often the case for babies of Asian origin. Also, occasionally, it may be linked to poor diet and health where the mother, living in a different culture, finds it difficult to obtain food she would normally enjoy.[36]

Due to poor nourishment from the placenta, the fetus is unable to lay down any spare stores of fat or glycogen and, once born, the baby will have difficulty in maintaining temperature and blood glucose levels.

- Although the baby will be small, his or her organs will be mature, especially if it is near to term.
- If the baby is also preterm, then the problems will be compounded by immaturity of the main organs and, depending on its gestation, this baby will also be at risk of the complications of prematurity and will need to be managed as a preterm baby (→ see Management of the preterm baby, p. 742).

Poor fetal growth may indicate placental failure and, without intervention, the fetus may die. A Caesarean section may be carried out when the fetus reaches a viable age.[37]

## Growth restriction

Growth of a fetus is referred to as symmetrical or asymmetrical, and is diagnosed using ultrasound scanning, when various measurements are taken:

- Biparietal diameter
- Head circumference
- Limb lengths
- Abdominal circumference.[36]

*Asymmetrical babies*

- Are diagnosed later in pregnancy.
- They have a normal-sized head and brain for gestation. The brain has received sufficient nutrients to grow normally. Referred to as 'brain-sparing syndrome'.
- The abdominal circumference is small because of depleted fat and glycogen stores in the liver.
- These babies normally make up their growth in the first 2 years and do not appear to have any adverse effects in the long term.

*Symmetrical babies*

- Are diagnosed early in the pregnancy from the first scan.
- The head and abdominal circumference are decreased but in proportion.
- This situation is more serious as it indicates a longer period of time without nutrition to the brain and major organs, and the baby will be slow to make up for the deficiency after birth.
- As the baby will have missed out on the biologically timed periods of brain growth and development, the long-term prognosis is guarded as to their intellectual development.[36]

## Congenital abnormalities

SGA may also be associated with some congenital abnormalities, such as trisomies (where there is an extra chromosome), leading to conditions such as Down's and Edwards' syndromes.[37]

## Congenital infections

Babies with congenital infections tend to be small-for-dates.

- These infections are usually transferred to the baby from the mother.
- They are viral and are the only infections capable of crossing the placenta.
- They can affect placental function, leading to diminished growth.
- Exposure to these infections can also lead to early miscarriage and fetal abnormalities.
- Handling babies born with these infections also presents a risk to the midwives, nurses, medical staff, and family.
- The use of universal precautions is recommended for all personnel handling newborn babies.[38]

Taking the first letter from each name of an infection in this group spells out the word TORCH:

- *Toxoplasmosis*
- *Others* (chickenpox, measles)
- *Rubella*
- *Cytomegalovirus*
- *Herpes*.

*TORCH screening* is the test carried out on the placenta and blood to detect these infections.[35]

### Characteristics of a small-for-gestational-age baby

At birth, the baby:

- Will probably be active and wide awake
- Tends to look anxious and wizened
- Has a loud cry, possibly fuelled by hunger
- Has lax, dry, and cracked skin
- Has a flat or scaphoid abdomen, due to poor liver storage of glycogen and a lack of subcutaneous fat
- Has a dull, yellow, thin, and stretchy cord
- May be jittery, due to a low blood sugar
- Has an apparently large head, disproportional to the body size
- Is at increased risk of meconium aspiration:
  - Due to poor oxygenation through the placenta, the fetus may have become distressed and passed meconium before birth
  - The baby's skin may also be stained with old meconium.[36,37]

### Management at birth

Taking the above factors into consideration, management will depend on the gestation and condition of the baby at birth.

- If the baby is also premature (<37 weeks' gestation), it may need to be admitted to the NICU or SCBU where he or she will receive full support.
- Babies near to term may require intensive care if they have major problems, e.g. meconium aspiration. If this has occurred, the baby must be taken to the NICU to clear the meconium from the lungs and to administer a course of antibiotics.
- If no major problems are apparent, then the baby can be managed in a transitional care setting where he or she can be observed by the midwife but can be kept with or near to the parents.

If on examination major problems are ruled out, care will entail the management of:

- Temperature
- Glucose homeostasis
- Nutrition
- Prevention of infection
- Care of the family.

### Glucose homeostasis

SGA babies have long been identified to be at risk of hypoglycaemia, due to:
- High brain-to-body mass ratio, with a corresponding increase in glucose consumption
- Reduced fat stores
- Failure of counter-regulation (the process that ensures the availability of glucose and other fuels, regulated by glucagon and adrenaline)
- Delayed gluconeogenesis
- Hyperinsulinism.

Some evidence suggests that babies with abnormal metabolic adaptation have had abnormal end-diastolic flow velocities (EDVs) in the umbilical artery.[37]

Not all SGA babies are at risk of hypoglycaemia. Those at risk:
- Are below the third percentile in weight, which is a weight two standard deviations from the mean for gestation
- Have an increased head-circumference-to-body-weight ratio (disproportionate)
- Have abnormal artery Doppler flow velocity profiles.[39]

Frequent blood sampling is not necessary to identify those at risk. Laboratory measurements of cord blood glucose and blood glucose at 4–6h of age (before the second feed) are recommended.[40]

Each maternity unit will have its own protocol for identifying and treating babies at risk of hypoglycaemia, based on the recommendations from the WHO.[40]

### Prevention of hypoglycaemia
- Avoid excessive infusions of glucose to the mother during labour.
- Dry and warm the baby immediately to avoid heat loss due to evaporation, which increases energy demands.[40]
- Provide skin-to-skin contact for maintenance of the baby's core temperature.

### Early enteral feeding
- Start at a rate of 90mL/kg as 3h feeds, increasing by 30mL/kg daily.[39]
- Breast milk is preferred as it promotes ketogenesis.
- Blood glucose levels are lower in formula-fed babies due to the insulinogenic effects of the protein in formula milks.[40,41]

### Temperature control
- The baby may need to be nursed in an incubator if temperature maintenance is difficult or if the baby is premature or ill with other problems.
- If the baby is otherwise well, he or she can be cared for in a cot near the mother once feeding is established and the blood sugar level is maintained.
- The parents can be encouraged to give skin-to-skin care to help the baby to maintain their temperature. This also helps to stimulate the mother's lactation and promotes bonding between the baby and the parents as the father can also provide skin-to-skin care.

*Prevention of infection*
• The baby may have been exposed to congenital infection. Depending on the baby's condition, a TORCH screening at birth will confirm or eliminate such infection.
• The baby's skin may be in a poor condition. If it is dry, cracked, and stained with meconium, the baby will be at increased risk of infection.
• Close observation of the baby's condition will detect any changes that indicate a developing infection. If suspected, this will be treated following a full infection screening.
• Breast milk from the baby's mother will help to give the baby some protection *against* infection. Breast milk confers some immunity due to its high IgA content (➔ see Neonatal infection, p. 706).

**Follow-up**
• If the baby is well and able to maintain its temperature and blood glucose level, then he or she will be discharged home as soon as possible.
• Those who are premature or who have other problems will stay in the NICU/SCBU until they have recovered.
• There may be a need for follow-up to assess the baby's future development.

**Parental support**
• If the baby is ill at birth and needs care within the NICU/SCBU, then the parents will need the same level of support as discussed in ➔ Management of the preterm baby, p. 742. Where congenital abnormality is confirmed, the parents will be referred for genetic counselling.

**References**
35 World Health Organization (1992). *International Statistical Classification of Diseases and Related Health Problems, 10th revision*. Geneva: World Health Organization.
36 Meeks M, Hallsworth M, Yeo H (eds.) (2010). *Nursing the Neonate*, 2nd edn. Oxford: Blackwell, pp. 1–17.
37 Rennie JM (ed.) (2012). *Textbook of Neonatology*, 5th edn. London: Churchill Livingstone, pp. 133–40.
38 Department of Health (1990). *Guidance for Clinical Health-care Workers: Protection against Infection with HIV and Hepatitis Viruses: Recommendations of Expert Advisory Group on AIDS*. London: HMSO.
39 Hawdon JM, Ward-Platt MP (1993). Metabolic adaptation in small for gestational age infants. *Arch Dis Child* **68**, 262–8.
40 World Health Organization (1997). *Hypoglycaemia of the Newborn: Review of the Literature*. Geneva: World Health Organization.
41 Beresford D, Connolly G (2010). Fluid and electrolyte balance. In: Boxwell G, ed. *Neonatal Intensive Care Nursing*, 2nd edn. London: Routledge, pp. 255–76.

# Management of the preterm baby

## Definitions
- A preterm baby is any baby born before 37 completed weeks of gestation.[42]
- The legal age of viability is 24 weeks.[43]

These definitions indicate a wide range of babies between 24 and 37 weeks of gestation who will potentially need specialist management in a NICU or SCBU.

## Main aims of management
- To provide an appropriate environment where normal homeostasis can be maintained and where emergencies can be responded to in an appropriate way.
- To support the physical, developmental, psychological, and emotional welfare of the babies.
- To provide support for the families of babies nursed within these contexts.

As there is a vast difference in maturity between a baby of 24 weeks' gestation and a baby of 37 weeks' gestation, the care provided will be tailored to each individual baby's needs.
- As the baby approaches 34–37 weeks, there is less need for intensive or invasive care, and these babies will be treated as normal term infants, provided they do not have any other problems.
- Babies of 24–34 weeks will need specialist care, with the smaller, sickest babies needing intensive care from birth.

## Management and care
Initially most preterm babies will be nursed in an incubator for:
- Temperature control
- Humidity control
- Easier observation
- Oxygenation
- Barrier to infection
- Cutting down on handling.

### Ventilation and surfactant replacement
A baby of 30 weeks or less will require ventilation and surfactant replacement from birth, due to surfactant deficiency and immaturity of the lungs (➜ see Respiratory distress syndrome in the newborn, p. 748). The need for ventilation will be assessed according to the baby's gestation and condition at birth. The main aim is to prevent the baby's condition from becoming worse because of tiredness.

Several different methods of ventilation are available, which have been developed especially for use with premature babies.

*Different techniques of ventilation*

- *High-frequency oscillation ventilation (HFOV)* has been developed to cut down on the use of high-pressure ventilation, which can lead to long-term damage to the immature lungs. HFOV provides breaths or cycles of 240–3000/min. It facilitates the diffusion of gases and improves ventilation and perfusion matching. It is used where there is poor gas exchange, as in RDS that has not responded to conventional ventilation.
- *Continuous positive airway pressure (CPAP)* delivers a predetermined continuous pressure and supplemental oxygen into the airways of a spontaneously breathing infant. It splints the chest, preventing collapse of the alveoli on expiration and maintaining a residual capacity that will improve ventilation and perfusion.
- *Patient-triggered ventilation (PTV) and synchronous intermittent ventilation (SIMV)* have been developed to provide ventilator breaths that will coincide with the infant's own breathing pattern.
  - In PTV, the ventilator rate is controlled by the baby. Every time the baby's breath exceeds a critical level, the machine will deliver a breath. If the infant does not breathe within a predetermined period, the machine will deliver a breath. Every breath initiated by the baby will be ventilator-assisted.
  - SIMV can help to prevent the problems caused by asynchronous breathing. The ventilator breaths can be delivered to coincide with the baby's breathing. A total number of breaths are decided and any further breaths that the baby takes will be unsupported by the ventilator.
- *Nitric oxide.* Inhaled nitric oxide is used as treatment for persistent pulmonary hypertension following meconium aspiration, and in babies with severe RDS. It produces localized vasodilatation in the pulmonary circulation and is used when the baby is not responding to conventional treatment or HFOV.[44]

## Temperature and blood sugar

As well as management of babies' ventilation needs, management of their temperature and blood sugar levels is fundamental to their survival.

## Nutrition

Provision of nutrition can be difficult due to:
- Poorly developed sucking and swallowing reflexes
- A lack of coordination.

Tube and IV feeding. Total parenteral nutrition may be required.

*Minimal enteral nutrition* is a small amount of milk given continuously via a nasogastric tube which will help to mature the gut and prepare it for receiving full milk feeds when the baby has matured enough to tolerate feeding.

Once the baby improves, breastfeeding or bottle-feeding can be introduced. Breastfeeding, or the provision of expressed breast milk, is preferred as it has many benefits for the premature baby, especially for protection against infection and the prevention of NEC. It has also been shown to improve the longer-term development of the brain.[45]

## Physiological jaundice

This occurs because of an immature liver and will probably need treatment with phototherapy and/or exchange transfusions (➔ see Neonatal jaundice, p. 712).

## Preventing infection

The baby's immune system will be immature, resulting in an increased susceptibility to infection.
- Early recognition and treatment with antibiotics is important.
- If infection is suspected, carry out a full infection screen and commence the baby on a 10-day course of antibiotics (➔ see Antibiotic therapies and sensitivities, p. 710).
- Scrupulous handwashing and drying by staff and visitors has been proved to be the most effective way of reducing the risk of infection.[46]
- All equipment is sterilized and used only for one baby.
- Each baby has its own personal equipment for day-to-day care.

*Visiting policies*
- These are in place to protect the baby from too many visitors.
- Parents are encouraged to be with the baby at all times.
- Other visitors are allowed at the discretion of the parents.
- Special arrangements are made for siblings to visit with parental support.

## Observations

Make constant observations of:
- Colour/activity
- Temperature/respirations/BP and oxygen saturation
- Incubator and inspired oxygen humidity and temperature
- Fluid intake
- Ventilator settings and oxygen concentrations.

Record all of these hourly over a 24h period. It is important to keep an accurate record of events, as even the slightest change can be very significant in detecting the problem as early as possible.

## Physiotherapy and suction

Whilst the baby is on ventilation, this is carried out by specialist physiotherapists who prescribe a daily treatment for each baby following individual assessment of its requirements.

The physiotherapist will advise the nursing staff and parents about how to correctly position the baby according to his or her gestation and medical needs. This is often referred to as 'supported positioning'.

*Importance of supported positioning*
- The muscle tone of premature babies is poor and their movement is limited because of underdeveloped muscles.
- They tend to lie in a 'frog-like' posture with the limbs extended.
- Being left to lie for long periods of time without a position change can lead to long-term musculoskeletal and developmental problems.
- Several supported positions are used, including prone, supine, and lateral.[47]

- The prone position is considered to be the best for preterm babies who are being monitored, as it promotes oxygenation and energy conservation.[48,49]
- Once the baby is ready to go home, advise the parents to use the supine position, as advocated by the Department of Health campaign for the prevention of cot death.[50]

## Environment

Babies can be affected by constant exposure to:
- Noise
- Light
- Pain from invasive procedure
- Excessive handling
- Separation from their parents.

Much research has been done into the possible short- and longer-term effects that these factors have on the baby and how to soften the nursery environment by reducing levels of noise and light, and ways of assessing and reducing the discomfort and distress caused by painful procedures.

## The use of therapeutic touch

Premature babies have a poor tolerance to the excessive handling to which they are often subjected, but they have been shown to have a positive response to parental handling.

Baby massage techniques have been modified for use for premature ill babies. These have become an important way of helping the parents to become involved with their baby by providing a positive loving touch.[51]

## Parental needs

The application of family-centred care for parents with a baby in the NICU or SCBU presents a challenge for the nursing and medical staff. These parents:
- Have yet to get to know their baby, and they may be parents for the first time
- Have to develop their relationship with their new baby in a very public way, in an alien environment which is also influenced by input from a variety of nursing and medical personnel
- Are faced with separation, which is not normal for most parents with a new baby
- Require a constant stream of up-to-date information and reassurance about their baby's progress
- Need an honest and realistic prognosis, which is difficult at first and can alter drastically if the baby develops any problems
- Need facilities for rest, sleeping, food, and drinks
- Need open visiting and a gradual involvement with the decision-making as their understanding of their baby increases
- Need access to other medical personnel such as health visitors and social workers
- Need help to give the baby its care and to take on more as their confidence increases
- Need to involve the baby's siblings and the support of their wider family.

## References

42 World Health Organization (1992). *International Statistical Classification of Diseases and Related Health Problems, 10th revision.* Geneva: World Health Organization.

43 Roberton NRC (1993). Should we look after babies less than 800 grams? *Arch Dis Child* **68**: 326–9.

44 Cameron J (2001). Management of respiratory disorders. In: Boxwell G, ed. *Neonatal Intensive Care Nursing*, 2nd edn. London: Routledge, pp. 101–3.

45 Wheeler J, Chapman C (2000). Feeding outcomes and influences within the neonatal unit. *Int J Nurs Pract* **6**: 196–206.

46 Yeo H (ed.) (2000). *Nursing the Neonate*, 2nd edn. Oxford: Blackwell.

47 Downs J (1991). The effect of intervention on development of hip posture in very preterm babies. *Arch Dis Child* **66**: 797–801.

48 Heimler R, Langlois J, Hodel DJ, Nelin LD, Sasidharan P (1992). Effects on the breathing pattern of preterm infants. *Arch Dis Child* **67**: 312–14.

49 Turrill S (1992). Supported positioning in intensive care. *Paediatric Nursing* **4**: 24–7.

50 Department of Health (1991). *Sleeping Position and the Incidence of Cot Death.* London: HMSO.

51 Appleton S (1997). 'Handle with care': an investigation of handling received by preterm infants in intensive care. *J Neonatal Nurs* **3**: 23–7.

# Respiratory distress syndrome in the newborn

- RDS is one of the main causes of morbidity and mortality in preterm infants.
- The lungs of babies born at 28 weeks or less will be immature, having few alveoli and reduced surfactant production.[52]

## Surfactant

- A substance produced in the type 2 alveolar cells in the lungs.
- It is composed of 95% lipid and 5% protein. The lipid adsorbs rapidly to the air–water interface and is responsible for the majority of the surface-active properties of pulmonary surfactant.
- Surfactant coats the entire surface of the lung.
- It equalizes the surface tension.
- It prevents collapse of the alveoli when breathing out.
- It stabilizes the size of the alveoli.
- It is produced in the fetal lungs from 20 weeks' gestation.
- It is present in small amounts from 24 weeks' gestation.
- It increases steadily up to 34 weeks, when there is a surge in production to prepare for birth.

RDS occurs because of a deficiency of surfactant, which in turn causes atelectasis, and high pressures are needed to reinflate the lungs.

In preterm babies, the diaphragm and intercostal muscles are still developing, so that the baby's efforts to breathe will often be inadequate and the baby will soon become tired, needing mechanical support to help with breathing.[52]

The lack of surfactant leads to:
- Alveolar collapse on expiration.
- The alveolar walls are thickened due to them not being fully expanded on inspiration, which leads to a decreased amount of oxygen diffusing into the blood, which further leads to hypoxia.

▶ The associated hypoxia can cause:
- Right-to-left shunting through the foramen ovale
- Left-to-right shunting through the ductus arteriosus
- Failure to make the transition from intrauterine to extrauterine life
- Pulmonary ischaemia
- Further damage to the developing lungs.[52]

## Onset of respiratory distress syndrome

Usually within 4h of birth as the baby becomes increasingly tired.

## Signs of respiratory distress syndrome

- Grunting on expiration caused by the baby trying to force air past a partially closed glottis. This effort can keep air in the alveoli at the end of each breath and prevent atelectasis.
- Increased rate of breathing.

- Intercostal, sternal, and subclavicular recession where the soft tissues around the clavicles, ribs, and sternum are sucked in on inspiration (chin tug).
- Nasal flair.
- Chin tug: where the baby's chin is pulled downwards on inspiration. This is related to the effort of breathing and the need to suck in the soft tissues around the neck and the ribs (known as recession) because the baby is unable to fully expand its lungs on inspiration due to the lack of surfactant. The soft tissues fill the vacuum left by the unexpanded lungs and as everything is connected from the trachea to the diaphragm the chin is tugged downwards.
- Cyanosis.
- Apnoea.
- Diminished breath sounds because of poor air entry.[52]

## Diagnosis

- A chest X-ray 4h after birth shows a 'ground glass' effect of contrasting white and black areas.
- The black areas are alveoli which have air in them, due to the presence of surfactant, in contrast to the white areas, which are collapsed due to the lack of surfactant.
- A chest X-ray before this time would probably be normal but may be carried out to rule out other respiratory problems, e.g. infection, which will be apparent at an earlier time.
- Babies who develop RDS are usually premature of <34 weeks.
- RDS is also associated with:
  - Perinatal asphyxia due to hypoxia
  - Acidosis
  - Hypothermia (a temperature of <35°C decreases surfactant production and efficiency even further).
- Maternal diabetes suppresses surfactant production and there is a higher risk of intrapartum asphyxia due to the size of the baby. Babies of diabetic mothers tend to be larger than normal due to the maternal fluctuating blood sugar levels, which allows higher than normal levels of sugar to be transferred to the fetus via the placenta.[52]

## Treatments

Include:

- The administration of maternal steroids prior to the baby being born, in an attempt to initiate a stress response in the fetus, which will mature the fetal lungs, stimulating an increase in normal surfactant production
- Surfactant replacement therapy at birth
- Ventilation at birth if the baby is <30 weeks' gestation.[52]

### Surfactant replacement

Most preterm babies of 28 weeks' gestation or less will be given surfactant at birth in measured doses directly down the endotracheal tube into the lower trachea.

- Exogenous surfactant therapy has been shown to reduce the severity of RDS.
- Early administration is more effective than rescue treatment.
- Animal surfactants are more effective than synthetic ones in reducing the need for ventilation.[53,54]

*Curosurf®*

This is an animal-based surfactant made from pigs' lungs and is one of only two licensed for use in the UK for the treatment of surfactant-deficient RDS, the other being Survanta® from calves' lungs.

Curosurf® is expensive; a single-dose vial of 1.5mL costs £281. The 3mL vial costs £547.

- The dose is 100–200mg/kg (1.25–2.5mL/kg).
- The baby must be lying supine and flat.
- The vials need to be warmed immediately prior to use, as they will have been stored in the fridge.
- Apply the surfactant directly down the endotracheal tube.
- Give the baby 1min of ventilation using a Neopuff® ventilation system (➲ see Neonatal resuscitation, p. 556) to disperse the surfactant as far as possible into the lungs, then reconnect to the ventilator.
- Give further doses in the same manner.
- If the baby has a closed suction device attached, give the surfactant through a catheter passed via the suction port. The baby can remain connected to the ventilator during this procedure.
- Following administration, pulmonary compliance can improve rapidly, requiring prompt adjustment of the ventilator settings and inspired oxygen concentrations to avoid hyperoxia.
- Avoid suction for at least 4h after administration.[53,54]

## Prophylaxis

If the baby is deemed suitable for prophylaxis, the surfactant is given immediately and a chest X-ray is obtained as soon as possible.

The aim is to give the surfactant within the first 30min after birth if the baby is <26 weeks' gestation.

The criteria for prophylaxis are:
- Gestational age 28 weeks or less
- Ventilated
- Receiving supplementary oxygen >30%
- Clinical judgement that the baby is unlikely to wean rapidly from the ventilator
- Chest X-ray compatible with RDS.

The criteria for rescue treatment are:
- Ventilated
- X-ray diagnosis of RDS
- Inspired oxygen >40%
- $PaO_2$ <7kPa.[53,54]

## Nursing care

- *Incubator care* provides warmth, humidification, observation, oxygen therapy, protection from infection, and easy access.
- *Vital signs*: monitor hourly.
- *Temperatures* of incubator and inhaled gases: monitor hourly, along with the baby's temperature.
- *BP and blood gases*: monitor via an arterial line 4–6h, backed up by continuous saturation monitoring.
- *Blood sugar*: check whenever blood samples are taken.
- *Fluid intake/output*: record hourly and evaluate every 24h.
- *Nutritional requirements*: work these out daily. This usually involves IV infusion of 10% glucose, followed by total parenteral nutrition if the baby's condition is unstable. When the baby's condition improves, commence continuous gastric feeding with breast milk or formula milk as soon as possible.
- *Early initiation of feeding* is important to stimulate the premature gut and digestive hormones.
- *Minimal enteral nutrition* is used where feeding is delayed. It stimulates the gut with small amounts of milk given continuously via a nasogastric tube.
- *Chest physiotherapy and suctioning* are not necessary for the first 24h. Assess after this time and give according to individual needs.
- *Minimal handling* and the reduction of light and noise help to promote periods of rest.
- *Supported positioning* helps to achieve flexion and support in a variety of positions. The premature baby has immature and weak muscles and skeleton, and will therefore need help with support, to prevent the development of longer-term problems.
- *Care for the family*: encourage them to visit and care for the baby with help and support from the nursing and medical staff. Provide constant explanation and reassurance, as well as practical support, such as 'rooming in' and facilities for food and drinks. Involve all family members in support of the parents.[52]

## Recovery from respiratory distress syndrome

- Usually occurs between 48h and 72h after birth, as surfactant production increases and the need for ventilation decreases.
- A very preterm baby will require specialized care and mechanical ventilation for some weeks, due to other complications of prematurity.[52]

## References

52 Jollye S, Summers D (2010). Management of respiratory disorders. In: Boxwell G, ed. *Neonatal Intensive Care Nursing*, 2nd edn. London: Routledge, pp. 121–7.
53 Ainsworth SB (2004). Exogenous surfactant and neonatal lung disease: an update on the current situation. *J Neonatal Nurs* **10**: 6–11.
54 OSARIS Collaborative Group (1992). Early versus delayed administration of synthetic surfactant—the judgment of OSARIS. *Lancet* **340**: 1363–9.

# Respiratory problems in the newborn

Respiratory problems manifesting as respiratory distress are the common-est cause of admission of newborns to the neonatal unit in the perinatal period.[55]

Respiratory distress is a general term used to describe respiratory symptoms and is not synonymous with RDS[56] (➜ see Respiratory distress syndrome in the newborn, p. 748). Respiratory distress arises from:

- Inadequate *in utero* maturation of the lungs and the mechanisms controlling respiration
- Disease processes present before or after birth which compromise respiratory function[55]

The clinical signs of respiratory distress are:

- Tachypnoea: respiration rate >60 breaths/min.
- Expiratory grunt: the baby expires against a closed glottis, which helps to maintain a higher lung residual lung volume preventing alveolar collapse at the end of expiration, thus improving oxygenation
- Central cyanosis
- Chest recession which can be intercostal, lower costal, sternal, or subclavicular
- Nasal flaring and chin tug: these along with chest recession represent the baby's use of accessory respiratory muscles
- These may be superseded by apnoea or acute collapse.[56]

Additional signs may include:
- Cardiac murmurs
- Abnormal peripheral pulses
- Signs of cardiac failure which may also be present if there is an underlying congenital heart defect.[55]

## Diagnosis

If two or more of the symptoms persist for 4h or more, then respiratory distress is the likely cause and a diagnosis will be made following:

- A full clinical history.
- A physical examination, including:
  - Observation
  - Vital signs
  - Auscultation of the lungs for air entry, symmetry, and breath sounds.
- Palpation for dextrocardia and hepatomegaly.
- Appropriate investigations (➜ see Investigations, p. 753), including a chest X-ray.
- Perinatal history, including:
  - Gestational age
  - The presence of poly-/oligohydramnios
  - Anomalies on ultrasound
  - Risk factors for sepsis
  - The passage of meconium
  - Respiratory depression at birth
  - Duration of membrane rupture.[56]

## Investigations

- Pulse oximetry to measure the arterial saturations. This gives an indication of the severity of hypoxia and the urgency of intervention.
- Temperature to exclude hypothermia or hyperthermia.
- Blood glucose to exclude hypoglycaemia.
- Arterial blood gases to determine the degree of respiratory failure and to decide on appropriate interventions such as the need for assisted ventilation and supplementary oxygen. A persistent metabolic acidosis may lead to a diagnosis of a metabolic disorder (➜ see Metabolic disorders and the neonatal blood spot test, p. 722).
- Chest X-ray to rule out:
  - Pneumothorax
  - Effusions
  - Pulmonary oedema
  - Abnormal cardiac silhouette
  - Congenital diaphragmatic hernia
  - Bell-shaped chest as seen in neuromuscular disorders
  - A 'ground glass' appearance seen with idiopathic RDS, congenital pneumonia, or aspiration.
- An FBC to detect infection suggested by a high or low white cell count and thrombocytopenia.
- Full infection screen where infection is suspected.
- ECG and echocardiogram where congenital heart disease is suspected.[55]

The causes and management of respiratory distress vary depending on the gestation and chronological age of the baby. The management is determined by the underlying diagnosis.[55,56]

## Causes

These include:
- RDS:
  - Surfactant deficiency seen in premature babies with RDS (➜ see Management of the preterm baby, p. 742).
- Pneumothorax:
  - Pneumomediastinum
  - Pulmonary interstitial emphysema
  - Pleural effusions.
- Pulmonary haemorrhage following:
  - Asphyxia
  - Hypothermia
  - Rh disease
  - Left-sided heart failure.
- Transient tachypnoea of the newborn:
  - Retained or slow absorption of fetal lung fluid at birth.
- Infection:
  - Pneumonia
  - Septicaemia
  - Meningitis.

- Aspiration syndromes:
  - MAS
  - Milk
  - Blood.
- Pulmonary hypoplasia: Potter's syndrome (renal agenesis and diminished amniotic fluid (oligohydramnios) leads to a lack of lung fluid which prevents the development of the lungs).
- Surgical conditions:
  - Choanal atresia
  - Pierre Robin syndrome
  - Diaphragmatic hernia
  - Lobar emphysema
  - Oesophageal atresia with tracheo-oesophageal fistula.
- Following birth asphyxia.
- Persistent fetal circulation (persistent pulmonary hypertension of the newborn (PPHN)).
- Congenital heart abnormalities leading to heart failure:
  - Hypoplastic left heart syndrome
  - Obstructed total anomalous pulmonary venous drainage
  - Severe coarctation of the aorta.
- Congenital lung malformation: cystic adenomatoid formation.
- Congenital malformations:
  - Pulmonary lymphangiectasia
  - Pulmonary hypoplasia
  - Congenital nasolacrimal duct obstruction (congenital dacryocystocele).
- Congenital surfactant protein B deficiency.
- Cold stress.
- Hypoglycaemia.
- Anaemia.
- Polycythaemia.
- Cerebral damage.
- Neuromuscular disorders:
  - Spinal muscular atrophy type 1
  - Myotonic dystrophy.
- Inherited metabolic disease (➔ see Metabolic disorders and the neonatal blood spot test, p. 722).
- Maternal drugs (e.g. opiates).
- Chronic causes of respiratory distress:
  - Bronchopulmonary dysplasia
  - Wilson–Mikity syndrome
  - Chronic pulmonary insufficiency of prematurity.[55,56]

## Management

The aims of management are to identify the underlying cause and to provide supportive care with appropriate interventions. The care needed is similar regardless of the aetiology.[55,56]

- Correct acid–base balance.
- Alleviate hypoxaemia and respiratory failure.
- Warm cold babies (➔ see Neonatal temperature control, p. 696).
- Correct hypoglycaemia.
- Give supplemental oxygen if needed.

- Intubate and give surfactant to premature babies with RDS (➔ see Respiratory distress syndrome in the newborn, p. 748).
- Provide mechanical ventilation or CPAP where necessary based on the blood gas results (➔ see Management of the preterm baby, p. 742).
- Site an arterial line for blood gas monitoring.
- Observe for the signs of infection and treat with broad-spectrum antibiotics (➔ see Neonatal infection, p. 706).
- Observe for the signs of pneumothoraces and effusions and provide drainage procedures.
- Chest and abdominal X-rays to monitor effectiveness of treatments and progress.
- Babies with congenital heart abnormalities requiring surgery need to be transferred to a specialist cardiac surgical unit as soon as they are stabilized.
- Babies with other abnormalities which require surgery need to be stabilized and transferred into a unit specializing in surgery.
- Provide appropriate fluids and nutrition.
  - IV infusion of 10% glucose for the first 24h during initial stabilization and assessment of the condition.
  - IV infusion of total parenteral nutrition may be used from 18h if the baby is very unstable or if there is an underlying abnormality which requires surgery.
  - If the condition stabilizes and does not require surgery, then early enteral nutrition via a nasogastric tube is recommended, preferably with expressed breast milk, especially if the baby is premature.
- Continuous monitoring and recording at regular intervals of:
  - Temperature
  - BP
  - Heart and breathing rates
  - Blood gases:
    - —Umbilical or radial arterial samples
    - —Pulse oximetry
    - —Transcutaneous $pO_2$ and $pCO_2$
  - Oxygen needs
  - Ventilation requirements
  - Fluid intake and output.
- Incubator care provides:
  - Thermal stability
  - Warmth and humidity
  - Administration of oxygen
  - Observation
  - Isolation
  - Protection from excessive handling.[55,56]

The parents will need to be given support and an explanation of the condition and treatment required. They will also need to be with or near to their baby during transfer and admission to the neonatal or surgical unit (➔ see Management of the preterm baby, p. 742).

## References

55 Mupanemunda RH, Watkinson M (2004). Key Topics in Neonatology, 2nd edn. Oxford: Bios Scientific.
56 Sinha S, Miall L (2012). Essentials Neonatal Medicine, 5th edn. London: Wiley Blackwell.

## Neonatal abstinence syndrome

- Neonatal abstinence syndrome results from prenatal exposure to opioids such as the morphine derivative heroin.
- Specific receptors in the CNS are associated with neurotransmitters called endorphins and encephalins, which are sometimes referred to as endogenous opioids, as they are produced naturally in the brain and activate analgesia. Long-term exposure to opioid drugs results in adaptation of these receptors, leading to tolerance.
- Physical dependence occurs as the CNS adapts and larger amounts of the drug are required to achieve the same physiological effects.
- Following birth, the baby is no longer exposed to maternal levels of the drug and therefore shows acute withdrawal. Physical symptoms are experienced, as the naturally occurring opioids have been suppressed.[57]
- The onset, duration, and severity of symptoms vary according to type of drug, length of the mother's dependency, timing and amount of the mother's last dose before birth, clearance of the drug by the baby, and his or her gestational age.[57]
- The symptoms are less severe if the mother has been on a methadone substitution programme during the pregnancy.[57]

### Common symptoms

Typically the symptoms involve the CNS and the respiratory, gastrointestinal, and vasomotor systems:

- Hyperactivity and hyperirritability
- High-pitched cry
- Increased muscle tone
- Exaggerated reflexes
- Tremors
- Hiccups and yawning
- Disorganized vigorous sucking, hyperphagia (wanting to feed very frequently)
- Vomiting/posseting
- Diarrhoea
- Drooling
- Excess secretions and stuffy nose
- Flushing of the skin and sweating.[57]

### Principles of care

- Withdrawal symptoms may appear between 24h and 3 weeks after the birth.
- A social model of care following birth, where mothers and babies can be cared for together on the postnatal wards, even if babies require medical support for neonatal abstinence syndrome, has been advocated. By following this model:
  - Mothers are encouraged to develop appropriate parenting skills
  - They receive support from midwives
  - They are not separated from their babies.

- ▶ Breastfeeding is not contraindicated as it aids the withdrawal process.
- Soothing interactions can help with some of the more distressing symptoms:
  - Cuddle the baby
  - Keep the baby wrapped up
  - Avoid overstimulation
  - Keep the baby in a quiet environment.
- Feed the baby slowly, with small, frequent amounts, allowing rest periods between feeds. This helps to overcome gastrointestinal symptoms.
- Medication may be required to relieve and control symptoms.
- Assess the baby's status regularly (2–3 times daily) and monitor the mother–baby interaction and bonding. Record-keeping is vital as this information is used to plan follow-up care.
  - Use score charts to monitor symptoms and their control. Some units have adapted or designed their own.
- The length of hospital stay will depend on the severity of withdrawal and the baby's response to interventions.
- The multidisciplinary team will decide whether the mother and baby go home together and whether the mother is adequately prepared and supported.
- The mother and baby will continue to receive extra support once transferred home. Care is coordinated between social services, the health visitor, and the community midwife.
- Child protection may be an issue and must be considered by the midwife (for further details, ➔ see Safeguarding children, p. 758).

## Reference

57 NHS Forth Valley (2011). *Management of neonatal abstinence syndrome*. NHS Forth Valley. Available at: ℘ www.nhsforthvalley.com/__documents/qi/ce_guideline_wcdneonatal/neonatalabstinencesyndrome.pdf.

## Further reading

Winklbaur AB, Jaqsch R, Peternell A, *et al.* (2007). Management of neonatal abstinence syndrome in neonates born to opioid maintained women. *Drug Alcohol Depend* 87: 131–8.

# Safeguarding children

### Definitions

- A number of terms are commonly used, i.e. child abuse (now outdated), child protection, safeguarding children, and children in need. 'Safeguarding children' is now the term used to cover all aspects.
- Legislation and guidance referred to here is that currently operating in the UK.
- The Children Act (2004) is an amendment of the Children Act (1989), largely as a result of the Victoria Climbié inquiry, to give boundaries and help for local authorities to better regulate official intervention in the interests of children. The Act also made changes to the laws pertaining to children, notably on adoption agencies, foster homes, babysitting services, and the handling of child-related crimes and crimes against children.
- A child is defined as a person <18 years (Children Act 1989). However, it is important to remember that a married woman >16 but <18 is not regarded as a child.
- In current British law, an individual has no legal entity until the moment of birth, i.e. the fetus has no legal rights. This is not the case in all parts of the world.

Safeguarding children is a complex topic and general principles are given here for guidance.[58]

- ▶The guiding principle in any consideration of the child's needs is that their welfare and interests are paramount. In other words, the current and future quality and safety of the child's physical, emotional, psychological, and cultural upbringing must be central to any decisions that may be made in this respect by a court.
- ▶ As a midwife, you must ensure personal familiarity with your national legislation and resulting local policies, procedures, and guidance in the child protection process, and update your understanding regularly.
- In the UK, each NHS trust has a specialist named nurse and midwife, who can be consulted and must be involved in all stages of child protection procedures, for specialist support, guidance, and leadership. A named midwife, usually the head of midwifery, is the named Midwife for Safeguarding Children within the local maternity service and must also be consulted and involved at all stages of the procedure in individual cases. Any midwife dealing with an established safeguarding children situation or who has concerns about any child's safety must make that concern known to these people in the first instance.
- A key, valuable role in safeguarding children situations is that of the SoM and the LSAMO in supporting the midwife and facilitating a system of tracing mothers of 'at-risk' newborn babies.
- The Local Safeguarding Children Board (LSCB) has overall responsibility for managing the interagency functioning, developing policies and procedures at senior management level, identifying training needs, and conducting reviews of difficult cases or where a child dies as a result of abuse or neglect in their area. The LSCB maintains the local child protection register.

## Key features of the Children Act

- A universal duty to promote and safeguard the welfare of the child. The child's welfare is paramount in all decisions made.
- Children are brought up with their own family, and local authorities have a duty to support and facilitate this, wherever possible.
- Wherever possible, professionals should work in partnership with parents, involving them in the care and decisions made about their children.
- The race, religion, culture, and language of the child are to be taken into account in the provision of services.
- Intervention by the statutory services should occur when it is in the child's best interest, and legal measures are only used as a last resort.
- The wishes and feelings of the child should be sought (depending on his/her age and level of understanding) and taken into account when decisions are made about his/her future.

## The midwife's role

- Current guidance requires all relevant agencies to work together with children and families. Midwives have a central role in this process, ensuring that the parents and families are involved in discussions and in the preparations for the care of the newborn baby.
- The midwife has an accepted role within society with pregnant mothers, their families, and their newborn babies, and will frequently undertake an advocacy role to support the parent(s) and baby, giving additional parenting education support, as necessary. In the case of teenage mothers, both the mother and her baby, and possibly the baby's father, may be regarded as children in need and require services in their own right.
- Within the multi-professional context, the midwife contributes significantly to the assessment, planning, and intervention required, particularly in pre-birth assessments and post-birth care, in terms of the child's development needs, parenting capacity, and family and environmental factors. The close contact with the mother, including home visiting, places the midwife in the ideal situation to be aware of the care of the newborn and other children in the family, conditions in the home, parenting, lifestyle, and injuries to the mother or children.
- A midwife working in an independent capacity should know how to seek advice, support, and training and should consult her SoM for guidance.

## Pre-birth assessment

Examples of issues that may trigger a pre-birth assessment or a referral to social services are:

- Young and vulnerable mothers who have no support mechanism—a girl herself 'in need', looked after by the local authority, recently left local authority care, or subject to a Care Order
- Extreme poverty or inadequate housing
- Social exclusion
- A mother with physical or learning disability, making it difficult for her to care for her baby

- Concern about the mental health of the mother or an adult likely to have care of the child
- Substance abuse: persistent use of illegal drugs or alcohol by the mother or within her environment
- The mother lives with, or has frequent social contact with, someone who has been convicted of an offence against children
- Families where a child has previously been placed on the child protection register
- Pregnancy as a result of rape.

**Making a referral**

You should identify vulnerable children and decide whether to refer them to social services for assessment, consulting the SoM and named midwife (safeguarding children) before taking any action.

**Assessment of risk and significant harm**

- Significant harm is defined in the Children Act (1989) as 'ill treatment or impairment of health or development'. Abuse and neglect are considered under the following categories:
  - Physical abuse
  - Emotional abuse
  - Sexual abuse
  - Neglect.
- The local authority has a duty to make enquiries, to decide whether or not any action to promote or safeguard the child's welfare is required. Each case is assessed individually. The decision as to whether or not the harm is significant is judged against what is reasonably expected for a child. A range of factors is considered and legal advice will normally be sought when the assessment determines that there is significant risk.
- Assessment is child-centred, so that the impact of parenting capacity, the family, and the environment on the child can be clearly identified. A quarter of the reasons identified refer to the child, whereas more than half relate to factors in respect of the parents.

**Emergency Protection Order (EPO)**

Section 44 of the Children Act (1989) allows emergency action if there is reasonable cause to believe that a child is likely to suffer harm unless the child is removed to other accommodation.

In respect of young babies, an EPO may be applied for at birth if there are concerns that the parent will remove the child. This usually applies when the baby is subject to *Safeguarding Children* proceedings and the parent(s) are threatening to remove the child.

Other powers allow the perpetrator to be removed from the home/baby's environment through an Exclusion Order attached to an EPO, or an Interim Care Order.

## Female genital mutilation

FGM has been illegal in the UK since 1985. The possibility of FGM is a legitimate reason for safeguarding children investigation and proceedings, as it constitutes physical injury and abuse and can take place any time from 1 week after birth to 12 years of age.

It can provide evidence for an EPO or a Care Order.

In 2015, it became a legal requirement in the UK for a midwife to report every case of FGM to the police.[59,60]

## Practice points

- The safety and welfare of the child are paramount.
- The Children Act protects the rights of children within society and provides the protection of children at risk.
- ▶ You must be aware of the context of working with vulnerable families and the impact on practice.
- You have a crucial and integral role in the interprofessional team, notably in pre-birth and post-birth assessments.
- ▶ Always seek guidance and support from the named professional nurse and midwife for child protection whenever dealing with actual or possible cases.
- Comply with the 2015 legislation requiring notification of all cases of FGM encountered in professional practice.[59,60]

## References

58 Department of Health (2015). *Working together to safeguard children*. Available at: ℬ www.gov. uk/government/uploads/system/uploads/attachment_data/file/419595/Working_Together_ to_Safeguard_Children.pdf.
59 Nursing and Midwifery Council (2015). *Additional information on female genital mutilation cases*. Available at: ℬ www.nmc.org.uk/standards/code/female-genital-mutilation-cases/.
60 Department of Health (2015). *Female genital mutilation (FGM)*. *Mandatory reporting duty*. Available at: ℬ www.gov.uk/government/uploads/system/uploads/attachment_data/file/472691/ FGM_guidance.pdf.

# Part 7
# Feeding

# Breastfeeding

# The Baby Friendly Initiative standards

The Baby Friendly Initiative (BFI) is a worldwide programme of the WHO and UNICEF. Its aim is to improve standards of care for breastfeeding within health-care settings. The UNICEF UK BFI has developed new standards for health-care settings which incorporate the previous standards specified in the 'Ten Steps to Successful Breastfeeding' and the 'Seven Point Plan for sustaining breastfeeding in the community'.[1]

## The Baby Friendly Initiative standards

*Stage 1: building a firm foundation*

- Have written policies and guidelines to support the standards.
- Plan an education programme that will allow staff to implement the standards according to their role.
- Have processes for implementing, auditing, and evaluating the standards.
- Ensure that there is no promotion of breast milk substitutes, bottles, teats, or dummies in any part of the facility or by any of the staff.

*Stage 2: an educated workforce*

- Educate staff to implement the standards according to their role and the service provided.

*Stage 3: parents' experiences of maternity services*

- Support pregnant women to recognize the importance of breastfeeding and early relationships for the health and well-being of their baby.
- Support all mothers and babies to initiate a close relationship and feeding soon after birth.
- Enable mothers to get breastfeeding off to a good start.
- Support mothers to make informed decisions regarding the introduction of food or fluids other than breast milk.
- Support parents to have a close and loving relationship with their baby.

*Parents' experiences of neonatal units*

- Support parents to have a close and loving relationship with their baby.
- Enable babies to receive breast milk and to breastfeed when possible.
- Value parents as partners in care.

*Parents' experiences of health visiting/public health nursing services*

- Support pregnant women to recognize the importance of breastfeeding and early relationships for the health and well-being of their baby.
- Enable mothers to continue breastfeeding for as long as they wish.
- Support mothers to make informed decisions regarding the introduction of food or fluids other than breast milk.
- Support parents to have a close and loving relationship with their baby.

*Parents' experiences of children's centres or equivalent early-years settings in Wales, Scotland, and Northern Ireland*

- Support pregnant women to recognize the importance of breastfeeding and early relationships for the health and well-being of their baby.
- Protect and support breastfeeding in all areas of the service.
- Support parents to have a close and loving relationship with their baby.

Full guidelines for the standards can be found at: ℰ www.unicef.org.uk/Documents/Baby_Friendly/Guidance/Baby_Friendly_guidance_2012.pdf.

## The UNICEF UK Baby Friendly Initiative University Standards programme

This is an accreditation programme aimed at university departments responsible for midwifery and health visitor/public health nurse education.

The purpose of the programme is to ensure that newly qualified midwives and health visitors are equipped with the knowledge and skills needed to support breastfeeding effectively. Accreditation is awarded to an individual course, not to the institution itself. Higher education institutions (HEIs) can apply for accreditation for each of the courses they provide for the training of midwives or health visitors/public health nurses.

Full guidelines for the standards can be found at: ℰ www.unicef.org.uk/BabyFriendly/Health-Professionals/going-baby-friendly/University/Old-standards/University-best-practice-standards/.

## Reference

1 UNICEF UK (2012). *Guide to the Baby Friendly Initiative Standards*. Available at: ℰ www.unicef.org.uk/Documents/Baby_Friendly/Guidance/Baby_Friendly_guidance_2012.pdf.

# Advantages of breastfeeding

An ever-increasing amount of quality research has demonstrated the advantages of breastfeeding for both the infant and mother.[2,3]

Advantages for the infant include:
- Optimal nutrition
- Reduced risk of mortality from NEC and sudden infant death
- Reduced infection: gastrointestinal, respiratory, urinary tract, ear, meningitis, intractable diarrhoea
- Reduced atopic disease: eczema, asthma
- Optimal brain development
- Reduced risk of autoimmune disease
- Enhanced immunity
- Reduction in childhood obesity.

Advantages for the mother include:
- Convenience, cost, and lack of contamination
- Reduced risk of maternal breast and ovarian cancer
- Reduced risk of hip fractures in women over 65
- Losing pregnancy weight gain if feeding for 6 months or longer.

For the infant, breastfeeding also may have positive effects on:
- Interpersonal relationships and sleep patterns[4]
- Reduced crying if they stay close to the mothers and breastfeed from birth.[5]

→ See also Health risks associated with formula feeding, p. 838.

## References

2  Horta BL, Bahl R, Martines JC, Victora CG (2007). *Evidence on the long-term effects of breast-feeding: systematic review and meta-analyses.* Available at: ℛ apps.who.int/iris/bitstream/10665/43623/1/9789241595230_eng.pdf.

3  The Baby Friendly Initiative (2015). *Breastfeeding research—an overview.* Available at: ℛ www.unicef.org.uk/BabyFriendly/News-and-Research/Research/Breastfeeding-research—An-overview/.

4  The Baby Friendly Initiative (2015). *Health benefits of breastfeeding.* Available at: ℛ www.unicef.org.uk/BabyFriendly/About-Baby-Friendly/Breastfeeding-in-the-UK/Health-benefits/.

5  Christensson K, Winberg J (1995). Separation distress call in the human neonate in the absence of maternal body contact. *Acta Pediatrica* **84**: 468–73.

# Constituents of breast milk

## Colostrum
- Provides complete nutrition for the healthy term baby until lactation is established, provided frequent feeds are offered and supplements are not considered medically necessary.
- Produced in the first 3 days after delivery.
- Volume: 2–10mL daily.
- Transparent and yellow, due to high β-carotene content.
- Easily digested and absorbed.
- Energy content: 58kcal/100mL.
- Rich in immunoglobulins responsible for passive immunity.
- Contains higher levels of protein and vitamins A and K than mature milk.
- Contains lower levels of sugar and fat than mature milk.
- The presence of lacto bifidus factor provides favourable (acidic) conditions, which encourage colonization of the infant's gut with the beneficial microbe *Lactobacillus bifidus*.
- Stimulates the passage of meconium.

## Breast milk
Breast milk is a complex fluid that contains above 200 known constituents[6] and changes to meet the needs of the infant from:
- Colostrum to transitional, then mature milk
- The beginning to the end of the feed
- Morning to evening.[7]

### Nutritional composition
- *Carbohydrate*: the main type being lactose, a disaccharide.
- *Fat*: the most variable constituent. Provides 50% of the energy supplied by breast milk. Linoleic and linolenic acids are converted into long-chain polyunsaturated fatty acids, which are essential for the development of the nervous system.
- *Protein*: in the form of whey protein, required for growth and energy. Consists of anti-infective factors, including lactalbumin, immunoglobulins, lactoferrin, lysozyme and other enzymes, hormones, and growth factors.[8]
- *Non-protein nitrogens*: the three most important are taurine, nucleotides, and carnitine. Taurine is important for bile acid conjugation and brain and retinal development.[7] Nucleotides are important for the function of cell membranes and for normal development of the brain.[7] Carnitine plays an important part in lipid metabolism and is thought to be important in thermogenesis and nitrogen metabolism.[9]
- *Minerals and trace elements*: the major ones are sodium, calcium, phosphorus, magnesium, zinc, copper, and iron. The quantities and ratios of these elements are species-specific; human and cow's milk differ significantly.

- *Vitamins*: human milk contains all the vitamins required for a term neonate, with the possible exception of vitamins D and K.
- *Enzymes*: breast milk contains at least 70 enzymes which contribute to digestion and development. Possibly the two most important are amylase and lipase.[8] Their presence in breast milk compensates for the limited pancreatic amylase and lipase activity in the newborn and therefore aids digestion.

For a comprehensive breakdown of the composition of breast milk, ➔ see References.[9]

*Immunological properties of breast milk*

Human milk also has a non-nutritive protective role for the infant and also for protecting the breasts from infection. Important constituents are as follows.

- *Immunoglobulins*: IgA, IgG, IgM, IgD, and IgE, which are active against specific organisms, e.g. *Salmonella* spp. and poliovirus.
- *Cells*: B lymphocytes, T lymphocytes, macrophages, and neutrophils. The actions of these cells include:
  - Production of antibodies against specific microbes
  - Killing of infected cells
  - Production of lysozyme and activation of the immune system
  - Phagocytosis of bacteria.
- *Lacto bifidus factor*: promotes an acidic environment suitable for the growth of *Lactobacillus bifidus* and inhibits the growth of pathogenic organisms.
- *Lactoferrin*: reduces iron availability for bacterial growth by binding to iron. It also acts as a bacteriostatic agent.
- *Binding proteins*: increase the absorption of nutrients, therefore reducing those available to be utilized by bacteria.
- Complement, lipids, fibronectin, gamma-interferon, mucins, oligosaccharides, bile salt-stimulated lipase, epidermal growth factor, and many more.[9]

The immunological properties of breast milk are increased with better maternal nutrition.[10]

## References

6 Jessen RG (ed.) (1995). *Handbook of Milk Composition*. London: Academic Press Inc.

7 Inch S (2014). Infant feeding. In: Marshall J, Raynor M, eds. *Myles Textbook for Midwives*, 16th edn. Edinburgh: Churchill Livingstone, pp. 703–36.

8 Czank C, Mitoulas LR, Hartmann PE (2007). Human milk composition—nitrogen and energy content. In: Hale TW, Hartmann PE, eds. *Textbook of Human Lactation*. Amarillo, TX: Hale Publishing LP, pp. 75–88.

9 Coad J (2011). *Anatomy and Physiology for Midwives*, 3rd edn. Edinburgh: Mosby.

10 Chang SJ (1990). Antimicrobial proteins of maternal and cord sera and human milk in relation to maternal nutritional status. *Am J Clin Nutr* 51: 183–7.

# Changes in the anatomy of the breast

The structure of the lactating breast was originally based on the interpretation of Cooper's detailed dissections in 1840. However, research by Ramsey et al. (2005) which was based on the results of ultrasound examination of the breasts of 21 lactating women highlighted the differences seen in Table 28.1.[11]

**Table 28.1** Differences between the classical anatomy of the breast and that of Ramsey et al. (2005)

| Classical | Ramsey et al. (2005) |
| --- | --- |
| Lobes approximately 20 | Lobes 8–12 |
| Ampulla/lactiferous sinuses present | No discernible lactiferous sinuses |
| Compression of the ampulla aids milk ejection | Lactiferous ducts near to the nipple branch, can be very small and compressible |
| | Ducts lined by contractile cells which open ducts widely to assist milk flow |

These differences, the lower number of patent ducts, superficial and compressible ducts that lack lactiferous sinuses, and ducts that do not store a large amount of milk impact upon our understanding of the process of lactation.

## Reference

11 Ramsey DT, Kent JC, Hartmann RA, Hartmann PE (2005). Anatomy of the lactating human breast redefined with ultrasound imaging. J Anat 206: 525–34.

# Contraindications to breastfeeding

- *Drugs.* Most drugs will pass into breast milk in a greater or lesser degree. The majority of drugs can be taken safely, but there are some drugs where breastfeeding is contraindicated.
- *Cancer.* Anticancer treatments are normally highly toxic and will make it impossible to breastfeed without harming the baby. The mother could, if she wishes, express and discard her milk for the duration of treatment and resume breastfeeding later. If the mother has had a mastectomy, she may successfully breastfeed from the other breast. If the mother has had a lumpectomy, she should seek advice from her surgeon as she may be able to feed from the treated breast.
- *Breast surgery.* Breast reduction and augmentation are not contraindications to breastfeeding, but this depends upon the surgical techniques used. Advice should be sought from the surgeon. Following unilateral mastectomy, it is perfectly possible to breastfeed using the other breast.
- *Breast injury.* Serious damage caused by burns and accidents may have caused scarring that makes breastfeeding impossible.
- *HIV infection.* HIV may be transmitted in breast milk.
  - Current WHO recommendations[12] are that when breast milk substitutes are acceptable, feasible, affordable, sustainable, and safe, then mothers should be advised not to breastfeed. Therefore, in the UK, mothers would be advised against breastfeeding.[13]
  - In developing countries or in countries where artificial feeding is a significant cause of infant mortality, exclusive breastfeeding may be less of a risk.
- Human T-cell lymphotropic virus (HTLV) type 1- or 2-positive mothers and in mothers who have herpes simplex lesions on the breast.[14] These mothers should be advised not to breastfeed.

## References

12 World Health Organization (2010). *Guidelines on HIV and infant feeding 2010: principles and recommendations for infant feeding in the context of HIV and a summary of evidence.* Available at: ℛ www.who.int/child_adolescent_health/documents/9789241599535/en/index.html.
13 BHIVA/CHIVA Writing Group on Infant Feeding in the UK (2014). *British HIV Association (BHIVA) and Children's HIV Association (CHIVA) position statement on infant feeding in the UK.* Available at: ℛ www.chiva.org.uk/files/3614/2900/9349/InfantFeeding.pdf.
14 ESPGHAN Committee on Nutrition, Agostoni C, Braegger C, Decsi T, et al. (2009). Breast-feeding: a commentary by the ESPGHAN Committee on Nutrition. *J Pediatr Gastroenterol Nutr* 49: 112–25.

# Preparation for infant feeding

All pregnant women should be informed about the benefits and management of breastfeeding.[15]
- Recording a woman's feeding intention at booking is questionable because:
  - She may feel that she cannot change this decision at a later date
  - Subsequent discussion may be more difficult if she has stated an intention to bottle-feed
  - Discussing breastfeeding when a woman has stated an intention to bottle-feed may seem unnecessary.

## Preparation for breastfeeding

No special care of the breasts is required in preparation for breastfeeding, but the following may be helpful:
- Bathing in the normal way is all that is necessary to keep the breasts and nipples clean
- Using soap may cause irritation as it removes the natural antiseptic lubricants (sebum) secreted from the Montgomery's tubercles
- It is useful to learn the skill of hand expression in the last month of pregnancy
- All women and their partners should have the opportunity to discuss breastfeeding during the antenatal period
- All women and their partners should have the opportunity to attend antenatal education classes/workshops related to breastfeeding.

## Preparation for artificial feeding, i.e. with infant formulas

If a mother has chosen to artificially feed her infant, the midwife should support her, but it is important to ensure that the mother has made an informed choice and is aware of the benefits of breastfeeding both for the baby and for herself.

Women should not receive instruction on how to make up bottles of infant formula as part of their antenatal group sessions; however, they should:
- Have the opportunity to discuss infant feeding individually with a health professional[16]
- Receive information and instruction on how to make up bottles,[16] if required, on a one-to-one basis or one-to-two basis with an appropriately trained health professional
- Receive information and instruction on how to sterilize equipment used in the preparation of infant feeds
- Receive information on artificial feeding, e.g. the different types of formulas.

## References

15 UNICEF UK (2012). *Guide to The Baby Friendly Initiative Standards*. London: UNICEF UK Baby Friendly Initiative.
16 National Institute for Health and Care Excellence (2006). *Routine postnatal care of women and their babies*. NICE guidelines CG37. Available at: ℜ www.nice.org.uk/guidance/cg37/evidence/full-guideline-485782237.

# Management of breastfeeding

### Initiation of breastfeeding

All mothers should '*have skin-to-skin contact with their baby after birth, at least until after the first feed and for as long as they wish. All mothers are encouraged to offer the first feed in skin contact when the baby shows signs of readiness to feed*'.[17]

The need to suckle is common to all mammalian young and the human baby is no different. If the mother and baby are given a peaceful, unhurried environment and the baby is placed on the mother's abdomen following delivery, it will crawl to the breast and initiate suckling.[18] This is termed 'breast crawl' (➔ see Breast crawl and skin-to-skin, p. 378) and has a positive effect on the initiation and duration of breastfeeding.

### Skin-to-skin contact
- Initiate as soon as possible after birth.
- Place the naked, dried baby against their mother's skin.
- Place a blanket around them both to ensure neither becomes cold.
- Very small babies may also need a hat.
- If the mother so wishes, place the baby inside her nightgown.
- Provide a calm, unhurried atmosphere.
- Ensure that the mother and baby are uninterrupted during this time.
- Skin-to-skin contact should last until after the first breastfeed or until the mother chooses to end it.[17]

The midwife is responsible for ensuring that the mother and infant have a successful first feed. It is also their responsibility to provide information about breastfeeding, although the timing of this should be decided on an individual basis.

### Positioning and attachment

Before commencing a feed, the comfort of the mother should be ensured. Talk the mother through the process as far as possible, to help develop her confidence and ability in breastfeeding. For the infant to suckle successfully at the breast, two processes need to be correct. These are positioning and attachment.

#### Positioning of the baby at the breast
Correct positioning is the secret of successful breastfeeding. Good positioning will enable the baby to achieve and maintain attachment at the breast. This, in turn, will enable the baby to feed effectively for as long as he or she needs. Good positioning is fundamental to successful breastfeeding and the prevention of problems. The mother should position the baby at the breast, although some mothers may need guidance.

#### Principles of effective positioning
- The baby's head and body should be in a straight line.
- The mother should hold the baby's body close to hers. 'Tummy to mummy' may not be the appropriate position for all babies, as this will depend upon the shape and size of the mother's breasts.

- The baby should face the breast with the nose opposite the nipple.
- The position should be sustainable for both the mother and the baby.

Support may sometimes be required to assist good positioning. This may be in the form of cushions to support a comfortable position for the mother or to raise the baby to the level of the breast.

The following should be avoided:

- Holding the back of the baby's head—this will cause the baby to push their head backwards away from the breast
- Holding the breast away from the baby's nose—this can disturb the attachment and also prevent drainage from some lobes of the breast
- Holding the baby in a bottle-feeding position—this necessitates the baby to turn their head, which can cause friction to the nipple
- Taking the breast down to the baby rather than bringing the baby to the breast—this alters the shape of the breast and can cause problems, including ineffective suckling by the baby and backache for the mother.

*Biological nurturing*

This is a new, non-prescriptive mother-centred breastfeeding approach that refers to a range of semi-reclined maternal breastfeeding postures and innate feeding behaviours.[19] The positions used are similar to those used in skin-to-skin contact. The baby is held instinctively and cuddled in a natural way. This can be done with the baby held longways, sideways, or slanting. The baby always has close contact with the breast and can have unrestricted access to the breast for feeding. This is a useful approach for many mothers and especially those encountering problems with latching on. The BFI recommends that those working towards BFI accreditation should inform themselves about biological nurturing and look for ways to incorporate this information within a framework of care that provides women with a range of skills to enable them to adapt their breastfeeding to a variety of situations.[20]

*Attachment of the baby at the breast*

Attachment is the term used to describe how the baby's mouth fits around the mother's nipple and areola to suckle at the breast.

The three main reflexes required for a baby to attach effectively are:

- Rooting reflex
- Sucking reflex
- Swallowing reflex.

If any of these reflexes is absent, the baby will not be able to attach and feed effectively. Premature babies frequently are unable to coordinate the reflexes.

*Process of attachment*

In order to attach correctly, the baby needs to:

- Open their mouth in a wide gape with their tongue down and forward (Fig. 28.1)
- The lower lip, then the tongue, should be the first point of contact
- The first contact should be well away from the base of the nipple
- They should then reach up and bring their mouth over the nipple, taking in a large portion of breast tissue to form the teat (Fig. 28.2).

Fig. 28.1 The baby should be encouraged to open their mouth widely.

Fig. 28.2 Baby correctly attached at the breast.

*Recognizing correct attachment*
- The baby's mouth is wide open (wider than 100°) and they have a large mouthful of breast
- The chin should indent the breast
- There should be more areola visible above his top lip than below the baby's bottom lip
- The nose should be close to the breast but not squashed
- The cheeks are round and full
- The whole of the lower jaw moves
- The lower lip is curled outwards, but this is not always easily visible if the baby is close to the breast
- The mother feels a strong, and sometimes uncomfortable, 'drawing' sensation as the baby scoops up the nipple and breast tissue, draws it into his or her mouth, and commences suckling
- Swallowing may be heard, but this only indicates that milk is flowing, not that the positioning and attachment are correct.

**Exaggerated attachment at the breast**
This is useful if:
- The baby is unable to attach and feed effectively
- The baby has a 'tongue tie' and has difficulty staying attached
- The baby has a cleft palate
- The baby is premature
- The nipples are sore or cracked and feeding is almost unbearable.

*How to attain an exaggerated attachment*
If the mother is going to feed from her left breast, she needs to cup the breast underneath with her left hand, keeping her fingers well away from the areola. There is always a tendency to want to move the fingers up, but this will affect the success of the attachment. The thumb should tilt the nipple back so it looks like it is pointing away from the baby. This will have the effect of making the breast under the nipple bulge forwards. The baby's bottom lip should make contact with the breast well away from the base of the nipple.

*Pattern of sucking*
Normally once the baby is attached, he or she will take a few quick sucks at the breast which will initiate the oxytocin reflex. As the milk begins to flow and fills the mouth, the baby's sucks will become slower and deeper. The baby will pause occasionally. If a baby continues to take frequent short sucks or there are audible 'smacking' noises as the baby sucks, this is a good indication that the attachment is incorrect.

*Recognizing incorrect attachment*
- The mouth is not wide open.
- The bottom lip is not curled outwards, or it is less curled than the upper lip.
- There is the same amount of areola below the bottom lip as above the top lip.
- There is a gap between the breast and the chin.

- The nose is either squashed into the breast or a wide distance from the breast.
- The cheeks are drawn in as the baby sucks.
- The breast tissue is puckered.
- The breast tissue moves in and out of the baby's mouth as he feeds.
- The baby makes little sucks as if he is sucking a dummy.
- There is no change in the rhythm of feeding.
- The baby will show frustration at not having his hunger satisfied by either becoming sleepy and ceasing to suck or by coming off the breast and crying.
- The colour of the stools may change back to green/brown from yellow.

*Results of ineffective attachment*

The mother may:
- Feel pain when feeding
- Experience sore nipples, especially cracks across the tip of the nipple or at the base of the nipple
- Experience engorgement of the breast.

The baby may:
- Appear unsatisfied
- Cry a lot and want frequent feeds, or may feed for protracted lengths of time
- Receive insufficient milk and fail to gain or even lose weight
- Become frustrated and refuse to feed
- Receive adequate nourishment for the first few weeks by feeding frequently if the oxytocin reflex works well but then will fail to thrive.

## Measures shown to enhance breastfeeding success

A comprehensive systematic review conducted by NICE[21] has identified what practices enable a mother to breastfeed for longer, and these should be used in conjunction with the following information.

*Responsive feeding*

Responsive feeding has replaced the terms 'baby-led feeding' and 'demand feeding' which have been often misunderstood. Responsive feeding is thought to more accurately describe the sensitive and symbiotic nature of breastfeeding.[22] It describes how the mother and baby respond to each other's needs and cues.

The BFI[22] explains how 'with responsive feeding a mother can offer her baby her breast:
- when he shows feeding cues
- when he appears unsettled
- when he seems lonely and just wants comfort
- when her breasts are full
- or when she just wants to have a sit down and spend time with her baby'.

There is substantial evidence that the timing and duration of breastfeeds should be responsive to the needs of the baby.[23] Babies will feed at the breast for very different lengths of time if left undisturbed, and it is thought that the length of a feed is determined by the rate of milk transfer between the mother and baby.[24]

Limiting the duration of the feed or removing a baby from the breast before they finish spontaneously may prevent the baby from receiving adequate calorific intake, causing failure to gain weight despite frequent feeds and an apparently good milk supply.

Unrestricted frequency of feeds is also advocated. Observation studies have demonstrated that the frequency of feeds in the first few weeks appears to be unpredictable and random, varying between 1h and 8h. Babies who regulate the length and frequency of feeds gain weight more quickly.

Advice to the mother to restrict or limit suckling time or frequency at the breast will not only do no good, but also could do harm. However, a baby that has protracted feeds without coming off spontaneously, or a baby that feeds very frequently, may be attached to the breast incorrectly. A baby that is poorly attached can also cause nipple trauma, which may give rise to engorgement and/or mastitis.[25]

### Night feeds

The advantages of night feeds include:
- Prolactin levels are higher at night, and a breastfeed at night will result in a greater prolactin surge than would occur with a feed given during the day. Night feeds therefore ensure good milk production[26]
- Exclusive breastfeeding that incorporates night feeds raises prolactin levels which, in turn, inhibits LH release; this prevents ovulation[27]
- Frequent feeds, including night feeds, help to prevent/reduce engorgement when the milk first comes in
- There is a soporific effect on the mother, which improves the quality of sleep. This results from the release of dopamine, which is believed to be involved in the mechanism of oxytocin release.[28]

### Rooming-in

Rooming-in, which allows mother and babies to remain together for 24h a day, has been shown to:
- Improve breastfeeding outcomes, especially the duration; this is partly because rooming-in facilitates responsive feeding[23]
- Improve mother–baby relationship, regardless of the feeding method
- Be preferable to nursery care for both the mother and baby.[23]

Common reasons to not room in, e.g. it interferes with the mother's sleep, do not appear to be valid.[23]

### Staff training

Health-care professionals who have not been trained in breastfeeding management cannot be expected to give mothers effective guidance and to provide skilled counselling. It is necessary to increase their skills to enable their knowledge to be used appropriately. Education and training sessions need to incorporate elements that enable health professionals to address bias that will hinder breastfeeding.[27]

In-service training needs to be mandatory to be successful and requires a strong policy supported by senior staff.

Inconsistent or conflicting information and advice disempowers women, reducing their self-confidence and ability to breastfeed successfully.[29]

## Breastfeeding and growth monitoring

NICE[30] recommends that GPs, paediatricians, midwives, health visitors, and community nursery nurses should:

- As a minimum, ensure babies are weighed (naked) at birth and at 5 and 10 days, as part of an overall assessment of feeding. After this, healthy babies should be weighed (naked) no more than fortnightly and at 2, 3, 4, and 8–10 months in their first year. Ongoing weekly weighing is unnecessary for healthy babies who give no cause for concern. Unnecessary weighing may lead to an inappropriate intervention and undermine parents' confidence
- Ensure infants are weighed using digital scales which are maintained and calibrated annually, in line with medical devices standards (spring scales are inaccurate and should not be used
- It is important that support staff are trained to weigh infants and young children and to record the data accurately in the child health record held by the parents.

### Breastfeeding patterns of growth

- Breastfed babies show a different pattern of growth from formula-fed babies.
- Growth rate is not constant and slowed growth is not always indicative of growth failure.
- Breastfed infants grow more quickly in the first few weeks and more slowly from about 4–5 months than formula-fed infants. The difference is on average half to one centile channel.[31]

New UK growth charts, based on breastfed babies, were introduced in May 2009 to plot the weight, height, and head circumference of children from birth to 4 years of age.[32] These charts should be used for all new births and new referrals to health professionals. The UK90 growth charts will continue to be used for children born before this date and for children over 4 years. Fact sheets about the new charts are available at the Royal College of Paediatrics and Child Health website (ℜ www.growthcharts.rcpch.ac.uk).

Weight loss of >7% in the first week of life is an indication of possible insufficient milk intake[32] and weight loss of >10% should be a cause for concern. Check that the baby is having plenty of wet and dirty nappies. Poor urine and stool output indicates the need for the baby to be weighed naked on digital scales, even if outside the recommended weighing guidelines. A breastfeeding history should be taken and a breastfeeding assessment form should be completed prior to advice being given for strategies to improve feeding. Weight loss of 15% or more requires urgent investigation, paediatric referral, and experienced breastfeeding support.

# References

17  UNICEF UK Baby Friendly Initiative (2012). Stage 3: Parents' experiences of maternity services: 2 Support all mothers and babies to initiate a close relationship and feeding soon after birth. In: UNICEF UK Baby Friendly Initiative. *Guide to the Baby Friendly Initiative standards.* Available at:  ℅  www.unicef.org.uk/Documents/Baby_Friendly/Guidance/Baby_Friendly_guidance_2012.pdf.

18  The Mother and Child Health and Education Trust (2016). *Breast crawl.* Available at:  ℅ www.breastcrawl.org/science.shtml.

19  Colson S (2007). A non-prescriptive recipe for breastfeeding. *Pract Midwife* 10: 42, 44, 46–7.

20  The Baby Friendly Initiative. *The Baby Friendly Initiative's position statement on biological nurturing.* Available at:  ℅ www.unicef.org.uk/BabyFriendly/News-and-Research/News/The-Baby-Friendly-Initiatives-position-on-Biological-Nurturing/.

21  Renfrew M, Dyson L, Wallace L, D'Souza L, McCormick F, Spiby H (2005). Breastfeeding for longer—what works? *J R Soc Promot Health* 125: 62–3.

22  UNICEF (UK) Baby Friendly Initiative (2014). *Breastfeeding and relationship building: a workbook.* London: Baby Friendly Initiative.

23  Renfrew MJ, Woolridge MW, McGill HR (2000). *Enabling women to breastfeed: a review of practices which promote or inhibit breastfeeding—with evidence-based guidance for practice.* London: The Stationery Office.

24  Woolridge MW, Baum JD, Drewett RF (1982). Individual patterns of human milk intake during breastfeeding. *Early Hum Dev* 7: 265–72.

25  National Institute for Health and Care Excellence (2015). *Mastitis and breast abscess. Clinical Knowledge Summaries.* Available at:  ℅ cks.nice.org.uk/mastitis-and-breast-abscess#!backgroundsub:2.

26  Czank C, Henderson JJ, Kent JC, Lai CT, Hartmann PE (2007). Hormonal control of the lactation cycle. In: Hale TW, Hartmann PE, eds. *Textbook of Human Lactation.* Amarillo, TX: Hale Publishing, pp. 89–111.

27  Battersby S (2006). Exploring attitudes towards breastfeeding. In: Moran VH, Dykes F, eds. *Maternal and Infant Nutrition and Nurture: Controversies and Challenges.* London: Quay Books, pp. 202–29.

28  Bourne MA (1982). Sleep in the puerperium. *Midwives Chronicle and Nursing Notes* March, 91.

29  Simmons V (2002). Exploring inconsistent breastfeeding advice. *Br J Midwifery* 10: 616–19.

30  National Institute for Health and Care Excellence (2008). *Maternal and Child Nutrition.* NICE guidelines PH11. London: National Institute for Health and Care Excellence.

31  Cole TJ, Paul AA, Whitehead RG (2002). Weight reference charts for British long-term breastfed infants. *Acta Paediatrica* 91: 1296–300.

32  Royal College of Paediatrics and Child Health (2015). *UK-WHO growth charts, 0–18 years.* Available at:  ℅ www.rcpch.ac.uk/improving-child-health/public-health/uk-who-growth-charts/uk-who-growth-charts-0-18-years.

# The infant's contribution to breastfeeding

Until recently, the infant's contribution to breastfeeding has received very little attention. However, like other baby mammals, the human baby has many instinctive or inborn abilities which assist it to find the mother's breast and initiate suckling.

## Breast crawl

Breast crawl or baby crawl are the terms used when a newborn baby is placed on the mother's abdomen immediately after birth and demonstrates their ability to find the mother's breast and initiate the first breastfeed unaided.[33] The instinctive or inborn abilities include sensory, central, motor and neuroendocrine components which both directly or indirectly help the baby's movement and facilitate its survival.

### Sensory inputs
- Olfactory.
- Visual.
- Taste.
- Auditory.
- Touch.

### Central component
- Following birth, the healthy newborn will undergo a quiet alert phase when they will become quiet and start exploring their environment. It is during this period of alertness that the baby is in optimal readiness to bring together the components and initiate the breast crawl. If not undertaken immediately following birth, the baby will become sleepy and the opportunity will be lost. Shortly following birth, the normal human infant will seek out the breast and this will commence with:
- Opening of the eyes
- Massage-like hand movement
- Hand to mouth
- Rooting
- Hand to nipple
- Tongue outside the mouth
- Licking movements
- Suckling.

### Motor components
- Orofacial.
- Lower limbs.
- Upper limbs.
- Salivation.

The three main reflexes required for a baby to attach effectively are:
- Rooting reflex
- Sucking reflex
- Swallowing reflex.

If any of these reflexes is absent, the baby will not be able to attach and feed effectively. Premature babies frequently are unable to coordinate the reflexes.

*Neuroendocrine component*
- Oxytocin.

*Benefits for the baby*
- Warmth.
- Comfort.
- Metabolic adaptation.
- Quality of attachment.

*Benefits for the mother*
- Expulsion of the placenta and reduction of PPH.

*Advantage for both the mother and baby*
- Bonding.

*Factors that facilitate breast crawl*
- Raising the mother's head on a pillow to assist mother–baby eye contact.
- Drying the baby thoroughly, except its hands.
- Covering the mother and baby to keep them warm whilst undergoing skin-to-skin.
- Continuing skin-to-skin until after the first feed.
- Delaying routine care until after the first feed, e.g. vitamin K, weighing and measuring, wrapping or dressing.
- Delaying the first bath for 24h.

*Factors that hinder breast crawl*
- Separation of mother and baby immediately following birth.
- Birth practices.
- Maternal drugs used in labour.
- Washing or wiping the breast.
- Moving the mother from the labour room before completion of the first feed.
- Oronasal suction.

## Reference

33 The Mother and Child Health and Education Trust (2016). *Breast crawl*. Available at: ℞ www. breastcrawl.org/science.shtml.

# Support for breastfeeding

The support the woman receives from her partner, family members, friends, health professionals, and support networks can affect the uptake and continuance of breastfeeding. Emotional support as well as practical support is needed to empower mothers to breastfeed successfully. Various levels of support may be required by breastfeeding mothers, depending upon their social circumstances. Caregivers may find it easier to support breastfeeding mothers effectively if they have had the opportunity to come to terms with their own breastfeeding experiences.[34]

## Partners

- The male partner may have a strong influence upon the choice of infant feeding method.[34]
- The partner's positive attitude to breastfeeding is important for the mother initiating and continuing to breastfeed.[35]
- Women need to talk to their partners antenatally about breastfeeding.
- Partners need to be informed of the benefits of breastfeeding for both the baby and mother.
- Partners should be involved in antenatal preparation for breastfeeding whenever possible.
- Partners are invaluable in providing emotional and practical support for breastfeeding mothers.
- Partners wishing to undertake shared care of the baby should be encouraged to look at alternatives to feeding, e.g. bathing the infant, skin-to-skin contact.

## Family and friends

- Family and friends exert a strong influence on a mother's decision about breastfeeding.
- About one in four mothers are helped by a relative or friend when they have problems breastfeeding.
- First-time mothers are more likely to turn to relatives and friends for assistance.
- Breastfeeding mothers who were breastfed themselves are more likely to be breastfeeding at 4 weeks than those who had been bottle-fed.
- Breastfeeding mothers whose friends mostly bottle-fed are more likely to discontinue in the first 2 weeks postnatally.[36]

## Peer support

NICE[37] recommends that there should be easily accessible breastfeeding peer support programmes and that appropriately trained breastfeeding peer supporters should be part of a multidisciplinary team. It also recommends that breastfeeding peer supporters should contact mothers directly within 48h of their transfer to the community and offer them ongoing support according to their individual needs. This could be via telephone, texting, face-to-face, local support groups, or the Internet.

Breastfeeding peer support projects have been shown to:

- Demonstrate a positive trend towards increasing continuation of breastfeeding
- Help mothers at a time when they were strongly considering stopping breastfeeding
- Empower those living in socially excluded communities.[36]

## Specialist infant feeding advisers

Many maternity units now employ specialist infant feeding advisers. Their role varies depending upon the needs of the local population and the requirements of the maternity units. There is very little research related to the role of the specialist feeding advisers, but they can improve the care and support that breastfeeding women receive by:

• Developing and monitoring infant feeding policies and guidelines
• Providing in-service training for health professionals and support workers
• Auditing infant feeding practices
• Ensuring up-to-date evidence-based practice related to infant feeding
• Ensuring that leaflets and information for women are accurate, in line with breastfeeding policies, and do not advertise formula milk companies
• Organizing and running breastfeeding workshops for women in the antenatal period
• Organizing and running breastfeeding drop-in services
• Supporting health professionals in their clinical area
• Supervising health professionals who are undertaking breastfeeding courses, e.g. BFI Breastfeeding Management Course
• Taking the lead role when maternity units and communities are working towards the BFI Award
• Liaising with local and national organizations to promote, protect, and support breastfeeding
• Providing a contact person for liaising with formula milk companies.

Their role is not to deskill the health professional by taking over the carer role for breastfeeding women, but to develop their skills and increase their knowledge base to ensure that all breastfeeding women are provided with evidence-based, sensitive, and consistent information and support.

## Voluntary groups

There are a number of breastfeeding voluntary organizations or organizations that have expertise in supporting breastfeeding mothers in special circumstances in the UK, including:

• National Childbirth Trust
• Breastfeeding Network
• Twins and Multiple Births Association
• La Leche League (Great Britain)
• Baby Milk Action
• Association of Breastfeeding Mothers.

These organizations supply information and support by telephone and in leaflets and books. Mothers should be offered leaflets or cards giving details about support organizations prior to leaving the postnatal ward.

## References

34 Battersby S (2006). Exploring attitudes towards breastfeeding. In: Moran VH, Dykes F, eds. *Maternal and Infant Nutrition and Nurture: Controversies and Challenges*. London: Quay Books, pp. 202–29.
35 McInnes RJ, Chambers JA (2008). Supporting breastfeeding mothers: qualitative synthesis. *J Adv Nurs* 62: 407–27.
36 McAndrew F, Thompson J, Fellows L, Large A, Speed M, Renfrew MJ (2012). *Infant Feeding Survey—UK, 2010 (NS)*. London: Health and Social Care Information Centre. Available at: ℬ www.hscic.gov.uk/catalogue/PUB08694.
37 National Institute for Health and Care Excellence (2008). *Maternal and child nutrition*. NICE guidelines PH11. Available at: ℬ www.nice.org.uk/guidance/ph11.

# Practices shown to be detrimental to successful breastfeeding

## Inconsistent information

Despite efforts to ensure that appropriate advice and information are given to breastfeeding mothers, there is still evidence that, for many mothers, difficulty in establishing breastfeeding is compounded by inconsistent advice.[38] Conflicting advice does exist and persist, mostly as inaccurate information and practice.

Conflicting advice and information:
• Reinforce a mother's lack of self-confidence in her ability to breastfeed
• Disempower women.[38]

In order to prevent inconsistent advice, midwives need to:
• Have in-depth knowledge and understanding of the physiology of lactation
• Be able to communicate effectively
• Acknowledge their own subjective bias
• Provide consistent information and support in line with the best available evidence.[38]

An authoritarian approach to communication is unhelpful and even detrimental.

## Use of pacifiers

The use of pacifiers (dummies) has become a widespread cultural practice in the UK. They are used to settle, soothe, or otherwise occupy a fretful or distressed baby.

The use of pacifiers has been implicated in:[39]
• Reducing the duration of breastfeeding
• Increasing the risk of otitis media
• Oral *Candida* infection
• Reduced jaw muscle activity
• Reduced intellectual attainment
• Greater incidence of abnormal jaw development.

### *Breastfeeding dummies and sudden infant death syndrome*

Some evidence suggests that the use of pacifiers can reduce the incidence of cot death.[40] This has been debated and further research is required. The recommendations at present are that they should:
• Not be used to replace breastfeeding
• Not be replaced after a baby has fallen asleep
• Not be given to a baby who does not want it.

The BFI (UK)[41] recommends that we must support parents to make informed decisions about using a dummy, based on their own personal circumstances. This should include a discussion of the benefits and risks of dummy use and the acknowledgement that we do not know everything about the issue.

## The use of nipple shields

The use of nipple shields is sometimes advocated as treatment for sore nipples; however, little evidence is currently available to support this practice.

The use of nipple shields:[42]
- Has been found to be unacceptable to mothers
- May lead to a conditioned rejection of the breast by the baby
- May adversely affect the mother's milk supply.

Clinical experience suggests that judicious use of a thin silicone shield may benefit mothers with severely traumatized nipples, but they should never be used as a substitute for teaching the mother how to correct the problem of sore nipples by improving positioning and attachment. They should never be used in the early postnatal days before the milk has 'come in'.

## Supplementary feeding

Supplementary feeding is the practice of giving extra feeds of formula, glucose, or water. A recent study found that 31% of breastfed babies were given supplementary feeds whilst in hospital.[43] This study also found that breastfeeding mothers whose babies were given bottles were more likely to discontinue breastfeeding in the first 2 weeks postnatally than were other mothers.

Supplementary feeds have been associated with:
- Interference with the supply and demand mechanism, therefore reducing milk supply
- Interference with the development of normal immunological mechanisms
- Allergic conditions in some babies
- Reactive hypoglycaemia
- 'Nipple confusion'
- Reduced maternal confidence.

## Extra fluids

Giving extra fluids, either in the form of water or dextrose, to babies with jaundice has not been shown to reduce peak serum bilirubin levels and may, in fact, cause levels to rise by reducing the milk intake and therefore delaying the evacuation of meconium.[44]

In a breastfed baby, filling the stomach with water will reduce the number of feeds and interfere with the establishment of breastfeeding. Women whose babies are given extra fluids are more likely to discontinue breastfeeding.

## References

38 McInnes RJ, Chambers JA (2008). Supporting breastfeeding mothers: qualitative synthesis. *J Adv Nurs* 62: 407–27.

39 La Leche League GB (2012). *Dummies and breastfeeding. Information Sheet No. 2706*. Nottingham: LLL Books Ltd.

40 Li DK, Willinger M, Petitti DB, Odouli R, Liu L, Hoffman HJ (2006). Use of a dummy (pacifier) during sleep and the risk of sudden infant death syndrome (SIDS): population based case-control study. *BMJ* 332: 18–22.

41 UNICEF UK (2006). *UNICEF UK statement on dummy use, SIDS and breastfeeding*. Available at: ⏎ www.unicef.org.uk/BabyFriendly/News-and-Research/News/UNICEF-UK-statement-on-dummy-use-sudden-infant-death-syndrome-and-breastfeeding1/.

42 Royal College of Midwives (2002). *Successful Breastfeeding*. Edinburgh: Churchill Livingstone.

43 McAndrew F, Thompson J, Fellows L, Large A, Speed M, Renfrew MJ (2012). *Infant Feeding Survey—UK, 2010 (NS)*. London: Health and Social Care Information Centre. Available at: ⏎ www.hscic.gov.uk/catalogue/PUB08694.

44 Gartner LM (2007). Hyperbilirubinemia and breast feeding. In: Hale TW, Hartmann PE, eds. *Textbook of Human Lactation*. Amarillo, TX: Hale Publishing LP, pp. 255–70.

# Expression of breast milk

## Why express?

Expression of breast milk should be taught to all mothers as it helps them to understand how the breasts work. It can aid the mother's understanding of effective attachment and may help her to recognize and overcome many breastfeeding complications.[45] Health professionals should be able to teach the skills of both hand expression and mechanical expression to breastfeeding mothers.

Expression of breast milk can be helpful in a variety of situations.[45]

- General breast comfort:
    - To relieve discomfort from overfull breasts if a feed has been missed
    - To prevent leakage if the mother and child are apart
    - To maintain healthy skin or to assist healing: if damage has occurred to the nipple, a small amount of breast milk may be applied to the nipple and areola.
- To assist a baby to breastfeed:
    - Expressing a small amount of breast milk will encourage a reluctant baby to breastfeed by enabling him to smell and taste the milk
    - By softening an overfull or engorged breast, enabling attachment
    - Milk may be expressed gently into the baby's mouth if he or she has a weak suck.
- To prevent or relieve breast conditions:
    - Overfull breasts due to a feed being missed
    - Engorgement
    - Blocked duct
    - Mastitis.
- To stimulate milk supply:
    - When the mother and baby are separated or the baby is unable to suckle
    - If additional stimulus is required to increase or induce lactation.
- To maintain milk supply:
    - When the mother and baby are separated, e.g. hospitalization, return to work
    - When the mother has to suspend breastfeeding temporarily, e.g. due to medication that may be harmful to the baby.

## Methods of expression

*Hand or manual expression*

- Hand expression is usually gentler than using a pump; it can be undertaken anywhere and no/minimal equipment is needed.
- Hand expression requires skill, and some mothers find it difficult and prefer to use a pump.
- The risk of cross-infection is reduced with hand expression as less equipment is required.
- Hand expression is useful as a self-help method if blocked ducts, engorgement, or mastitis occurs.
- Inform the mother that when she first starts to express her breasts, only small amounts will be expressed, but with practice it will become easier and she will be able to express more.

*How to hand express*

The mother should:
- Wash her hands
- Use a wide-mouthed sterile container to collect the milk
- Sit comfortably in a warm, peaceful, and relaxing environment if possible
- Lean very slightly forward.
- Encourage the let-down reflex by:
  - Relaxing with a warm drink, music, or TV
  - Being near the baby or a photo of the baby
  - Warming the breasts
  - Gently pulling or rolling the nipples
  - Gently massaging the breasts by stroking with the fingertips, rolling with the knuckles, or using circular movements.

The mother should then:
- Make a 'C' shape with her thumb above and her fingers below the breast near the edge of the areola but away from the nipple (Fig. 28.3).
- Gently press her thumb and fingers together, release the fingers, and repeat in a rhythmic pattern (Fig. 28.4).
- Sometimes it is helpful to press inwards and back towards the chest wall whilst squeezing gently.
- The fingers should be repositioned at intervals to allow drainage from all the lactiferous ducts.

The length of time for expressing depends on the reason why the mother is expressing. If she wants to express all the milk she can from the breast, she should continue until the flow subsides.

The mother may express from the second breast by repeating the above process. A mother who wishes to express as much milk as possible should continue to switch between breasts for as long as milk is being obtained.[45,46]

**Fig. 28.3** Make a C-shape with the finger and thumb.

**Fig. 28.4** Expressing breast milk.

*Breast pumps*
Mothers who use a mechanical pump may find they are able to express larger volumes, especially if using an electrical pump.[45]

Numerous pumps are available to hire or buy, but they fall into three types:
- *A hand pump* that is mainly for relieving the breasts. These are usually of simple design and work on a simple vacuum principle. They are not suitable for expressing milk which is to be stored and given to a baby because they cannot be sterilized effectively[45]
- *Battery-operated pumps* vary widely in design; all produce a rhythmic vacuum, although some are also designed to give a degree of compression. Some mothers find these pumps useful if they are expressing on a regular basis, as they are less tiring than a hand pump
- *Electric pumps* are usually heavy and bulky and therefore less portable. As they are efficient, they are commonly used within hospitals, but they are usually shared by several mothers and therefore maintenance and cleanliness are essential. Ideally all mothers should be given their own equipment for the machine, which should include a collection beaker, tubing, and sterilizing equipment.[45]

*Using breast pumps*
Women may find that their let-down reflex is more difficult to induce with a pump than with hand expressing. Massaging the breast and hand expressing for a short time prior to using the pump may help. A photograph, an item of the baby's clothing, or a toy may also help.

## Dual pumping

Dual pumping is when both breasts are expressed at the same time. This can be done either by hand expression or using a pump. It has been shown to shorten the time required for expressing and increases the mother's prolactin levels.[45] If using a pump, a Y coupling is required. It is particularly helpful if a large amount of milk is required, e.g. with twins and multiple births, or if there is a need to increase the milk supply rapidly.

## Principles of expression

Establishment of lactation:
• Expression should commence as soon as possible after the birth
• Express frequently, 6–8 times in 24h, more if possible
• Express at least once during the night
• Avoid set patterns of expressing; instead aim to imitate the irregular feeding pattern adopted by most babies.

If lactation is already established, and there is a need to express to maintain lactation because of separation of the mother and baby, the last three of the above principles should be applied. It is important to remember that expressing does not provide the same stimulus to the breast as the baby suckling, and the milk supply may begin to diminish. If this is the case, the mother should be encouraged to increase the number of expressions.

To increase the milk supply, e.g. if the baby is not feeding sufficiently or if the mother wishes to build up a milk supply before returning to work, the mother should be encouraged to:
• Express after and/or between feeds or, if the baby is not feeding, to increase the number of expressions
• Express at least once in the night
• Avoid set patterns of expressing; rather, expressing whenever she can.

It takes appropriately 24h for the supply to increase.

## Recommendations for storage of breast milk

*For use in the home*
• Fresh breast milk can be:
  • Kept for up to 5h at room temperature
  • Stored in a refrigerator at a temperature 2–4°C for up to 5 days.
• If milk is not to be used within 24h, freezing is recommended:
  • Milk can be kept frozen in an ice-making compartment for 2 weeks
  • Milk can be kept safely for up to 6 months in a domestic freezer.
• Any plastic container that can be sterilized and made airtight is suitable for storing breast milk. Many commercial products are available.[47]

*Storing breast milk for use in hospital*
• Some types of plastic are not suitable for storing breast milk for preterm or sick babies.
• Use up-to-date guidelines, e.g. NICE (2010) Donor Milk Banks—the operation of Donor Milk Bank Services.[48]
• Hospitals often pasteurize milk for use in a milk bank, but this is not usually necessary if the milk is for the mother's own baby.

## Reheating expressed breast milk at home

- Frozen milk can be:
  - Thawed slowly in a refrigerator but must be used within 24h or discarded
  - Thawed at room temperature and used immediately
- Frozen milk should never be thawed or heated in a microwave.[49]
- Some prefer to warm the milk to body temperature.
- Never refreeze breast milk.

## References

45 UNICEF UK (2004). *Breastfeeding Management Course*. London: UNICEF UK Baby Friendly Initiative.

46 Breastfeeding Network (2009). *Expressing and Storing Breast Milk Leaflet*. Paisley: Breastfeeding Network.

47 UNICEF UK/Department of Health (2010). *Off to the best start*. Available at: ℘ www.unicef.org.uk/Documents/Baby_Friendly/Leaflets/otbs_leaflet.pdf.

48 National Institute for Health and Care Excellence (2010). *Donor milk banks: service operation*. NICE guidelines CG93. Available at: ℘ www.nice.org.uk/guidance/cg93.

49 The Breastfeeding Network (2014). *Breastfeeding information: expressing and storing*. Available at: ℘ www.breastfeedingnetwork.org.uk/breastfeeding-help/expressing-storing/.

# Breastfeeding and returning to work

Mothers who are returning to work may find this a stressful time, especially if they are breastfeeding. The longer a mother breastfeeds, the more benefits there are for both the mother and baby. Mothers may wish to consider different working options, e.g. part-time work, job sharing, working different hours, working partly at home. Health professionals should give mothers information and assistance to try to make the return to work as easy as possible.

Three practical ways to combine breastfeeding and work are:

- Expression of breast milk whilst at work
- Childcare near the mother's place of work
- Partial breastfeeding.

There are advantages and disadvantages to all three options and it will depend upon the mother's circumstances which option is most appropriate for her.

If the mother decides to express breast milk at work, she will need to:

- Practise expressing milk prior to returning to work (if possible, she should wait until breastfeeding is fully established, when the baby is about 2 months old). The EBM can be stored in the freezer to give the mother a backup supply
- Ensure she has equipment for expressing at work, which will include a pump, storage containers, sterilizing equipment, spare breast pads, and a cool bag for transportation (many commercial products are being produced now to make this easier for mothers)
- Consider dual pumping, as this reduces the time required to express
- Have spare batteries and vacuum seals at work if using a pump
- Speak to her employer about where and when she can express milk
- Ask at work for the following facilities:
  - Use of a room that is warm and clean, and has a lockable door
  - Facilities for handwashing
  - Somewhere clean to leave the equipment for sterilizing
  - Use of a fridge to store the EBM
  - A low comfortable chair.
- Store milk safely.

## The law relating to breastfeeding at work

In the UK, mothers do not have statutory rights to paid breastfeeding breaks but do have certain legal protection under the health and safety and sex discrimination laws.[50] Whilst breastfeeding, she and her baby have special health and safety protection, the same as that for a pregnant woman. However, to use this protection, she must inform her employers in writing. Employers are also obliged to provide 'suitable facilities' where breastfeeding employees can 'rest'. If the woman is working with hazardous substances, the employer should take appropriate actions to make the job safe. If this is not possible, an alternative job should be offered or she should be suspended on full pay.[50]

## When to express

This will depend upon the individual and the type of work, but also upon the employer's attitude. It is not essential to have regular breaks, as it is better to aim to imitate the irregular feeding pattern that most babies adopt.

## Childcare near the mother's workplace

If the baby is in childcare near the mother's place of work, the mother could visit the baby during breaks and breastfeed normally. Although this is the best option, it may prove difficult to responsively feed around working hours, and the baby may be upset by the mother coming and going.

## Partial breastfeeding

This is when the mother breastfeeds normally when at home, but the baby receives formula milk whilst the mother is at work. This can work very well when the mother is unable to express or visit the baby. However, her milk supply may diminish and she may still have to continue with formula feeds for those feeds that are normally missed when working. Partial breastfeeding is not possible before the milk supply is fully established at around 2 months.

## Reference

50 Maternity Action (2016). *Continuing to breastfeed when you return to work.* Information Sheet. London: Maternity Action. Available at: ℜ www.maternityaction.org.uk/advice-2/mums-dads-scenarios/6-breastfeeding-rights/continuing-to-breastfeed-when-you-return-to-work/.

# Discontinuation of breastfeeding

The Department of Health recommends exclusive breastfeeding for the first 6 months (26 weeks) of an infant's life, and 6 months is the recommended age for the introduction of solid foods for infants.[51] However, the time when mothers discontinue breastfeeding is very variable and depends upon many factors. Sudden cessation should be avoided, if possible, to maximize the mother's comfort and to avoid mastitis. The mother should be advised to slowly drop one feed at a time, to allow several days before dropping a further feed, and to feed on alternate days when down to one feed. This helps the milk supply to adjust and allows the milk to diminish naturally. There are circumstances that need special consideration.

## Mother going into hospital

- If possible, arrange for the baby to accompany the mother and continue feeding.
- A family carer may need to assist the mother with baby care if the hospital cannot provide assistance.
- If this is known in advance, the mother can express and freeze the EBM, especially if she is to undergo a general anaesthetic.
- The mother needs to ask about equipment and facilities for expressing, sterilizing, and storing breast milk. She may need to take in her own pump.
- If a mother has to stop feeding temporarily due to medication, the supply can be maintained by expressing.
- The mother should ask if safe alternative drugs are available.

## Baby going into hospital

- If possible, the mother should accompany the baby.
- If not possible, e.g. because of other children at home, the mother should express and send the milk to the hospital.
- If the baby is unable to suckle and/or receive breast milk, the mother should express to maintain the supply and reduce the risk of mastitis.
- If stopping breastfeeding, this should be done gradually.

## Sudden cessation due to cot death or illness

- A small amount should be expressed, just to relieve pressure.
- Support the breasts well with a firm bra; binding has not been shown to help and may increase the risk of mastitis.
- Use cold compresses.
- Mild analgesics, e.g. paracetamol, may help relieve the discomfort.
- Slightly reduce fluids, but do not drastically reduce fluids as this may temporarily increase the supply.
- Pharmacological suppression using cabergoline may be considered.

## Reference

51 Department of Health (2011). *Introducing solid foods—giving your baby a better start in life*. Available at: ℘ www.gov.uk/government/publications/introducing-solid-foods-giving-your-baby-a-better-start-in-life.

# Breastfeeding problems

A problem-solving approach should be taken when managing common breastfeeding problems. This should include:

- Listening to the mother
- Taking a breastfeeding history; use of the UNICEF BFI Breastfeeding Assessment Form is advised[52]
- Observing a breastfeed
- Offering information on appropriate solutions and alternatives to enable a mother to make her own decision
- Offering the ongoing support of a breastfeeding peer supporter.

## Sleepy/non-feeding baby

There are a number of reasons why a baby will not feed in the first few days following delivery and these include:

- Drugs given to the mother in labour, e.g. pethidine and epidural
- Unpleasant experience at the breast, e.g. force applied to the head when fixing
- Frustration as a result of not obtaining nourishment due to poor fixing at the breast
- Jaundice
- If lethargic when awake, the baby may not be receiving adequate nutrition
- The baby is ill.

### Actions

The first two actions should be addressed with all babies and the following actions acted upon as relevant to the history.

- A breastfeeding history should be taken to see if the reason can be identified.
- A breastfeed should be observed, and positioning and attachment improved.
- If necessary, wake the baby and give additional feeds (EBM or colostrum if possible) until the situation has improved.
- If the baby is jaundiced, encourage the baby to feed as frequently as possible.
- Feed the baby when he or she is half asleep.
- Encourage the baby to stay awake whilst feeding by keeping the baby cooler during feeds.
- Switch feed, i.e. change the baby from one breast to the other as the baby becomes sleepy.
- Change the baby's position whilst feeding to stimulate the baby to suckle more vigorously.
- Encourage the mother to adopt skin-to-skin as much as possible—do not offer the breast; let the baby find it.
- Change the nappy to wake the baby.
- Bathe the baby.
- Sit in a warm bath to feed the baby.
- Breast compression:[53]
  - If the baby starts to doze at the breast, this process will help them breastfeed more actively and take more milk

- Support the breast with one hand—thumb on one side, fingers on the other
- Wait until the baby feeds actively, his jaw moving all the way to the ear. When he stops swallowing, compress the breast firmly. Hold it squeezed until he stops actively nursing, then release the hand
- Rotate the hand around the breast and repeat step 2 on different areas of the breast as needed. Go gently—this should not hurt.

## Sore/cracked nipples

Breastfeeding should be comfortable and pain-free, although some mothers may experience some discomfort at the beginning of the feed for the first few days. This usually resolves spontaneously. However, 22% of mothers who discontinue breastfeeding in the first week postnatally do so because of sore or cracked nipples.[54] It is very likely that the majority of sore nipples could be prevented and treated by correct positioning and attachment of the baby at the breast.

The causes of sore and cracked nipples include:

- Poor positioning and attachment of the baby at the breast
- Engorgement, which may prevent good attachment
- Physiological causes that include a baby with a short tongue or tongue tie, a high palate, or a mismatch between the size of the mother's nipple and the baby's mouth
- Pulling the baby off the breast without first breaking the seal between the baby's mouth and the mother's breast
- The use of substances that may trigger a skin reaction or increase its susceptibility to damage, e.g. soap and scented bath products, antiseptic sprays
- Thrush infections (➔ see *Candida* (thrush) infection, p. 807)
- Expressing too vigorously with a breast pump.

*Actions*

- Observe a feed and assist the mother to attain better positioning and attachment.
- Provide emotional support to the mother.
- If engorgement is present, express a small amount of milk to soften the area immediately behind the nipple area.
- If the baby has a short tongue or tongue tie, an exaggerated fix may help (➔ see Exaggerated attachment at the breast, p. 779). This is where the mother slightly compresses the breast in the same direction as the baby's mouth, thus narrowing the width of the breast to enable the baby to attach easier. It may be appropriate to refer the baby for separation of the frenulum.[55]
- Avoid the use of soap and similar products, which remove the natural oils.
- Teach the mother how to break the suction by inserting a finger gently into the baby's mouth before removing the baby from the breast.
- Alter the position of the baby at different feeds.
- If the nipple is cracked, correct positioning usually enables the mother to feed without severe pain. In severe cases, short-term topical treatment may assist healing and be soothing for the mother. Moist wound healing promotes granulation and the use of an oil-based preparation may be advocated, e.g. highly purified lanolin.

## Inverted nipples

Nipples usually protrude, but approximately 10% of pregnant women who wish to breastfeed have inverted or non-protractile nipples. Currently there is no evidence that any antenatal nipple treatment or preparation contributes to successful breastfeeding. No prediction of success of breastfeeding should be made on antenatal inspection.

### Actions

- The mother should be reassured that the baby breastfeeds, and not nipple-feeds.
- Skilled help with attachment is important for these women in the first few days post partum.
- If difficulty is encountered attaching the baby, expressing a small amount of milk to soften the area around the areola can sometimes be helpful.
- Lactation can be initiated and sustained with a breast pump and further attempts at attaching are made when the milk has 'come in' and the breasts are softer.
- Dummies and nipple shields should be avoided as they require a different action and may confuse the baby.
- Mothers with inverted nipples can be as successful at breastfeeding as mothers with protractile nipples.

## Engorgement

There are two types of engorgement:
- Milk arrival engorgement
- Secondary engorgement.

### Milk arrival engorgement

This occurs usually around the second to fourth days postnatally as the milk 'comes in'. It can result from poor attachment, restricting feeds in the early days or not waking the baby enough. It is caused by increased blood supply to the breasts and extra lymph fluid. The mother will have red, painful, and swollen breasts. She may also have a mild pyrexia and flu-like symptoms. If action is not taken, it may result in mastitis.

### Secondary engorgement

The mother presents with the same symptoms of painful, swollen breasts, but this can occur at any time and is due to the ineffective drainage of the breasts. It may result from a variety of causes, including:
- The mother missing a feed
- Reduced appetite in the baby
- Overstimulation of the supply
- Too rapid weaning
- Baby sleeping through the night.

### Actions

The actions taken are the same in both types of engorgement:
- Warm flannels can be used to aid the milk flow
- Expressing a small amount of milk will also help to get the milk flowing and make it easier for the baby to attach
- Improve positioning and attachment

- Encourage the baby to feed frequently
- Analgesia may be required (paracetamol is usually the drug of choice).

Reassure the mother that it is a temporary situation.

## Blocked duct/s

The woman will generally feel well, but she will present with a localized tender lump or a feeling of bruising. It usually occurs in one breast and can occur at any time during the breastfeeding period. The woman's temperature is not usually raised.

*Actions*
- Ensure effective positioning and attachment.
- Feed from the affected side first for the next two feeds, then alternate.
- Ensure the baby feeds frequently.
- Use warm flannels, the shower or bath to bathe the breast in warm water.
- Massage the lump gently towards the nipple during a feed, after a feed, or whilst in the bath.
- Remove any white spot from the nipple.
- Use alternate positions.
- Feed the baby with its chin on the same side as the affected duct.
- Avoid bras that dig into the breast.

## Mastitis

Mastitis means inflammation of the breast. The term should not be regarded as synonymous with 'breast infection' because although inflammation may be the result of infection, in over 50% of cases of mastitis it is not. Mastitis can be the result of milk leaking into the breast tissue because of a blocked duct or engorgement. The body's defence mechanism reacts in the same way as it would for an infection by increasing the blood supply, which in turn is responsible for the redness and inflammation. Therefore, antibiotics may not be required if self-help measures are initiated promptly.

*Signs*
- A red, swollen, usually painful area on the breast, often the outer upper area.
- A lumpy breast that feels hot to touch.
- The whole breast may ache and become red.
- Flu-like symptoms which arise very quickly and rapidly get worse.

*Predisposing factors*
There are a number of factors that may make non-infective mastitis more likely; these include:
- Incorrect positioning and attachment, which may lead to inadequate draining of the breast
- Restriction of the breast as a result of tight clothing or by pressing the fingers too firmly into the breast when feeding
- Engorgement
- Blocked duct/s
- Stress and tiredness
- Sudden changes in the baby's feeding pattern.

*Prevention of non-infective mastitis*

The condition is often a consequence of engorgement and the following simple measures can help to avoid or reduce the risk of mastitis:

- Ensure correct positioning and attachment
- Avoid suddenly going longer between feeds—reduce gradually if possible
- Avoid pressure on the breasts by either clothing or the fingers
- Commence self-help measures as soon as symptoms occur.

*Self-help measures*

These measures will help to relieve engorgement and blocked ducts as well as mastitis:

- Breastfeeding must be continued if possible; it is the most effective way to reduce the symptoms
- Reassure the mother that her milk will not harm the baby
- Ensure correct positioning and attachment
- Increase the frequency of feeds, and if the breasts are uncomfortably full, express between feeds
- Ensure adequate drainage of the breasts and express gently following feeds until resolved
- Feed from the affected breast first
- Try using different positions for feeding
- Prior to feeding, apply warmth to the breast and gently express to soften the breast, enabling the baby to attach more effectively
- If necessary, express breast milk by hand or pump until breastfeeding can be resumed
- Gently massage the breast towards the nipple to help the milk flow whilst feeding
- Check positioning of the fingers when feeding and check to see if clothing is restrictive
- Rest
- Plenty of fluids
- An anti-inflammatory agent may help, e.g. ibuprofen. Aspirin should not be taken by breastfeeding mothers. It can result in rashes, platelet abnormalities, bleeding, and the potentially fatal Reye's syndrome in nursing infants; 4–8% of the maternal dose can be transferred.

If no improvement has occurred 12–24h after onset of symptoms or infective mastitis is suspected, refer to the doctor.

*Infective mastitis*

Bacterial infections result from organisms breaching the preventative barrier of the skin and multiplying in spite of the body's defence system. The epithelium of the breast and nipple may be damaged by:

- Incorrect positioning and attachment
- Sensitivity to creams, lotions, and sprays.

*Treatment of infective mastitis*

- The self-help measures above should be initiated.
- Systemic antibiotics compatible with breastfeeding should be commenced. This may be needed for 10–14 days. However, there is very little evidence on the effectiveness of antibiotic therapy, and more research is needed.[56]

- Beneficial bacteria killed by the antibiotics can be restored by taking live yoghurt or *Acidophilus*.
- Bacteriotherapy—this is a new development that looks at the use of beneficial bacteria to prevent or treat colonization of the host by pathogens. It can be used as an alternative or complement to antibiotic therapy.[57]

Abrupt discontinuation of feeding increases the chances of a breast abscess, as will unresolved mastitis.

## Breast abscess

This is a rare, but serious, medical condition. The mother will be pyrexial and have severe flu-like symptoms, and the affected area will be very painful and swollen. It presents as a localized breast infection with the presence of pus. The pus is not considered harmful to the baby, but if blood is also present, the baby may vomit. It may occur without prior symptoms but often results from unresolved mastitis.

*Actions*

- Refer immediately to a doctor who will prescribe antibiotics.
- Aspiration of the abscess or surgical drainage may be required.
- The mother should continue to feed on the unaffected breast.
- It is preferable for the mother to continue breastfeeding on the affected breast, but she may prefer to express and discard the milk, especially if the baby is vulnerable, e.g. on the SCBU.
- The mother may need to boost the milk supply on the affected side once the infection has cleared.

## Insufficient milk supply

This is one of the most commonly quoted reasons for women discontinuing breastfeeding. In the UK, it was the cause in 66% of women who discontinued breastfeeding in the first 2 weeks after birth.[58] The mother may express concern that she has an insufficient milk supply because the baby is not settling after a feed or is waking frequently for feeds, or the baby is not gaining weight. The most common cause of insufficient milk supply is the low intake by the baby which leads to a decrease in the production of milk.

*Actions*

- Reassure the mother that this can usually be dealt with because actual insufficient milk is extremely rare.
- A breastfeed should be observed and the positioning and attachment improved as necessary.
- There should be no time limit on the frequency or duration of feeding.
- The baby should drain one breast before being offered the second.
- Different feeding positions may be suggested, as this will assist drainage of all areas of the breast.
- Women should be encouraged and supported to continue breastfeeding. Supplementary feeds should not be suggested.
- If after the above action has been taken, the baby fails to gain weight, refer to a breastfeeding adviser or a breastfeeding clinic.

**Breast refusal**

There are two types of breast refusal: the baby who has never had a successful breastfeed and the baby who has breastfed well but then starts to refuse to go to the breast. Twenty-seven per cent of mothers who discontinue breastfeeding within the first week postnatally do so because the baby would not suck or rejected the breast;[54] therefore, it is important for midwives to have the knowledge to help mothers overcome this problem.

*Causes when breastfeeding not established*

Breast refusal in the initial stages of establishing breastfeeding may be caused by a number of factors, including:

• Pain relief the mother received in labour
• Breast engorgement as the milk 'comes in'
• The baby being forced on to the breast
• Incorrect positioning and attachment
• Powerful let-down
• Let-down inhibited
• The baby prefers bottles.

*Actions*

• Reassure the mother and try to establish a relaxed environment.
• Observe a feed and check positioning and attachment.
• If the breasts are overfull, express a small amount to soften the area around the areola to enable the baby to attach easier.
• Stimulate the let-down reflex by massaging the breast prior to attaching the baby.
• Express some breast milk onto the nipple or drip the EBM in the baby's mouth to encourage him or her to suckle.
• Attempt to put the baby to the breast before they are fully awake.
• Try skin-to-skin stimulation and do not offer the breast; let the baby find it.
• Co-bathing—where the mother and baby bathe together, this is thought to re-create the birth experience for the baby and has been shown to help. The baby needs to be kept warm by a helper pouring warm water over the baby as it lies on the mother's chest.
• If supplements of EBM are given to the baby, this should be given by either a cup or a spoon.

*Breast refusal once feeding is established*

The following are various factors that may cause a baby to refuse the breast, but a cause may not be found:

• Baby ill
• Hormonal changes in the mother, e.g. menstruation, ovulation, contraceptive pill, pregnancy
• Mother using different toiletries or mother eating spicy or garlicky food
• If the mother has undertaken prolonged, vigorous exercise, lactic acid may alter the taste of the milk—but this is usually short-lived
• If the mother has had mastitis, the milk may taste saltier for a short time afterwards.

*Actions*
- Check the baby's health. If he or she appears ill, refer to the doctor.
- If thrush is present, ➔ see *Candida* (thrush) infection, p. 807 below for action.
- If the baby is teething, offer a cool toy to chew on.
- Continue to offer the breast.
- Change the setting in which the baby is fed.
- Try feeding when the baby is sleepy.
- Check whether the mother wishes to continue feeding or if she had thought of discontinuing.
- If the baby is ill and refusing the breast, offer EBM. The baby may take it better by a spoon or cup.

## *Candida* (thrush) infection

This is an occasional cause of sore nipples, although the incidence appears to be increasing. It is caused by a microorganism *Candida*, which is a fungus. It commonly occurs after the mother has received antibiotic treatment. It often occurs after a period of trouble-free feeding and is commonly bilateral.

*Signs*
- Hypersensitive or itchy nipples even when wearing loose clothing.
- Pink and shiny nipples and areola.
- Burning sensations in nipples, especially after feeds.
- Shooting pains deep in the breast after feeding which may continue for up to an hour.
- Cracked nipples that will not heal.
- Loss of colour in the nipple or areola.
- Pain in both breasts.

The baby may also exhibit signs of a thrush infection such as:
- Creamy white spots in the mouth which do not rub off
- Baby keeps pulling away from the breast, which may be a result of a sore mouth
- A windy unsettled baby
- Nappy rash.

*Action*
- Ensure correct positioning and attachment.
- Continue breastfeeding.
- Refer to the GP for treatment. Effective treatment enables the mother to continue pain-free breastfeeding. When left untreated, many mothers find the severity of pain difficult to deal with and will discontinue feeding earlier than they wish.
- Both the mother and baby need to be treated simultaneously to prevent reinfection, even if only one shows signs of infection.
- Surface infection on the nipple is treated by application of an antifungal cream (usually miconazole 2%) which is prescribed. If the nipples are very inflamed, hydrocortisone cream 1% may be used or a combination cream of both hydrocortisone and miconazole.

- Oral treatment is required for infected milk ducts (usually nystatin or fluconazole 150–300mg as a single dose followed by 50–100mg twice a day for 10 days is prescribed). Poor absorption of nystatin in the gut can delay resolution of symptoms. Fluconazole is not licensed for lactating mothers, although the WHO recognizes it as compatible with breastfeeding.[59]
- Persistent or systemic/ductal *Candida* may require treatment for longer (14–28 days).[60]
- Babies are usually prescribed nystatin drops or miconazole oral gel. However, due to a change in the manufacturer's licence, use of miconazole oral gel is no longer considered suitable for use in babies <4 months old due to being a potential choking risk. Responsibility for use in a baby <4 months remains the responsibility of the person who prescribes or recommends its use.
- Any teats, dummies, or nipple shields used should be sterilized.
- Strict hygiene should be observed—washing of hands and use of separate towels for each member of the family.
- Any EBM collected during the infected period is best discarded to prevent reinfection.
- The mother taking *Acidophilus* capsules may help restore the normal, healthy bacterial flora which helps prevent thrush infections.
- Painkillers may help the mother to cope with the pain.

## References

52 UNICEF UK Baby Friendly Initiative (2014). *Breastfeeding assessment form*. Available at: ℘ www.unicef.org.uk/Documents/Baby_Friendly/Guidance/breastfeeding_assessment_tool_mat.pdf?epslanguage=en.
53 La Leche League GB (2011). *Sleepy Baby—Why and What to do. Information sheet no. 3101*. Nottingham: LLL Books Ltd.
54 McAndrew F, Thompson J, Fellows L, Large A, Speed M, Renfrew MJ (2012). *Infant Feeding Survey—UK, 2010 (NS)*. London: Health and Social Care Information Centre. Available at: ℘ www.hscic.gov.uk/catalogue/PUB08694.
55 National Institute for Health and Care Excellence (2005). *Division of ankyloglossia (tongue-tie) for breastfeeding*. NICE interventional procedure guidance IPG149. Available at: ℘ www.nice.org.uk/guidance/ipg149.
56 Jahanfar S, Ng CJ, Teng CL. Antibiotics for mastitis in breastfeeding women. *Cochrane Database Syst Rev* 2: CD005458. Available at: ℘ onlinelibrary.wiley.com/doi/10.1002/14651858.CD005458.pub3/abstract.
57 Arroyo R, Martín V, Maldonado A, Jiménez E, Fernández L, Rodríguez JM (2010). Treatment of infectious mastitis during lactation: antibiotics versus oral administration of Lactobacilli isolated from breast milk. *Clin Infect Dis* 50: 1551–6.
58 Renfrew MJ, Dyson L, Wallace L (2005). *The Effectiveness of Public Health Interventions to Promote the Duration of Breastfeeding: Systematic Reviews of the Evidence (Report)*. London: National Institute for Health and Care Excellence.
59 World Health Organization (2002). *Breastfeeding and maternal medication. Recommendations for drugs in the eleventh WHO model list of essential drugs*. Geneva: World Health Organization. Available at: ℘ whqlibdoc.who.int/hq/2002/55732.pdf.
60 National Institute for Health and Care Excellence (2013). *Candida—oral: management*. Clinical Knowledge Summaries. Available at: ℘ cks.nice.org.uk/candida-oral#!management.

# Breastfeeding in special situations

## Twins and higher multiples

The production of breast milk is based on a demand and supply system; therefore, provided the infants are suckling effectively, nature will supply the milk. In the early days postnatally, the mother will require a lot of reassurance and assistance to get breastfeeding established.

There are no rights and wrongs for whether the babies should be fed separately or together. The RCM[61] advocates that in the early days the babies should be fed separately, so that common early problems can be resolved, whereas the Twins and Multiple Births Association[62] believes that feeding the babies together in the early days will help to stimulate the milk supply, and feeding them together at night will ensure that the mother gets more sleep. Ultimately, the decision is up to the mother and the babies, as the infants' feeding patterns may not synchronize. One option is to mix and match so that at some feeds the babies are fed together and at others separately. The mother may decide that each baby has its own breast, or she may wish to swap breasts at each feed.

### Positions for breastfeeding twins

When breastfeeding both babies at the same time, positioning of the babies at the breast may take some time and practice to get it right. The mother should:

- Ensure she has adequate cushions to provide support for both herself and the babies
- Use a footstool under her feet, if necessary, to create a lap
- Find a position in which she feels comfortable to feed the babies. This may be the 'double football position' where the babies are tucked under the mother's arms and their heads are opposite each other at the front. This enables the mother to support each baby's head. Alternatively, one baby could be held conventionally in the cradle hold and the other held in the football position, so that the babies are parallel to each other. Another position is the criss-cross where both babies could be held conventionally, one lying across the other.

A mother who is breastfeeding twins must remember her own needs; she should eat well and try to obtain some rest each day to prevent exhaustion.

## Cleft lip and palate

Cleft lip and palate are congenital malformations that result in the incomplete fusion of the upper lip and jaw.

Cleft lip should not present any problems for breastfeeding. Following surgery, some surgeons encourage breastfeeding soon afterwards, whilst others prefer an initial period of spoon-feeding.

A cleft palate, however, may present major difficulties. The baby is unable to form an effective seal between the mouth and the breast, so that the breast and nipple cannot be formed into a teat. There are feeding plates/palate seals (palatal obturator), which can assist in 'closing' the defect. A baby with a cleft palate will not usually stimulate the breast effectively, which will result in a diminished milk supply. A mother with large, elastic breasts and a ready milk ejection reflex may succeed in breastfeeding, but normally mothers will need to supplement with a nursing supplementer (➔ see Alternative methods of giving expressed breast milk/formula, p. 813). Alternatively, mothers may wish to express breast milk and feed it to the baby with a special bottle, teat, or spoon. Breastfeeding is both possible and beneficial following surgical repair, but the mother will need practical and accurate support from appropriately skilled professionals.

## Breastfeeding and HIV

Mother-to-child transmission of HIV can occur through breastfeeding. The WHO[63] advises that HIV-infected pregnant mothers should consider their infant feeding options. It stipulates that 'when replacement feeding (formula milk) is acceptable, feasible, affordable, sustainable, and safe, HIV infected mothers should avoid breastfeeding completely'. This view is endorsed by the Department of Health through BHIVA and Children's HIV Association (CHIVA) position statement on infant feeding in the UK, which recommends that HIV-infected women should avoid breastfeeding.[64] Advice and counselling should be given to mothers during the antenatal period. If a mother decides to breastfeed once she has received advice, there may be a child protection issue, especially if she has a high viral load, which will place the baby at severe risk.

## Breastfeeding and diabetes

Diabetes is not a contraindication to breastfeeding. It can be advantageous to the mother's and baby's health.
- For the mother it can facilitate better management of diabetes and improve the mother's long-term health; this is because breastfeeding is a natural response to childbirth and the hormones responsible for lactation allow the physiological changes that follow childbirth to occur more gradually.
- For the baby it may reduce the risk of developing diabetes.[65]

### Considerations for diabetic mothers when breastfeeding
- Mothers may require extra carbohydrate to facilitate breastfeeding. An extra 50g of carbohydrate per day has been suggested. These extra carbohydrates are best spread equally over the day, remembering especially to increase the supper snack to cover the night-time feeds.
- Warnings should be given to all diabetic mothers about the possibility of hypoglycaemia, especially when breastfeeding. They should be advised to eat before breastfeeding the baby or have a snack handy whilst feeding.[66]
- Mothers who are breastfeeding are at an increased risk of mastitis and *Candida* (thrush), especially if their blood sugar levels are poorly controlled.[67] Therefore, they should be informed of the symptoms of mastitis and thrush, how they can help themselves, and where help is available, e.g. midwife, health visitor, breastfeeding peer supporter, National Childbirth Trust, etc.
- Diabetic mothers may find a delay in their milk production (lactogenesis II) and the milk may not 'come in' until the fourth or fifth postnatal day. Expressing (if mother and baby are separated) or breastfeeding every 2–3h during the first few days following delivery can help reduce the delay.[67]

*Care of the newborn infant of a diabetic mother*

- Babies of diabetic mothers are more prone to hypoglycaemia; this is because in intrauterine life the hypertrophic islets of Langerhans produce more insulin in response to the maternal blood sugar levels. After birth, the pancreas initially continues to produce excess insulin, thus causing hypoglycaemia.
- Preparation for prevention of neonatal hypoglycaemia can commence in pregnancy with the expressing and storage of colostrum for use in the immediate postnatal period. Expression and storage of colostrum should be discussed with the hospital during the antenatal period.[67]
- The baby should be given its first feed as soon as possible (within 30min of birth) and then 2–3h until pre-feeding blood glucose levels are maintained at 2mmol/L or more.[66]
- The baby's blood glucose levels should be monitored until stabilized. The frequency and timing of testing neonatal blood glucose levels may vary according to hospital policies.
- The mother and baby should not be transferred to community care until the baby is at least 24h old and the baby's blood sugar levels have stabilized and feeding is established.
- The mother should be given the opportunity for peer support with breastfeeding.[68]

## Breastfeeding and epilepsy

All women and girls with epilepsy should be encouraged to breastfeed, except in very rare circumstances.[69] Breastfeeding for most women and girls taking AEDs is generally safe and should be encouraged. However, each mother needs to be supported in the choice of feeding method that best suits her and her family.

Prescribers should consult individual drug advice in the Summary of Product Characteristics (SPC) and the *British National Formulary* (BNF) (available at ℀ bnf.org) when prescribing AEDs for women and girls who are breastfeeding. The decision regarding AED therapy and breastfeeding should be made between the woman or girl and the prescriber, and be based on the risks and benefits of breastfeeding against the potential risks of the drug affecting the child.[70]

## Separation

There are many reasons why a baby may be separated from its mother. The usual cause of separation of the mother and baby immediately following delivery is that the baby requires specialist care in a SCBU, neonatal surgical unit, or paediatric ward. Alternatively, the mother may be seriously ill, requiring care in either an ICU or an HDU. Whenever possible, mothers and babies should be cared for together.

If the mother intends to breastfeed, expression of breast milk should commence as soon as her condition allows (if the mother is ill) or as soon as possible following delivery (if the baby is on a SCBU). The mother should be encouraged to express breast milk and will need extra reassurance and support in these circumstances, especially if the baby is in a unit where there are no midwives to assist and support her. For detailed guidance on expression and storage of breast milk, ➔ see Expression of breast milk, pp. 790–4.

## Breast surgery

- Advice should be sought from the surgeon prior to surgery if the woman is of an age where she may wish to breastfeed.
- There are two types of breast reduction—pedicle and free-nipple. With the former, the mother may be able to breastfeed, but with the latter, it is not possible.
- Augmentation is not a contraindication to breastfeeding, but if a peri-areolar surgical technique has been used, then the mother may find she has an insufficient milk supply.
- Women can breastfeed successfully following unilateral mastectomy.

## Alternative methods of giving expressed breast milk/formula

Breastfeeding is the natural way to feed infants, but occasionally some infants may not be able to breastfeed immediately or the mother may require assistance to help improve her milk supply. The method of choice will depend upon the individual situations, and the aim of any alternative method of feeding should be to attain full breastfeeding as soon as possible. The alternative methods of feeding include cup, syringe, dropper, spoon, pipette, Lact-Aid®, and nasogastric feeding. The means used will depend upon the age of the baby and the reason for not breastfeeding. The main methods discussed in this text are nasogastric feeding, cup feeding, and supplementing with a Lact-Aid® device.

### Nasogastric feeding

- Sometimes, if a baby is so premature, ill, or weak that oral feeding is not possible, the option is to tube-feed the baby.
- A baby requiring nasogastric feeds would usually be cared for in a SCBU.
- Staff require training in the technique.
- Encourage the mother to express breast milk so that the baby can receive it via the nasogastric tube.
- A baby that has been fed via a nasogastric tube may present with sensory defensiveness and aversive behaviour once oral feeding commences, thought to be a result of a sore throat or irritated nasal passages.

### Cup feeding

- Cup feeding prevents exposure of the baby to artificial teats.
- In some countries, where teats are difficult to obtain and to clean, cup feeding is widely practised.
- Once the skill of cup feeding is mastered, then it is no more stressful than bottle-feeding.
- Cup feeding is very useful to promote the early acquisition of oral skills.
- Cup feeding also accelerates the transition from nasogastric feeding to established functional breastfeeding by providing a positive way to learn suck/swallow/breathing coordination.
- Caution needs to be taken with premature or compromised babies if their cough reflex is immature. This could lead to an increased risk of aspiration.

- There is also a higher level of spillage when cup feeding, and this needs to be taken into account if trying to calculate the amount taken.
- It is important that mothers are taught the correct technique.

*Technique for cup feeding*
- Stabilize the baby's head and body.
- Place the baby in an upright position on your lap.
- Have the cup at least half full (if possible).
- Place the rim of the cup at the corners of the baby's mouth. Rest the side of the cup lightly on the lower lip. Do not apply pressure to the lower lip.
- Tilt the cup so that the milk just touches the upper lip.
- The baby can then control the intake, pausing as necessary.
- In effect, the baby laps from the cup, rather than milk being poured into the baby's mouth.
- It is important that the milk is offered but never poured.

*Nursing supplementers*
- This is a feeding tube device that allows the infant to be supplemented at the breast with either EBM or formula.[71]
- The aim of these devices is to deliver a faster flow of milk to the baby whilst he or she is still suckling at the breast.
- Feeding tube devices are helpful for mothers who have a very poor milk supply, are trying to re-establish lactation, or are attempting to induce lactation for an adopted baby.
- Mothers need supervision when first using these devices.
- They are more effective if the baby is able to latch onto the breast, although an augmented flow may assist a baby to suck better because he or she is being rewarded for their efforts.

*Technique*
- The tube is usually positioned on the nipple so that it enters the baby's mouth centred along the palate. However, the positioning of the tube may need to be adapted to enable the baby to obtain the flow of milk more effectively.
- The flow of milk from the receptacle is determined by a combination of the baby's suck and its position/height.
- Adjustments will be required to establish the correct flow for the baby.

# References

61 Royal College of Midwives (2002). *Successful Breastfeeding*. Edinburgh: Churchill Livingstone.
62 Twins and Multiple Births Association (2014). *Breastfeeding more than one*. Guildford: Tamba. Available at: ℅ www.tamba.org.uk/document.doc?id=44.
63 World Health Organization (2010). *Guidelines on HIV and infant feeding 2010: principles and recommendations for infant feeding in the context of HIV and a summary of evidence*. Geneva: World Health Organization. Available at: ℅ www.who.int/child_adolescent_health/documents/9789241599535/en/index.html.
64 British HIV Association, Children's HIV Association (2010). *British HIV Association (BHIVA) and Children's HIV Association (CHIVA) position statement on infant feeding in the UK*. Available at: ℅ www.chiva.org.uk/files/3614/2900/9349/InfantFeeding.pdf.
65 Jackson W (2004). Breastfeeding and type 1 diabetes. *Br J Midwifery* 12: 158–65.
66 Sadauskaite-Kuehne V, Ludvigsson J, Padaiga Z, Jasinskiene E, Samuelsson U (2004). Longer breastfeeding is an independent protective factor against development of type 1 diabetes in childhood. *Diabetes Metab Res Rev* 20: 150–7.
67 National Institute for Health and Care Excellence (2015). *Diabetes in pregnancy: management from preconception to the postnatal period*. NICE guidelines NG3. Available at: ℅ www.nice.org.uk/guidance/ng3.
68 Finigan V (2012). Breastfeeding and diabetes: part 2. *Pract Midwife* 15: 33–34, 36.
69 National Institute for Health and Care Excellence (2008). *Improving the Nutrition of Pregnant and Breastfeeding Mothers and Children in Low-income Households*. NICE public health programme guidance 11. London: National Institute for Health and Care Excellence.
70 National Institute for Health and Care Excellence (2012). *Epilepsies: diagnosis and management*. NICE guidelines CG137. Available at: ℅ www.nice.org.uk/guidance/cg137.
71 La Leche League GB (2011). *Nursing Supplementers. Information Sheet no. 3105*. Nottingham: LLL Books Ltd.

# Lactation and nutrition

New mothers do not need to eat anything special when breastfeeding.[72] However, all new mothers need to eat a healthy diet for their own well-being and to help them to replenish stores of certain nutrients that become depleted during pregnancy. They also need a healthy diet to assist them to cope with the demands of a new baby and possibly older siblings. Even if eating a suboptimal diet, either in calories or content, they will still produce high-quality milk which will satisfy their infant's nutritional requirements.

A healthy diet should be based on the five food groups and a breastfeeding mother should include:

- Group 1—carbohydrates: a portion of bread, rice, potatoes, pasta, or other starchy food should be eaten with each meal. Wholegrain should be eaten whenever possible.
- Group 2—fruit and vegetables: should be included in each meal, aiming for five portions a day.
- Group 3—dairy products: 2–3 portions of milk, cheese and yoghurt should be eaten a day and they can be of low-fat varieties if desired.
- Group 4—protein: meat, fish, nuts, and pulses should be included in two meals per day. Non-meat eaters should ensure they include eggs, nuts, and pulses in their diet on a regular basis.
- Group 5—high-fat and sugar foods and drinks: these should be kept to a minimum and the diet basically based on the other four food groups.

## Fluids and breastfeeding

Breastfeeding mothers do not need to drink excessive amounts of fluid but should drink to their thirst. A minimum of eight drinks a day is recommended and can include a range of sources, including water, fruit juice, milk, tea, coffee, and soups. Milk is not necessary to produce breast milk. In hot weather, more fluid may be required to quench the mother's thirst.

## Food to avoid whilst breastfeeding

Generally women who are breastfeeding do not need to avoid certain foods; however, there are several recommendations:

- Oily fish—can be included in the diet but no more than two servings a week.
- Large fish—shark, swordfish, and marlin should be avoided altogether as they contain large amounts of mercury.
- Alcohol—passes into the bloodstream and levels peak at 30–90min after consumption. The recommendation is that daily consumption should not exceed 1 unit per day.
- Peanuts—mothers are advised to avoid eating peanuts if they, the infant's father, or siblings suffer from allergic conditions such as hay fever, asthma, or eczema. If there are no known allergies and the mother wishes to eat peanuts or foods containing peanuts, she may do so as part of a balanced diet.
- Caffeine—in tea, coffee, cola, energy drinks, and chocolate should be limited as it can make some babies restless and may cause breast pain in some women.

Mothers who are overweight or obese should not embark on very low-calorie diets whilst breastfeeding but should eat a balanced diet and limit high-fat and high-sugar foods. Once breastfeeding is established, some regular physical activity of at least 30min on all or most days of the week will help weight loss and women can still breastfeed successfully and lose about 450g (1lb) in weight each week.

Even with a healthy diet, it is difficult to get an adequate intake of vitamin D in the UK. Breastfeeding mothers are therefore advised to take 10 micrograms of vitamin D each day to prevent vitamin D deficiency in both them and their baby. Vitamin D is needed for bone health and the immune system. Babies of mothers who did not take vitamin D supplements during pregnancy may be born with low levels of vitamin D. There is a very small chance that these babies may have fits due to low levels of calcium. Older babies and toddlers with very low levels of vitamin D can develop rickets.

The NHS Healthy Start vitamins for women contain 10 micrograms of vitamin D along with 400 micrograms of folic acid and some vitamin C, and are ideal for breastfeeding mothers. The vitamins are free for mothers included within the Healthy Start Scheme (see ℘ www.healthystart. nhs.uk). Vegan mothers may need a supplement containing vitamin $B_{12}$ and calcium, in addition to vitamin D.

### Reference

72  NHS Choices (2016). *Breastfeeding and diet.* Available at: ℘ www.nhs.uk/conditions/pregnancy-and-baby/pages/lifestyle-breastfeeding.aspx#close.

# Artificial feeding

# Introduction

Although breastfeeding is best for the mother and infant, the 2010 Infant Feeding Survey[1] showed that 19% of mothers chose to formula-feed their infants from birth. This is usually for social, psychological, or cultural reasons, but there will be some cases where breastfeeding is contraindicated for medical reasons (→ see Contraindications to breastfeeding, p. 773). There will also be mothers who commence breastfeeding but, for a variety of reasons, discontinue earlier than they intended.

All pregnant women should be informed of the benefits of breastfeeding, but ultimately it is the mother's choice which feeding method she adopts. If the mother decides to formula-feed, give her guidance to ensure that she does so safely, but do not give her the impression that formula milk is equivalent to breastfeeding or that it is without risk.[2]

## References
1 McAndrew F, Thompson J, Fellows L, Large A, Speed M, Renfrew MJ (2012). *Infant Feeding Survey—UK, 2010 (NS)*. London: Health and Social Care Information Centre. Available at: ℜ www.hscic.gov.uk/catalogue/PUB08694.
2 Royal College of Midwives (2002). *Successful Breastfeeding*. Edinburgh: Churchill Livingstone.

# International Code of Marketing of Breast Milk Substitutes

In May 1981, the World Health Assembly approved an International Code of Marketing of Breast Milk Substitutes.[3] The purpose of this code was to protect the practice of breastfeeding and to help control the marketing of products for the artificial feeding of infants. Nowhere does it seek to enforce breastfeeding, and the code does not prevent mothers from bottle-feeding if that is what they choose to do. At present, the code is voluntary in the UK, but some countries have chosen to enshrine it in law. Employees in Baby Friendly hospitals and community health-care facilities are required to ensure that their practice is in line with the International Code, and not just with the UK law.[4] The code has major implications for the work of the midwife. The major recommendations are included in Box 29.1.

Midwives have a responsibility to ensure safe infant feeding practices as per UNICEF and NICE guidelines.

## Box 29.1 Recommendations of the International Code of Marketing of Breast Milk Substitutes

- No advertising or promotion of these products in hospital or shops, or to the general public.
- No free samples of breast milk substitutes to be given to mothers or members of their families.
- No free gifts relating to the products within the scope of the code to be given to the mothers.
- No promotion of products in health-care facilities.
- No gifts or personal samples to be given to health workers, nor any free or subsidized supplies to hospitals or maternity wards.
- No words or pictures idealizing bottle-feeding, including pictures of infants on product labels.
- All information on infant feeding, including product labels, should explain the benefits of breastfeeding and the costs and hazards associated with bottle-feeding.
- Information provided by manufacturers to health-care workers should include only scientific and factual material and should not create or imply that bottle-feeding is equivalent or superior to breastfeeding.
- Unsuitable products (i.e. sweetened condensed milk) should not be promoted for babies.
- All products should be of a high quality and should take into account the climate and storage conditions of the country where they are to be used.
- Health-care workers should encourage and protect the practice of breastfeeding.

## References

3 World Health Organization (1981). *International Code of Marketing of Breast Milk Substitutes*. Geneva: World Health Organization.
4 UNICEF UK Baby Friendly Initiative (2008). *Three-day Course in Breastfeeding Management: Participant's Handbook*. London: UNICEF UK.

# Suppression of lactation

If a mother does not wish to breastfeed her infant and has a late miscarriage or a stillbirth, lactation will still occur and she may experience discomfort for several days.

## Aetiology

- The classical theory is that milk secretion is controlled principally by the maternal hormones prolactin and oxytocin.
- However, removal of milk from the breasts has also been found to be a crucial element in milk secretion.
- If milk is not removed from the breast, a chemical (autocrine inhibitor) in the whey protein fraction prevents further production by exerting a negative feedback control. This is known as the feedback inhibitor of lactation.
- A build-up of this autocrine inhibitor then accelerates the breakdown of milk components already produced.

## Management

- If unstimulated, the breasts will naturally stop producing milk.
- The breasts should be well supported, but binding has not been shown to contribute towards suppression of lactation.
- If there is severe discomfort with engorgement, encourage the mother to express very small amounts of milk once or twice. This can help relieve the discomfort without interfering with the regression of lactation. Also anti-inflammatory drugs may be useful and so may cold compresses.
- Give mild analgesics to assist in relieving the pain and discomfort felt.
- Do not restrict fluids.
- Pharmacological suppression using dopamine receptor agonists is effective but is not advised for routine use.[5]

## Reference

5 Inch S (2009). Infant feeding. In: Fraser DM, Cooper MA, eds. *Myles Textbook for Midwives*, 15th edn. Edinburgh: Churchill Livingstone, pp. 758–816.

# Nutritional requirements of formula-fed babies

Three areas need to be taken into consideration:
- Energy requirements
- Fluid requirements
- Balance of ingredients.

## Energy requirements

- An average healthy baby will thrive on 440kJ/kg of body weight per day.
- Breast milk and infant formula milk contain approximately 90kJ/30mL.
- A 3.5kg baby would therefore require 1540kJ in 24h = approximately 525mL of milk.

This is only a guide, and individual babies will take as much as they require at each feed to satisfy their needs. This amount may vary from feed to feed and the overall picture should be considered, e.g. the general health and weight gain of the baby.

## Fluid requirements

- An average healthy baby requires 150–165mL of fluid per kg of body weight per day to remain hydrated.
- A 3.5kg baby would therefore require approximately 525–575mL per day.

## Balance of ingredients

Infant formula feeds can be developed from cow's or goat milk, which is balanced to meet the needs of calves or kids and therefore requires modification for human infants. 'Modified milks' are those that have had the balance of ingredients adjusted to resemble human milk as closely as possible.

Cow's milk formula modifications include:
- Most of the casein removed and replaced by whey protein
- Some of the milk fat removed and replaced by vegetable fat
- Lactose added to increase the energy value
- Vitamins added to resemble levels in human milk
- Minerals adjusted to resemble levels in human milk
- Higher levels of iron required as it is less bioabsorbable from formulas than from breast milk.

Goat milk formula modifications include:
- Using whole milk
- Lactose supplemented with refined lactose
- Vitamins and minerals supplemented
- Fatty acids supplemented with essential fatty acids from selected vegetable oils
- No added whey proteins
- Does not require supplementing with synthetic nucleotides as natural levels are sufficient.

# Selecting an appropriate infant formula

All infant formula milks are highly processed, factory-produced products. Under UK law, it is an offence to sell any infant formula milk as being suitable from birth unless it conforms to the compositional and other criteria set out in the Infant Formula and Follow-on Formula Regulations 2013.[6]

- There is no scientific basis for recommending one brand over another.
- Health professionals must not recommend one brand of infant formula over another.
- First milk is recommended for the first year of life.
- There is no reason for a mother to remain with one brand.
- All common baby milks suitable for home use are supplied in dried powder form so they can be stored and transported without risk of deterioration.
- Many manufacturers also supply individual feed sachets and ready-to-feed cartons, but these tend to be more expensive.
- In 2013, in England, the Infant Formula and Follow-on Formula Regulations have been amended to allow goat milk as the source of protein in formula milks from March 2014.[6]
- The Department of Health recommends that soya formula should only be used for babies who are intolerant of cow's milk or lactose, and only with medical guidance.
- For babies and infants who are intolerant of standard infant formulas, alternative formulas, such as extensively hydrolysed and amino acid-based formulas, are medically prescribed.

## Examples of specific types of formulas

This is not a comprehensive list of all infant formulas. There may be other specific types of formulas that have not been included as brand names change frequently due to constant research and rebranding by formula companies.

*Examples of whey- and casein-dominant formulas*
See Table 29.1.

Table 29.1 Examples of whey- and casein-dominant formulas

| Whey-dominant formula | Casein-dominant formula |
|---|---|
| (60% whey, 40% casein) | (80% casein, 20% whey) |
| Aptamil 1 First Milk® | Aptamil Hungry Milk® |
| Aptamil Profurtura 1 First Infant Milk® | |
| Babynat 1 Infant Milk® | |
| Cow & Gate 1 First Milk® | Cow & Gate for Hungrier Babies® |
| HIPP Organic Combiotic First Infant Milk® | HIPP Organic Combiotic Hungry Infant Milk® |
| Holle Organic Infant formula® | |
| SMA First Infant Milk® | SMA Extra Hungry® |

*Examples of goat milk formulas suitable from birth*
- Kabrita Gold 1®.
- NANNYcare First Infant Milk®.

*Examples of soya infant formulas suitable from birth*
- Wysoy (SMA)®.

*Examples of specially modified formulas*
- Aptamil Comfort®.
- Cow & Gate Comfort®.
- SMA Comfort®.
- SMA HA®.

*Examples of follow-on milks*
- Aptimil 2 Follow-on Milk®.
- Babynat 2 Optima Follow-on Milk®.
- Cow & Gate 2 Follow-on Milk®.
- HIPP Organic Combiotic Follow-on Milk 2®.
- SMA Follow-on Milk®.

*Examples of goat milk follow on milks*
- Kabrita Gold 2®.
- NANNYcare Follow-on Milk®.

*Examples of pre-thickened formulas*
- Aptamil Anti-reflu®.
- SMA Stay Down®.

*Examples of 'good night milks'*
- HIPP Organic Good Night Milk®.

## Reference

6 Gov.UK (2013) *Statutory Instruments 2013 No. 3243 Food, England. The Infant Formula and Follow-on Formula (England) (Amendment) Regulations 2013.* Available at: ✆ www.legislation.gov.uk/uksi/2013/3243/pdfs/uksi_20133243_en.pdf.

# Types of cow's milk infant formula

Whey and casein are proteins found in milk. Formulas are modified to vary the ratio of these proteins. There are two main types—whey-dominant and casein-dominant formulas.

## Whey-dominant formulas

- Whey is the dominant protein in human milk.
- Whey-based formulas have been modified so that the whey:casein ratio (60:40) is closer to that of human milk.
- These formulas are more easily digested, which affects gastric emptying times and leads to feeding patterns similar to those of breastfed babies.
- These formulas are suitable for use from birth to 1 year.

## Casein-dominant formulas

- Casein is the dominant protein in cow's milk.
- Casein-dominant formulas have been modified so that the whey:casein ratio is 20:80 and is nearer to the type found in cow's milk.
- These formulas are not comparable to breast milk.
- Such feeds form large, harder-to-digest curds in the stomach, which are intended to make the infant feel full for longer. However, there is little evidence to support this.[7]
- They are advertised for the hungrier bottle-fed baby and can be used from birth to 1 year.
- There may be an even greater metabolic demand on the infant when these formulas are given.[8]
- Babies who are settled and gaining weight on whey-dominant formulas will not need casein-dominant formulas.

## Additional ingredients

Whey- and casein-dominant formulas may also have additional ingredients, e.g. long-chain polyunsaturated fatty acids (LCPs), nucleotides, β-carotene, and selenium. The ingredients and their sources vary from one brand to another.

### Long-chain polyunsaturated fatty acids

- Occur naturally in breast milk.
- Aid brain, eye, and CNS development.
- Are added to formulas in the form of fish oils or egg yolk.

Research into both the long- and short-term effects of adding LCPs to formulas is continuing.

### β-carotene

- Occurs naturally in breast milk.
- Can be metabolized by the baby to produce vitamin A.

### Nucleotides

- Nucleotides are present in breast milk.
- Assist with the development of the baby's immune system.
- Aid adsorption of other nutrients from breast milk.

*Selenium*
- An antioxidant found in breast milk.

## Specially modified formula

Several formula manufacturers have recently introduced specially modified formulas which they claim aids digestion and helps reduce some of the common problems associated with formula feeding, e.g. constipation, colic. These products are available over the counter, but their efficacy needs further research.

## Follow-on milks

These milks are made from slightly modified cow's milk and they have added vitamin D and iron.
- They are *not* to be given to infants <6 months old.[7]
- The large amounts of iron may make some babies constipated.
- Full-fat cow's milk has low levels of iron and vitamin D and should *not* be used as a main drink for an infant under 1 year of age. However, it can be used for preparing baby weaning foods from 4 to 6 months of age.
- If an infant tolerates a well-balanced and varied diet, full-fat cow's milk can be used from the age of 1 year.

## 'Good night milks'

- 'Good night milks' have added starch and rice flakes and are represented as helping to settle babies at bedtime and are promoted for use as a bedtime liquid feed from a bottle or feeding cup.
- The Scientific Advisory Committee on Nutrition[9] has identified no scientific evidence that demonstrates 'good night' milk products offer any advantage over the use of currently available infant formulas.
- Concern expressed that their promotion will encourage parents to believe that it is desirable for a baby to sleep longer at an age when healthy infants show considerable variation in normal sleeping patterns.
- There is a potential risk that mothers may consider the product suitable for 'settling' their infant more than once a day and use these products on occasions additional to bedtime.
- An even greater concern is that they may be used to 'settle' infants <6 months. Such unintended use would be contrary to advice that gluten-containing products should not be given to infants <6 months of age.[9]

## Thickened formulas

- Pre-thickened formulas are advertised for infants with reflux or posseting.
- They are casein-based infant formulas with added pre-gelatinized starch. They thicken when in contact with the acid in the stomach and this increases the feed thickness whilst still flowing easily through the teat.
- Infants taking these formulas should not be prescribed thickeners or antireflux medication such as Gaviscon®.
- Can be purchased over the counter or they may be prescribed.

- Most infants do not need this sort of preparation once solids have been established as part of their diet. However, they are suitable for use up to the age of 1 year.
- Extra care is needed when making up some of these feeds as they require cooled boiled water. Water at 70°C will cause the feed to thicken in the bottle.

## References

7  UNICEF UK (2014). *A guide to infant formula for parents who are bottle feeding: the health professionals' guide*. Available at: ℘ www.unicef.org.uk/Documents/Baby_Friendly/Leaflets/HP_Guide_for_parents_formula_feeding.pdf.

8  Inch S (2009). Infant feeding. In: Fraser DM, Cooper MA, eds. *Myles Textbook for Midwives*, 15th edn. Edinburgh: Churchill Livingstone, pp. 785–816.

9  Scientific Advisory Committee on Nutrition (2008). *Consideration of the place of 'good night' milk products in the diet of infants aged 6 months and above*. London: Scientific Advisory Committee on Nutrition. Available at: ℘ www.gov.uk/government/uploads/system/uploads/attachment_data/file/339388/SACN_Statement_on_Good-Night_Milks_2008.pdf.

# Alternatives to modified cow's milk formulas

## Goat milk formula

- UK regulations were changed from 2 February 2014 to allow goat milk proteins to be used in the manufacture of infant formula. Therefore, using goat milk formula is an acceptable alternative to modified cow's milk formula.
- Goat milk formula is not an alternative to cow's milk formula if there is an allergy to cow's milk as the protein content of goat milk is very similar.
- Based on whole goat milk.
- Supplemented with refined lactose and relevant minerals and vitamins added.
- Fatty acids supplemented with essential fatty acids vegetable oils.
- Does not have any added whey proteins and therefore does not require supplementation with synthetic nucleotides.

## Specialized formula milks

These are available for parents who wish their baby to have vegetarian feeds. These should only be given under the direction of a dietitian.

## Soya formulas

- Are not recommended for infants under 6 months.[10]
- It is recommended by the Department of Health that these milks should only be used if a baby/infant is intolerant to cow's milk or lactose and only under medical guidance. There are now other alternatives that are more suitable.[10]
- There are concerns about the possible effects of oestrogen-like compounds produced by soya beans (phyto-oestrogens) and unacceptable levels of manganese and aluminium in such formulas.[11]
- Soya-based infant formula contains glucose, a type of sugar. Glucose is more harmful to babies' and small children's teeth than the lactose in infant formula made with cow's milk.[10]
- They may contain genetically modified ingredients.

## Specialist formulas for babies intolerant to standard infant formulas

Predicting allergies is an inexact science. The likelihood has been estimated to be:[12]

- Almost one in 12 young children will suffer from a food allergy
- Prevalence of cow's milk allergy is between 2% and 3%
- Food allergies are more common among children who come from families where other members suffer from allergies
- A baby with severe eczema before 3 months is very likely to suffer from food allergies.

*Lactose-free formulas*
- Appropriate for infants who are intolerant to lactose but can tolerate the milk protein.
- Cow's milk protein-based with lactose replaced by glucose.
- Prescribable or may be purchased in pharmacies.
- Glucose in these formulas may be dangerous to teeth.

*Extensively hydrolysed formulas*
- Used if breastfeeding is not possible.
- Prescription only.
- Some are designed to treat an existing allergy; some are designed to prevent an allergy.
- Prescribing guidelines: some extensively hydrolysed formulas need proven intolerance, whereas others do not.

*Amino acid-based formulas*
- Have a completely synthetic protein base.
- Are very expensive.

## References

10 NHS Choices (2015). *Can I give my baby soya-based infant formula?* Available at: ℘ www.nhs.uk/chq/Pages/can-I-give-my-baby-soya-based-infant-formula.aspx?CategoryID=62&SubCategoryID=63.
11 UNICEF UK (2014). *A guide to infant formula for parents who are bottle feeding: the health professionals' guide.* Available at: ℘ www.unicef.org.uk/Documents/Baby_Friendly/Leaflets/HP_Guide_for_parents_formula_feeding.pdf.
12 AllergyUK (2013). *Food allergy in babies and children.* Allergy UK Factsheet. Available at: ℘ www.allergyuk.org/downloads/factsheets/childhood-allergy/food-allergy-in-children.pdf.

# Management of formula feeding

## Sterilization of infant feeding equipment

All infant feeding equipment must be completely clean and sterilized prior to use. This includes any equipment used for breastfed babies or for storing EBM, e.g. bottles, teats, breast pumps, and nipple shields. This is to protect babies against any potential sources of infection. Due to their immature immune system, babies are at risk of infection, particularly gastroenteritis (potentially life-threatening for newborn babies) and fungal infections (which can be difficult to treat).

Demonstrations of sterilization of equipment are best given on a one-to-one basis in the mother's home environment.

### Types of sterilization

- Boiling.
- Chemical sterilization.
- Steam sterilization.
- Microwave sterilization using a microwave sterilization unit. This is not suitable for metal items or certain types of plastic.

### For all types of sterilization

*Before sterilization*

- Wash all bottles and other equipment thoroughly in hot, soapy water, using a bottle brush. Scrub both inside and outside to remove fatty deposits. Pay special attention to the rim.
- Clean the teat by:
  - Either using a small teat brush
  - Or turning inside out and washing in hot, soapy water.
- Rinse all the washed equipment thoroughly with non-soapy water before sterilizing.

*After sterilization*

- Always wash your hands before removing equipment from the sterilizer.

### To sterilize by boiling

- Put the equipment in a large pan filled with water, ensuring that there is no air trapped in the bottles or teats. Cover the pan with a lid and bring to the boil.
- *Boil for 10min*, ensuring that the pan does not boil dry.
- Allow the water to cool and store the equipment in the covered pan until required. Use the equipment within 12h (if longer, repeat the process).
- Remove equipment from the saucepan carefully to avoid desterilization.
- Check bottles and teats regularly for any signs of deterioration. If this is detected, discard them. Prolonged boiling of teats may destroy them.

### To sterilize using chemicals (cold water sterilization)

- Use the liquid or tablets to make up the solution following the manufacturer's instructions.
- Use either a sterilizing tank or a large container with a well-fitting lid.

- Submerge the equipment, ensuring that no air bubbles are trapped in the bottles or teats.
- Keep all the equipment under the water, using the plunger provided or a plate.
- Leave in the solution for a minimum of 30min.
- Discard the solution and make up fresh every 24h.
- Wash the container before making up new solution.
- Use cooled boiled water if you wish to rinse the equipment prior to use.

*Sterilization using a steam or microwave sterilizer*
- Follow the manufacturer's instructions.
- Sterilizing in a microwave without a microwave sterilizer is not advisable.

## Preparing a formula feed

The correct preparation of infant formula feeds is important to prevent conditions such as dehydration, constipation, and gastroenteritis. The Food Standards Agency and the Department of Health[13] have produced guidelines on the safe preparation of infant formulas to reduce the risk of gastroenteritis. Powdered infant formula is not a sterile product and may contain bacterial contaminants. *Enterobacter sakazakii* and *Salmonella* are those of greatest concern. Both NICE and UNICEF UK recommend that all mothers who are artificially feeding their infants should be shown the correct method of preparing a formula feed prior to discharge from hospital.[14,15]

## Methods of making up formula feeds
- Scoop method.
- Individual feed sachets.
- Ready-to-feed cartons.

*Scoop method*
- A fresh bottle should be made up for each feed. This is because bacteria multiply quickly at room temperature and may survive and multiply slowly in some fridges; therefore storing formula milk can increase the risk of gastroenteritis.
- The feed should be made up with water above 70°C as this will destroy most bacterial contaminants. This means boiling 1L of water in the kettle and leaving it to cool for no longer than 30min. Do *not* use bottled artificially softened water or previously boiled water.
- There is now equipment on the market that can be used to ensure feeds are made up at the correct temperature and in a short timescale. The manufacturer's instructions should be followed carefully.
- Read the tin or pack to find out how much water and formula you require.
- Clean a surface on which to prepare the feed. Wash your hands thoroughly with soap and water, and dry on a clean towel.
- All equipment used for making up the feed must have been freshly sterilized.
- If using a sterilizer, remove the lid; turn upside down and place the teat(s) and cap(s) in it. If using a chemical (cold water) sterilizer, rinse with cool boiled water (not tap water) if wished.

- Remove the bottle, rinse with cooled boiled water (if wished) and stand on a clean, flat surface. Pour cool boiled water, which should still be hot, into the bottle, up to the required mark. This is better if undertaken at eye level.
- Measure the exact amount of formula using the scoop provided. Level the formula in the scoop using the knife or spatula provided.
- Do *not* compress or compact the formula in the scoop.
- Add the formula to the water in the bottle, *never* the other way round. In the UK, all baby formulas use one scoop to 1oz (30mL) of water.
- Do *not* add anything else to the feed unless medically prescribed.
- Apply the top or teat and cover. Shake the bottle well until all the formula is dissolved.
- Cool the feed down to the required temperature by holding the bottle with the cap in place under cold running water.
- Check the temperature of the formula prior to feeding the baby by dripping a little onto the inside of your wrist; it should be lukewarm but not hot.
- Discard any formula that has not been used within 2h; clean and resterilize the bottle.

*When it is not practical to make up feeds just before feeding*
It is best to make up feeds individually as required, but this may not always be practical. Ready-to-use formula is the safest option, but this is more expensive.

*Feeding the baby away from home*
It is safest to carry a measured amount of formula powder in a small clean, dry container, a flask of hot water that has been boiled, and an empty sterilized feeding bottle. The feed is then made up fresh as required. The water should still be hot when used, and therefore the bottle will need to be cooled before giving to the baby.

*Making up and transporting feeds for later use*
If the above advice is difficult to follow, e.g. if preparing and transporting feeds either to a nursery or child minder, the following steps should be adopted.
- Prepare feeds individually, not in one large container.
- Make the feeds up on the day they are required, not the night before. This reduces storage time and therefore reduces the risk.
- Once prepared, store at the back of a fridge at below 5°C.
- Ensure the feed has been in the fridge for at least 1h before transporting.
- Store for the minimum of time.
- Remove from the fridge just before leaving home and transport in a cool bag with ice packs.
- Use within 4h. If arriving at the destination in <4h, remove from the cool bag and store in the back of a fridge below 5°C.
- Never store reconstituted feeds for >24h.
- Re-warm before use.

*Re-warming stored feeds*
- Only remove the feed from the fridge just before it is needed.
- Re-warm using a bottle-warmer or placing in a container of warm water.
- *Never* use a microwave to re-warm a feed.
- *Never* warm for >15min.
- Shake the bottle to ensure even heating of the feed.
- Check the temperature before feeding the baby.

## Principles of artificial feeding
- Feed the baby when he or she is hungry.
- Let him or her take as little or as much as desired.
- Ideally, the minimum of caregivers should feed the baby and he or she should not be passed from person to person for feeding.
- *Never* feed babies by 'bottle propping' and *never* leave them unattended when feeding from a bottle.
- Make up feeds individually as required whenever possible.
- Test the temperature of the feed on the inside of your wrist before offering it to the baby.
- Feeding times should be enjoyable and relaxed.
- Hold the baby securely and close to your body, in a similar position to that used in breastfeeding.
- Maintain eye contact.
- Ensure that the teat covers the baby's tongue, and tip the bottle up sufficiently so that air is excluded from the teat.
- The baby will suck and pause whilst retaining the teat in their mouth.
- During the feed, when necessary, sit the baby in an upright position so he or she can bring up wind; this may be once or twice.
- It is normal for babies to regurgitate small amounts (posseting).
- If the baby is sucking but the feed does not appear to be reducing, check the teat for blockages.
- The baby will stop feeding when he or she has had enough.
- If the baby is draining the full amount offered, the amount should be increased.
- Any feed left at the end of the feed should be discarded after 2h and should *never* be reheated.

## References
13 Food Standards Agency/Department of Health (2007). *Guidance for Health Professionals on Safe Preparation, Storage and Handling of Powdered Infant Formula*. London: Food Standards Agency.
14 National Institute for Health and Care Excellence (2008). *Improving the Nutrition of Pregnant and Breastfeeding Mothers in Low-income Households*. London: National Institute for Health and Care Excellence.
15 UNICEF UK (2014). *A guide to infant formula for parents who are bottle feeding: the health professionals' guide*. Available at: ℛ www.unicef.org.uk/Documents/Baby_Friendly/Leaflets/HP_Guide_for_parents_formula_feeding.pdf.

# Problems associated with formula feeding

## Constipation

It is the consistency, not the frequency, of bowel movements that should be considered when discussing constipation. Babies may go several days without a bowel movement, but if the stools are soft and yellow, then no treatment is required. Constipation results from reabsorption of water from the stools and stools present as hard, round pellets.

### Management

- Check that the condition is constipation, and not just infrequent stools.
- Ensure that the feeds are being prepared correctly, i.e. the water is being placed in the bottle prior to the formula, the powder in the scoop is not being compressed, and extra scoopfuls are not being added.
- Offer the baby cooled boiled water between feeds. There should be *no* additives to the water, e.g. brown sugar or orange juice.
- Try an alternative make of formula; not all formulas suit all babies.
- If the above strategies do not work, seek a medical opinion.

## Posseting

It is normal for a baby to regurgitate a small amount of milk following a feed. Reassure the mother that it is normal and take no action unless it becomes persistent or projectile vomiting, in which case medical aid should be sought immediately.

## Colic

Colic is the name for excessive, frequent crying in a baby who appears to be otherwise healthy. It is a common problem that affects up to one in five babies.

Colic tends to begin when a baby is a few weeks old. It normally stops by 4 months of age or by 6 months at the latest.

### Techniques that may help

There is no method that works for all babies with colic, but the following may help:

- Holding the baby during a crying episode
- Preventing the baby from swallowing air by sitting or holding them upright during feeding
- Burping the baby after feeds
- Gently rocking the baby over your shoulder
- Bathing the baby in a warm bath
- Gently massaging the baby's tummy.

# Disadvantages associated with formula feeding

The following disadvantages for the formula-fed infant have been identified.[16]
Formula milk is deficient in:
- Some nutrient compounds (e.g. epidermal growth factors)
- Cells (e.g. leucocytes, macrophages) which are important in protecting the infant from a wide variety of pathogens
- Antibodies, antibacterial and antiviral factors (e.g. IgA, IgG, IgM, lactoferrin)
- Hormones (e.g. prolactin, thyroid hormones)
- Enzymes (e.g. mammary amylase, milk lipase, lysozyme)
- Prostaglandins.

These deficiencies are important to the infant's immunological and hormonal responses, as well as neonatal development and cell maturation.
The formula-fed infant may be further compromised by:
- The presence of cow's milk or soya proteins
- The possibility of errors during manufacture, including incorrect manufacture, bacterial contamination, foreign bodies, etc.[16]
- The addition of new ingredients on an uncertain scientific basis
- Frequent errors in the preparation of feeds, which alter their concentration[17]
- Variability of the mineral and trace element content in the water used to reconstitute feeds.
- Formulas which may be contaminated with bacteria and/or pathogens:
  - During manufacture
  - Whilst preparing feeds at home with unclean utensils and/or contaminated water.

## References

16 Crawley H, Westland S (2016). *Infant milks in the UK: a practical guide for health professionals.* Available at: ℘ firststepsnutrition.org/newpages/Infants/infant_feeding_infant_milks_UK.html.
17 McAndrew F, Thompson J, Fellows L, Large A, Speed M, Renfrew MJ (2012). *Infant Feeding Survey—UK, 2010 (NS).* London: Health and Social Care Information Centre. Available at: ℘ www.hscic.gov.uk/catalogue/PUB08694.

# Health risks associated with formula feeding

The RCM[18] stated that, taking breastfeeding as the 'gold standard', bottle-feeding has been shown to be associated with certain health risks.

For the infant:

- Increased risk of gastrointestinal infections
- Increased risk of respiratory infections
- Increased incidence of otitis media
- Increased risk of urinary infections
- Increased risk of atopic disease in families where there is a history of this disease
- Increased risk of sudden infant death
- Increased risk of insulin-dependent diabetes mellitus
- Reduced cognitive development
- Decreased visual acuity
- Reduced IQ in preterm infants
- Increased risk of NEC.

Some risks that manifest in later life have been demonstrated, including:

- Cardiovascular disease
- Obesity
- Some childhood cancers.

For the mother:

- Increased risk of ovarian and premenopausal breast cancer. The exact mechanisms whereby breastfeeding affords protection against these cancers are not fully understood. However, in the case of breast cancer, it is thought to be linked with increased circulating hormones, which result in systemic metabolic effects as well as structural changes in the breast, whereas in the case of ovarian cancer, it is believed that breastfeeding may afford a protective effect as a result of inhibition of ovulation[19]
- Increased risk of hip fractures and reduced bone density. Prolactin, which is released during breastfeeding, increases the rate at which vitamin D is converted to its active form, and this enhances calcium utilization.[20]

For full reference sources and details of further associated risks, see Appendix 5 in RCM's *Successful Breastfeeding* (2002)[18] and the UNICEF UK Baby Friendly website (℘ www.babyfriendly.org.uk).

## References

18 Royal College of Midwives (2002). *Successful Breastfeeding*. Edinburgh: Churchill Livingstone.
19 Collaborative Group on Hormonal Factors in Breast Cancer (2002). Breast cancer and breast feeding: collaborative reanalysis of individual data from 47 epidemiological studies in 30 countries, including 50302 women with breast cancer and 96973 without the disease. *Lancet* **360**: 187–95.
20 Palmer G (2009). *The Politics of Breastfeeding: When Breasts Are Bad for Business*. London: Pinter and Martin Ltd.

# Index